T0205312

Jerry L. Prince   Dzung L. Pham
Kyle J. Myers (Eds.)

Information Processing in Medical Imaging

21st International Conference, IPMI 2009
Williamsburg, VA, USA, July 5-10, 2009
Proceedings

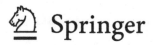 Springer

Volume Editors

Jerry L. Prince
Johns Hopkins University, Department of Electrical and Computer Engineering
3400 North Charles Street, Baltimore, MD 21218, USA
E-mail: prince@jhu.edu

Dzung L. Pham
Johns Hopkins University, Department of Radiology
600 North Wolfe Street, Baltimore, MD 21287, USA
E-mail: pham@jhu.edu

Kyle J. Myers
U.S. Food and Drug Administration
Division of Imaging and Applied Mathematics, OSEL
10903 New Hampshire Avenue, Silver Spring, MD 20993, USA
E-mail: kyle.myers@fda.hhs.gov

Library of Congress Control Number: Applied for

CR Subject Classification (1998): I.4, I.5, I.2.5-6, J.1, J.3, I.3

LNCS Sublibrary: SL 6 – Image Processing, Computer Vision, Pattern Recognition, and Graphics

ISSN   0302-9743
ISBN-10   3-642-02497-1 Springer Berlin Heidelberg New York
ISBN-13   978-3-642-02497-9 Springer Berlin Heidelberg New York

springer.com

© Springer-Verlag Berlin Heidelberg 2009
Printed in Germany

Typesetting: Camera-ready by author, data conversion by Scientific Publishing Services, Chennai, India
Printed on acid-free paper   SPIN: 12700561   06/3180   5 4 3 2 1 0

Preface

The 21st International Conference on Information Processing in Medical Imaging (IPMI) was held July 5–10, 2009 at the College of William and Mary in Williamsburg, Virginia, USA. The conference was the latest in a series of biennial scientific meetings, the last being held in July of 2007 in the south of The Netherlands, during which new developments in the acquisition, analysis, and use of medical images were presented. IPMI is one of the longest running conferences devoted to these topics in medical imaging. The first IPMI conference was held in 1969, when a group of young scientists working in nuclear medicine gathered to discuss the current problems in their field. Since that time the conference has expanded into other medical imaging acquisition modalities, including ultrasound, optics, magnetic resonance, and x-ray imaging techniques. IPMI is now widely recognized as one of the most exciting and influential meetings in medical imaging, with a unique emphasis on active participation from all attendees and a strong commitment to vigorous discussion and open debate.

A wide variety of topics are covered at IPMI meetings, all within a single-track format. This year 150 full-length manuscripts were submitted to the conference. Of these, 26 papers were selected for oral presentation and 33 were accepted as posters. Submissions were carefully reviewed by at least three members of the Scientific Review Committee, who evaluated the novelty, methodological development, and scientific rigor of each manuscript. A Paper Selection Committee, comprising the conference co-chairs and three senior investigators, took on the difficult task of creating a meeting program. Using the rankings and detailed comments of the reviewers of each manuscript, and adding to that their own judgment of the merits of each manuscript, they designed the meeting program represented in this volume. The many high-quality manuscripts submitted for consideration made the selection process extremely difficult, and many excellent papers did not make it into the final program. This is an unfortunate inevitability of the high selectivity for which IPMI is known.

A key goal of IPMI is to encourage active participation of the most talented and promising young investigators in the field, in an environment that also fosters in-depth interactions with senior researchers. To achieve this goal, all IPMI participants were involved in small study groups where they prepared for the conference presentations. After reading their assigned papers, graduate students, post-docs, and young faculty members discussed their understanding of related work in the field with senior investigators and together formulated both clarifying and probing questions for the oral presenters. The study groups thus led off the discussion of each paper, ensuring a lively and vigorous dialogue. Further emphasis on the young researcher was made through the competition for the prestigious Erbsmann award. The Francois Erbsmann Prize is awarded for the best contribution by a young scientist who is the first author of a paper and a first-time IPMI oral presenter. This year 21 of the 26 oral presenters were eligible for the Erbsmann Prize.

IPMI 2009 featured a keynote lecture by Jonathan S. Lewin, an internationally renowned expert in interventional and intra-operative magnetic resonance imaging who currently serves as the Martin W. Donner Professor and director of the Russell H. Morgan Department of Radiology and Radiological Science at Johns Hopkins University. Dr. Lewin spoke on "Information-Intensive Minimally Invasive Intervention: Concepts and Applications". Dr. Lewin has developed minimally invasive procedures for the treatment of cancer, vascular disease, and other disorders. His lecture gave the IPMI audience a unique opportunity to hear the perspective of an active clinician-researcher in this important application area that relies so heavily on information extracted from medical images.

The IPMI 2009 conference featured the traditions that past IPMI attendees have come to expect as part of the unique character of the meeting. Most importantly, each oral presentation was allowed unlimited time for discussion to give the audience the opportunity to resolve all questions regarding the methods and results. IPMI discussions can go on for hours, involving virtually every attendee in the room! Session Chairs play a key role at IPMI as they strive to ensure that these extended discussions are productive and continuing to add to the group's understanding of the nature and significance of each presentation's original contribution.

IPMI is traditionally held in a small and sometimes remote location. This year's venue, the campus of the College of William and Mary, is located in the heart of the historical town of Williamsburg, Virginia, USA. Chartered in 1693, the college claims many honors; it is the second oldest college in America and counts among its alumni presidents Thomas Jefferson, James Monroe, and John Marshall. Attendees to the meeting were housed in the college's dorm rooms, enjoyed communal meals in a college dining hall, and enjoyed late-night conversations at the nearby taverns reminisicent of 18th century America. On Wednesday afternoon, participants were able to explore adjacent Colonial Williamsburg, a living museum dedicated to preserving the memory of life at the time of the American Revolution, visit the Jamestown Settlement, ride the Colonial Parkway on bike, or browse the shops of the Williamsburg Pottery Factory. Later that evening, a conference banquet was held in the College of William and Mary's Alumni House. On Thursday afternoon, the traditional IMPI soccer match was held, pitting the American team against "the rest of the world." At the time of this writing the outcome of the latest match in this long-standing rivalry is uncertain. What is known, however, is that the refereeing will be a major factor in deciding the outcome and there will be deeply held opinions on all sides regarding the fairness of this aspect of the game!

These proceedings contain the IPMI 2009 papers in the order they were presented at the meeting. We hope that this volume serves as a valuable source of information for the participants, as well as a reminder of the great conference experience that we had. For those who were not able to attend the conference, we hope that these proceedings provide you with an excellent summary of the latest research contributions to the medical imaging field. We look forward to the next IPMI conference, which is currently planned for 2011 in Germany. More information will be posted on www.ipmi-conference.com as it becomes available.

April 2009

Jerry L. Prince
Dzung L. Pham
Kyle J. Myers

Acknowledgements

The organization of the 21st IPMI conference was only possible through the efforts and contributions of several organizations and many individuals. First of all, the IPMI 2009 Co-chairs would like to thank the members of the Scientific Review Committee for providing so many high-quality reviews within a very limited time frame; because of these reviews, we were able to make a fair selection of the best papers for the final program. We also express our gratitude to the Paper Selection Committee members—Nico Karssemeijer, Richard Leahy, and Guido Gerig—who each read many papers and their reviews and traveled to Baltimore for a marathon organizational meeting that resulted in an outstanding final program. We would also like to thank previous IPMI organizers, particularly Chris Taylor, Gary Christensen, and Nico Karssemeijer, for sharing their experiences and insights with us.

We are very grateful to Laura Libertini at Johns Hopkins University for her expert handling of countless administrative tasks including gathering much information for the original conference proposal, preparing the conference budget, coordinating all meetings, handling the conference registrations, supervising student and staff help, and many other administrative tasks too numerous to count. For expert help in managing mailing lists and our IPMI website, we are grateful to Jonathan Boswell at the U.S. Food and Drug Administration. Thanks as well to Simon Jackson for his assistance with the Web-based CAWS conference management system.

We are grateful to the College of William and Mary for hosting the IPMI 2009 conference and particularly to Lois Parker for enthusiastically supporting our conference proposal and to both Lois and Elizabeth Keiwiet for expertly managing all of our requests for services before and during the conference. We thank our students for volunteering to spend a week during the hot 2009 summer working at the numerous odd jobs that are essential to maintaining a smooth and effective program.

Finally, we are grateful to the following organizations for their generous financial support:

National Institute of Biomedical Imaging and Bioengineering (NIBIB)
National Cancer Institute (NCI)
National Institute of Neurological Disorders and Stroke (NINDS)
National Institute on Aging (NIA)
Johns Hopkins University

Francois Erbsmann Prizewinners

1987 (Utrecht, The Netherlands): **John M. Gauch**, University of North Carolina, Chapel Hill, NC, USA.
J.M. Gauch, W.R. Oliver, S.M. Pizer: Multiresolution shape descriptions and their applications in medical imaging.

1989 (Berkeley, CA, USA): **Arthur F. Gmitro**, University of Arizona, Tucson, AZ, USA.
A.F. Gmitro, V. Tresp, V. Chen, Y. Snell, G.R. Gindi: Video-rate reconstruction of CT and MR images.

1991 (Wye, Kent, UK): **H. Isil Bozma**, Yale University, New Haven, CT, USA.
H.I. Bozma, J.S. Duncan: Model-based recognition of multiple deformable objects using a game-theoretic framework.

1993 (Flagstaff, AZ, USA): **Jeffrey A. Fessler**, University of Michigan, Ann Arbor, MI, USA.
J.A. Fessler: Tomographic reconstruction using information-weighted spline smoothing.

1995 (Brest, France): **Maurits K. Konings**, University Hospital, Utrecht, The Netherlands.
M.K. Konings, W.P.T.M. Mali, M.A. Viergever: Design of a robust strategy to measure intravascular electrical impedance.

1997 (Poultney, VT, USA): **David Atkinson**, Guys Hospital, London, UK.
D. Atkinson, D.L.G. Hill, P.N.R. Stoyle, P.E. Summers, S.F. Keevil: An autofocus algorithm for the automatic correction of motion artifacts in MR images.

1999 (Visegrad, Hungary): **Liana M. Lorigo**, Massachusetts Institute of Technology, Cambridge, MA, USA.
L.M. Lorigo, O. Faugeras, W.E.L. Grimson, R. Keriven, R. Kikinis, C.-F. Westin: Codimension 2 geodesic active contours for MRA segmentation.

2001 (Davis, CA, USA): **Viktor K. Jirsa**, Florida Atlantic University, FL, USA.
V.K. Jirsa, K.J. Jantzen, A. Fuchs, J.A. Scott Kelso: Neural field dynamics on the folded three-dimensional cortical sheet and its forward EEG and MEG.

2003 (Ambleside, UK): **Guillaume Marrelec**, INSERM, France.
G. Marrelec, P. Ciuciu, M. Pelegrini-Issac, H. Benali: Estimation of the hemodyamic response function in event-related functional MRI: directed acyclic graphs for a general Bayesian inference framework.

2005 (Glenwood Springs, Colorado, USA) **Duygu Tosun**, Johns Hopkins University, Baltimore, USA.
D. Tosun, J.L. Prince: Cortical surface alignment using geometry-driven multispectral optical flow.

2007 (Kerkrade, The Netherlands) **Ben Glocker**, Technische Universität München, Garching, Germany.
B. Glocker, N. Komodakis, N. Paragios, G. Tziritas, and N. Navab: Inter-and intra-modal deformable registration: continuous deformations meet efficient optimal linear programming.

Conference Committees

Chairs

Jerry L. Prince	Johns Hopkins University, USA
Dzung L. Pham	Johns Hopkins University, USA
Kyle J. Myers	U.S. Food and Drug Administration, USA

Paper Selection Committee

Guido Gerig	University of Utah, USA
Nico Karssemeijer	Radboud University Nijmegan Medical Center, The Netherlands
Richard Leahy	University of Southern California, USA

Scientific Committee

Craig K. Abbey	University of California, Davis, USA
Amir A. Amini	University of Louisville, USA
Stephen R Aylward	KITWARE Inc., USA
Christian Barillot	IRISA/CNRS, France
Pierre-Louis Bazin	Johns Hopkins University, USA
Djamal Boukerroui	Université de Technologie de Compiègne, France
Mike Brady	University of Oxford, UK
Aaron B. Brill	Vanderbilt University, USA
Elizabeth Bullitt	University of North Carolina, USA
Gary E. Christensen	University of Iowa, USA
Ela Claridge	University of Birmingham, UK
Eric Clarkson	University of Arizona, USA
Alan Colchester	University of Kent, UK
Timothy F. Cootes	University of Manchester, UK
Christos Davatzikos	University of Pennsylvania, USA
Marleen de Bruijne	University of Copenhagen, Denmark
Herve Delingette	INRIA, France
James S. Duncan	Yale University, USA
Alejandro F. Frangi	Universitat Pompeu Fabra, Spain
James C. Gee	University of Pennsylvania, USA
Maryellen Giger	University of Chicago, USA
Polina Golland	Massachusetts Institute of Technology, USA
Michael L. Goris	Stanford University School of Medicine, USA
Kenneth R. Hoffmann	State University of New York at Buffalo, USA
Michael Insana	University of Illinois at Urbana-Champaign, USA
Sarang C. Joshi	University of Utah, USA

IPMI 2009 Board

Table of Contents

Space Curves

Tractography

Poster Session I

Microscopy

Exploratory Analyses

Features and Detection

Image Guided Surgery

Shape Analysis

Poster Session II

Motion

Segmentation and Validation

Diffusion Propagator Imaging: Using Laplace's Equation and Multiple Shell Acquisitions to Reconstruct the Diffusion Propagator

Maxime Descoteaux[1], Rachid Deriche[2], Denis Le Bihan[1],
Jean-François Mangin[1], and Cyril Poupon[1]

[1] NeuroSpin, IFR 49 CEA Saclay, France
[2] INRIA Sophia Antipolis - Méditerranée, France

Abstract. Many recent single-shell high angular resolution diffusion imaging reconstruction techniques have been introduced to reconstruct orientation distribution functions (ODF) that only capture angular information contained in the diffusion process of water molecules. By also considering the radial part of the diffusion signal, the reconstruction of the ensemble average diffusion propagator (EAP) of water molecules can provide much richer information about complex tissue microstructure than the ODF. In this paper, we present diffusion propagator imaging (DPI), a novel technique to reconstruct the EAP from multiple shell acquisitions. The DPI solution is analytical and linear because it is based on a Laplace equation modeling of the diffusion signal. DPI is validated with *ex vivo* phantoms and also illustrated on an *in vivo* human brain dataset. DPI is shown to reconstruct EAP from only two b-value shells and approximately 100 diffusion measurements.

1 Introduction

One of the quest of diffusion-weighted (DW) imaging is the reconstruction of the full three-dimensional (3D) ensemble average propagator (EAP) describing the diffusion process of water molecules in biological tissues. Many recent high angular resolution diffusion imaging (HARDI) techniques have been proposed to recover complex diffusion orientation distribution functions (ODF) of the white matter geometry. However, these orientation functions derived from HARDI only capture the angular structure of the diffusion process on a single shell and are therefore mostly useful for fiber tractography applications. The EAP can capture richer information by considering both radial and angular information part of the q-space diffusion signal. Thus, the EAP might provide means to infer axonal diameter and also be sensitive to white matter anomalies [1].

In order to relate the observed diffusion signal to the underlying tissue microstructure, we need to understand how the diffusion signal is influenced by the tissue geometry and its properties. Under the narrow pulse assumption, the relationship between the diffusion signal, $E(\mathbf{q})$, in q-space and the EAP, $P(\mathbf{R})$, in real space, is given by an inverse Fourier transform (IFT) [3] as

J.L. Prince, D.L. Pham, and K.J. Myers (Eds.): IPMI 2009, LNCS 5636, pp. 1–13, 2009.

$$P(\mathbf{R}) = \int_{\mathbf{q} \in \Re^3} E(\mathbf{q}) e^{-2\pi i \mathbf{q} \cdot \mathbf{R}} d\mathbf{q}, \tag{1}$$

where $E(\mathbf{q}) = S(\mathbf{q})/S_0$ is the diffusion signal measured at position $\mathbf{q}$ in q-space and S_0 is the baseline image acquired without any diffusion sensitization ($q = 0$). We denote $q = |\mathbf{q}|$ and $\mathbf{q} = q\mathbf{u}$, $\mathbf{R} = R_0\mathbf{r}$, where $\mathbf{u}$ and $\mathbf{r}$ are 3D unit vectors, and $q, R_0 \in \Re$. The wave vector $\mathbf{q}$ is $\mathbf{q} = \gamma\delta\mathbf{G}/2\pi$, with γ the nuclear gyromagnetic ratio and $\mathbf{G}$ the applied diffusion gradient vector.

Various methods already exist to reconstruct the EAP [4,5,6,7,8,9,10,11,12]. Among the most commonly used methods, diffusion tensor imaging (DTI) [4] is limited by the Gaussian assumption of the free diffusion model, which excludes observed *in vivo* phenomena such as restriction, heterogeneity, anomalous diffusion, and finite boundary permeability. Diffusion spectrum imaging (DSI) [5] can account for DTI limitations. The technique has the advantage of being model-free but requires hundreds of DW measurements sampled on a dense Cartesian grid, which requires strong gradient fields, in order to evaluate the Fourier transform of Eq. 1. DSI was also shown to be possible on a non-Cartesian grid in [11] using less measurements on multiple spherical shells. More recently, inspired by computed tomography, another technique was proposed to perform measurements along many radial lines before computing 1D tomographic projections to reconstruct the 3D EAP [10]. This technique also requires hundreds of samples on a few radial lines of q-space to recover the EAP. The results are promising but have not yet been applied on an *in vivo* brain. Other techniques suggest using multiple spherical shell acquisitions in order to reconstruct the features of the EAP, such as generalized high order tensors [6] based on cumulant expansions; or the composite and hindered restricted model of diffusion (CHARMED) [7]; or the diffusion kurtosis [8]; or the diffusion orientation transform (DOT) [9]; or hybrid diffusion properties of the EAP [11]; or a fourth order Cartesian tensor representation of the probability profile [12]. Unfortunately, for most of these methods, many DW measurements are needed. Moreover, it remains unclear what is the right number of spherical shells needed and most of the results lack validation. Of all the mentioned techniques, DOT is in closer spirit to our approach and will be revisited later.

In this paper, we develop diffusion propagator imaging (DPI), a novel technique for analytical EAP reconstruction from multiple shell acquisitions. Our solution is simple, linear and compact. DPI is based on a 3D Laplace equation modeling of the q-space diffusion signal, which greatly simplifies the solution to Eq. 1 and allows one to obtain an analytical solution. An important part of this paper is dedicated to validate DPI, both the signal fitting with Laplace equation and the EAP reconstruction, on real datasets from *ex vivo* phantoms [13]. We also illustrate DPI on a real *in vivo* human brain.

2   Diffusion Propagator Imaging (DPI)

q-Space Signal Approximation with Laplace's Equation. Modeling the 3D q-space diffusion signal to recover the EAP and capture complex fiber crossing configurations was proposed before in CHARMED [7] and DOT [9], where the diffusion signal was modeled with multiple fiber compartments; in CHARMED, with a mixture of restricted and hindered compartements and in DOT, with a mixture of exponential decay functions (mono-, bi or tri-exponential). In our approach, we do not want to assume any mixture models *a priori*. We seek a simpler representation of the diffusion signal that will naturally capture multiple shell measurements and allow for an analytical EAP solution.

Our main assumption is that the diffusion signal attenuation can be estimated using the 3D Laplace Equation. Under this assumption, we express the q-space diffusion signal $E(\mathbf{q}) = S(\mathbf{q})/S_0$ in terms of any radius using the general or *total* solution of the Laplace equation in spherical coordinates, which gives

$$E(\mathbf{q}) = E(q\mathbf{u}) = \sum_{j=0}^{\infty} \left[\frac{c_j}{q^{\ell(j)+1}} + d_j q^{\ell(j)} \right] Y_j(\mathbf{u}) \quad \text{for} \quad q > 0, \tag{2}$$

where $\ell(j)$ is the order associated with element j of the spherical harmonic (SH) basis Y_j, which is defined to be real and symmetric, and c_j and d_j are the unknown SH coefficients describing the signal. Also, for $q = 0$, $E(\mathbf{q}) = 1$.

The Laplace equation requires boundary conditions. In our problem, we need at least two shell measurements and more diffusion measurements N than unknown coefficients to properly constrain Eq. 2. Intuitively, our Laplace equation modeling can be seen as the heat equation between each given shell measurements, i.e. the solution is obtained when the heat does not change between the temperature measurements given at each shell.

Analytical Diffusion Propagator Reconstruction. Under this Laplace equation modeling assumption, we prove, in Appendix A, that the EAP can be reconstructed as

$$P(R_0\mathbf{r}) = 2 \sum_{j=0}^{\infty} \frac{(-1)^{\ell(j)/2} 2\pi^{\ell(j)-1} R_0^{\ell(j)-2}}{(2\ell(j) - 1)!!} c_j Y_j(\mathbf{r}) \quad \text{for} \quad R_0 > 0, \tag{3}$$

where $(n - 1)!! = (n - 1) \cdot (n - 3) \cdot \ldots \cdot 3 \cdot 1$. This expression is analytical and quite simple to compute. Note also that the EAP expression is linear and only depends on the c_j coefficients, but the d_j coefficients are nonetheless important in the diffusion signal fitting/modeling procedure of Eq. 2. We finally note that if $R_0 = 0$, $P(0) = \int_{\mathbf{q} \in \Re^3} E(\mathbf{q}) d\mathbf{q}$, the average diffusion signal in q-space.

3   Methods

As a starting point, we are given n HARDI shell datasets with the same number of diffusion measurements N per shell. It is now standard in HARDI processing techniques to use a modified real and symmetric SH basis of order ℓ with elements Y_j, where $j := j(k, m) = (k^2 + k + 2)/2 + m$ is defined from the order ℓ and phase m standard SH Y_ℓ^m (see [14,15,16,17]).

We can then generate the linear system associated with the Laplace equation signal estimation given in Eq. 2. We let $\mathbf{S}_n$ be the N x 1 vector representing the diffusion signal of shell number n at each of the N diffusion encoding gradient direction. We also let $\mathbf{C}$ and $\mathbf{D}$ represent the R x 1 vectors of unknown SH coefficients, c_j and d_j in Eq. 2, where $R = 1/2(\ell+1)(\ell+2)$. Next, we let $\mathbf{B}$ represent the N x R matrix constructed with the modified SH basis (as ine [14,15,16,17]). Finally, we define $R_\ell(q) = r^\ell$ and $I_\ell(q) = r^{-\ell-1}$ to capture the regular and irregular radial part of the total Laplace equation. We can then construct the matrices of coefficients for each shell, $\mathbf{F}_n$ and $\mathbf{G}_n$, as two R x R diagonal square matrices with diagonal entries $R_{\ell(j)}(q_n)$ and $I_{\ell(j)}(q_n)$ respectively. As before, q_n is the q-value of shell n and $\ell(j)$ is the order of the jth SH coefficient[1].

Lastly, for each of the n shell, we have the linear system $\mathbf{S}_n = \mathbf{BG}_n\mathbf{C}+\mathbf{BF}_n\mathbf{D}$. Combining all n systems, we obtain the general linear system representing Eq. 2, $\mathbf{S} = \mathbf{AX}$. This system of over-determined equations is solved with a standard least-square solution yielding the vector $\mathbf{X}' = [\mathbf{C}'\,\mathbf{D}']^T$, given by $\mathbf{X}' = (\mathbf{A}^T\mathbf{A})^{-1}\mathbf{A}^T\mathbf{S}$. Therefore, the estimated signal, $\mathbf{S}'$, can be recovered simply with $\mathbf{AX}'$. We can then report the mean and standard deviation (std) of the Euclidean error $|\mathbf{S}_n - \mathbf{S}'_n|$ percentage between the original and estimated diffusion signal for each of the n shell and over all N diffusion measurements.

Finally, taking the first part of the estimated vector $\mathbf{X}'$, we can extract the $\mathbf{C}'$ coefficients needed to compute the EAP. The spherical function $\mathbf{P}_{R_0}$ representing the EAP for given R_0, can be obtained with a simple matrix multiplication

$$\mathbf{P}_{R_0} = \mathbf{B} \left(\begin{matrix} \cdots \\ 2(-1)^{\ell(j)/2}2\pi^{\ell(j)-1}R_0^{\ell(j)-2}/(2\ell(j)-1)!! \\ \cdots \end{matrix} \right) \mathbf{C}', \qquad (4)$$

$\mathbf{P}_{R_0}$ can then be visualized for different values of R_0.

Data Acquisition. DPI was used to estimate the diffusion signal and the associated EAP on *ex vivo* phantoms with fibers crossing at $90°$ and $45°$ designed in [13] with parameters: FOV=32cm, matrix 32x32, TH=14mm, TE=130ms, TR=4.5s,12.0s ($45°,90°$), BW=200KHz and b-values of 2000, 4000, 6000, 8000 s/mm^2 and 4000 uniformly distributed orientations. The number of directions were also resampled to $N = 15, 25$ and 60 to test DPI under lower and more realistic sampling schemes.

DPI was also applied on data acquired from a 3T Trio MR Siemens system, equipped with a whole body gradient (40 mT/m and 200 T/m/s) and an 32 channel head coil. The acquisition parameters were TE/TR = 147ms/11.5s, BW=1680Hz/pixel, 96x96 matrix, isotropic 2mm resolution, and 60 axial slices. We acquired a b=0 diffusion image followed by four b-values acquisitions with 64 uniform directions, at b = 1000, 2000, 4000 and 6000 s/mm^2.

4 Results

Diffusion Propagator Imaging of the *Ex Vivo* Phantom. DPI is applied on the 90 and 45 degree phantoms shown in Figure 1. We pick the center

---

[1] For $j = \{1, 2, 3, 4, 5, 6, 7, 8, ...\}$, $\ell_j = \{0, 2, 2, 2, 2, 2, 4, 4, ...\}$.

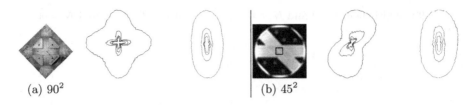

(a) 90^2 (b) 45^2

Fig. 1. Physical phantoms designed in [13]. (a) 90° (photograph), and (b) 45° (fast spin-echo map and ROI)) phantoms. We also show the original diffusion signal equators perpendicular to the z (in blue, axial view) and x (in red, sagittal view) axes, from $b = 2000, 4000, 6000$, and 8000 s/mm^2, showing the diffusion signal decay.

Table 1. Mean and standard deviation of the percentage error in the multi-shell signal fit depending on the order ℓ and number of measurements N used (sampling scheme)

(a) Estimation order ℓ, multi-shell experiment with $N = 4000$

shell	90° crossing			45° crossing		
s/mm^2	$\ell = 2$	$\ell = 4$	$\ell = 16$	$\ell = 2$	$\ell = 6$	$\ell = 16$
2000	9.4±2.5%	2.6±0.3%	2.5±0.3%	13±3.3%	2.0±0.2%	2.0±0.3%
4000	16±3.9%	4.3±1.0%	4.3±1.1%	13±3.4%	3.9±0.7%	3.7±0.9%
6000	18±4.4%	5.1±1.6%	4.5±1.1%	14±3.8%	5.2±1.2%	5.2±1.4%
8000	20±6.5%	8.5±2.8%	8.5±3.0%	15±6.6%	8.5±2.7%	8.4±3.1%

(b) Sampling scheme N, multi-shell experiment

shell	90° crossing, $\ell = 4$			45° crossing, $\ell = 6$		
s/mm^2	$N = 4000$	$N = 60$	$N = 15$	$N = 4000$	$N = 60$	$N = 28$
2000	2.6±0.3%	2.7±0.3%	2.8±0.4%	2.0±0.2%	2.1±0.2%	2.3±1.0%
4000	4.3±1.0%	4.3±1.0%	5.1±1.4%	3.9±0.7%	4.0±0.8%	4.0±1.1%
6000	5.1±1.6%	5.2±1.8%	6.2±2.6%	5.2±1.2%	5.3±1.3%	6.3±2.0%
8000	8.5±2.8%	8.5±2.7%	8.6±3.2%	8.5±2.7%	8.5±2.5%	8.5±2.8%

voxel of the phantom, which contains approximately equal proportion of the two fiber branches of the crossing. The diffusion signal attenuation is also shown in Figure 1. In this visualization, red and blue lines illustrate equators of the original diffusion signal perpendicular to the x and z plan respectively, whereas later, black lines illustrate the associated estimated signal in the signal fit experiments.

Can Laplace's Equation be used for diffusion signal estimation? Table 1 quantitatively shows that the diffusion signal can be modeled using Laplace's equation, on both *ex vivo* phantoms. This is qualitatively confirmed in Figure 2. From Table 1, we first see that estimation is accurate and that there is less than 10% mean signal fitting error with a small standard deviation at every shell, for every estimation order ℓ and every sampling scheme N. We also see that the mean percentage error is increasing with increasing b-value. The most significant error systematically occurs at shell $b = 8000$ s/mm^2. This is due to the intrinsic smoothness of the diffusion signal fit with Laplace's equation. As

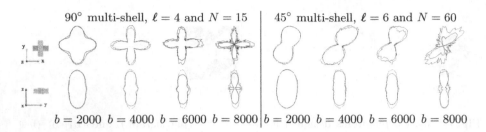

$90°$ multi-shell, $\ell = 4$ and $N = 15$ | $45°$ multi-shell, $\ell = 6$ and $N = 60$

$b = 2000$ $b = 4000$ $b = 6000$ $b = 8000$ | $b = 2000$ $b = 4000$ $b = 6000$ $b = 8000$

Fig. 2. Multi-shell signal fit experiment on the 90 and 45 degree crossing phantoms. We show original (colored) and estimated (black) diffusion signal equators perpendicular to the z (in blue) and x (in red) axes respectively.

seen in curves of Figure 2, a desired smoothing occurs in the diffusion signal estimation, which for high b-values, increases the mean error between the more jagged original signal curves in color and the smooth estimated curves in black.

What is the right estimation SH order? From Table 1, we note that the signal estimation accuracy is more or less equivalent for SH order $\ell \geq 4$. Under the simple geometrical phantom configuration, increasing estimation order does not significantly reduce the mean percentage error nor the standard deviation.

What is the right number of diffusion measurements? We do not need hundreds of diffusion measurements for accurate diffusion signal fit. From Table 1, we note that the diffusion signal estimation accuracy remains relatively stable for all sampling schemes N. No significant error increase is observed as one decreases the number of measurements, down to $N = 15$ and 28 for order $\ell = 4$ and 6 respectively.

Can we recover fiber crossings? Because we can accurately estimate the diffusion signal, we can obtain EAP reconstructions that recover fiber crossing information. First, we note in Figure 3a) that a SH order of 2 is insufficient to discriminate the fiber crossing. This is in fact reflected in the first column ($\ell = 2$) of Table 1 with large percentage errors in the diffusion signal estimation. A DPI reconstruction of order 2 is similar to a DTI reconstruction of the "Gaussian" diffusion propagator. Next, we also note in Figure 3b)-f), that a SH order 4 is sufficient to discriminate the 90 degree crossing but insufficient for the 45 degree crossing. One must use SH order $\ell \geq 6$ or higher to discriminate the crossing fibers in the 45 degree crossing example, at the cost of having some small spurious peaks appearance for higher radii R_0. Hence, even though increasing SH order does not significantly improve the signal fitting accuracy (seen in Table 1), increasing SH order does improve the angular resolution of the EAP reconstruction. However, higher SH order EAP reconstruction have higher frequency coefficients that are more perturbed by noise and thus, they can have spurious peaks. We therefore choose $\ell = 4$ in the 90 crossing phantom and $\ell = 6$ in the 45 degree crossing phantom in the rest of our experiments.

What is the right number of shells? Figure 4 shows that two-shell diffusion signal fitting is also possible using Laplace's equation. We see that the diffusion signal estimation remains relatively accurate even if one uses only

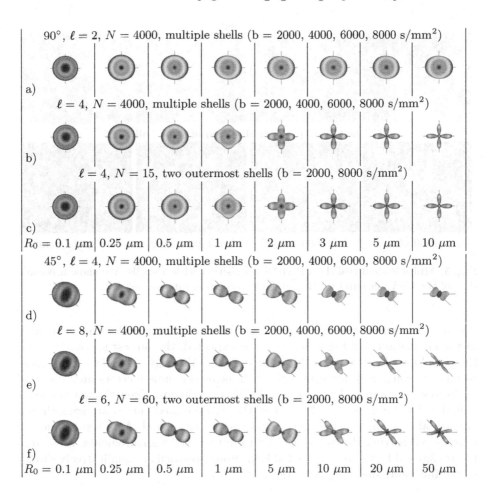

Fig. 3. EAP reconstruction on the 90° and 45° crossing phantom for different SH order ℓ, sampling scheme N, number of shells, and radius R_0

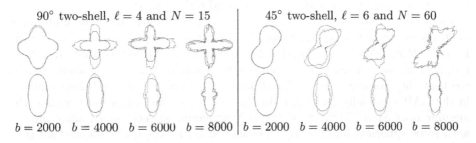

Fig. 4. Two-shell signal fit experiment on the 90° and 45° crossing phantoms using shells $b = 2000$ and 8000 s/mm^2

GFA map

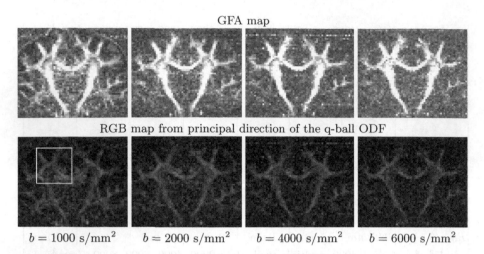

RGB map from principal direction of the q-ball ODF

$b = 1000 \text{ s/mm}^2$ $b = 2000 \text{ s/mm}^2$ $b = 4000 \text{ s/mm}^2$ $b = 6000 \text{ s/mm}^2$

Fig. 5. Multiple shell real data HARDI acquisition with 4 shells. We show a coronal slice of the GFA map and RGB map with a region of interest.

two-shell measurements. We also see that the best fit occurs for the shells used in the estimation. On the other hand, as expected, the largest errors occur for the signal associated to the extrapolated shells. Although not shown here, these results are confirmed quantitatively with mean percentage errors and standard deviations as computed for the multi-shell experiment. Even though the error is higher for the unused shell's signal, the extrapolated curves are smooth and are still able to capture the angular contrast of the signal. As a result, one can reliably reconstruct the diffusion EAP from two shell measurements. As seen in Figure 3c) and f), the reconstructed EAP from two-shell are qualitatively similar to the full multi-shell reconstruction.

Diffusion Propagator Imaging of the Human Brain. We now apply DPI on the *in vivo* brain dataset illustrated in Figure 5. Based on the previous section, we choose SH order $\ell = 4$ and use all measurements, either in a full multi-shell DPI reconstruction, using all four shells, or in a two-shell DPI reconstruction using the two outermost shells ($b = 1000$ and 6000 s/mm^2).

Figure 6 first shows that the EAP reconstructions agree with the underlying anatomy in the ROI shown in Figure 5. The extracted spherical functions of the EAP, $P(R_0\mathbf{r})$, emphasize directionality of the EAP and we see that the CC in red, CST in blue and SLF in green are well identified. Most importantly, we also see that the crossing fiber configurations are recovered and well discriminated in the EAP, especially for high radii R_o. In fact, as the radius R_0 increases, the angular resolution improves, at the cost of having slightly more noisy profiles with some spherical function that become spiky. Figure 6 also shows that two-shell DPI closely agrees with the full multi-shell DPI. This confirms the *ex vivo* phantom results that DPI can be done reliably with only two different shells.

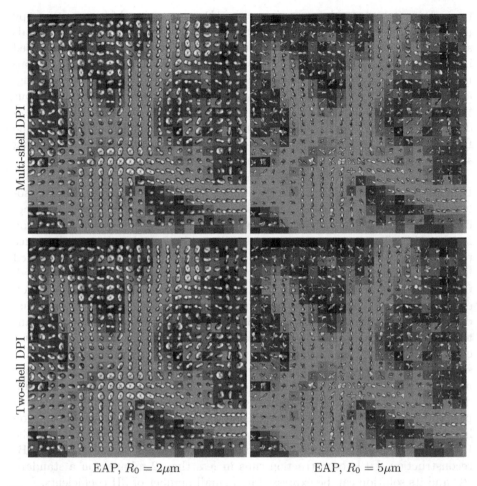

Multi-shell DPI

Two-shell DPI

EAP, $R_0 = 2\mu m$ EAP, $R_0 = 5\mu m$

Fig. 6. DPI on the human brain dataset in the same crossing region as Figure 5. In the first row, a multi-shell DPI reconstruction and in the second row, a two-shell DPI was done using the two outermost shells $b = 1000$ and 6000 s/mm^2.

5   Discussion and Conclusions

The Laplace equation was successfully used to model the diffusion signal and reconstruct the EAP but *a priori*, there is no physical reason why this should be. There might exist other possible model and family of functions to do so. In fact, [16] and [18] recently proposed new orthogonal bases to estimate the diffusion signal. In [16], the Spherical Polar Fourier (SFP) basis is used to extract features of the EAP. The basis is composed of an angular part using spherical harmonics and a radial part using an orthonormal radial basis function called the Gaussian-Laguerre polynomials. However, [16] do not have the full analytical EAP reconstruction itself as we do. Only EAP features such as the ODF or other angular functions of the EAP can be computed. Separately, [18] proposed to use Hermite polynomials to estimate the 1D q-space signal from spectroscopy imaging. While forming a complete orthogonal basis, the Hermite polynomials also have the important property that their Fourier transform can be expressed in terms of themselves. This property could potentially be very powerful to evaluate Eq. 1. Although the Hermite polynomials were used for 1D q-space imaging, an extension to the 3D problem seems conceivable. One now has to think about the best way to sample q-space (with Cartesian points, spherical shells, or radial lines) in order to have sufficient measurements to robustly reconstruct the EAP and avoid the necessity for hundreds of measurements. Different sampling schemes might be better adapted depending on the chosen basis functions.

Our Laplace equation assumption also has several positive aspects that make DPI an appealing technique. The advantages of DPI are threefold: i) The solution is analytical. ii) The signal modeling performs some level of smoothing. iii) The solution is linear and compact. First, having an analytical expression for the EAP allows one to estimate probability values outside the actual q-space range prescribed by the acquisition. In comparison, the DSI technique is limited by the boundaries of q-space and thus, the reconstructed EAP is also bounded. Our approach is in closer spirit in with the DOT technique, where an expression of $P(R_0 \mathbf{r})$ is also obtained based on an exponential assumption of the signal decay. A systematic comparison of DSI, DOT and DPI thus seems important to highlight the limitations of the modeling and numerical versus analytical reconstructions. Next, as seen in the *Result* section, DPI performs some level of smoothing in the estimation. We believe this intrinsic smoothing of the Laplace modeling is actually desired. Again, in comparison, DSI [5] uses a Hanning window to smooth the signal before Fourier transform computation. No such low-pass filtering is needed for robust diffusion estimation and EAP reconstruction in DPI. Finally, the DPI solution is linear and quite compact, which makes the EAP reconstruction extremely fast; as fast as a simple least-square DTI or QBI reconstruction. DPI reconstruction runs in less than 2 minutes on a standard PC and its solution can be expressed in a small number of SH coefficients.

To conclude, we have introduced diffusion propagator imaging, a novel technique for reconstructing the diffusion propagator from multiple shell acquisitions. We have shown that DPI can provide a new and efficient framework to study characteristics of the diffusion EAP, which opens interesting perspectives for tissue microstructure investigation. We now need to exploit DPI in clinical acquisitions and clinical settings. Future work will focus on new measures that integrate radial part of the diffusion signal, to lead to the development of new biomarkers sensitive to white-matter anomalies, brain development and aging, and might also provide means to infer axonal diameter.

Acknowledgments. The authors are thankful to A. Ghosh and the diffusion MRI group of NeuroSpin for insightful discussion on the diffusion propagator estimation. Moreover, thanks to K-H. Cho, Y-P. Chao and Pr. C-P. Lin for their participation in he data acquisition. This work was supported by *Programme Hubert Curien Orchid 2008 franco-taiwanais*, l'Ecole des Neurosciences Paris-Ile de France (ENP), and l'Association France Parkinson for the NucleiPark project.

References

1. Cohen, Y., Assaf, Y.: High b-value q-space analyzed diffusion-weighted mrs and mri in neuronal tissues - a technical review. NMR Biomed. 15, 516–542 (2002)
2. Tuch, D.S.: Diffusion MRI of Complex Tissue Structure. PhD thesis, Massachusetts Institute of Technology (2002)
3. Callaghan, P.T.: Principles of nuclear magnetic resonance microscopy. Oxford University Press, Oxford (1991)
4. Basser, P., Mattiello, J., LeBihan, D.: Estimation of the effective self-diffusion tensor from the nmr spin echo. J. Magn. Reson. B 103(3), 247–254 (1994)
5. Wedeen, V.J., Hagmann, P., Tseng, W.Y.I., Reese, T.G., Weisskoff, R.M.: Mapping complex tissue architecture with diffusion spectrum magnetic resonance imaging. Magn. Reson. Med. 54(6), 1377–1386 (2005)
6. Liu, C., Bammer, R., Acar, B., Moseley, M.E.: Characterizing non-gaussian diffusion by using generalized diffusion tensors. Magn. Reson. Med. 51, 924–937 (2004)
7. Assaf, Y., Freidlin, R.Z., Rohde, G.K., Basser, P.J.: New modeling and experimental framework to characterize hindered and restrcited water diffusion in brain white matter. Magn. Reson. Med. 52, 965–978 (2004)
8. Jensen, J.H., Helpern, J.A., Ramani, A., Lu, H., Kaczynski, K.: Diffusional kurtosis imaging: The quantification of non- gaussian water diffusion by means of magnetic resonance imaging. Magn. Reson. Med. 53, 1432–1440 (2005)
9. Özarslan, E., Shepherd, T., Vemuri, B., Blackband, S., Mareci, T.: Resolution of complex tissue microarchitecture using the diffusion orientation transform (dot). NeuroImage 31(3), 1086–1103 (2006)
10. Pickalov, V., Basser, P.: 3-D tomographic reconstruction of the average propagator from MRI data. In: IEEE ISBI, pp. 710–713 (2006)
11. Wu, Y.C., Alexander, A.L.: Hybrid diffusion imaging. NeuroImage 36, 617–629 (2007)
12. Barmpoutis, A., Vemuri, B.C., Forder, J.R.: Fast displacement probability profile approximation from hardi using 4th-order tensors. In: IEEE ISBI, pp. 911–914 (2008)
13. Poupon, C., Rieul, B., Kezele, I., Perrin, M., Poupon, F., cois Mangin, J.F.: New diffusion phantoms dedicated to the study and validation of hardi models. Magn. Reson. Med. 60, 1276–1283 (2008)
14. Hess, C., Mukherjee, P., Han, E., Xu, D., Vigneron, D.: Q-ball reconstruction of multimodal fiber orientations using the spherical harmonic basis. Magn. Reson. Med. 56, 104–117 (2006)
15. Tournier, J.D., Calamante, F., Connelly, A.: Robust determination of the fibre orientation distribution in diffusion mri: Non-negativity constrained super-resolved spherical deconvolution. NeuroImage 35(4), 1459–1472 (2007)
16. Assemlal, H.E., Tschumperlé, D., Brun, L.: Efficient computation of pdf-based characteristics from diffusion mr signal. In: Metaxas, D., Axel, L., Fichtinger, G., Székely, G. (eds.) MICCAI 2008, Part II. LNCS, vol. 5242, pp. 70–78. Springer, Heidelberg (2008)
17. Descoteaux, M., Angelino, E., Fitzgibbons, S., Deriche, R.: Regularized, fast, and robust analytical q-ball imaging. Magn. Reson. Med. 58(3), 497–510 (2007)
18. Özarslan, E., Koay, C.G., Basser, P.J.: Simple harmonic oscillator based estimation and reconstruction for one-dimensional q-space mr. In: ISMRM, p. 35 (2008)

A   Proof of the Analytical Diffusion Propagator Solution

We want to prove that, under the Laplace equation assumption (Eq. 2), $P(R_0\mathbf{r})$ is given by Eq. 3. We need the following four identities: (1) The pointwise convergent expansion of the plane wave in spherical coordinates is given by

$$e^{\pm 2\pi i \mathbf{q} \cdot \mathbf{R}} = 4\pi \sum_{j=0}^{\infty} (\pm i)^{\ell(j)} j_{\ell(j)}(2\pi q R_0) Y_j(\mathbf{u}) Y_j(\mathbf{r}),$$

where j_n is the spherical Bessel function (also used in the DOT derivation [9]). (2) We also need the following definite integral involving the Bessel function $\int_0^\infty x^m J_n(x) dx = 2^m (\Gamma(n/2 + m/2 + 1/2))/(\Gamma(n/2 - m/2 + 1/2))$. Note however that this integral blows up when the denominator is *undefined*, which occurs in the specific case $m = n + 1$ because $\Gamma(0)$ is undefined. (3) Hence, we need to solve property (2) in the special case that we have $\int_0^\infty x^n J_{n-1}(x) dx$. To do so, we need the following recurrence relation $J_{n-1}(x) = 2n/x J_n(x) - J_{n+1}(x)$. It is straightforward to show that the integral is zero. (4) Finally, $\Gamma(n + 1/2) = \sqrt{\pi}(2n - 1)!!/2^n$ for $n = 1, 2, 3, ...,$ where $(2n - 1)!! = 1 \cdot 3 \cdot 5 \cdots (2n - 1)$. For $n = 0$, $\Gamma(1/2) = \sqrt{\pi}$.

Now, we first write the 3D Fourier integral (Eq. 1) in spherical coordinates

$$P(R_0\mathbf{r}) = \int E(\mathbf{q}) e^{-2\pi i R_0 \mathbf{q} \cdot \mathbf{r}} d\mathbf{q} = \int_{q=0}^{\infty} \int_{|\mathbf{u}|=1} q^2 E(q\mathbf{u}) e^{-2\pi i R_0 q \mathbf{u} \cdot \mathbf{r}} dq d\mathbf{u}. \quad (5)$$

Using the pointwise convergent expansion of property (1) above, it implies that

$$P(R_0\mathbf{r}) = 4\pi \sum_{j=0}^{\infty} (-i)^{\ell(j)} Y_j(\mathbf{r}) \int_{q=0}^{\infty} \int_{|\mathbf{u}|=1} q^2 E(q\mathbf{u}) j_{\ell(j)}(2\pi q R_0) Y_j(\mathbf{u}) dq d\mathbf{u} \quad (6)$$

Next, we replace $E(\mathbf{q})$ by the Laplacian equation given in Eq. 2 to obtain $P(R_0\mathbf{r})$

$$4\pi \sum_{j=0}^{\infty} (-i)^{\ell(j)} Y_j(\mathbf{r}) \int \int q^2 \sum_{k=0}^{\infty} \left[\frac{c_k}{q^{\ell_k+1}} + d_k q^{\ell_k} \right] Y_k(\mathbf{u}) Y_j(\mathbf{u}) j_{\ell(j)}(2\pi q R_0) dq d\mathbf{u}$$

Because the SH basis is orthonormal, $\int Y_k(\mathbf{u}) Y_j(\mathbf{u}) d\mathbf{u} = \delta_{kj}$. Also, since $\ell(j)$ is even in our basis, $(-i)^{\ell(j)} = (-1)^{\ell(j)/2}$. Finally, we use $j_n(x) = \sqrt{\pi/2x} J_{n+1/2}(x)$.

$$P(R_0\mathbf{r}) = \frac{2\pi}{\sqrt{R_0}} \sum_{j=0}^{\infty} (-1)^{\frac{\ell(j)}{2}} Y_j(\mathbf{r}) \underbrace{\int_0^\infty \left(\frac{c_j}{q^{\ell(j)-\frac{1}{2}}} + d_j q^{\ell(j)+\frac{3}{2}} \right) J_{\ell(j)+\frac{1}{2}}(2\pi q R_0) dq}_{I_{\ell(j)}}$$

$$(7)$$

$$I_{\ell(j)} = \underbrace{\int_0^\infty c_j q^{1/2 - \ell(j)} J_{\ell(j)+1/2}(2\pi q R_0) dq}_{P1} + \underbrace{\int_0^\infty d_j q^{\ell(j)+3/2} J_{\ell(j)+1/2}(2\pi q R_0) dq}_{P2}$$

From property (3), we see that $P2$ is zero. For $P1$, we do the change of variable $x = 2\pi q R_0, dx = 2\pi R_0 dq$, and use properties (2) and (4) to obtain

$$P1 = c_j (2\pi R_0)^{\ell(j)-\frac{3}{2}} 2^{\frac{1}{2}-\ell(j)} \frac{\Gamma(\ell(j) + \frac{1}{4} + \frac{1}{4} - \frac{\ell(j)}{2} + \frac{1}{2})}{\Gamma(\frac{\ell(j)}{2} + \frac{1}{4} - \frac{1}{4} + \frac{\ell(j)}{2} + \frac{1}{2})} = c_j \sqrt{\frac{2}{\pi}} \frac{(2\pi R_0)^{\ell(j)-\frac{3}{2}}}{(2\ell(j) - 1)!!}$$

We insert $P1$ and $I_{\ell(j)}$ back into Eq. 7 and we obtain the desired result of Eq. 3 with some algebra. This completes the proof.   ∎

Clustering of the Human Skeletal Muscle Fibers Using Linear Programming and Angular Hilbertian Metrics[*]

Radhouène Neji[1,2,3], Ahmed Besbes[1,2], Nikos Komodakis[4],
Jean-François Deux[5], Mezri Maatouk[5], Alain Rahmouni[5], Guillaume Bassez[5],
Gilles Fleury[3], and Nikos Paragios[1,2]

[1] Laboratoire MAS, Ecole Centrale Paris, Châtenay-Malabry, France
[2] Equipe GALEN, INRIA Saclay - Île-de-France, Orsay, France
[3] Département SSE, Ecole Supérieure d'Electricité, Gif-sur-Yvette, France
[4] Department of Computer Science, University of Crete, Crete, Greece
[5] Centre Hospitalier Universitaire Henri Mondor, Créteil, France

Abstract. In this paper, we present a manifold clustering method for
the classification of fibers obtained from diffusion tensor images (DTI) of
the human skeletal muscle. Using a linear programming formulation of
prototype-based clustering, we propose a novel fiber classification algorithm over manifolds that circumvents the necessity to embed the data
in low dimensional spaces and determines automatically the number of
clusters. Furthermore, we propose the use of angular Hilbertian metrics
between multivariate normal distributions to define a family of distances
between tensors that we generalize to fibers. These metrics are used to
approximate the geodesic distances over the fiber manifold. We also discuss the case where only geodesic distances to a reduced set of landmark
fibers are available. The experimental validation of the method is done
using a manually annotated significant dataset of DTI of the calf muscle
for healthy and diseased subjects.

1 Introduction

Diffusion Tensor Imaging (DTI) has started to become more ubiquitous in other
fields than brain white matter study [1]. Indeed, this modality has been used for
other anatomical regions such as the tongue [2] and the human skeletal muscles
[3]. The latter are of particular interest because they present an architecture
of elongated myofibers with well known anatomy. Furthermore, the study of
the effects of myopathies (neuromuscular diseases) on water diffusion in muscle
tissues is essential to assess the possibility of the use of DTI in a diagnosis
procedure and early detection of diseases. Since myopathies result in an atrophy
and weakness of the muscle, we expect an alteration of the diffusion properties

---

[*] This work was partially supported by Association Française contre les Myopathies
(AFM: http://www.afm-france.org) under the DTI-MUSCLE project.

J.L. Prince, D.L. Pham, and K.J. Myers (Eds.): IPMI 2009, LNCS 5636, pp. 14–25, 2009.

among diseased subjects. It is therefore important to cluster fiber tracts for local statistical analysis of diffusion information.

DTI previous studies of the human skeletal muscle [3,4] provided a comparative study between subjects and different muscle regions of scalar values derived from tensors like trace, fractional anisotropy, etc. They also evaluated experimentally the physiological cross-sectional area (PCSA), which is an important measure of muscle architecture since it is related to the maximum muscle force. However little emphasis was put on muscle segmentation in comparison with brain white matter, where several approaches were proposed. The use of graph theory and manifold learning has been extensively explored in the previous literature. For instance, in [5] the distribution of points along each fiber tract is considered to be Gaussian, which allows to derive a Euclidean distance between each pair of fibers. Fiber bundling is done using a normalized cut. In [6], the affinity between fibers is based on the symmetrized Hausdorff distance and spectral clustering is achieved using an eigenanalysis of the affinity matrix and k-means in the embedding space. The method presented in [7] relies on Laplacian Eigenmaps and similarity between fibers is determined using their end points. In [8], the authors construct a graph-based distance between fiber tracts where both local and global dissimilarities are taken into account. The considered distance is then incorporated in a Locally Linear Embedding framework and clustering is done using k-means. Curve modeling has attracted attention and was handled in [9] by defining a spatial similarity measure between curves and using the Expectation-Maximization algorithm for clustering. The method proposed in [10] considers the simultaneous use of medoid-shift clustering and Isomap manifold learning and proposed to include prior knowledge in the segmentation process using a white matter fiber atlas. Mean-shift was also used in [11] where each fiber is first embedded in a high dimensional space using its sequence of points, and kernels with variable bandwidths are considered in the mean-shift algorithm. More recently, fibers were represented in [12] using their differential geometry and frame transportation and a consistency measure was used for clustering. Another class of methods suggested to circumvent the limitation of unsupervised clustering where the obtained segmentation may not correspond to anatomical knowledge. They opt for supervised algorithms that try to achieve a clustering consistent with a predefined atlas. Expert manual labeling of the fibers for one subject provides an atlas in [13]. This is followed by the registration of B0 images and a hierarchical classification of fibers where the B-spline coefficients of the curves are considered to measure curve similarity. In [6], a Nystrom approximation of the out-of-sample extension of the spectral embedding is considered to build an atlas of fibers.

We can note that the existing literature puts a lot of emphasis on manifold embeddings. They are considered crucial to reflect faithfully the diffusion process modeled by tensors and fibers, and proved to be useful for a more accurate analysis of DTI information [14]. However, the use of embeddings and common clustering techniques like k-means requires to choose the dimension of the embedding and the number of clusters. It would be preferable to obtain the number of clusters as a result of the clustering algorithm, especially when the inter-subject variability (which is rather important for skeletal muscles) may require the use of different numbers of clusters across patients. Moreover, selecting the embedding dimension is an issue since a too low dimension will result in information loss and a too high dimension will include an important dispersion in the data. Furthermore, clustering on the manifold directly is a tricky issue since one has to compute intrinsic means on submanifolds where an explicit expression of geodesic distances is not necessarily available. Another issue is the sensitivity of methods like k-means to initialization and the possible failure of the medoid-shift technique to determine correctly the modes of a density[15]. Besides, when dealing with fiber similarities, the prior art seems to discard the information provided by the tensor field when considering metrics between fibers. In [16], we proposed a kernel between tensors primarily, generalized it to fiber tracts and used k-means clustering after kernel PCA and Isomap embedding. In this paper, we propose a method that performs manifold clustering of fibers without resorting to manifold embeddings or computations of intrinsic means. It is based on a linear programming (LP) technique [17] and uses the geodesic distances from the fibers to a reduced set of landmark fibers to perform the clustering. Unlike k-means, the algorithm provides automatically the number of clusters, is not sensitive to initialization and the class centers are chosen as examplars from the dataset. As far as fiber similarity is concerned, we develop the viewpoint that we proposed in [16] and build Hilbertian angular metrics between fibers. These are derived from their counterparts between tensors, providing a more general and much simpler formulation than [16]. The metrics are incorporated afterwards in the Dijkstra algorithm to approximate the geodesic distances along the manifold of fibers.

The remainder of the paper is organized as follows: in section 2, we present the clustering method and develop the landmark-based geodesic clustering costs. In section 3, we discuss and derive the family of Hilbertian angular metrics between tensors and propose their extension to fiber tracts. Section 4 is dedicated to the experimental results and we discuss the perspectives of this work in section 5.

2   Manifold Clustering via Linear Programming

Clustering refers to the process of organizing a set of objects into groups such that the members of each group are as similar to each other as possible. A common way of tackling this problem is to formulate it as the following optimization task: given a set of objects $\mathcal{V} = \{p_1, \ldots, p_n\}$, endowed with a distance function $d(\cdot, \cdot)$ that measures dissimilarity between objects, the goal of clustering is to choose K objects from $\mathcal{V}$, say, $\{q_1, \ldots, q_K\}$ (these will be referred to as cluster centers hereafter) such that the obtained sum of distances between each object and its nearest center is minimized, or:

$$\min_{q_1, \ldots, q_K \in \mathcal{V}} \sum_{p \in \mathcal{V}} \min_i d(p, q_i) \ . \tag{1}$$

An important drawback of the above formulation is that it requires the number of clusters K to be provided beforehand, which is problematic as this number is very often not known in advance. Note that a wrong value for K may have a very negative effect on the final outcome. One would thus prefer K to be automatically estimated by the algorithm as a byproduct of the optimization process. To address this issue, we will let K be a variable here, and, instead of (1), we will use the following modified objective function, which additionally assigns a penalty $g(q_i)$ to each one of the chosen cluster centers q_i:

$$\min_{K} \min_{q_1,\ldots,q_K \in \mathcal{V}} \left(\sum_{p \in \mathcal{V}} \min_{i} d(p, q_i) + \sum_{i=1}^{K} g(q_i) \right) . \tag{2}$$

But, even if K is known, another serious drawback of many of the existing optimization-based techniques for clustering is that they are particularly sensitive to initialization and thus may get easily trapped in bad local minima. For instance, K-means (one of the most commonly used clustering methods) is doomed to fail if its initial cluster centers happen not to be near the actual cluster centers. To deal with that, here we will rely on a recently proposed clustering algorithm [17], which has been shown to yield approximately optimal solutions to the NP-hard problem (2). This algorithm relies on reformulating (2) as an equivalent integer program, whose LP-relaxation (denoted as PRIMAL hereafter) has the following form:

$$\text{PRIMAL} \equiv \min_{\mathbf{x}} \sum_{p,q \in \mathcal{V}, p \neq q} d(p, q) x_{pq} + \sum_{q \in \mathcal{V}} g(q) x_{qq} \tag{3}$$

$$\text{s.t.} \sum_{q \in \mathcal{V}} x_{pq} = 1, \ x_{pq} \leq x_{qq}, \ x_{pq} \geq 0 \tag{4}$$

If constraints $x_{pq} \geq 0$ are replaced with $x_{pq} \in \{0,1\}$, then the resulting integer program is equivalent to clustering problem (2). In this case, each binary variable x_{pq} with $p \neq q$ indicates whether object p has been assigned to cluster center q or not, while binary variable x_{qq} indicates whether object q has been chosen as a cluster center or not. Constraints $\sum_{q \in \mathcal{V}} x_{pq} = 1$ simply express the fact that each object must be assigned to exactly one center, while constraints $x_{pq} \leq x_{qq}$ require that if p has been assigned to q then object q must obviously be chosen as a center. The most crucial issue for tackling this integer LP is setting the variables x_{qq} correctly, ie, deciding which objects will be chosen as centers. To this end, the so-called *stability* of an object has been introduced in [17]. This is a measure which tries to quantitatively answer the following question: *how much does one need to further penalize an object to ensure that it will never be selected as an optimal cluster center?* Intuitively, the greater the stability of an object, the more appropriate that object is to become a cluster center. For having a practical algorithm based on object stabilities, an efficient way of estimating them is required. It turns out that this can indeed be done very fast by moving to the dual domain and appropriately updating a solution of a dual relaxation to PRIMAL. Since each dual cost provides a lower bound to the cost of the optimal clustering, an additional advantage of working in the dual domain is the ability to provide online optimality guarantees and to avoid bad local minima. We refer the reader to [17] for more details.

We now discuss the case where the objects lie on a manifold. This implies the use of the geodesic distance as a similarity measure. Ideally this distance should correspond to the pairwise cost $d(p, q)$ for $p \neq q$ in the linear programming formulation proposed in (3). A first possible choice is to compute the geodesic distances between all the pairs of points using the Dijkstra algorithm in an Isomap-like fashion, as suggested in [10]. The shortest path is found using a local approximation of the geodesic distance, for example a Euclidean distance. The pairwise cost $d(p, q)$ is set to $d(p, q) = d_g(p, q)$ where d_g is the corresponding geodesic distance. However, inspired by the landmark Isomap algorithm [18], we can compute the geodesic distances from all the data points to a reduced set of randomly selected landmarks. This will reduce the computational load that a full computation of the geodesic distances between every pair of data points would entail. Let $(l_m)_{m=1\ldots n_l}$ be a set of such chosen n_l landmarks. We would like to replace $d_g(p, q)$ by a reasonable approximation. Given that the geodesic distance between two points is the length of the shortest path linking these points, we note the following $\forall m \in [1 \ldots n_l]$, $|d_g(p, l_m) - d_g(q, l_m)| \leq d_g(p, q) \leq d_g(p, l_m) + d_g(q, l_m)$, which implies

$$\sup_m |d_g(p, l_m) - d_g(q, l_m)| \leq d_g(p, q) \leq \inf_m (d_g(p, l_m) + d_g(q, l_m)) \qquad (5)$$

This provides a lower bound and an upper bound to the cost $d_g(p, q)$ in the case where only the geodesic distances to some landmarks are computed. Note that in the particular case where p and q are landmarks $d_g(p, q) = \sup_m |d_g(p, l_m) - d_g(q, l_m)| = \inf_m (d_g(p, l_m) + d_g(q, l_m))$. On the other hand we can also note that

$$\inf_m (d_g(p, l_m) + d_g(q, l_m)) - 2\eta \leq \quad d_g(p, q) \qquad (6)$$

$$d_g(p, q) \leq \quad \sup_m |d_g(p, l_m) - d_g(q, l_m)| + 2\eta \qquad (7)$$

where $\eta = \inf_m \min(d_g(p, l_m), d_g(q, l_m))$. Therefore it makes sense to replace the cost $d_g(p, q)$ whether by its upper bound or its lower bound, since both approximate the cost up to 2η. A byproduct of inequalities (6) and (7) is that both approximations are exact if p or q are landmarks, since in that case we have $\eta = 0$.

It is interesting to note in this setting that the lower bound is the L^∞ norm between the distance-to-landmarks representation of p and q. Indeed, let $\mathbf{u_p}$ (resp. $\mathbf{u_q}$) be the n_l-dimensional vector of geodesic distances of p (resp. q) to the landmarks

$$\mathbf{u_p} = [d_g(p, l_1), \ldots, d_g(p, l_{n_l})]^t, \ \mathbf{u_q} = [d_g(q, l_1), \ldots, d_g(q, l_{n_l})]^t \qquad (8)$$

By definition, $\sup_m |d_g(p, l_m) - d_g(q, l_m)| = ||\mathbf{u_p} - \mathbf{u_q}||_\infty$. Thus the lower bound approximation has the advantage of defining a metric cost. Intuitively, for a number of landmarks sufficiently larger than the intrinsic dimension of the manifold, the distance vector representation will provide a good characterization of the points on the manifold.

In order to apply the clustering framework to fiber tracts, we will define a Euclidean structure over the fiber domain. For this purpose, we show in the next section how to map the fibers to a Hilbert space and derive corresponding metrics that will provide a local approximation of the geodesic distance.

3   From Metrics on Tensors to Metrics on Fibers

In this section, we build a family of Hilbertian metrics between fibers that will be incorporated in the Dijkstra algorithm to find the shortest path (and thus d_g) between two elements of the fiber set. The starting point is to consider angular distances between diffusion tensors based on Gaussian probability densities and generalize these distances to the fiber domain.

3.1   Multivariate Normals: A Subset of the Exponential Distributions Family

The structure of the set of multivariate normal distributions $\mathcal{M}$ as a statistical manifold endowed with the Fisher information geometry was discussed in [19], where a closed-form solution of the geodesic distance over this manifold is available for the particular case of Gaussian distributions with common mean. Here we view the multivariate normal distributions as a subset of the exponential distributions family. Let us consider a normal probability density p. In this context, given the exponential decay of the distribution, it is interesting to notice that not only p is an element of the Hilbert space L^2 of square integrable functions but any power p^α, with α a strictly positive real number is also square integrable. This motivates the use of normalized probability product kernels [20] to define a family of angular similarities between multivariate normal distributions. Indeed, considering two elements p_1 and p_2 of $\mathcal{M}$ and $\alpha \in \mathbb{R}_+^*$, we can define the following similarity $C_\alpha(p_1, p_2)$ between p_1 and p_2 as follows:

$$C_\alpha(p_1, p_2) = \frac{\int p_1(\mathbf{x})^\alpha p_2(\mathbf{x})^\alpha d\mathbf{x}}{\sqrt{\int p_1(\mathbf{x})^{2\alpha} d\mathbf{x}}\sqrt{\int p_2(\mathbf{x})^{2\alpha} d\mathbf{x}}} \tag{9}$$

C_α is simply the normalized L^2 inner product between p_1^α and p_2^α. It is therefore the cosine of the angle between p_1^α and p_2^α. It defines a Mercer kernel over the space of multivariate normal distributions, i.e. for any subset $(p_i)_{i=1...N}$ of $\mathcal{M}$, the Gram matrix G of C_α with entries $G_{ij} = C_\alpha(p_i, p_j)$ is semi-definite positive. The Mercer property allows the construction of a mapping ϕ_α associated with the kernel C_α that provides an embedding of $\mathcal{M}$ in the Reproducing Kernel Hilbert Space (RKHS) $\mathcal{H}_\alpha$ such that $C_\alpha(p_1, p_2) = <\phi_\alpha(p_1), \phi_\alpha(p_2)>_{\mathcal{H}_\alpha}$, where $< .,. >_{\mathcal{H}_\alpha}$ is the inner product of $\mathcal{H}_\alpha$. Given that C_α is a normalized scalar product, i.e. $C_\alpha(p, p) = 1$, we can define the following Hilbertian metric $d_{\alpha|\mathcal{H}_\alpha}$:

$$d_{\alpha|\mathcal{H}_\alpha}(p_1, p_2) = \sqrt{C_\alpha(p_1, p_1) - 2C_\alpha(p_1, p_2) + C_\alpha(p_2, p_2)} = \sqrt{2 - 2C_\alpha(p_1, p_2)} \tag{10}$$

In the following subsection, we derive the closed-form expression of C_α and $d_{\alpha|\mathcal{H}_\alpha}$ for normal distributions that model a local diffusion process.

3.2   Explicit Derivation of the Angular Distances

Let us consider the Gaussian distribution p that models the motion distribution of water protons at a location $\mathbf{x}$ with a tensor $\mathbf{D}$. Given a diffusion time t, the probability of displacement from the position $\mathbf{x}$ to the position $\mathbf{y}$ is provided by the following equation:

$$p(\mathbf{y}|\mathbf{x}, t, \mathbf{D}) = \frac{1}{\sqrt{\det(\mathbf{D})(4\pi t)^3}} \exp\left(-\frac{(\mathbf{y}-\mathbf{x})^t \mathbf{D}^{-1}(\mathbf{y}-\mathbf{x})}{4t}\right) \qquad (11)$$

We now consider two normal distributions p_1 and p_2 with parameters $(x_1, \mathbf{D}_1)$ and $(x_2, \mathbf{D}_2)$ respectively. Based on [20] and (11), we can see that C_α is the product of two terms:

$$C_\alpha(p_1, p_2) = C_\alpha^{tensor}(\mathbf{D}_1, \mathbf{D}_2) C_\alpha^{spatial}(p_1, p_2) \qquad (12)$$

where

$$C_\alpha^{tensor}(\mathbf{D}_1, \mathbf{D}_2) = 2\sqrt{2}\, \frac{\det(\mathbf{D}_1)^{\frac{1}{4}} \det(\mathbf{D}_2)^{\frac{1}{4}}}{\sqrt{\det(\mathbf{D}_1 + \mathbf{D}_2)}}$$

$$C_\alpha^{spatial}(p_1, p_2) = \exp\left(-\frac{\alpha}{4t}(\mathbf{x}_1^t \mathbf{D}_1^{-1}\mathbf{x}_1 + \mathbf{x}_2^t \mathbf{D}_2^{-1}\mathbf{x}_2)\right) \times$$
$$\exp\left(\frac{\alpha}{4t}(\mathbf{D}_1^{-1}\mathbf{x}_1 + \mathbf{D}_2^{-1}\mathbf{x}_2)^t (\mathbf{D}_1^{-1} + \mathbf{D}_2^{-1})^{-1}(\mathbf{D}_1^{-1}\mathbf{x}_1 + \mathbf{D}_2^{-1}\mathbf{x}_2)\right) \quad (13)$$

We notice that $C_\alpha^{spatial}$ has a much simpler expression. Indeed, using the following inversion properties

$$(\mathbf{D}_1 + \mathbf{D}_2)^{-1} = \mathbf{D}_1^{-1} - \mathbf{D}_1^{-1}(\mathbf{D}_1^{-1} + \mathbf{D}_2^{-1})^{-1}\mathbf{D}_1^{-1} \qquad (14)$$

$$(\mathbf{D}_1 + \mathbf{D}_2)^{-1} = \mathbf{D}_2^{-1} - \mathbf{D}_2^{-1}(\mathbf{D}_1^{-1} + \mathbf{D}_2^{-1})^{-1}\mathbf{D}_2^{-1} \qquad (15)$$

we obtain the following compact expression for $C_\alpha^{spatial}$:

$$C_\alpha^{spatial}(p_1, p_2) = \exp\left(-\frac{\alpha}{4t}(\mathbf{x}_1 - \mathbf{x}_2)^t (\mathbf{D}_1 + \mathbf{D}_2)^{-1}(\mathbf{x}_1 - \mathbf{x}_2)\right) \qquad (16)$$

We can see that C^{tensor} is a tensor similarity term and is independent of the parameter α while $C_\alpha^{spatial}$ is a spatial connectivity term where appears the Mahalanobis distance between the locations $\mathbf{x}_1$ and $\mathbf{x}_2$ with respect to the sum of tensors $(\mathbf{D}_1 + \mathbf{D}_2)$. Therefore C_α takes into account the tensor affinity as well as the spatial position. This is crucial since the combination of spatial and diffusion information allows for a better modeling of the interactions between tensors and favors a generalization to the fiber domain, as will be discussed in the next subsection. The diffusion time t is important to weight the contribution of each term and $t \to \infty$ corresponds to the case where the spatial interaction is not taken into account. Furthermore, there is a striking similarity between the proposed family of measures since α appears as a scale parameter in the exponential function. Given the present formulation, we can conclude that changing the parameter α amounts to a rescaling of the diffusion time t. The derivation of the metrics $d_{\alpha|\mathcal{H}_\alpha}$ is handily done using (10).

In the next subsection, we show how the Mercer property of C_α allows the definition of angular similarities between fiber tracts.

3.3   Angular Similarities between Fibers

A fiber tract is obtained by following the principal directions of diffusion of the tensor field starting from an initial location. It is therefore natural to represent a fiber $\mathbf{F}$ as a sequence of Gaussian probability measures $(p_i)_{i=1...N}$ where N is the number of points of the fiber. Every probability measure (p_i) has a pair of parameters $(\mathbf{x}_i, \mathbf{D}_i)$ where $\mathbf{x}_i$ is the spatial location and $\mathbf{D}_i$ is the tensor at $\mathbf{x}_i$ when the tensor field is supposed to be continuous. When considering the mapping ϕ_α of these measures in the RKHS $\mathcal{H}_\alpha$, we can represent $\mathbf{F}$ as a weighted average of $(\phi_\alpha(p_i))_{i=1...N}$, i.e. $\mathbf{F} = \sum_{i=1}^{N} w_i \phi_\alpha(p_i)$. A straightforward choice of weights is $\forall i, w_i = \frac{1}{N}$.

Let us consider a fiber $\mathbf{F}_1$ (resp. $\mathbf{F}_2$) represented using a set of probabilities $(p_i^{(1)})_{i=1...N_1}$ (resp. $(p_i^{(2)})_{i=1...N_2}$) and weights $w_i^{(1)}$ (resp. $w_i^{(2)}$). The angular similarity $\widehat{C}_\alpha$ between $\mathbf{F}_1$ and $\mathbf{F}_2$ is defined as follows:

$$\widehat{C}_\alpha(\mathbf{F}_1, \mathbf{F}_2) = \frac{< \sum_{i=1}^{N_1} w_i^{(1)} \phi_\alpha(p_i^{(1)}), \sum_{j=1}^{N_2} w_j^{(2)} \phi_\alpha(p_j^{(2)}) >_{\mathcal{H}_\alpha}}{\left\| \sum_{i=1}^{N_1} w_i^{(1)} \phi_\alpha(p_i^{(1)}) \right\|_{\mathcal{H}_\alpha} \left\| \sum_{j=1}^{N_2} w_j^{(2)} \phi_\alpha(p_j^{(2)}) \right\|_{\mathcal{H}_\alpha}} \tag{17}$$

Using the bilinearity of the inner product $< .,. >_{\mathcal{H}_\alpha}$, we can express $\widehat{C}_\alpha$ using C_α :

$$\widehat{C}_\alpha(\mathbf{F}_1, \mathbf{F}_2) = \frac{\sum_{i=1}^{N_1} \sum_{j=1}^{N_2} w_i^{(1)} w_j^{(2)} C_\alpha(p_i^{(1)}, p_j^{(2)})}{\left\| \sum_{i=1}^{N_1} w_i^{(1)} \phi_\alpha(p_i^{(1)}) \right\|_{\mathcal{H}_\alpha} \left\| \sum_{j=1}^{N_2} w_j^{(2)} \phi_\alpha(p_j^{(2)}) \right\|_{\mathcal{H}_\alpha}} \tag{18}$$

where $\left\| \sum_{i=1}^{N_k} w_i^{(k)} \phi_\alpha(p_i^{(k)}) \right\|_{\mathcal{H}_\alpha} = \sqrt{\sum_{i=1}^{N_k} \sum_{j=1}^{N_k} w_i^{(k)} w_j^{(k)} C_\alpha(p_i^{(k)}, p_j^{(k)})}$ for $k = \{1, 2\}$. Again the corresponding Hilbertian metric between fibers is derived in a similar way to (10). Note that the present formulation endows the fiber domain with an Euclidean structure without resorting to a dimensionality reduction step.

4   Experimental Validation

Thirty subjects (twenty healthy subjects and ten patients affected by myopathies) underwent a diffusion tensor imaging of the calf muscle using a 1.5 T MRI scanner with the following parameters : repetition time (TR)= 3600 ms, echo time (TE) = 70 ms, slice thickness = 7 mm and b value of 700 $s.mm^{-2}$ with 12 gradient

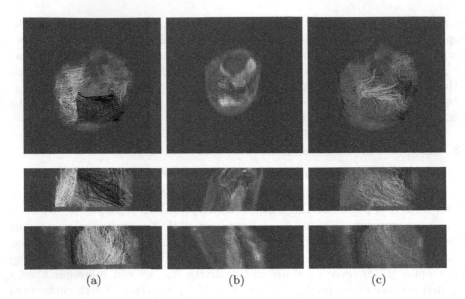

(a)   (b)   (c)

Fig. 1. Axial, coronal and sagittal views of fiber segmentation obtained with the lower bound approximation for (a) a healthy subject in 10 classes (b) a diseased subject in 3 classes. The parameter β was set to 10 in both cases. In (c) the ground truth segmentation of (a) with the following muscles: the soleus (cyan), lateral gastrocnemius (red), medial gastrocnemius (magenta), posterior tibialis (yellow), anterior tibialis (green), extensor digitorum longus (purple), and the peroneus longus (blue).

directions and 13 repetitions. The size of the obtained volumes is $64 \times 64 \times 20$ voxels with a voxel resolution of $3.125mm \times 3.125mm \times 7mm$. T1-weighted volumes were simultaneously acquired, so they are naturally registered to the diffusion images. They were afterwards manually segmented by an expert in 7 classes [Fig.1 (c)].

Fiber tracts were reconstructed using [21], based on a manual region of interest. To obtain the ground-truth class of each fiber, we counted the number of voxels belonging to each muscle group that the fiber crosses and assigned the latter to the majority class. In our experiments we set the diffusion time to $t = 2\,10^4$ and the parameter α in the fiber metric to $\alpha = 1$. To compute the Hilbertian metrics between fiber tracts, the weights w_i of each fiber $\mathbf{F}$ in (18) were chosen as the inverse of the number of points in $\mathbf{F}$. We selected 30% of the fibers as landmarks and for the computation of the geodesic distances using the Dijkstra algorithm, we considered a k-NN graph where k was set to $k = 12$. The cost $g(\mathbf{F})$ of choosing a fiber $\mathbf{F}$ as a class center in (3) was set to a constant $g = \beta\,\mu_{\frac{1}{2}}\,(d_g(\mathbf{F}_i, \mathbf{F}_j)_{i \neq j})$ where $\mu_{\frac{1}{2}}$ is the statistical median. We tested the following values of β: $\{7, 10, 13\}$. For a quantitative assessment of the method, we measure the dice overlap coefficient between the obtained segmentation using the proposed method and the ground-truth segmentation provided by the expert. For the sake of comparison, we evaluate also the performance of k-means clustering using the same metric and a manifold embedding. The dimensionality of the embedding is chosen to be the number

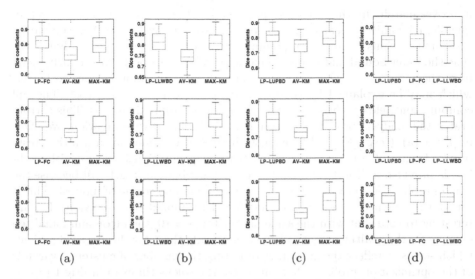

Fig. 2. Boxplots of dice overlap coefficients for the thirty subjects. Each row corresponds to a value of β, from top to bottom β takes the following values 7 , 10 and 13. (a) LP clustering using full computation of distances (LP-FC), comparison is done with respect to the average score of k-means (AV-KM) and the score of the k-means clustering with least distortion (MAX-KM) after manifold embedding. (b) LP clustering using lower bound approximation (LP-LLWBD). (c) LP clustering using upper bound approximation (LP-LUPBD). (d) Comparison between LP-FC, LP-LLWBD and LP-LUPBD.

of clusters obtained by our method, which is a common choice in embedding-based approaches. The k-means algorithm is run 50 times and each time we compute the dice overlap of the clustering result with the ground-truth segmentation. We consider both the average dice coefficients over the restarts of the k-means algorithm and the dice coefficient of the clustering with the least distortion. We run the following experiments:

1. We compute all the geodesic distances between every pair of points and use them for linear programming clustering. We compare the obtained result with an Isomap embedding followed by k-means.
2. We compute the geodesic distances to a set of landmarks and use the lower (resp. upper) bound approximation for linear programming clustering. We compare the obtained result with a landmark-Isomap embedding followed by k-means.

We provide in [Fig.2 (a), (b), (c)] the boxplots showing the distributions of the dice coefficients for the thirty subjects using different values of β for our algorithm, compared with k-means after manifold embedding. We can note that linear programming clustering performs significantly better than the average score achieved by k-means both for a full and landmark-based computation of the geodesic distances. Furthermore, it achieves results equivalent to the best k-means with an average dice coefficient of approximately 0.8 and in some cases it

improves marginally the dice overlap. The advantage is that our result is reproducible, i.e. unlike k-means it is not sensitive to initialization. When comparing
the three versions of linear programming clustering, we can see in [Fig.2 (d)]
that the lower bound and upper bound approximations perform similarly apart
from the case $\beta = 10$ where the lower bound approximation performed better,
which may be explained by the metricity of the corresponding cost. The full
computation yields slightly better results than the approximations. This corrob-
orates the analysis provided is section 2. For qualitative evaluation, we show
in [Fig.1 (a)] (resp. [Fig.1 (b)]) a clustering result obtained for a healthy (resp.
diseased) subject for $\beta = 10$. Ground truth segmentation for the healthy subject is provided in [Fig.1 (c)]. There are too few fibers in [Fig.1 (b)] because the
tractography fails to recover fibers through the manual region of interest. This is
due to the presence of tensors with very low determinant (low diffusion). It is interesting to note that with the same parameter $\beta = 10$, the algorithm found ten
clusters for the healthy subject while it found only three for the diseased patient,
which seems to reflect the advantage of letting the number of clusters a variable
of the optimization problem. Note also how the soleus (in cyan in [Fig.1 (c)]) is
subdivided in an anterior and a posterior part in [Fig.1 (a)], which is consistent
with its anatomy of oblique fibers converging towards a central aponeurosis.

5   Conclusion

In this paper, we proposed a novel manifold-based fiber clustering approach
where there is no need to perform an embedding in a low dimensional space or
to select the number of clusters. We applied the method to the bundling of the
fibers of the human skeletal muscle. We also developed the theoretical aspects
of angular distances between multivariate normal distributions that model local
diffusion processes and showed that the RKHS formulation allows for the definition of corresponding metrics between fiber tracts. These metrics were used
to approximate the geodesic distances on the fiber manifold using the Dijkstra
algorithm. A procedure of landmark selection should be investigated based on
the bounds tightness in (6) and (7), as well as other metrics and structures over
the fiber domain. Based for example on the metric in (10), the method can also
be used for a clustering at the tensor level.

References

1. Bihan, D.L., Mangin, J.F., Poupon, C., Clark, C.A., Pappata, S., Molko, N.,
   Chabrait, H.: Diffusion tensor imaging: Concepts and applications. Journal of Magnetic Resonance Imaging 13, 534–546 (2001)
2. Gilbert, R.J., Napadow, V.J.: Three-dimensional muscular architecture of the human tongue determined in vivo with diffusion tensor magnetic resonance imaging.
   Dysphagia 20, 1–7 (2005)
3. Galban, C.J., Maderwald, S., Uffmann, K., de Greiff, A., Ladd, M.E.: Diffusive sensitivity to muscle architecture: a magnetic resonance diffusion tensor imaging study
   of the human calf. European Journal of Applied Physiology 93(3), 253–262 (2004)

4. Damon, B., Ding, Z., Anderson, A., Freyer, A., Gore, J.: Validation of diffusion tensor MRI-based muscle fiber tracking. Magnetic Resonance in Medicine 48, 97–104 (2002)
5. Brun, A., Knutsson, H., Park, H.J., Shenton, M.E., Westin, C.F.: Clustering fiber traces using normalized cuts. In: Barillot, C., Haynor, D.R., Hellier, P. (eds.) MICCAI 2004. LNCS, vol. 3216, pp. 368–375. Springer, Heidelberg (2004)
6. ODonnell, L., Westin, C.F.: Automatic tractography segmentation using a high-dimensional white matter atlas. IEEE TMI 26(11), 1562–1575 (2007)
7. Brun, A., Park, H.J., Knutsson, H., Westin, C.F.: Coloring of DT-MRI fiber traces using laplacian eigenmaps. In: Moreno-Díaz Jr., R., Pichler, F. (eds.) EUROCAST 2003. LNCS, vol. 2809, pp. 518–529. Springer, Heidelberg (2003)
8. Tsai, A., Westin, C.F., Hero, A.O., Willsky, A.S.: Fiber tract clustering on manifolds with dual rooted-graphs. In: CVPR (2007)
9. Maddah, M., Grimson, W., Warfield, S., Wells, W.: A unified framework for clustering and quantitative analysis of white matter fiber tracts. Medical Image Analysis 12(2), 191–202 (2008)
10. Wassermann, D., Deriche, R.: Simultaneous manifold learning and clustering: Grouping white matter fiber tracts using a volumetric white matter atlas. In: MICCAI 2008 Workshop - Manifolds in Medical Imaging: Metrics, Learning and Beyond (2008)
11. Zvitia, O., Mayer, A., Greenspan, H.: Adaptive mean-shift registration of white matter tractographies. In: ISBI (2008)
12. Savadjiev, P., Campbell, J.S.W., Pike, G.B., Siddiqi, K.: Streamline flows for white matter fibre pathway segmentation in diffusion MRI. In: Metaxas, D., Axel, L., Fichtinger, G., Székely, G. (eds.) MICCAI 2008, Part I. LNCS, vol. 5241, pp. 135–143. Springer, Heidelberg (2008)
13. Maddah, M., Mewes, A.U.J., Haker, S., Grimson, W.E.L., Warfield, S.K.: Automated atlas-based clustering of white matter fiber tracts from DTMRI. In: Duncan, J.S., Gerig, G. (eds.) MICCAI 2005. LNCS, vol. 3749, pp. 188–195. Springer, Heidelberg (2005)
14. Verma, R., Khurd, P., Davatzikos, C.: On analyzing diffusion tensor images by identifying manifold structure using isomaps. IEEE TMI 26(6), 772–778 (2007)
15. Vedaldi, A., Soatto, S.: Quick shift and kernel methods for mode seeking. In: Forsyth, D., Torr, P., Zisserman, A. (eds.) ECCV 2008, Part IV. LNCS, vol. 5305, pp. 705–718. Springer, Heidelberg (2008)
16. Neji, R., Paragios, N., Fleury, G., Thiran, J.P., Langs, G.: Classification of tensors and fiber tracts using Mercer-kernels encoding soft probabilistic spatial and diffusion information. In: CVPR (2009)
17. Komodakis, N., Paragios, N., Tziritas, G.: Clustering via LP-based stabilities. In: NIPS (2008)
18. de Silva, V., Tenenbaum, J.B.: Global versus local methods in nonlinear dimensionality reduction. In: NIPS (2002)
19. Deriche, R., Tschumperlé, D., Lenglet, C., Rousson, M.: Variational Approaches to the Estimation, Regularization and Segmentation of Diffusion Tensor Images. In: Paragios, Chen, Faugeras (eds.) Mathematical Models of Computer Vision: The Handbook. Springer, Heidelberg (2005)
20. Jebara, T., Kondor, R., Howard, A.: Probability product kernels. Journal of Machine Learning Research 5, 819–844 (2004)
21. Fillard, P., Toussaint, N., Pennec, X.: Medinria: DT-MRI processing and visualization software Similar Tensor Workshop (2006)

High-Resolution Adaptive PET Imaging*

Jian Zhou and Jinyi Qi

Department of Biomedical Engineering, University of California-Davis, California, USA

Abstract. While the performance of small animal PET systems has been improved impressively in terms of spatial resolution and sensitivity, demands for further improvements remain high with growing number of applications. Here we propose a novel PET system design that integrates a high-resolution detector into an existing PET system to obtain higher-resolution images in a target region. The high-resolution detector will be adaptively positioned based on the detectability or quantitative accuracy of a feature of interest. The proposed system will be particularly effective for studying human cancers using animal models where tumors are often grown near the skin surface and therefore permit close contact with the high resolution detector. It will also be useful for the high-resolution brain imaging in rodents. In this paper, we present the theoretical analysis and Monte Carlo simulation studies of the performance of the proposed system.

1 Introduction

The performance of small animal PET systems has been improved impressively in terms of spatial resolution and sensitivity since their first development in the mid 1990s. Most current systems use scintillator-based detectors because of the ability to achieve high performance with a relatively compact geometry and at an acceptable cost [1]. Some research systems have reported a sub-mm spatial resolution in animal studies using arrays of small scintillator elements [2,3,4]. However, the resolution of these systems is still mainly limited by the physical size of the scintillator elements and the intrinsic spatial resolution of the detectors [5]. Therefore, placing detectors with much smaller scintillator elements in close proximity to the object is useful to obtain higher spatial resolution and higher sensitivity. Successful instances have been presented [6,7,8,9], where high-resolution detectors are inserted into an existing whole body PET scanner to improve the system performance in a smaller field of view (FOV). Recently, Tai *et al* [10] has developed a so-called virtual-pinhole PET scanner which is built on a commercial microPET scanner including an entire ring insert using smaller detector elements to improve the spatial resolution.

While these approaches have been successful, room for improvement remains. For instance, most PET-insert scanners still require a large number of high-resolution detectors (either partial or full ring) to be placed within the gantry of an existing system, which significantly increases the number of electronic channels and cost. Secondly, most existing PET inserts use short detectors (e.g., 3.75 mm for the virtual-pinhole PET)

---

* This work is supported by the US Department of Energy under Grant No. DE-FG02-08ER64677.

J.L. Prince, D.L. Pham, and K.J. Myers (Eds.): IPMI 2009, LNCS 5636, pp. 26–37, 2009.

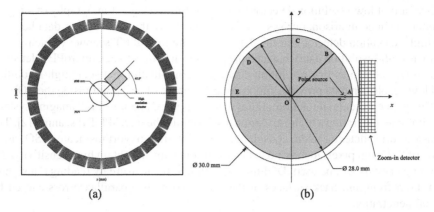

Fig. 1. (a) The proposed PET system shown with a high resolution detector positioned inside a scanner at angle $45°$. (b) A phantom used for resolution measurements.

to avoid the depth of interaction (DOI) effect, so the sensitivity of the high-resolution detector is fairly low, which limits the potential improvement. In addition, the detectors are in a ring at a fixed radius, so it may not be possible to position animals right up against the high-resolution detectors to take full advantage of the resolution available.

Here, we propose a new PET system that integrates a single high-resolution detector into an existing PET scanner that acts somewhat analogously to a "magnifying glass" and is expected to provide much higher resolution and sensitivity in a small region around the face of this detector (see Fig. 1). It will be particularly effective for studying human cancers using animal models where tumors are often grown near the skin surface and therefore permit close contact with the high resolution detector. The proposed system then provides high-resolution and high-sensitivity images that can reveal the heterogeneity inside a tumor, which permits better understanding of tumor progression and response to therapies. It will also be useful for high-resolution brain imaging in rodents.

The advantage of using a single high-resolution detector as compare to a half- or full-ring insert is three folds. First, it is much easier to build a single detector module than a full-ring PET with a large number of modules. For some detector designs, it may even be cost-prohibitive to build a large number of detector modules in near future. Thus, the proposed design offers an innovative solution to take the advantage of a single available high-resolution detector and to obtain high-resolution images well before a full-ring system can be built. Second, the electronics and system integration can be significantly simplified because only one high-resolution detector module is used. Third, a single high-resolution detector also provides greater flexibility. A novel feature of our design is that the high-resolution detector can be adaptively positioned with respect to the subject being imaged to provide the optimal image quality in a target region. In our initial implementation, we plan to allow the high-resolution detector to rotate about the animal in the transaxial plane. A combination with the axial and vertical bed movement can position this detector optimally at close contact with most part of animal. Huh *et al* [11] presented a PET imaging probe where a high-resolution detector is used in coincidence with an arc of low-resolution detector to perform limited angle tomography of a region of interest. In comparison, our system collects not only the coincidence data between the high-resolution detector and the detectors in the microPET scanner (which we refer to as high-resolution data), but also the projection data between microPET detectors (which we refer to as low-resolution data). The combination between high-resolution and low-resolution data provides full angular coverage of any point inside the FOV.

This paper presents simulation studies of the proposed adaptive PET imaging system. We simulate integrating a high-resolution detector into the microPET II scanner [2]. The high-resolution detector under consideration is a lutetium oxyorthosilicate (LSO) array made of 0.25 mm pixels to maximize the resolution gain. To obtain high sensitivity, 20-mm long crystals will be used. DOI information will be measure by reading out signals from both front and back surfaces of the crystal to reduce parallax errors caused by crystal penetration.

The paper is organized as follows. Section 2 describes image reconstruction method for the proposed system and theoretical analysis on resolution and noise properties, and lesion detectability of the MAP reconstruction. Section 3 presents Monte Carlo (MC) simulation studies to verify the theoretical predictions and to demonstrate the feasibility of adaptively positioning the high-resolution detector for lesion discrimination tasks. Finally, discussion and conclusion are given in Section 4.

2 Theory

2.1 Imaging Model

The data from the proposed PET system consist of both high-resolution data from the high-resolution detector and low-resolution data from the microPET II scanner. These emission data are well modeled as a collection of independent Poisson random variables with the expectation $\bar{y} = [\bar{y}_1, \ldots, \bar{y}_N]' \in \mathbb{R}^N$ (where N is the total number of detector pairs, and $''$ denotes the vector or matrix transpose), related to the unknown image $x \in [x_1, \ldots, x_M]'$ (where M is the number of voxels) by an affine transform:

$$\bar{y} = Px + r, \tag{1}$$

where $P \in \mathbb{R}^{N \times M}$ is the system matrix with the (i, j)th element representing the probability of detecting an event from voxel j by detector pair i, and $r = [r_1, \ldots, r_N] \in \mathbb{R}^N$ is the mean contribution of background events such as randoms and scatters. The system matrix can be factorized as follows [12]

$$P = P_{\text{det.sens}} P_{\text{attn}} P_{\text{sys}}. \tag{2}$$

$P_{\text{det.sens}} \in \mathbb{R}^{N \times N}$ is a diagonal detector normalization matrix. $P_{\text{attn}} \in \mathbb{R}^{N \times N}$ is a diagonal matrix containing attenuation factors for each line of response (LOR). In the proposed PET system, the attenuation effects of the high-resolution detector on the low-resolution data are also included in this matrix. $P_{\text{sys}} \in \mathbb{R}^{N \times M}$ is the system matrix modeling the probability that a photon pair emitted from one voxel is detected by a detector pair in the absence of photon attenuation and detector efficiency variations.

It includes both the solid angle effect and crystal penetration effect. Here we used a numerical method previously proposed in [13] which is capable of handling arbitrary geometry. It models the block structure of the PET scanner and takes into account the photon penetration and gaps between detectors.

For comparison with the original microPET scanner, we divide the system matrix of the proposed system as

$$P = [(P^{\text{low}})', (P^{\text{high}})']', \tag{3}$$

where P^{low} concerns the LORs formed by the microPET II detectors, and P^{high} models the LORs between the microPET II detectors and the high-resolution detector. Similarly, we also partition the data as

$$\bar{y} = [(\bar{y}^{\text{low}})', (\bar{y}^{\text{high}})']', \tag{4}$$

where $\bar{y}^{\text{low}}$ and $\bar{y}^{\text{high}}$ represent the low- and high-resolution data, respectively.

2.2 MAP Image Reconstruction

A MAP reconstruction is found by

$$\hat{x} = \arg\max_{x \geq 0} \{L(y|x) - \beta U(x)\} \tag{5}$$

where $L(y, x)$ is the Poisson log-likelihood function with $y = [y_1, \ldots, y_N]' \in \mathbb{R}^N$ as measured sinogram data, $U(x)$ is the prior energy function, and β is the smoothing parameter that controls the resolution of a reconstructed image. The Poisson log-likelihood is given by

$$L(y|x) = \sum_{i=1}^{N} \{y_i \log(\bar{y}_i) - \bar{y}_i - \log y_i!\}. \tag{6}$$

The prior we use here are Gaussian priors whose energy function has the form

$$U(x) = \frac{1}{2} \sum_{m=1}^{M} \sum_{k \in \mathcal{N}_m} \omega_{mk}(x_k - x_m)^2 \tag{7}$$

where $\mathcal{N}_m$ represents the neighborhood of voxel m, and ω_{mk} is a weighting factor that is chosen to be the reciprocal of the Euclidean distance between voxels m and k.

2.3 Theoretical Analysis of Resolution and Noise Properties

Theoretical analysis is used to obtain insights into the performance of the system. It also allows fast predictions of image quality without using time-consuming Monte Carlo simulations and thus is very important for the adaptive PET imaging. We follow the same approaches that have been used in previous works [14,15,16,17]. Specifically, image properties are analyzed at the fixed-point solution of MAP reconstruction and the first-order Taylor series expansion is used to approximate the solution under a low-noise assumption. Using the results derived in [17], the local impulse response at the jth voxel and the covariance can be written as

$$l_j(\hat{x}) \approx (F + \beta R)^{-1} F e_j, \tag{8}$$
$$\Sigma \approx (F + \beta R)^{-1} F (F + \beta R)^{-1}. \tag{9}$$

where $F \triangleq P' \text{diag}\{1/\bar{y}_i\} P \in \mathbb{R}^{M \times M}$ is the Fisher information matrix with $\text{diag}\{1/\bar{y}_i\}$ being a diagonal matrix whose (i,i)th element is $1/\bar{y}_i$, R is the Hessian matrix of the energy function $U(x)$, and e_j is the jth unit vector.

By assuming local shift invariance, it has been shown that the local impulse response can be evaluated using the fast Fourier transform as [17,18]

$$l_j(\hat{x}) \approx Q' \text{diag} \left\{ \frac{\lambda_m(j)}{\lambda_m(j) + \beta \mu_m(j)} \right\} Q e_j, \tag{10}$$

and the jth column of the covariance matrix as

$$\Sigma_j \approx Q' \text{diag} \left\{ \frac{\lambda_m(j)}{(\lambda_m(j) + \beta \mu_m(j))^2} \right\} Q e_j, \tag{11}$$

where $Q \in \mathbb{C}^{M \times M}$ is the Kronecker form of the Fourier transform, $\{\lambda_m(j) \geq 0, m = 1, \ldots, M\}$ and $\{\mu_m(j) \geq 0, m = 1, \ldots, M\}$ are the Fourier transform of the jth column of F and R, respectively, i.e. $\{\lambda_m(j)\} = QFe_j$ and $\{\mu_m(j)\} = QRe_j$. [1] Note that throughout the paper we use index j to denote the point of interest (e.g., location of a lesion) and the vectors that are being put along the diagonal in (10) and (11) are indexed by m.

For a given image prior, $\{\mu_m(j)\}$ is fixed. Therefore, it is the quantities $\{\lambda_m(j)\}$, which depends on the system matrix and noise in sinogram data, that characterizes the performance of MAP reconstruction for different PET scanners.

2.4 Theoretical Analysis of Lesion Detection

Lesion detection is one major application of PET imaging. Here we analyze the performance of a "signal-known-exactly, background-known-exactly" (SKE-BKE) detection task using computer observers. One observer that we studied is the prewhitening (PW) observer, which computes the test statistic by

$$\eta_{\text{PW}}(\hat{x}) = (\mathcal{E}\{\hat{x}|H_1\} - \mathcal{E}\{\hat{x}|H_0\})' \Sigma^{-1} \hat{x} \tag{12}$$

In previous work [20], it has been shown that for MAP reconstruction, the SNR of PW observer can be approximated by

$$\text{SNR}^2_{\text{PW}}(\eta(\hat{x})) \approx \bar{f}_l' Q' \text{diag}\{\lambda_m(j)\} Q \bar{f}_l \tag{13}$$

---

[1] When computing $\{\lambda_m\}$ and $\{\mu_m\}$, we assumed symmetry of Fe_j and Re_j so that the spectrums are real valued. The negative spectrums were truncated to zero to fulfill the positivity definite of matrices F and R.

where $\bar{f}_l$ is the true lesion profile and centered at the jth pixel, and $\lambda_m(j)$ represents the local Fourier spectrums of F around the lesion location. Note that the PW observer SNR depends only on the system matrix and is independent of the prior function and parameter β.

From (3) and (4), we have

$$F = F^{\text{low}} + F^{\text{high}} \triangleq (P^{\text{low}})' \text{diag}\left\{1/\bar{y}_\ell^{\text{low}}\right\}(P^{\text{low}}) + (P^{\text{high}})'\text{diag}\left\{1/\bar{y}_p^{\text{high}}\right\}(P^{\text{high}}),$$
$$(14)$$

where F^{low} and F^{high} are essentially the Fisher information matrices of the low- and high-resolution data, respectively. We can then define

$$\{\lambda_m^{\text{low}}(j)\} = QF^{\text{low}}e_j \quad \text{and} \quad \{\lambda_m^{\text{high}}(j)\} = QF^{\text{high}}e_j,$$

and thus we have

$$\lambda_m(j) = \lambda_m^{\text{low}}(j) + \lambda_m^{\text{high}}(j) \tag{15}$$

for $m = 1, \ldots M$. Substituting (15) into (13), we get

$$[\text{SNR}_{\text{PW}}(\eta(\hat{x}))]^2 \approx \bar{f}_l' Q' \text{diag}\left\{\lambda_m^{\text{low}}(j)\right\} Q\bar{f}_l + \bar{f}_l' Q' \text{diag}\left\{\lambda_m^{\text{high}}(j)\right\} Q\bar{f}_l. \tag{16}$$

Ignoring the attenuation of the high-resolution detector, the PW observer SNR of the original PET system can be approximate by

$$[\text{SNR}_{\text{PW}}^{\text{orginal}}(\eta(\hat{x}))]^2 \approx \bar{f}_l' Q' \text{diag}\left\{\lambda_m^{\text{low}}(j)\right\} Q\bar{f}_l.$$

Because $Q'\text{diag}\left\{\lambda_m^{\text{high}}(j)\right\}Q$ is nonnegativity definite, the above expressions indicate

$$\text{SNR}_{\text{PW}}(\eta(\hat{x})) > \text{SNR}_{\text{PW}}^{\text{original}}(\eta(\hat{x})), \tag{17}$$

i.e., the PW observer performance of the proposed PET is always superior to that of the original PET. The SNR gain is approximately equal to $\bar{f}_l' Q' \text{diag}\left\{\lambda_m^{\text{high}}(j)\right\} Q\bar{f}_l$, which comes from the contribution of the high-resolution detector. One can also show that (17) still holds when the attenuation of the high-resolution detector is considered with the following two assumptions: (i) Any photon that is attenuated by the high-resolution detector is detected by the high-resolution detector, i.e. the total number of detected events is not reduced by the insertion of the high-resolution detector; 2) An event detected by the high-resolution detector carries more information than a similar event detected by a low-resolution detector because the former has higher intrinsic resolution. The improvement in lesion detectability is demonstrated by computer simulations, even though the second assumption may not be satisfied for photons entering the high-resolution detector from the side in our configuration.

We also studied channelized Hotelling observers (CHOs) [21,22], which have been shown to have good correlation with human performance. The CHO test statistic is calculated by

$$\eta_{\text{CHO}}(\hat{x}) = (\mathcal{E}\{\hat{x}|H_1\} - \mathcal{E}\{\hat{x}|H_0\})'U'K^{-1}(U\hat{x} + n) \tag{18}$$

where $U \in \mathbb{R}^{l \times M}$ represents l frequency-selective channels that mimic the human visual system, $K \in \mathbb{R}^{l \times l}$ is the covariance of channel outputs, and n is the internal channel noise with mean zero and covariance K_N that models the uncertainty in human detection process. Using the results derived in [23], the SNR of a CHO can be computed by

$$\mathrm{SNR}^2_{\mathrm{CHO}} \approx \left[\sum_m \frac{\tilde{U}_{k,m} \lambda_m(j) \xi_m}{\lambda_m(j) + \beta \mu_m(j)} \right]' K^{-1} \left[\sum_m \frac{\tilde{U}_{k,m} \lambda_m(j) \xi_m(j)}{\lambda_m(j) + \beta \mu_m(j)} \right], \quad (19)$$

and

$$K \approx \tilde{U} \mathrm{diag} \left\{ \frac{\lambda_m(j)}{(\lambda_m(j) + \beta \mu_m(j))^2} \right\} \tilde{U}' + K_N, \quad (20)$$

where $\tilde{U} = UQ'$ are the Fourier coefficients of the channel functions, $\{\xi_m, \ m = 1, \dots, M\}$ is the Fourier transform of $\bar{f}_l$, and $[c_k]$ denotes a column vector with the kth element being c_k.

The above theoretical expressions allow fast evaluation of image quality and will be used to guide the positioning of the high-resolution detector based on the imaging task. Since the theoretical analysis is general, the above results are not only applicable to our proposed system but also useful for other PET-insert systems such as the virtual-pinhole PET scanner.

3 Simulation Study

3.1 Materials

We simulated the microPET II scanner operating in two-dimension mode, which has 30 LSO detectors in a 16 cm diameter ring, with each detector module containing 14×1 individual LSO crystals of size $1.0 \times 1.0 \times 12.5$ mm^3. For the high-resolution detector, we considered a multilayer LSO array. Each layer has a thickness of 2.5 mm and 64×1 LSO crystals of size $0.25 \times 0.25 \times 2.5$ mm^3. A total of 8 layers were used to simulate a 20-cm long detector. The FOV is restricted to a circular region of diameter 30 mm, which is large enough for small animals such as mouse. The high-resolution detector was placed outside this FOV, 15 mm away from the center of the scanner transaxially. It can perform 360° rotation around the FOV. A combination with vertical bed movement can position the high-resolution detector optimally at close contact with most part of the animal. The transaxial view of our target PET system is shown in Fig. 1.

3.2 Spatial Resolution

We measure the spatial resolution of the proposed PET system by simulating a point source on a uniform disc phantom as shown in Fig. 1(b). A point source of 0.1 mm in diameter was positioned at various radial offsets along five line segmentations: OA, OB, OC, OD, and OE. The activity ratio between the point source and the background disc was 100 : 1. The high resolution detector was positioned at angle 0°. Noise-free data were used for resolution measurements. For resolution measurements, we set $\beta = 0$ in MAP reconstruction (equivalent to ML reconstruction). To reduce computation time, images were reconstructed using OSEM algorithm with 14 subsets and 75 iterations.

Table 1. Spatial resolution of the proposed PET system (radial FWHM, tangential FWHM) (unit in mm)

radial distance	OA	OB	OC	OD	OE	microPET II
0mm	(0.52,0.26)	(0.28,0.34)	(0.26,0.52)	(0.34,0.28)	(0.52,0.26)	(0.49,0.51)
2mm	(0.58,0.22)	(0.28,0.31)	(0.24,0.60)	(0.31,0.28)	(0.66,0.22)	(0.60,0.53)
4mm	(0.58,0.22)	(0.28,0.31)	(0.24,0.58)	(0.31,0.28)	(0.58,0.26)	(0.54,0.54)
6mm	(0.54,0.22)	(0.25,0.31)	(0.24,0.54)	(0.34,0.28)	(0.58,0.26)	(0.56,0.51)
8mm	(0.56,0.22)	(0.25,0.28)	(0.24,0.54)	(0.34,0.31)	(0.66,0.26)	(0.57,0.47)
10mm	(0.56,0.22)	(0.25,0.31)	(0.30,0.48)	(0.37,0.31)	(0.66,0.26)	(0.58,0.46)
12mm	(0.50,0.22)	(0.25,0.31)	(0.36,0.48)	(0.40,0.31)	(0.68,0.26)	(0.63,0.45)

The FWHM of each reconstructed point source was measured by using linear interpolation after subtracting the uniform background. For comparison, the spatial resolution of the microPET II (without the high-resolution detector) was also measured by reconstructing the low-resolution data only.

The measured FWHM values are shown in Table 1. It is clear that the proposed system offers higher resolution than the original microPET II scanner. Note that the resolution of the proposed system is not isotropic because LORs are not uniformly spread in the FOV with only one high-resolution detector. Greater resolution improvement is often found along the direction parallel to the face of the high-resolution detector.

To demonstrate the effect of the resolution improvement on resolving small features, we created a phantom which consists of a warm disc background (diameter of 28.0 mm) and five sets of 3×3 tiny round spots located at the ends of the five line segments

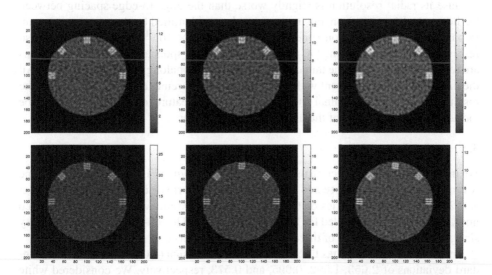

Fig. 2. Reconstructed images of the hot spots phantom for the microPET II (top row) and the proposed system (bottom row). Images from left to right were reconstructed with β values of 1×10^{-4}, 1×10^{-3}, and 1×10^{-2}, respectively.

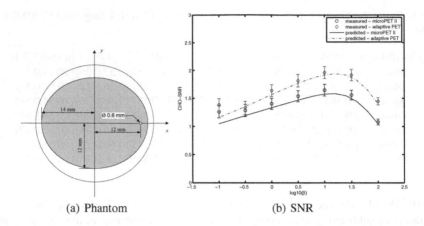

(a) Phantom   (b) SNR

Fig. 3. Comparison of CHO-SNR between the proposed PET and the microPET II scanner

(OA-OE). The diameter of each hot spot is 0.3 mm, and the center-to-center spacing between adjacent spots is 0.8 mm. The activity ratio of the hot spots to the background is 40 : 1. A noisy sinogram was generated with the expected total number of events equal to one million.

Fig. 2 shows MAP reconstructed images of the phantom for the proposed system and the microPET II with different β values. The second-order neighborhood was used in the prior, which contains eight nearest pixels in 2D. Clearly it is difficult to distinguish individual hot spots along radial directions from microPET II reconstructed images, because its radial resolution is slightly worse than the edge-to-edge spacing between the hot spots. In comparison, the hot spots are better identified by the proposed system, in particular, at 45° position (line OB). With $\beta = 1 \times 10^{-4}$, the 3×3 array is also resolved at 90° position (line OC). The two sets of hot spots at 0° and 180° positions are resolve sharply along the tangential direction, but not along the radial direction. All the these results are consistent with the resolution measurements shown in Table 1. The result indicates that the optimal target region for small feature identification may not be located exactly at the face of the high-resolution detector.

3.3 Lesion Detectability

We investigated lesion detection using the phantom shown in Fig. 3(a). The background was a uniform activity ellipse and the lesion was a uniform disc of 0.6 mm in diameter at (12.0 mm, 0.0 mm). The lesion to background activity ratio was 1.5 : 1. Two hundred noisy data sets were generated for both lesion-absent and lesion-present cases. All noisy sinograms have an average of three million photon counts.

The CHO that we used has three difference-of-Gaussian (DOG) channels with standard deviations of 2.653, 1.592, 0.995, and 0.573, respectively. We considered white channel noise with variance 1×10^{-4}. The CHO-SNR were estimated using both theoretical expression (19) and Monte Carlo reconstructions. The results are shown in Fig. 3(b) with comparison to those of the microPET II scanner. The theoretical predictions match with the Monte Carlo results very well. The results also demonstrate that the

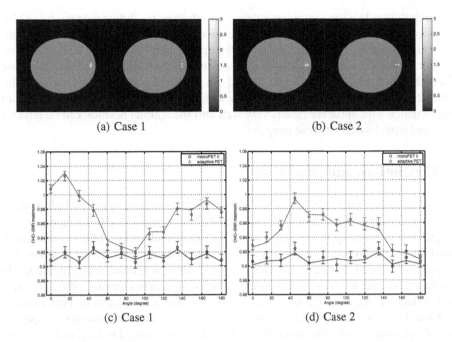

(a) Case 1   (b) Case 2

(c) Case 1   (d) Case 2

Fig. 4. Predicted CHO-SNR maximum changes as a function of the position angle of the high-resolution detector. The solid lines are the results based on noisefree data. The diamonds and circles are predictions based on low-count scout images. The error bars indicate plus and minus one standard deviation.

proposed system has higher SNR for lesion detection than the microPET II scanner at all β values.

3.4 Adaptive Positioning of the High-Resolution Detector

To demonstrate that the high-resolution detector should be adaptively positioned based on specific imaging tasks, we simulated two scenarios (Fig. 4 (a) and (b)) in which the tasks were to distinguish a solid tumor (left images) from a tumor with small features (right images). The difference between the two cases is the orientation of the features. We positioned the high-resolution detector at different angular positions and calculated the SNR of the CHO. For a fair comparison between different positions, the maximum SNR among all possible β values was used. The results are plotted in Fig. 4 (c) and (d) (solid lines). It shows that for the first task, the optimal position of the high-resolution detector is at 15°, while for the second task the optimal position is at 45°. Interestingly, 45° is almost the worst position for the first task. These results clearly show the importance of adaptively positioning the high-resolution detector.

In real applications, information about the features and the background will be obtained using both prior knowledge of the tumor model and an initial scout image of the animal. To evaluate the feasibility of predicting the optimal position of the high-resolution detector using a low-count scout image, we generated 100 independent identically distributed noisy sinograms with an average of 50k detected events in each sinogram to simulate low-count scout data. Only the low-resolution data were used for reconstructing the scout images. For each scout image, we plugged it into the theoretical formula as the true image and calculate the maximum SNR at every high-resolution detector position. From 100 realizations, we calculated the mean and standard deviation of the predicted maximum SNR and plotted the results also in Fig. 4 (c) and (d) (diamonds and circles). It shows that in both cases the predicted SNR from low-count scout images match with noisefree results very well and the optimal position can be reliably estimated from low-count scout images.

4   Conclusions and Discussions

We have proposed a novel PET system design that integrates one high-resolution detector into an existing PET scanner. Unlike other PET systems with a full-ring insert, our design aims at zooming-in at a target area. We have developed a MAP reconstruction algorithm for the proposed system with an accurate system model. The performance of the proposed system has been analyzed theoretically and verified using Monte Carlo simulation. The results show that the proposed system achieves significantly higher resolution than the original PET system and also improves lesion detection performance. We have shown that the optimal position of the high-resolution depends on the specific task of an imaging study. The theoretical expressions can be used to adaptively position the high-resolution detector to maximize the task-performance.

The theoretical analysis and simulations in this work were done in 2D. Both the high-resolution low-resolution detectors have one layer in the axial direction. In practice, the axial dimension of the high-resolution detector will be the same as its transaxial dimension, so we can expect a similar improvement in the axial resolution and further improvement in sensitivity and lesion detectability. Extension of this work to 3D imaging is currently underway.

References

1. Chatziioannou, A.: PET Scanners dedicated to molecular imaging of small animal models. Molecular Imaging and Biology 4, 47–63 (2002)
2. Tai, Y., Chatziioannou, A., Yang, Y., Silverman, R., Meadors, K., Siegel, S., Newport, D., Stickel, J., Cherry, S.: MicroPET II: design, development and initial performance of an improved microPET scanner for small-animal imaging. Phys. Med. Biol. 48, 1519–1537 (2003)
3. Rouze, N., Schmand, M., Siegel, S., Hutchins, G.: Design of a small animal PET imaging system with 1 microliter volume resolution. IEEE Transactions on Nuclear Science 51, 757–763 (2004)
4. Miyaoka, R., Janes, M., Lee, K., Park, B., Gillispie, S., Kinahan, P., Lewellen, T.: Development of a single detector ring micro crystal element scanner: quickPET II. Molecular Imaging 4, 117–127 (2005)
5. Stickel, J., Cherry, S.: High-resolution PET detector design: modelling components of intrinsic spatial resolution. Phys. Med. Biol. 50, 179–195 (2005)
6. Clinthorne, N., Sangjune, P., Rogers, W., Chiao, P.: Multiresolution image reconstruction for a high-resolution small animal PET device. In: IEEE Nuclear Science Symposium Conference Record, pp. 1997–2001 (2003)

7. Janecek, M., Wu, H., Tai, Y.: A simulation study for the design of a prototype insert for whole-body PET scanners. IEEE Transactions on Nuclear Science 53, 1143–1149 (2006)
8. Pal, D., O'Sullivan, J., Wu, H., Janecek, M., Tai, Y.: 2D linear and iterative reconstruction algorithms for a PET-insert scanner. Phys. Med. Biol. 52, 4293–4310 (2007)
9. Park, S., Rogers, W., Clinthorne, N.: Design of very high-resolution small animal PET scanner using a silicon scatter detector insert. Phys. Med. Biol. 52, 4653–4677 (2007)
10. Tai, Y., Wu, H., Pal, D., O'Sullivan, J.: Virtual-pinhole PET. Journal of Nuclear Medicine 49, 471–479 (2008)
11. Huh, S., Rogers, W., Clinthorne, N.: On-line sliding-window list-mode PET image reconstruction for a surgical PET imaging probe. In: IEEE Nuclear Science Symposium and Medical Imaging Conference (2008)
12. Qi, J., Leahy, R., Cherry, S., Chatziioannou, A., Farquhar, T.: High-resolution 3D Bayesian image reconstruction using the microPET small-animal scanner. Phys. Med. Biol. 43, 1001–1013 (1998)
13. Hu, J., Qi, J., Huber, J., Moses, W., Huesman, R.: MAP image reconstruction for arbitray geometry PET systems with application to a prostate-specific scanner. In: International Meeting on Fully Three-Dimensional Image Reconstruction in Radiology and Nuclear Medicine, pp. 210–416 (2005)
14. Fessler, J., Rogers, W.: Spatial resolution properties of penalized-likelihood image reconstruction: Space-invariant tomographs. IEEE Transactions on Image Processing 9, 1346–1358 (1996)
15. Fessler, J.: Mean and variance of implicitly defined biased estimators (such as penalized maximum likelihood): Applications to tomography. IEEE Transactions on Image Processing 5, 493–506 (1996)
16. Qi, J., Leahy, R.: A theoretical study of the contrast recovery and variance of MAP reconstructions for PET data. IEEE Transactions on Medical Imaging 18, 293–305 (1999)
17. Qi, J., Leahy, R.: Resolution and noise properties of MAP reconstruction for fully 3D PET. IEEE Transactions on Medical Imaging 19, 493–506 (2000)
18. Stayman, J., Fessler, J.: Regularization for uniform spatial resolution properties in penalized-likelihood image reconstruction. IEEE Transactions on Medical Imaging 19, 601–615 (2000)
19. Stayman, J., Fessler, J.: Efficient calculation of resolution and covariance for penalized-likelihood reconstruction in fully 3-D SPECT. IEEE Transactions on Medical Imaging 23, 1543–1556 (2004)
20. Qi, J.: Theoretical study of lesion detectability of MAP reconstruction using computer observers. IEEE Transactions on Medical Imaging 20, 815–822 (2001)
21. Myers, K., Barrett, H.: Addition of a channel mechanism to the ideal-observer model. J. Opt. Soc. Amer. A 4, 2447–2457 (1987)
22. Yao, J., Barrett, H.: Predicting human performance by a channelized Hotelling model. SPIE Math. Meth. Med. Imag. 1768, 161–168 (1992)
23. Qi, J.: Analysis of lesion detectability in Bayesian emission reconstruction with nonstationary object variability. IEEE Transactions on Medical Imaging 23, 321–329 (2004)
24. De Pierro, A.: A modified expectation maximization algorithm for penalized likelihood estimation in emission tomography. IEEE Transactions on Medical Imaging 14, 132–137 (1995)
25. Hudson, H., Larkin, R.: Accelerated image reconstruction using ordered subsets of projection data. IEEE Transactions on Medical Imaging 13, 601–609 (1994)

Dynamic Dual-Tracer PET Reconstruction

Fei Gao[1], Huafeng Liu[1], Yiqiang Jian[1], and Pengcheng Shi[2]

[1] State Key Laboratory of Modern Optical Instrumentation,
Zhejiang University, HangZhou, Zhejiang, China
[2] Golisano College of Computing and Information Science,
Rochester Institute of Technology, Rochester, NY, USA

Abstract. Although of important medical implications, simultaneous dual–tracer positron emission tomography reconstruction remains a challenging problem, primarily because the photon measurements from dual tracers are overlapped. In this paper, we propose a simultaneous dynamic dual–tracer reconstruction of tissue activity maps based on guidance from tracer kinetics. The dual–tracer reconstruction problem is formulated in a state–space representation, where parallel compartment models serve as continuous–time system equation describing the tracer kinetic processes of dual tracers, and the imaging data is expressed as discrete sampling of the system states in measurement equation. The image reconstruction problem has therefore become a state estimation problem in a continuous–discrete hybrid paradigm, and H_∞ filtering is adopted as the estimation strategy. As H_∞ filtering makes no assumptions on the system and measurement statistics, robust reconstruction results can be obtained for the dual-tracer PET imaging system where the statistical properties of measurement data and system uncertainty are not available *a priori*, even when there are disturbances in the kinetic parameters. Experimental results on digital phantoms, Monte Carlo simulations and physical phantoms have demonstrated the superior performance.

1 Introduction

Positron emission tomography (PET) is a functional molecular imaging technology which uses compounds labelled with positron emitting radioisotopes as molecular probes to image and measure biochemical processes of mammalian biology *in vivo*. Molecular probes for PET are developed by first identifying a target process to be studied and then synthesizing a positron labelled molecule, injected intravenously, through which an assay can be performed. With the increasingly wider availability of radiotracers, i.e. 18F–2-fluoro-2deoxy-D-glucose (FDG), 13N-ammonia, 11C–dihydrotetrabenazine(DTBZ) and 11C–WIN35,428, there have been many clinical and biomedical research applications in imaging various molecular *interactions* of biological processes.

Because of the complicated nature of the disease, the importance of multi–tracer PET imaging is well recognized yet seldom addressed because of paramount technical difficulties. Typically, multi–tracer imaging are treated as sequential problems, which are not well qualified for real time comparison in neuropharmcologic

J.L. Prince, D.L. Pham, and K.J. Myers (Eds.): IPMI 2009, LNCS 5636, pp. 38–49, 2009.

measurements and dynamic imaging between tracers. More crucially, the increased scanning time and suffering of patients hinder its practical applications. Hence, simultaneous multi–tracer imaging is of great recent interest.

Several attempts do try to tackle the dual-tracer imaging problem based on double–injection single–scan strategy[1,2,3,4,5]. However, all these works have been based upon the activity images are reconstructed as *a priori* using FBP or EM algorithm, and the aim is to use these maps to perform kinetic parameters estimation in some optimal sense. It is recognized that the recovery of activity maps of individual radio tracer is not a completely solved problem yet, and the great challenge here is that there is no direct way of separating signals from two different tracers as the modality based on measuring the 511 keV emitted by positron annihilations[1,2,6].

In this paper, we focus on simultaneous dynamic PET reconstruction of dual–tracer activity maps. The state–space representation is used to formulate the double–injection, single–scan protocol, where parallel compartment models for dual–tracer are coupled into state equations, while the mixed photon acquisition is integrated into measurement equations. The reconstruction problem therefore becomes a state estimation problem, and H_∞ filtering is applied to achieve robust estimation. Finally, respective dynamic reconstructed images for each tracer from digital Zubal phantom, Monte Carlo simulations and real phantom scan are presented as validations.

2   Methodology

2.1   Modeling of PET Measurement

In PET imaging, once radiopharmaceutical is injected or inhaled, it is transported and absorbed by the tissue of interests. An emitted positron meets a free electron and their annihilation produces two gamma ray photons traveling in opposite directions. If two photons are detected within the coincidence time window, an event is recorded along the line of response (LOR), and summing many of such events results in quantities that approximate line integrals (or equivalently projections and sinograms) through the radioisotope distribution.

Dynamic PET imaging involves a sequence of contiguous acquisition with different temporal resolutions, and a time series of activity images need to be reconstructed from the measurement data. The procedure can be formulated as a projection transform from image to data:

$$Y(t) = DX(t) + e(t) \qquad (1)$$

$$X(t) = \Lambda\varphi(t) \qquad (2)$$

here $Y(t)$ is the projection sinogram acquired from time frame 0 to time frame t, system probability matrix D is constructed from the physical and geometrical structure of PET acquisition system, $e(t)$ is the overall measurement errors in system, $\varphi(t)$ is a $n \times 1$ matrix representing the activity concentration in one

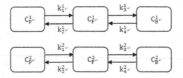

Fig. 1. Parallel dual–tracer two–tissue compartment model

tissue and Λ is a block $4n \times n$ diagonal matrix with blocks $[1 \quad 1 \quad 1 \quad 1]$ that help to extend to dual–tracer reconstruction simultaneously. To be in accordance with time configuration in dynamic PET imaging, The measurement equation is expressed as:

$$Y(t_k) = DX(t_k) + e(t_k) \tag{3}$$

here t_k $(k = 1, 2, \cdots, M.$ M is the total number of the time frames) is the time point at the end of the kth time frame.

2.2 Modeling of Tracer Kinetics

Due to their simple implementation and biological plausibility, compartment models have been widely employed to quantitatively describe regional tracer kinetics in PET imaging. Model–driven tracer kinetics use a particular compartmental structure to describe the behavior of the tracer and allow for an estimation of either micro or macro system parameters [9]. The discrete nature of a compartment is what allow one to reduce the complex biological system into a finite number of discrete compartments and pathways [10].

In this paper, a parallel dual–tracer two–tissue compartment model is used to model the dual–tracer kinetic processes, with the structure shown in Fig. 1. The superscripts 1 and 2 correspond to parameters for the 1st tracer and the 2nd tracer respectively. C_P^1/C_P^2(pmol/ml) is arterial concentration of radiotracer 1/2. C_F^1/C_F^2(pmol/ml) is the concentration of non–specific binding tracer 1/2 in tissue. C_B^1/C_B^2(pmol/ml) is the concentration of specific binding tracer 1/2 in tissue. The parameters k_1^1/k_1^2, k_2^1/k_2^2, k_3^1/k_3^2 and k_4^1/k_4^2 are first–order rate constants specifying the tracer exchange rates between compartments for tracer 1/2. The two tissue compartment model satisfies many radioligand tracers well. Those include tracers such as 18F–FDG for the quantitative measurement of glucose metabolism, 11C–acetate for measurement of myocardial oxidative metabolism and monitor of tumor growth, and 62Cu–pyruvaldehyde bis[N4–methyl–thiosemicarbazone] (PTSM) for imaging blood flow. Note that two arterial input functions C_P^1 and C_P^2 are introduced into the tracers delivery process,

Table 1. Kinetic parameters for different tissue regions in Zubal thorax phantom

	k_1^{FDG}	k_2^{FDG}	k_3^{FDG}	k_4^{FDG}	$k_1^{acetate}$	$k_2^{acetate}$	$k_3^{acetate}$	$k_4^{acetate}$
ROI a	0.55951	2.75288	0.44793	0.01101	0.65188	0.22766	0.05311	0.03882
ROI b	0.37811	1.04746	0.13483	0.00857	0.45044	0.22871	0.07253	0.01417
ROI c	0.78364	1.15641	0.11200	0.02706	0.70372	0.53690	0.17755	0.01425

and each compartment model performs independently without interfering with the other. Using the model in Fig. 1, the time variation of kinetic model in an individual voxel can be denoted by the following first–order differential equations:

$$\frac{dC_{Fi}^1}{dt} = k_{1i}^1 C_P^1(t) + k_{4i}^1 C_{Bi}^1(t) - (k_{2i}^1 + k_{3i}^1)C_{Fi}^1(t) \tag{4}$$

$$\frac{dC_{Bi}^1}{dt} = k_{3i}^1 C_{Fi}^1(t) - k_{4i}^1 C_{Bi}^1(t) \tag{5}$$

$$\frac{dC_{Fi}^2}{dt} = k_{1i}^2 C_P^2(t) + k_{4i}^2 C_{Bi}^2(t) - (k_{2i}^2 + k_{3i}^2)C_{Fi}^2(t) \tag{6}$$

$$\frac{dC_{Bi}^1}{dt} = k_{3i}^2 C_{Fi}^2(t) - k_{4i}^2 C_{Bi}^2(t) \tag{7}$$

with subscript i representing a single voxel in reconstructed images. Equation(4)–Equation(7) can also be expressed in vector–space denotation as:

$$\begin{bmatrix} \dot{C}_{Fi}^1(t) \\ \dot{C}_{Bi}^1(t) \\ \dot{C}_{Fi}^2(t) \\ \dot{C}_{Bi}^2(t) \end{bmatrix} = \begin{bmatrix} -(k_{2i}^1 + k_{3i}^1) & k_{4i}^1 & 0 & 0 \\ k_{3i}^1 & -k_{4i}^1 & 0 & 0 \\ 0 & 0 & -(k_{2i}^2 + k_{3i}^2) & k_{4i}^2 \\ 0 & 0 & k_{3i}^2 & -k_{4i}^2 \end{bmatrix} \begin{bmatrix} C_{Fi}^1(t) \\ C_{Bi}^1(t) \\ C_{Fi}^2(t) \\ C_{Bi}^2(t) \end{bmatrix} + \begin{bmatrix} k_{1i}^1 & 0 \\ 0 & 0 \\ 0 & k_{1i}^2 \\ 0 & 0 \end{bmatrix} \begin{bmatrix} C_P^1(t) \\ C_P^2(t) \end{bmatrix} \tag{8}$$

The above equation can be expressed in a compact form as

$$\dot{x}_i(t) = a_i x_i(t) + b_i \tilde{C}_P(t) \tag{9}$$

where

$$x_i(t) = [\int_0^t C_{Fi}^1(\tau)d\tau, \int_0^t C_{Bi}^1(\tau)d\tau, \int_0^t C_{Fi}^2(\tau)d\tau, \int_0^t C_{Bi}^2(\tau)d\tau]$$

$$\tilde{C}_P(t) = [\int_0^t C_P^1(\tau)d\tau, \int_0^t C_P^2(\tau)d\tau]$$

$$a_i = \begin{bmatrix} -(k_{2i}^1 + k_{3i}^1) & k_{4i}^1 & 0 & 0 \\ k_{3i}^1 & -k_{4i}^1 & 0 & 0 \\ 0 & 0 & -(k_{2i}^2 + k_{3i}^2) & k_{4i}^2 \\ 0 & 0 & k_{3i}^2 & -k_{4i}^2 \end{bmatrix} \quad b_i = \begin{bmatrix} k_{1i}^1 & 0 \\ 0 & 0 \\ 0 & k_{1i}^2 \\ 0 & 0 \end{bmatrix}$$

The standard state transition equation for all the voxels can be constructed from Equation(9):

$$\dot{X}(t) = AX(t) + B\tilde{C}_P(t) + v(t) \tag{10}$$

where state vector $X(t) = [x_1(t)^T, x_2(t)^T, \cdots, x_n(t)^T]^T$ (n is the total number of voxels), A is a $4n \times 4n$ block diagonal matrix with block a_i, B is a $4n \times 2$ row block matrix with block b_i and $v(t)$ is a $4n \times 1$ vector describing model errors.

2.3   State Space Representation of PET Imaging

The state–space representation is introduced into the dynamic dual–tracer PET reconstruction problem, Equation(3) and Equation(10) form the state–space representation of dynamic dual–tracer PET reconstruction, in which parallel compartment models serve as a continuous time state equation to describe the tracer kinetic processes, and the projection data is expressed as discrete sampling of observation in a measurement equation. With given measurement $Y(t_k)$, the target of our dynamic dual–tracer reconstruction is to obtain the separate distribution of activity concentration for each tracer :

$$X_k^1 = \Lambda_1[X(t_{k+1}) - X(t_k)] \tag{11}$$

$$X_k^2 = \Lambda_2[X(t_{k+1}) - X(t_k)] \tag{12}$$

here Λ_1 and Λ_2 are $4n \times n$ block diagonal matrices with respective blocks [1 1 0 0] and [0 0 1 1]. A robust H_∞ filtering algorithm described in the following section will be used for estimation in this state–space framework.

2.4   Robust Estimation of Dual Tracer Activity Maps

Since PET data after attenuation correction is not Poisson distributed, and have even more complicated statistics due to scatter events, scanner sensitivity and dead time correction. Instead of imposing certain distribution (Poisson or Shifted Poisson) on the data, the mini-max H_∞ estimation criterion is adopted in our filtering framework, which minimizes the worst possible effects of the disturbances on the state estimation errors, and requires no priori knowledge of noise statistics, making it an appropriate choice for PET reconstruction where the noise statistics is complicated. The H_∞ filtering strategy has been applied to static PET reconstruction [7] and dynamic single–tracer reconstruction [8] in previous efforts. Following this spirit, similar procedure is used in our work, while more sophisticated setting on parameters must be considered in dual–tracer situation. The state Equation(10) contains the separate components of each tracer, and thus the state noise and estimation error in respective kinetic process need to be estimated simultaneously during parallel calculation. Besides, the measurement equation(3) describes overlap sinogram data in dynamic time frames, so the mixed measurement noises should be incorporated into filtering strategy.

The objective function of H_∞ filtering is given by

$$\sup \frac{||X(t) - \tilde{X}(t)||_{Q(t)}^2}{||v(t)||_{V(t)^{-1}}^2 + ||e(t)||_{W(t)^{-1}}^2 + ||X_0 - \tilde{X}_0||_{H_0^{-1}}^2} \leqslant \gamma^2 \tag{13}$$

where $\tilde{X}(t)$ is the estimation of $X(t)$ at time t, the subscripts $Q(t)$, $V(t)^{-1}$, $W(t)^{-1}$ and H_0^{-1} denote the weighting matrices for the estimation error, the state error, the measurement error and the initial value error, and γ^2 is a constant describing the disturbance level. Equation(13) defines the supremum of estimation error over all possible disturbances of noise energy. H_∞ criterion is a robust strategy to deal with the noise uncertainty in real situation. It is a game theory where the internal estimator plays against the external disturbances [11]. The complicated statistics of noises are not a required priori in this framework, and instead, we have only to maintain the small estimation errors with small disturbances, and vice versa. The minimum disturbance $\gamma^* \le \gamma^2$ in equation(13) can also be expressed as a min-max problem:

$$\min_{X} \max_{V(t),W(t),X_0} \gamma^* = ||X(t)-\tilde{X}(t)||^2_{Q(t)} - \gamma^2(||v(t)||_{V(t)^{-1}} + ||e(t)||^2_{W(t)^{-1}} + ||X_0-\tilde{X}_0||^2_{H_0^{-1}})$$

(14)

A complete solution to the H_∞ estimation problem for state–space model was present in [11], and the iterative equation is given as:

$$\tilde{X}(t_k) = A\tilde{X}(t_k^-) + H(t_k)[Y(t_k) - D\tilde{X}(t_k^-)]$$

(15)

$$H(t_k) = H(t_k^-)[I + C^T V(t)^{-1} C H(t_k^-)]^{-1} C^T V(t)^{-1}$$

(16)

where $H(t_k)$ is the filtering gain which satisfies the Riccati equation:

$$\dot{H}(t) = AH(t) + H(t)A^T + \frac{H(t)Q(t)H(t)}{\gamma^2} + N(t) \quad \text{with} \quad H(0) = H_0 \quad (17)$$

There are many numerical algorithms that solve this Riccati equation by successive integration. We adopt the scheme proposed in [12] to avoid the singularity during the process of iteration and obtain the stable solution.

3   Experiments

3.1   Experiments on Digital Phantoms

Simulation experiments are used to evaluate the accuracy and robustness of the simultaneous dual–tracer activity map reconstruction framework. Fig. 2 left shows a schematic representation of the Zubal thorax phantom, which has three distinctive tissue regions and a background region. The phantom is digitized at 32×32 pixels . Two regular tracers are used to simulate the injection and metabolic process: 18F-FDG for glucose metabolism and 11C-acetate for tumor growth monitor. The kinetic parameters of different regions are set from some known values in tracer kinetic research on FDG and acetate, as presented in Table 1. The plasma input function for 18F-FDG is simulated as:

$$C_P^{FDG}(t) = (A_1 t - A_2 - A_3)e^{-\lambda_1 t} + A_2 e^{-\lambda_2 t} + A_3 e^{-\lambda_3 t}$$

(18)

the parameters λ_i and A_i were selected for each tracer to match blood curves appearing in the literatures, here the value chosen were $A_1 = 851.1225\mu Ci/mL/$

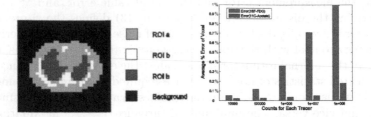

Fig. 2. Left: Zubal thorax phantom with multiple tissue regions indicated by different colors. Right: The APE of reconstructed images in the first group of experiments with different counting levels: 10^4, 10^5, 10^6, 10^7 and 10^8. For every pair, the left one is 18F, the right one is 11C.

$min, A_2 = 20.8113 \mu Ci/mL, A_3 = 21.8798 \mu Ci/mL$, $\lambda_1 = 4.133859 min^{-1}$, $\lambda_2 = 0.01043449 min^{-1}$ and $\lambda_3 = 0.1190996 min^{-1}$. The plasma input function for 11C-acetate is obtained by correcting the whole-blood for circulating metabolites as [3]:

$$C_P^{acetate}(t) = [1 - 0.88(1 - e^{-(\frac{2\ln 2}{15}t)})]C_P^{FDG}(t) \qquad (19)$$

With both input functions coupled into state equation(10), 18 frames of activity images were obtained from above compartment model simulations, sampled as $4 \times 0.5min$, $4 \times 2min$ and $10 \times 5min$. The system probability matrix in equation(1) was computed by using MATLAB toolbox developed by Prof. J.Fessler

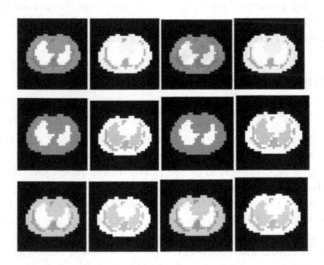

Fig. 3. The original and reconstructed activity images of 18F-FDG and 11C-acetate with perfect kinetic parameters and total 10^6 counts for time frame 2nd (top), 5th (middle) and 8th (bottom). 1st column: original 18F-FDG activity images; 2nd: original 18C-acetate activity images; 3rd: reconstructed 18F-FDG activity images; 4th: reconstructed 18C-acetate activity images.

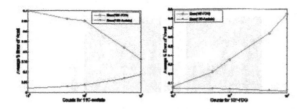

Fig. 4. The APE of reconstructed images with 18F and 11C of different count level. Left: the total counts of 18F-FDG were set to 10^6, and the counts of 11C-acetate varied from 10^5 to 10^7. Right: the total counts of 11C-acetate were set to 10^6, and the counts for 18F-FDG varied 10^5 to 10^7.

et al.. Then the activity images were projected into sinograms using a poisson model to generate raw data. Poisson-distributed random events were simulated and online subtracted. Two groups of simulation data were generated to evaluate the reconstruction performance. In every simulation, noise photons in simulated data was set to be about 30%. To analysis the reconstruction accuracy, we define a average percentage error(APE) for each tracer as:

$$APE = \frac{1}{N} \sum_i |\psi_{ik} - \tilde{\psi}_{ik}|/\psi_{ik} \qquad (20)$$

here N is the total number of pixels, ψ_{ik} is the reconstructed activity values, $\tilde{\psi}_{ik}$ is the true values. In the first group of simulation data, We generated sinograms with the count levels of 18F and 11C being similar. 5 different count levels: 10^4, 10^5, 10^6, 10^7 and 10^8 were used in the data generation, which represent the total counts of the simulated data. The purpose here is to see the different reconstruction results at different count levels. Fig. 2 right presents the APE of reconstructed results in these five groups of experiments, the APE of reconstructed images for each pair of tracers increased with the overall counts increasing. The comparison between the original images and reconstructed images of count level 10^6 is shown in Fig. 3, where the APE for simulated 18F-FDG reconstruction is 0.360%, and the APE for simulated 11C-acetate reconstruction is 0.037%. The second group of simulations was performed with 18F and 11C of different count level. The purpose here is to see the interaction between the

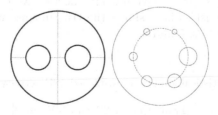

Fig. 5. The transverse view of phantoms. Left: the phantom used for Monte Carlo simulation; Right: the 6-sphere phantom used for real PET scan.

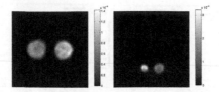

Fig. 6. The EM reconstruction of simulation data and real phantom scan data. Left: Monte Carlo simulation data; Right: real phantom scan data.

two tracers. As shown in Fig. 4 left, the total counts of 18F-FDG were set to 10^6, and the counts for 11C-acetate varied from 10^5 to 10^7 with an interval of 5×10^5. The APE of 11C-acetate reconstructed images increased from 0.022% to 0.085%, and the APE of 18F-FDG images decreased from 0.400% to 0.161%. Fig. 4 right gives an analogous result by setting the total counts of 11C-acetate as 10^6 and that for 18F-FDG varied from 10^5 to 10^7. In this experiment, the APE for 18F-FDG images increased from 0.075% to 0.850%, and the APE for 11C-acetate images decreased from 0.045% to 0.021%.

3.2   Experiments with Data from Monte Carlo Simulations

The second data set used for validation in this study was acquired by Monte Carlo simulations [13]. The simulated scanner is Concord microPET R4, and a 6cm diameter cylindrical phantom with 2 hot regions was used. The transverse view of the phantom is shown in Fig. 5 left, the phantom was filled with pure water, two hot regions were filled with 18F–FDG solutions and 11C–acetate solutions respectively, the initial activity concentration was set to 2.315kBq/ml. A simulation of a dynamic sequence of 10 frames over 160 minutes(10 × 16min) from the mixed effect of dual tracers was performed, the final generated sinogram data set has 128 × 128 projections for every slice. First several static reconstruction were performed, then the kinetic parameters k_1^1/k_1^2, k_2^1/k_2^2, k_3^1/k_3^2 and k_4^1/k_4^2 in the parallel compartment models used here were calculated using these static reconstruction results by COMKAT [14]. Since this is a Monte Carlo simulation, we can get the true activity concentration at every time frame. The reconstructed images at time frame 1 by traditional EM algorithm is shown in Fig. 6 left, the activity concentrations of 18F and 11C can not be separated. The respective images of 18F–FDG and 11C–acetate were reconstructed by our framework simultaneously, Fig. 7 shows the true images and the reconstructed images at time frame 1, 2, 5 and 8.

Table 2. Statistical studies of estimated 18F activity distribution

	Frame1	Frame2	Frame5	Frame8
bias	-0.0343	-0.0313	-0.0812	0.2432
std	0.2378	0.3664	0.2878	0.4461

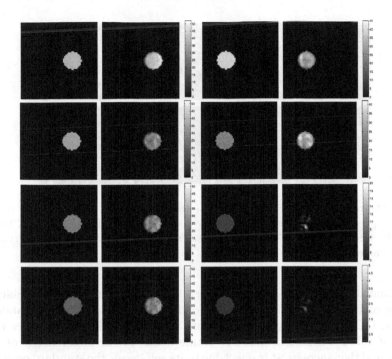

Fig. 7. The true and reconstructed activity images of 18F-FDG and 11C-acetate with data set from Monte Carlo simulations, from top to bottom, 4 rows correspond to the 1st, 2nd, 5th and 8th time frame. The 1st column is the true 18F-FDG activity images; the 2nd column is reconstructed 18F-FDG activity images; the 3rd column is the true 11C-acetate activity images; the 4th column is reconstructed 11C-acetate activity images.

A statistical analysis on reconstructed images against true values in the hot regions is performed. Let N_p be the total number of pixels and XR_i be the final reconstruction result of pixel i respectively, and XT_i be true value of corresponding pixel i, then we have the following error definitions:

$$bias = (1/N_p) \sum_i (XR_i - XT_i)/XT_i \qquad (21)$$

$$std = (1/(N_p - 1)) \sum_i ((XR_i - XT_i)/XT_i)^2)^{0.5} \qquad (22)$$

The calculated bias and standard derivation values of the reconstruction images from different time frames are summarized in Table 2 and Table 3, Table 2 is bias and standard derivation values for 18F–FDG reconstruction and Table 3

Table 3. Statistical studies of estimated 11C activity distribution

	Frame1	Frame2	Frame5	Frame8
bias	-0.2983	0.1979	-0.7256	-0.7894
std	0.3445	0.4016	0.9053	0.8930

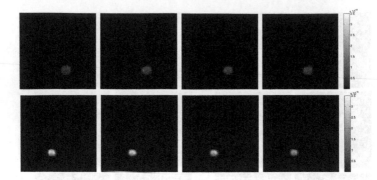

Fig. 8. The reconstructed activity images of 18F-FDG and 11C-acetate with data set from real phantom scan. The 1st row is the reconstructed 18F-FDG images, the 2nd row is the reconstructed 11C-acetate images. From left to right, 4 columns correspond to time frame 1, 2, 5 and 8 respectively.

is bias and standard derivation values for 11C–acetate reconstruction. Since the half–life of 18F–FDG is 110 minutes and that of 11C-acetate is only about 20 minutes, 11C–acetate decayed faster than 18F–FDG, so the standard derivation values of 18F–FDG first decrease at frame 5 due to the faster decay of 11C–acetate, and then increase at frame 8 due to its self-decay, the standard derivation values of 11C-acetate increase continuously though all former frames due to its fast decay, after frame 5, the standard derivation values keep high because the low concentration of 11C–acetate in the phantom.

3.3 Experiments with Physical Phantom Scanning Data

The real data set used in this study was acquired on the Hamamatsu SHR-22000 scanner using a 6 – spheres phantom, which is usually used to measure the recovery coefficient. The SHR-22000 is designed as a whole body imaging system. It has a 838mm detector ring diameter with a patient aperture of 600mm, an axial field of view (FOV) of 224mm, can operate in 2D or 3D mode. For the phantom, there are six circular regions of different diameters. These sphere objects have diameters of 37mm, 28mm, 22mm, 17mm, 13mm, 10mm and are inserted in a circular cylinder with diameter of 200mm corresponding to a volume of 9300ml, as shown in Fig. 5 right. The phantom filled with pure water was located at the center of both transaxial and axial FOV in the scanner using the patient bed. We injected 22mCi 11C–acetate solution into the 28mm diameter sphere and 5 minutes later injected 8mCi 18F–FDG solution into the 37mm diameter sphere. Acquirement of a dynamic sequence of 10 frames over 20 minutes(10 × 2min) from the mixed effect of dual tracers was performed, the final generated sinogram data has 192 × 192 projections for every slice. The kinetic parameters used were also calculated by COMKAT like above section. The reconstructed image at time frame 1 by EM algorithm is shown in Fig. 6 right for comparison. The respective images of 18F–FDG and 11C–acetate were reconstructed by our framework simultaneously, Fig. 8 shows the reconstructed images at frame 1, 2, 5 and 8. The two tracers are correctly reconstructed respectively, it is evident that this framework is effective for double–injection single–scan PET reconstruction of dual–tracer activity maps.

Acknowledgements

This work is supported in part by the National Natural Science Foundation of China(No: 60772125), and by a Development Project of Zhejiang Province (NO: 2008C23060).

References

1. Huang, S.C., Carson, R.E., Hoffman, E.J.: An investigation of a double-tracer technique for positron computerized tomography. Journal of Nuclear Medicine 23, 816–822 (1982)
2. Koeppe, R.A., Raffel, D.M., Snyder, S.E.: Dual-[11C] Tracer Single-Acquisition Positron Emission Tomography Studies. Journal of Cerebral Blood Flow & Metabolism 21, 1480–1492 (2001)
3. Kadrmas, D.J., Rust, T.C.: Feasibility of rapid multi-tracer PET tumor imaging. Nuclear Science Symposium Conference Record 4, 2664–2668 (2004)
4. Rust, T.C., Dibella, E.V., McGann, C.J.: Rapid dual-injection single-scan (13) N-ammonia PET for quantification of rest and stress myocardial blood flow. Physics in Medicine and Biology 51, 5347–5362 (2006)
5. Hayashi, T., Kudomi, N., Watabe, H.: A rapid CBF/CMRO2 measurement with a single PET scan with dual-tracer/integration technique in human. Journal of Cerebral Blood Flow & Metabolism 25, S609 (2005)
6. Black, N.F., McJames, S., Rust, T.C.: Evaluation of rapid dual-tracer 62Cu-PTSM + 62Cu-ATSM PET in dogs with spontaneously occurring tumors. Physics in Medicine and Biology 53, 217–232 (2008)
7. Liu, H., Tian, Y., Shi, P.: PET image reconstruction: A robust state space approach. In: Christensen, G.E., Sonka, M. (eds.) IPMI 2005. LNCS, vol. 3565, pp. 197–209. Springer, Heidelberg (2005)
8. Tong, S., Shi, P.: Tracer kinetics guided dynamic PET reconstruction. In: Karssemeijer, N., Lelieveldt, B. (eds.) IPMI 2007. LNCS, vol. 4584, pp. 421–433. Springer, Heidelberg (2007)
9. Gunn, R.N., Gunn, S.R., Turkheimer, F.E.: Positron Emission Tomography Compartmental Models: A Basis Pursuit Strategy for Kinetic Modeling. Journal of Cerebral Blood Flow & Metabolism 21, 635–652 (2001)
10. Cobelli, C., Foster, D., Toffolo, G.: Tracer Kinetics in Biomedical Research: From Data to Model. Kluwer Academic/Plenum Publishers, New York (2000)
11. Shen, X., Deng, L.: A dynamic system approach to speech enhancement using the H1 filtering algorithm. IEEE Transactions on Speech and Audio Processing 7(4), 391–399 (1997)
12. Schiff, J., Shnider, S.: A natural approach to the numerical integration of Riccati differential equations. SIAM Journal on Numerical Analysis 36, 1392–1413 (1996)
13. Jan, S.: GATE: a simulation toolkit for PET and SPECT. Physics in Medicine and Biology 49, 4543–4561 (2004)
14. Muzic, R.F., Cornelius, S.: COMKAT: Compartment Model Kinetic Analysis Tool. Journal of Nuclear Medcine 42, 636–645 (2001)

DRAMMS: Deformable Registration via Attribute Matching and Mutual-Saliency Weighting

Yangming Ou and Christos Davatzikos

Section of Biomedical Image Analysis (SBIA),
University of Pennsylvania, Philadelphia, PA, 19104
{Yangming.Ou,Christos.Davatzikos}@uphs.upenn.edu

Abstract. A *general-purpose* deformable registration algorithm referred to as "DRAMMS" is presented in this paper. DRAMMS adds to the literature of registration methods that bridge between the traditional voxel-wise methods and landmark/feature-based methods. In particular, DRAMMS extracts Gabor attributes at each voxel and selects the optimal components, so that they form a highly distinctive morphological signature reflecting the anatomical context around each voxel in a multi-scale and multi-resolution fashion. Compared with intensity or mutual-information based methods, the high-dimensional optimal Gabor attributes render different anatomical regions relatively distinctively identifiable and therefore help establish more accurate and reliable correspondence. Moreover, the optimal Gabor attribute vector is constructed in a way that generalizes well, i.e., it can be applied to different registration tasks, regardless of the image contents under registration. A second characteristic of DRAMMS is that it is based on a cost function that weights different voxel pairs according to a metric referred to as "mutual-saliency", which reflects the uniqueness (reliability) of anatomical correspondences implied by the tentative transformation. As a result, image voxels do not contribute equally to the optimization process, as in most voxel-wise methods, or in a binary selection fashion, as in most landmark/feature-based methods. Instead, they contribute according to a continuously-valued mutual-saliency map, which is dynamically updated during the algorithm's evolution. The general applicability and accuracy of DRAMMS are demonstrated by experiments in simulated images, inter-subject images, single-/multi-modality images, and longitudinal images, from human and mouse brains, breast, heart, and prostate.

1 Introduction

Deformable registration is the building block for a variety of medical image analysis tasks, such as multi-modality information fusion, atlas-based image segmentation and computational anatomy. Existing deformable registration methods can be generally classified into two main categories: voxel-wise methods (e.g., [1,2,3,4,5,6,7]) and landmark/feature-based methods (e.g., [8,9,10,11,12,13,14]).

J.L. Prince, D.L. Pham, and K.J. Myers (Eds.): IPMI 2009, LNCS 5636, pp. 50–62, 2009.
© Springer-Verlag Berlin Heidelberg 2009

While landmark/feature-based methods are more intuitive (in the sense that they often explicitly detect and establish correspondence on those anatomically salient regions), they often suffer from the inevitable errors in the landmark/feature detection and matching processes. Moreover, they only utilize a small subset of imaging data (e.g., corner, boundary, line intersection), in a way that is often *ad hoc* and dependent on the specific image contents under registration. For those reasons, recent literature on general-purpose registration has mostly focused on voxel-wise methods, which usually equally utilize all imaging data and maximize the overall similarity on certain voxel-wise attributes (e.g., intensities, intensity distributions). However, voxel-wise methods usually have limitations in the following two respects.

First, the attributes used for characterizing voxels are often not optimal. Since the matching between a pair of voxels is usually determined by the matching between their attributes, suboptimal attributes often lead to ambiguities in matching [15,30]. Ideally, an optimal set of attributes should satisfy two conditions: 1) discriminative, i.e., attributes of voxels from the two images should be similar if and only if those voxels are anatomically corresponding to each other, therefore leaving minimum ambiguity in matching; 2) generally applicable, i.e., they can be extracted from any image while satisfying the first condition, regardless of the image contents under registration. However, most voxel-wise methods only use the simple attribute of image intensity, which is generally applicable for diverse registration tasks but often not sufficiently discriminative for matching (for instance, hundreds of thousands of gray matter voxels in a brain image would have similar intensities; but they may all correspond to different anatomical regions). Other methods attempt to reduce matching ambiguities (e.g., [11,30]) by using a richer set of attributes, such as sulci, organ boundaries, tissue membership and tensor orientations. Those attributes, although more discriminative for matching, are often task- and parameter- specific.

Second, equally utilizing all imaging data may undermine the performance of the optimization process. Actually, different anatomical regions/voxels usually have different abilities to establish unique correspondence [16,17,18]. An ideal optimization process should weight more on those regions/voxels having higher abilities to establish unique correspondences across images. For instance, Fig. 1 shows three similarity maps (Fig. 1(c)(d)(e)) between one specific voxel (red, blue or orange) in the subject image and all the voxels in the template image. An ideal optimization process should rely more on the red point, then the blue point, and lastly the orange point. Unfortunately, most voxel-wise methods treat all voxels equally, ignoring such differences; other approaches (e.g. [11]) attempted to address this issue, by driving the registration adaptively/hierarchically using certain anatomically salient regions, however, in their approaches voxels are often utilized in a heuristic and binary way, ignoring the potential contributions from other voxels that are not utilized.

This paper presents a *general-purpose* image registration framework referred to as "DRAMMS" – Deformable Registration via Attribute Matching and Mutual-Saliency weighting. To overcome the first limitation, DRAMMS extracts a rich set

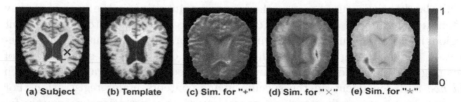

(a) Subject   (b) Template   (c) Sim. for "+"   (d) Sim. for "×"   (e) Sim. for "*"

Fig. 1. Demonstration of the importance of weighting voxels continuously, as they often have different abilities to establish unique correspondence. Similarity maps (c-e) are generated between one specific voxel in image (a) to all voxels in image (b). The red point should have higher weight than the blue point, then the orange point.

of multi-scale and multi-orientation Gabor attributes at each voxel and automatically selects the optimal attribute components. The optimal Gabor attributes render it relatively robust in attribute-based image matching and are also constructed in a way that is generalizable to diverse problems, organs and image modalities. To overcome the second limitation, DRAMMS continuously weights voxels during the optimization process, based on a function referred to as "mutual-saliency", which measures the uniqueness (hence reliability) of a tentative correspondence implied by the transformation. Instead of equally treating voxels or isolating voxels that have more distinctive attributes, this mutual-saliency based continuous weighting mechanism utilizes all imaging data with appropriate and dynamically-evolving weights and leads to a more effective optimization process. DRAMMS is elaborated in Section 2 and demonstrated in Section 3. The whole paper is concluded in Section 4.

2   Methods

2.1   Formulation

Given two intensity images $I_1 : \Omega_1 \mapsto \mathbb{R}$ and $I_2 : \Omega_2 \mapsto \mathbb{R}$ in the 3D image domains $\Omega_i(i = 1, 2) \subset \mathbb{R}^3$, DRAMMS seeks a transformation T that maps every voxel $\mathbf{u} \in \Omega_1$ to its counterpart $T(\mathbf{u}) \in \Omega_2$, by minimizing an overall cost function $E(T)$,

$$\min_{T} E(T) = \int_{\mathbf{u} \in \Omega_1} w\left(\mathbf{u}, T(\mathbf{u})\right) \cdot \left\| A_1^{\star}(\mathbf{u}) - A_2^{\star}\left(T(\mathbf{u})\right) \right\|^2 d\mathbf{u} \; + \; \lambda R(T) \qquad (1)$$

where $A_i^{\star}(\cdot)$ $(i = 1, 2)$ is the optimal attribute vector that reflects the geometric and anatomical context around each voxel. By minimizing $\| A_1^{\star}(\mathbf{u}) - A_2^{\star}\left(T(\mathbf{u})\right) \|^2$, we seek a transformation T that minimizes the *dissimilarity* between a pair of voxels $\mathbf{u} \in \Omega_1$ and $T(\mathbf{u}) \in \Omega_2$. The derivation of the optimal attribute vector $A_i^{\star}(\cdot)$ $(i = 1, 2)$ will be discussed in Sections 2.2 and 2.3.

$w\left(\mathbf{u}, T(\mathbf{u})\right)$ is a continuous weight that is calculated from the mutual-saliency of $\mathbf{u} \in \Omega_1$ and $T(\mathbf{u}) \in \Omega_2$ – higher uniqueness of their matching in the neighborhood indicates higher mutual-saliency, and hence higher weight in the optimization process. In contrast, most traditional voxel-wise methods use equal weights $(w(\cdot) \equiv 1)$. The definition of mutual-saliency will be discussed in Section 2.4.

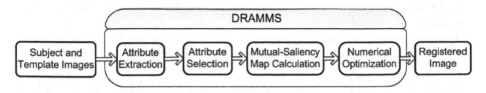

Fig. 2. The components of DRAMMS

$R(T)$ is a smoothness/regularization term usually corresponding to the Laplacian operator, or the bending energy[19], of the deformation field T, whereas λ is a balancing parameter that controls the extent of smoothness.

Fig. 2 illustrates the components of DRAMMS. Details for each component are elaborated in the subsequent sections.

2.2 Attribute Extraction

DRAMMS extracts Gabor attributes at each voxel by convolving the images under registration with Gabor filter banks. The use of Gabor attributes is mainly motivated by the following three properties of Gabor filter banks:

1) General applicability and successful application in numerous tasks. As a general-purpose registration framework, DRAMMS must extract attributes that are generally applicable to different registration tasks, regardless of the image contents. Fortunately, almost all anatomical images have texture information, at some scale and orientation, reflecting the underlying geometric and anatomical characteristics. This texture can be effectively captured by Gabor attributes, as demonstrated in a variety of studies, including texture segmentation [21], image retrieval [23], cancer detection [22] and prostate tissue differentiation [24]. Recently, Gabor attributes have been successfully used in [25][26][27] to register different images, showing their promise for diverse image registration tasks. These methods have also noted the high computational cost required by the high-dimensional Gabor attributes and the need for optimally using Gabor attributes. These challenges are dealt with in DRAMMS by an attribute selection method, as discussed in Section 2.3.

2) Suitability for single- and multi-modality registration tasks. The multi-scale Gabor filter banks often cover a wide range of frequencies, where low frequency filters often serve as local image smoothers, and high frequency filters often serve as edge-detectors. The detected edge information is, to some extent, independent from the underlying intensity distributions, and is therefore suitable for multi-modality registration tasks, even when intensity distributions in the two images no longer follow consistent relationship, in which case mutual-information [7] based methods may fail [25];

3) Multi-scale and multi-orientation nature. As scale and orientation are closely related to the distinctiveness of attributes [28], the multi-scale and multi-orientation attributes are more likely to render each voxel distinctively identifiable, therefore reducing ambiguities in attribute-based voxel matching.

Following the work in [24], the 3D Gabor attributes at each voxel are approximated by convolving the 3D image with two 2D Gabor filter banks in two orthogonal planes (x-y and y-z), so as to save computational cost. Mathematically, the two 2D Gabor filter banks in two orthogonal planes are

$$g_{m,n}(x,y) = a^{-m} g\left(a^{-m} x_g', a^{-m} y_g' \right), \; h_{m,n}(y,z) = a^{-m} h\left(a^{-m} y_h', a^{-m} z_h' \right) \quad (2)$$

where a is the scale factor, $m = 1, 2, \ldots, M$ is the scale index, with M being the total number of scales; $x_g' = x \cos\left(\frac{n\pi}{N}\right) + y \sin\left(\frac{n\pi}{N}\right)$, $y_g' = -x \sin\left(\frac{n\pi}{N}\right) + y \cos\left(\frac{n\pi}{N}\right)$], $y_h' = y \cos\left(\frac{n\pi}{N}\right) + z \sin\left(\frac{n\pi}{N}\right)$ and $z_h' = -y \sin\left(\frac{n\pi}{N}\right) + z \cos\left(\frac{n\pi}{N}\right)$ are rotated coordinates, where $n = 1, 2, \ldots, N$ is the orientation index, with N being the total number of orientations. $g(x,y)$ and $h(y,z)$, known as the "mother Gabor filters", are complex-valued functions in the spatial domain and are each obtained by modulating a Gaussian envelope with a complex exponential,

$$g(x,y) = \frac{1}{2\pi\sigma_x\sigma_y} \exp\left[\underbrace{-\frac{1}{2}\left(\frac{x^2}{\sigma_x^2} + \frac{y^2}{\sigma_y^2}\right)}_{\text{Gaussian Envelope}} + j2\pi f_x \right]; \quad (3)$$

$$h(y,z) = \frac{1}{2\pi\sigma_y\sigma_z} \exp\left[\underbrace{-\frac{1}{2}\left(\frac{y^2}{\sigma_y^2} + \frac{z^2}{\sigma_z^2}\right)}_{\text{Gaussian Envelope}} + j2\pi f_y \right] \quad (4)$$

where σ_x, σ_y and σ_z are the semi-axes lengths of the Gaussian envelope in the spatial domain; f_x and f_y are modulating (shifting) factors in the frequency domain (often known as "central frequencies"). Therefore, at each voxel (x, y, z) in the image $I_i (i = 1, 2)$, the approximated 3D Gabor attributes are assembled into a $D = M \times N \times 4$ dimensional attribute vector $\tilde{A}_i(x, y, z)$, from which we can select the optimal components.

$$\tilde{A}_i(x, y, z) = \left[\; (I_i * g_{m,n})_{\text{Re}}(x, y), \; (I_i * g_{m,n})_{\text{Im}}(x, y), \right. \quad (5)$$
$$\left. (I_i * h_{m,n})_{\text{Re}}(y, z), \; (I_i * h_{m,n})_{\text{Im}}(y, z) \right]_{m=1,2,\ldots,M; \; n=1,2,\ldots,N}.$$

2.3 Attribute Selection

A disadvantage of Gabor attributes is the redundancy among attributes, which is caused by the non-orthogonality among Gabor filters at different scales and orientations. This redundancy not only increases computational cost, but more importantly, it may reduce the distinctiveness of attribute representation, causing ambiguities in the attribute matching [23]. It is therefore important to design a learning-based method to select a set of optimal Gabor attributes so that voxels from the two images can be *accurately* and *reliably* matched.

To design such a learning-based attribute selection method, we would ideally need some *a priori* knowledge of a number of anatomically corresponding voxel pairs to serve as ground-truth, or training voxel pairs. However, in the context of a general-purpose algorithm, this kind of *a priori* knowledge is often absent. Therefore, DRAMMS first automatically selects training voxel pairs, then based on them selects the optimal attributes. These two steps are respectively described below.

Selecting Representative Training Voxel Pairs
The training voxel pairs should 1) be representative of all other voxels in the entire image domain; and 2) offer examples of good correspondence. Accordingly, DRAMMS regularly partitions the subject image into a number of J regions $\Omega_1^{(j)} (j = 1, 2, \ldots, J)$ and selects from each region a voxel pair $(\mathbf{p}_j^\star \in \Omega_1^{(j)}, \mathbf{q}_j^\star \in \Omega_2)$ that is most *reliably* matched to each other, as illustrated in Fig. 3 and mathematically described in Eqn. 6. Here regular partition is used instead of more complicated organ/tissue segmentation,

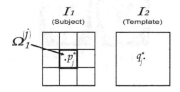

Fig. 3. Illustration of the selection of representative training voxel pairs. Please refer to text for details.

in order to keep DRAMMS as a general-purpose registration method that can be applied to different registration tasks without assumptions on segmentation. Note also that the template image I_2 is not partitioned because at this stage, no transformation is performed and no corresponding regions should be assumed.

$$(\mathbf{p}_j^*, \mathbf{q}_j^*) = \arg \max_{\substack{\mathbf{p} \in \Omega_1^{(j)} \subset \Omega_1, \\ \mathbf{q} \in \Omega_2}} \left[\underbrace{w(\mathbf{p}, \mathbf{q})}_{\text{Reliability}} \cdot \underbrace{sim\left(\tilde{A}_1(\mathbf{p}), \tilde{A}_2(\mathbf{q}) \right)}_{\text{Similarity}} \right] \qquad (6)$$

In Eqn. 6, $sim\left(\tilde{A}_1(\mathbf{p}), \tilde{A}_2(\mathbf{q}) \right) = \frac{1}{1 + \frac{1}{D} \| \tilde{A}_1(\mathbf{p}) - \tilde{A}_2(\mathbf{q}) \|^2} \in [0, 1]$ reflects the attribute-wise similarity between the two points, with D being the number of attributes. $w(\mathbf{p}, \mathbf{q})$, the mutual-saliency, is elaborated in Section 2.4. For now, the bottom line is that $w(\mathbf{p}, \mathbf{q})$ reflects the uniqueness (hence reliability) of the matching between $\mathbf{p} \in \Omega_1$ and $\mathbf{q} \in \Omega_2$.

Selecting Optimal Attributes. DRAMMS selects a subset of optimal attributes, $A_1^\star$ and $A_2^\star$, such that they maximize the overall *reliability* and *similarity* of the matching on those selected training voxel pairs,

$$\max_{A_1 \subset \tilde{A}_1, A_2 \subset \tilde{A}_2} \sum_{j=1}^{J} \left[\underbrace{w(\mathbf{p}_j^\star, \mathbf{q}_j^\star)}_{\text{Reliability}} \cdot \underbrace{sim\left(A_1(\mathbf{p}_j^\star), A_2(\mathbf{q}_j^\star) \right)}_{\text{Similarity}} \right] \qquad (7)$$

In implementation, DRAMMS adopts an iterative backward elimination and forward inclusion strategy for attribute selection, which are commonly used for attribute/variable selection in the machine learning community [29]. Note that, in order to make the quantity in Eqn. 7 comparable for different numbers of attributes, the difference between two attribute vectors $\|A_1(\mathbf{p}^\star) - A_2(\mathbf{q}^\star)\|^2$ in the definition of $sim\left(A_1(\mathbf{p}_j^\star), A_2(\mathbf{q}_j^\star) \right)$ is normalized by the number of attributes.

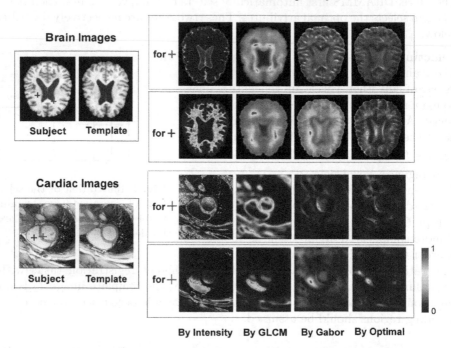

Fig. 4. Role of attribute selection in reducing matching ambiguities, as illustrated on special voxels (red crosses) and ordinary voxels (blue crosses) in brain and cardiac images of different individuals. Similarity maps are generated between a voxel (red or blue) in the subject image and all voxels in the template image. "GLCM", gray-level co-occurrence matrix [20], is another commonly used texture attribute descriptor.

Role of Optimized Gabor Attributes. Fig. 4 shows that the optimized Gabor attributes lead to highly distinctive attribute similarity maps between the subject and the template brain and cardiac images, for two voxels in each case. This reduces the computational cost and the ambiguities in matching. In particular, since the similarity function for a given voxel now looks more like a delta function, the optimal Gabor attributes are likely to reduce local minima and therefore assist the optimization process to converge to the global minimum.

2.4   Using Mutual-Saliency Map to Modulate Registration

As addressed in the introduction, an ideal optimization process should utilize all voxels but assign a continuously-valued weight to each voxel, based on whether a reliable correspondence could be established at this voxel.

Previous work [30][31] assumed that more *salient* regions could establish more *reliable* correspondence and hence should be assigned with higher weights. They have reported improved registration accuracies. However, this assumption does not always hold, as regions that are salient in one image are not necessarily salient in the other image, or do not necessarily have unique correspondence across images, especially in convoluted and complex structures such as the human brain cortex. In other words, saliency in one image does not necessarily indicate matching reliability between two images.

To measure matching reliability (uniqueness) between two images, DRAMMS extends the concept of *saliency*, which is often observed in one image, to the concept of *mutual-saliency*, which, as manifested in Fig. 5, is directly defined on a pair of voxels in the two images under registration. In particular, a pair of voxels $\mathbf{u} \in \Omega_1$ and $T(\mathbf{u}) \in \Omega_2$ is defined to have high mutual-saliency $ms(A_1(\mathbf{u}), A_2(T(\mathbf{u})))$ and hence should be assigned with high weight $w(\mathbf{u}, T(\mathbf{u}))$, if $\mathbf{u}$ has high similarity to voxels in the core neighborhood of $T(\mathbf{u})$ and low similarity to voxels far away from $T(\mathbf{u})$,

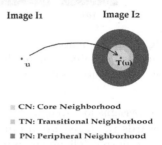

Image I₁   Image I₂

■ CN: Core Neighborhood
■ TN: Transitional Neighborhood
■ PN: Peripheral Neighborhood

Fig. 5. Illustration of the definition of mutual-saliency function. Refer to text for details.

$$w(\mathbf{u}, T(\mathbf{u})) = ms(A_1(\mathbf{u}), A_2(T(\mathbf{u}))) = \frac{MEAN_{\mathbf{v} \in CN(T(\mathbf{u}))} \left[sim(A_1(\mathbf{u}), A_2(\mathbf{v})) \right]}{MEAN_{\mathbf{v} \in PN(T(\mathbf{u}))} \left[sim(A_1(\mathbf{u}), A_2(\mathbf{v})) \right]}$$

(8)

where $sim(\cdot, \cdot)$ is defined in the same way as in Eqns. 6 and 7. Note that voxels in between the core and peripheral neighborhoods of $T(\mathbf{u})$ are ignored because there is typically a smooth transition from high to low similarities, especially for coarse-scale Gabor attributes. For the same reason, the radii of those neighborhoods are adaptive to the scale in which Gabor attributes are extracted.

Roles of Mutual-Saliency Maps. 1) *Missing data*: the mutual-saliency map effectively identifies regions in which no good correspondence can be found and reduces their negative impact. In Fig. 6, motivated by our work on matching histological sections with MRI, we have simulated cross-shaped tears in the subject image, which are typical when sections are stitched together. Mutual-saliency

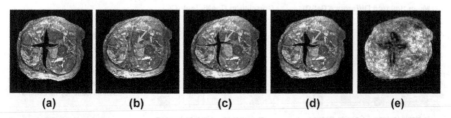

(a)   (b)   (c)   (d)   (e)

Fig. 6. Role of mutual-saliency map in accounting for partial loss of correspondence. (a) Subject image, with simulated deformation and tears from (b) template image. (c, d) Registered images without and with using mutual-saliency map; (e) Mutual-saliency map associated with (d). Red points denote the same spatial locations in all sub-figures.

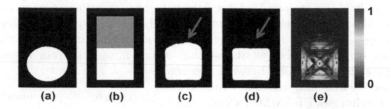

Fig. 7. Role of mutual-saliency map in reducing the negative impact of matching ambiguities. (a) Subject image; (b) Template image; (c,d) Registered images, without and with using mutual-saliency map; (e) Mutual-saliency map associated with (d).

map assigns low weights to the tears, therefore reducing their negative impacts towards the registration process. On the contrary, registration process without using mutual-saliency map tends to fill in the tears by aggressively pulling other regions, causing inaccurate results, as pointed out by the arrows in Fig. 6(c); 2) *Matching ambiguities*: even without loss of correspondences, mutual-saliency map can accurately identify regions having matching ambiguities and reduce their negative impact. In Fig. 7, the mutual saliency map assigns highest weights to those regions that have minimum ambiguity in matching (e.g., the center, the left, right and bottom edge of the circular plate in Fig. 7(a)). Meanwhile, regions that have considerable ambiguity in matching (e.g., the top edge of the circular plate) are correctly assigned with low weights; therefore their negative impact is minimized and a desirable registration result is obtained, as shown in Fig. 7(d).

2.5   Numerical Optimization

DRAMMS was optimized using free form deformation (FFD) model, which has been widely used in deformable registration community, and was implemented using gradient descent and line search strategies in a multi-resolution fashion, so as to reduce the risk of being trapped at local minima. Following standard FFD model, the transformation field is regularized by its "bending energy" [6,19], and the distance between the control points is chosen at 7 voxels in $x - y$ directions and 2 voxels in z direction. All experiments were operated in C code on a 2.8

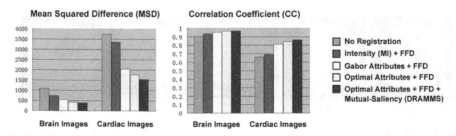

Fig. 8. Quantitative evaluation of the registration accuracies of inter-subject brain and cardiac images, in terms of MSD and CC between registered and template images. Each of DRAMMS' components provides additive improvement over MI-based FFD.

G Intel Xeon processor with UNIX operation system. Registering two 2D slices (256 × 256) typically costs about 80 seconds and registering two 3D images (256 × 256 × 30) typically costs about 25 minutes.

3   Results

As a general-purpose registration method, DRAMMS has been tested extensively in diverse registration tasks and on different organs, and has been compared with mutual information (MI)-based FFD, another commonly used general-purpose registration method. Note that, the default set of parameters is used for MI-based FFD as provided in MIPAV, a public software package [32]. To be fair, DRAMMS also used a single set of parameters throughout the comparisons.

3.1 Simulated Images. Registration results for simulated images have already been shown in Figs. 6 and 7. Largely due to the mutual-saliency component, DRAMMS outperforms MI-based FFD in both experiments.

3.2 Inter-Subject Registration. Brain and cardiac images of different individuals (the ones shown in the left column of Fig. 4) have been registered by different methods. Registration results are quantitatively compared in terms of mean squared difference (MSD) and correlation coefficient (CC) between the registered and the template images. Since the images under registration are of the same modality, high registration accuracy normally corresponds to decreased MSD and increased CC. As shown in Fig. 8, each of DRAMMS' components provides additive improvement of registration accuracy over MI-based FFD.

3.3 Multi-modality Registration. In Fig. 9, histological images of mouse brain and human prostate are registered to MR images of the same subject in order to map histologically-defined tumor ground truth onto MR space. Due

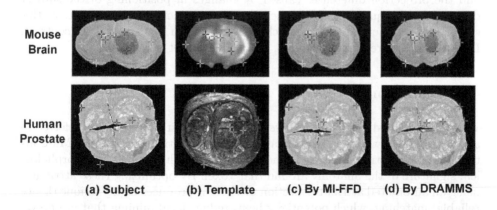

Fig. 9. Multi-modality registration on mouse brain and human prostate between (a) histological and (b) MR images, by (c) MI-based FFD and (d) DRAMMS. In each case (row), crosses of the same color denote the same spatial locations in all images.

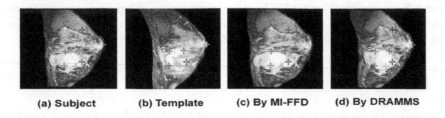

(a) Subject   (b) Template   (c) By MI-FFD   (d) By DRAMMS

Fig. 10. Longitudinal registration of breast images, between (a) subject (baseline) and (b) template (follow-up) images, with results generated by (c) MI-based FFD and (d) DRAMMS. Crosses of the same color denote the same locations in all images

to the greatly different imaging characteristics between the two modalities, their intensity distributions do not follow consistent relationship, violating the underlying assumption of MI-based methods, so theoretically it is not surprising that MI-based methods tend to fail. To make things worse, registration is also challenged by the partial loss of correspondence caused by the stitching effects in the histology (as in the prostate case). For the same reasons, registration accuracy could no longer be evaluated by MSD or CC. Instead, crosses of the same colors have been placed at the same spatial locations in each sub-figure, in order to visually reveal whether the anatomical structures have been successfully aligned. Compared with MI-based FFD, DRAMMS is able to align tumor and other complicated structures.

3.4 Longitudinal Registration. In Fig. 10, a baseline MR image is registered to a follow-up MR image of the same breast to study the tumor change. Even though the two images are of the same modality, it is not difficult to observe that their intensity distributions, to some extent, no longer follow a consistent relationship, largely due to the unpredictable changes of tumor in size and shape, and the projection differences caused by changes in positioning of the subject during image acquisition. Consequently, it is also not surprising that, in this case, MI-based method is severely challenged or even tends to fail. In contrast, DRAMMS captures tumor changes, although still not perfectly.

4   Conclusions

We have presented a *general-purpose* deformable registration method referred to as "DRAMMS", which makes primarily two contributions. First, DRAMMS attaches a Gabor attribute vector to each image voxel, which serves as a morphological signature of the anatomy around that voxel. By optimizing these attributes using an automated attribute selection method, it produces highly unique (hence reliable) matching, which potentially helps reduce local minima that are prevalent in intensity-based matching methods. Second, DRAMMS modulates the optimization process by a continuously-valued weighting function derived from "mutual-saliency". Mutual-saliency maps assign lower weights to regions having difficulties establishing reliable correspondences, therefore reducing the negative impacts caused by the matching ambiguities and/or the partial loss of correspondence. The general applicability and accuracy of DRAMMS are demonstrated in diverse registration tasks, including simulated images, inter-subject images, single- and multi-modality images and longitudinal images, on human and mouse brains, heart, breast and prostate. In images that the traditional mutual information-based free form deformation (MI-based FFD) method could register, DRAMMS has obtained slightly higher registration accuracy; while in images where the MI-based FFD method tended to fail, DRAMMS has provided significant improvement.

References

1. Glocker, B., et al.: Dense image registration through MRFs and efficient linear programming. Medical Image Analysis 12(6), 731–741 (2008)
2. Vercauteren, T., et al.: Non-parametric Diffeomorphic Image Registration with the Demons Algorithm. In: Ayache, N., Ourselin, S., Maeder, A. (eds.) MICCAI 2007, Part II. LNCS, vol. 4792, pp. 319–326. Springer, Heidelberg (2007)
3. Christensen, G.E., Rabbitt, R.D., Miller, M.I.: 3D brain mapping using a deformable neuroanatomy. Phys. Medicine Biol. 39, 609–618 (1994)
4. Collins, D.L., et al.: Automatic 3D intersubject registration on MR volumetric data in standardized talairach space. J. Comput. Assist. Tomogr. 18(2), 192–205 (1994)
5. Thirion, J.-P.: Image matching as a diffusion process: An analogy with maxwells demons. Med. Image Anal. 2(3), 243–260 (1998)
6. Rueckert, D., et al.: Nonrigid registration using free-form deformations: Application to breast MR images. IEEE Trans. Med. Imag. 18(8), 712–721 (1999)
7. Wells III, W.M., et al.: Multi-modal volume registration by maximization of mutual information. Medical Image Analysis 1(1), 35–51 (1996)
8. Davatzikos, C., Prince, J.L., Bryan, R.N.: Image registration based on boundary mapping. IEEE Trans. on Med. Imag. 15(1), 112–115 (1996)
9. Thompson, P., Toga, A.: Anatomically-driven strategies for high-dimensional brain image warping and pathology detection. Brain Warping, 311–336 (1998)
10. Rohr, K., et al.: Landmark-based elastic registration using approximating thin-plate splines. IEEE Trans. Med. Imaging 20(6), 526–534 (2001)
11. Shen, D., Davatzikos, C.: HAMMER: Hierarchical Attribute Matching Mechanism for Elastic Registration. IEEE Trans. Med. Imaging 21(11), 1421–1439 (2002)
12. Joshi, S.C., Miller, M.I.: Landmark matching via large deformation diffeomorphisms. IEEE Trans. Image Processing 9, 1357–1370 (2000)
13. Chui, H., Rangarajan, A.: A new point matching algorithm for non-rigid registration. Computer Vision Image Understanding 89, 114–141 (2003)
14. Zhan, Y., et al.: Registering Histologic and MR Images of Prostate for Image-based Cancer Detection. Academic Radiology 14(11), 1367–1381 (2007)
15. Xue, Z., Shen, D., Davatzikos, C.: Determining correspondence in 3-D MR brain images using attribute vectors as morphological signatures of voxels. IEEE Trans. Med. Imag. 23(10), 1276–1291 (2004)
16. Anandan, P.: A computational framework and an algorithm for the measurement of visual motion. Int. J. Comput. Vision 2, 283–310 (1989)
17. McEachen II, J.C., Duncan, J.: Shape-Based Tracking of Left Ventricular Wall Motion. IEEE Trans. Med. Imaging 16(3), 270–283 (1997)

18. Wu, G., Qi, F., Shen, D.: Learning Best Features and Deformation Statistics for Hierarchical Registration of MR Brain Images. In: Karssemeijer, N., Lelieveldt, B. (eds.) IPMI 2007. LNCS, vol. 4584, pp. 160–171. Springer, Heidelberg (2007)
19. Bookstein, F.L.: Principal warps: Thin-Plate splines and the decomposition of deformations. IEEE Trans. Pattern Anal. Mach. Intell. 11(6), 567–585 (1989)
20. Haralick, R.M.: Statistical and structural approaches to texture. Proc. IEEE 67(5), 786–804 (1979)
21. Jain, A.K., Farrokhnia, F.: Unsupervised texture segmentation using Gabor filters. Pattern Recognition 24(12), 1167–1186 (1991)
22. Zhang, J., Liu, Y.: Cervical Cancer Detection Using SVM Based Feature Screening. In: Barillot, C., Haynor, D.R., Hellier, P. (eds.) MICCAI 2004. LNCS, vol. 3217, pp. 873–880. Springer, Heidelberg (2004)
23. Manjunath, B.S., Ma, W.Y.: Texture features for browsing and retrieval of image data. IEEE Trans. Pattern Anal. Mach. Intell. 18(8), 837–842 (1996)
24. Zhan, Y., Shen, D.: Deformable Segmentation of 3D Ultrasound Prostate Images Using Statistical Texture Matching Method. IEEE TMI 25, 256–272 (2006)
25. Liu, J., Vemuri, B.C., Marroquin, J.L.: Local frequency representations for robust multimodal image registration. IEEE Trans. on Med. Imag. 21, 462–469 (2002)
26. Verma, R., Davatzikos, C.: Matching of Diffusion Tensor Images using Gabor Features. In: ISBI, pp. 396–399 (2004)
27. Elbakary, M., Sundareshan, M.K.: Accurate representation of local frequency using a computationally efficient Gabor filter fusion approach with application to image registration. Pattern Recognition Letters 26(14), 2164–2173 (2005)
28. Kadir, T., Brady, M.: Saliency, scale and image description. Int. J. Comput. Vision 45(2), 83–105 (2001)
29. Fan, Y., et al.: COMPARE: Classification of Morphological Patterns Using Adaptive Regional Elements. IEEE Trans. Med. Imaging 26(1), 93–105 (2007)
30. Wu, G., Qi, F., Shen, D.: Learning-based deformable registration of MR brain images. IEEE Trans. Med. Imaging 25(9), 1145–1157 (2006)
31. Mahapatra, D., Sun, Y.: Registration of dynamic renal MR images using neurobiological model of saliency. IEEE ISBI, 1119–1122 (2008)
32. McAuliffe, M., et al.: Medical image processing, analysis and visualization in clinical research. In: Proc. 14th IEEE Comp. Based Med. Sys., pp. 381–386 (2001)

Simultaneous Consideration of Spatial Deformation and Tensor Orientation in Diffusion Tensor Image Registration Using Local Fast Marching Patterns

Hai Li[1,2], Zhong Xue[1], Lei Guo[2], and Stephen T.C. Wong[1]

[1] The Center for Biotechnology and Informatics, The Methodist Hospital Research Institute and Department of Radiology, The Methodist Hospital, Weill Cornell Medical College, Houston, TX, USA
[2] School of Automation, Northwestern Polytechnical University, China
{hli, zxue}@tmhs.org, lguo@nwpu.edu.cn, stwong@tmhs.org

Abstract. Diffusion tensor imaging (DTI) plays increasingly important roles in surgical planning, neurological disease diagnosis, and follow-up studies in recent years. In order to compare the tractography obtained from different subjects or the same subject at different timepoints, a key step is to spatially align DTI images. Different from scalar or multi-channel image registration, tensor orientation should be considered in DTI registration. Several DTI registration methods have been proposed before, and some of them are based on first extracting the orientation-invariant features and then registering images using traditional scalar or multi-channel registration techniques followed by tensor reorientation. They essentially do not fully use the tensor information. Other methods such as the piece-wise affine transformation and the diffeomorphic non-linear registration algorithms use analytical gradients of the registration objective functions by considering the reorientation of tensor during the registration. However, only local tensor information such as voxel tensor similarity is utilized in these algorithms, which can be regarded as a counterpart of the traditional intensity similarity-based image registration in the DTI case. This paper proposes a novel DTI image registration algorithm, called fast marching-based simultaneous registration. It not only considers the orientation of tensors but also utilizes the neighborhood tensor information of each voxel, which is extracted from a local fast marching algorithm around voxels of interest. Compared to the voxel-wise tensor similarity-based registration, richer and more distinctive tensor features are used in this algorithm to better define correspondences between DTI images. Thus, more robust and accurate registration results can be obtained. In the experiments, comparative results using the real DTI data show the advantages of the proposed algorithm.

Keywords: Diffusion tensor imaging, image registration, tensor reorientation, fast marching.

1 Introduction

Diffusion tensor imaging (DTI) enables visualization and quantitative characterization of white matter tracts in 3D human brain magnetic resonance imaging (MRI), and can

J.L. Prince, D.L. Pham, and K.J. Myers (Eds.): IPMI 2009, LNCS 5636, pp. 63–75, 2009.
© Springer-Verlag Berlin Heidelberg 2009

be used to study the white matter architecture to distinct the normal and diseased brains [1,2]. Applications include multiple sclerosis, stroke, aging, dementia, schizophrenia, epilepsy, brain tumor and others. During the last 15 years, it has been one of the most popular MRI techniques in brain research, and is becoming more popular in clinical practice.

Using special techniques the diffusion tensor for each voxel can be measured in MR brain images. With the 3D tensor information new insight on the brain structures can be studied. Recent clinical studies mostly focus on regional statistics of fractional anisotropy (FA), apparent diffusion coefficient (ADC), and mean diffusivity (MD) derived from such tensors. Neuroimaging researchers are focusing more on the orientation and patterns of the nerve fibers extracted from DTI [2]. In order to compare DTI images from different subjects and from the same subject at different timepoints, inter-subject and intra-subject registrations are required to spatially align the images. Such a registration operation is also essential to construct the DTI atlas of human brain of different groups [3].

Many new distance/similarity measures and deformation mechanisms are being developed based on the tensor information contained in DTI. The basic method is to globally align the DTI images, and it is especially useful for motion correction during multiple acquisitions. Because of the relatively low resolution of DTI and less advanced alignment techniques previously, global brain registration is also applied in quantitative analysis of various diseases, and parameters such as FA and ADC are used for such an analysis based on the voxel-based morphometry (VBM) framework or region of interest (ROI)-based methods. Typical methods used for global registration include multi-channel DTI features [4,5] and tensor similarities [6,7]. Noticeable differences of these methods are that in [6], the voxel-wise tensor similarity measures are used and in [7] image correspondence is measured by the mutual information criterion.

In deformable registration of DTI images, many traditional scalar or multi-channel image registrations have been applied for first registering the feature maps such as FA and then reorienting the tensors based on the resultant deformation fields. For example, in [8] the HAMMER algorithm [4] has been applied, and a principal direction preserving reorientation algorithm is proposed to align tensors. In [9] the geometry and orientation-invariant features are integrated into a hierarchical matching framework. Similarly various tensor features are extracted for registration. Irfanoglu *et al.* [10] proposed a novel method for deformable tensor-to-tensor registration by modeling the distances between the tensors with Geodesic-Loxodromes, and the multidimensional scaling algorithm is used to unfold the manifold with this metric. Ziyan *et al.* [11] used fiber bundles extracted from DTI images for nonlinear registration with a poly-affine transformation model. Other registration algorithms include [12-14]. Although compared to simple features such as FA, the tensor orientation-invariant features improve the matching of the WM fiber tracts by taking into account the statistical information of underlying fiber orientations, these algorithms are essentially traditional multi-channel image registration, and full tensor information has not been used in the registration procedure.

Other recent exciting methods such as the piece-wise affine transformation [15,16] and the diffeomorphic non-linear registration [17] algorithms use analytical gradients of the registration objective functions by considering the reorientation of tensor during the registration. In [16] an explicit analytic optimization of tensor reorientation during the optimization is proposed, and the algorithm seeks a piecewise affine trans-formation that divides the image domain into uniform sub-regions and transforms each of them using affine transformation. Yeo *et al.* [17] used a diffeomorphic non-linear registration algorithm using an analytical gradient of the registration objective function. In [18] Zhang *et al.* evaluated different registration approaches including low and high-dimensional normalization using the FA-based registration and high-dimensional normalization using full tensor information (piece-wise affine tensor registration). The results suggested that high-dimensional approaches utilizing full tensor features instead of tensor-derived indices can further improve the alignment of WM tracts.

These deformable DTI image registration algorithms can be regarded as the coun-terparts of the traditional intensity-based image registration: the former is in the DTI space using tensor similarity by considering orientation while the latter is in the inten-sity or scalar space, wherein no orientation is needed. In the scalar or multi-channel image registration domain, various richer and distinctive image features have been proposed to better define image correspondences and hence the registration is more robust and accurate. But to our knowledge DTI registration embedding fiber reorien-tation is still in the image similarity-based registration domain due to the difficulty of extracting neighborhood tensor features of each point in DTI images.

In this paper, we propose a novel DTI image registration algorithm, referred to as fast marching (FM)-based simultaneous registration. The algorithm not only considers the orientation of tensors in the registration procedure but also uses the tensor infor-mation of the neighborhood of each voxel as distinctive attributes in the registration. Such tensor features can be extracted from a local fast marching algorithm executed around each voxel of interest. Compared to the tensor similarity-based methods, richer and more distinctive tensor features can be extracted using the FM-based si-multaneous registration, and they can better define point correspondences between images. Thus, more robust and accurate registration results can be obtained.

Two sets of experiments are performed in order to evaluate the proposed algo-rithm. The first set uses simulated DTI images to evaluate the accuracy of registration by comparing with the known deformation ground truth, and the FA-based free-form deformation is compared. In the second experiment we apply the proposed algorithm to real diffusion tensor MRI images from normal subjects to demonstrate its perform-ance. Both visualization results of real data and the quantitative comparison using simulated data indicate the advantages of the FM-based simultaneous registration.

2   Methods

2.1   Problem Formulation

The formulation of our DTI registration algorithm is similar to the common image registration framework, and the objective is to solve a deformation field $\mathbf{f}$ in order to align the template DTI image D_T and the subject image D_S. The energy function can be defined as follows,

$$E(\mathbf{f}) = E_{sim}(D_T, D_S, \mathbf{f}) + \lambda E_{con}(\mathbf{f}), \tag{1}$$

where $E_{sim}(D_T, D_S, \mathbf{f})$ stands for the similarity measure between the two images based on the current deformation $\mathbf{f}$, and $E_{con}(\mathbf{f})$ is the smoothness constraint of the deformation field. In our study, the deformation field $\mathbf{f}$ is modeled using the cubic B-Spline registration model [5], thus the smoothness of the deformation is guaranteed and the second term is omitted. So the detailed energy function, $E = E_{sim}$, is,

$$E = \sum_{\mathbf{x} \in \Omega} \| A[D_S(\mathbf{f}(\mathbf{x}) + \mathbf{x})] - A[Q(\mathbf{f}(\mathbf{x}))D_T(\mathbf{x})Q^T(\mathbf{f}(\mathbf{x}))] \|^2 , \qquad (2)$$

where $\mathbf{x}$ is a voxel in the template image domain Ω. $D_T(\mathbf{x})$ is the tensor at voxel $\mathbf{x}$ in the template image, and $D_S(\mathbf{f}(\mathbf{x}) + \mathbf{x})$ is the tensor at the corresponding voxel in the subject image. $Q(\mathbf{f}(\mathbf{x}))$ is the rotation matrix calculated from the deformation field at voxel $\mathbf{x}$. Thus the tensor in the template image needs to be reoriented in order to be compared with the corresponding tensor in the subject image. $A[]$ represents the feature extraction operator of the diffusion tensors centered on a voxel, and $\| A[D_1] - A[D_2] \|^2$ gives the distance between two sets of feature vectors. If $A[] = I$, the feature of the diffusion tensor image at a voxel is the tensor itself, and hence $\| A[D_1] - A[D_2] \|^2 = \| D_1 - D_2 \|^2$ becomes one of the tensor distances defined in [1]. In this case the above formulation in Eq.(2) is similar to the tensor similarity-based registration, wherein the overall similarity between two images is based on a summation of the voxel-wise tensor differences.

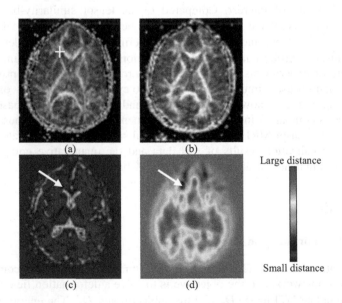

Fig. 1. Comparison of the distance maps using tensor similarity and FM-based tensor features. (a) the template image (FA) and a picked point; (b) the subject image (FA); (c) the distance map using tensor similarity; and (d) the distance map using the FM-based tensor features.

Notice that the voxel-wise tensor distance only reflects relatively local similarity and can be stuck into local minima. Following the idea in scalar image registration, the features of all the tensors around a voxel **x** can be used in the registration, which reflects not only the tensor at the voxel but also its neighboring patterns in the tensor space. This is the reason of using $A[]$ in the formulation.

In our work, the neighborhood tensor feature $A[]$ is defined by the arrival time maps of the evolving fronts through performing a local tensor-based fast marching. Clearly although the tensors within a neighborhood of a voxel is a high dimensional system, a simple fast marching starting from that voxel can extract the tensor patterns around it. Thus the major idea of this paper is to use local fast marching tensor features for more accurate DTI registration.

In addition to the FM-based tensor features, the FA values are also included as one element of the feature vectors in order to emphasize more about the current tensor point. To illustrate why FM-based tensor features are more distinctive, Figure 1 shows the distance maps calculated from the tensor distance and the FM-based tensor features, respectively. In this case the local fast marching is performed within a sphere with radius $16mm$ around each point of the subject image. It can be seen that if only the tensor distance is used, for the selected voxel from the template image there are a large number of voxels that are similar to that voxel, whereas the FM-based tensor feature is more distinctive. Therefore, such distinctive features can be used in the registration for more robust results. Next, we introduce the local fast marching algorithm and describe the FM-based simultaneous registration in details.

2.2 Local Fast Marching for Diffusion Tensor Feature Extraction

In DTI images, the diffusivity of water molecules at a location is characterized by a tensor. Although FA, ADC, and other factors can be used as the diffusion features in the registration, they only reflect the local tensor features and do not reflect the diffusion patterns around the voxel of interest. In this work, we apply the local fast marching algorithm [19] to capture the diffusion patterns around a voxel. First the evolution of a front starts from the current voxel **x** and marches according to the neighboring tensors within a neighborhood of that voxel. Suppose at a timepoint the evolving front comes to point $\mathbf{y}'$, then the marching speed from $\mathbf{y}'$ to another neighboring candidate point **y** outside the evolving front can be defined as,

$$v_{\mathbf{y}}(\mathbf{r}) = v_{\mathbf{y}}^{\text{tensor}}(\mathbf{r}) + \eta v_{\mathbf{y}}^{\text{inertia}}(\mathbf{r}),\qquad(3)$$

where $v_{\mathbf{y}}^{\text{tensor}}(\mathbf{r})$ is the major evolution speed calculated from the tensor at the current point $\mathbf{y}'$ toward point **y** along direction $\mathbf{r}: \mathbf{y}' \to \mathbf{y}$, and,

$$v_{\mathbf{y}}^{\text{tensor}}(\mathbf{r}) = w\mathbf{r}^{T}D_{\mathbf{y}}\mathbf{r},\qquad(4)$$

where w is the coefficient to eliminate fast evolution within cerebrospinal fluid (CSF). w is small if FA value is small, and vise versa. Thus w can be calculated by $w = 1/(1 + \exp(-\alpha \cdot (FA - \beta)))$, where α and β are constants to control the effects of FA. The second term in Eq. (3) is the inertia term to make the evolution smooth,

$$v_y^{\text{inertia}}(\mathbf{r}) = v_{y'}(\mathbf{r}_{y'} \cdot \mathbf{r}), \tag{5}$$

where $\mathbf{r}_{y'}$ and $v_{y'}$ are the evolution direction and the speed of the current front point $\mathbf{y}'$, respectively, and "." stands for dot product or two vectors. According to the fast marching method the arrival time of the evolution front and the evolution speed are associated by the Eikonal equation [20],

$$|\nabla T| V = d, \tag{6}$$

where ∇T is the time needed for the evolution from one point to another, V stands for the marching speed between them, and d represents the distance between these points. Thus the arrival time t_y of the front at point $\mathbf{y}$ is,

$$t_y = t_{y'} + d / v_y. \tag{7}$$

$t_{y'}$ is the arrival time at point $\mathbf{y}'$, and v_y is the marching speed determined in Eq. (3). For each neighboring point of $\mathbf{y}'$ outside the evolving front, we calculate its arriving time using Eq.(7), and the one with the least arrival time is then updated to be the new front point. In this way the front evolves away from voxel $\mathbf{x}$, and the arrival times within the neighborhood around $\mathbf{x}$ form a map that characterizes its neighborhood tensor information. In this paper, η is set as 0.9, α as 50 and β as 0.3.

Figure 2 shows an example of the time map calculated around a given voxel. It can be seen that the time map patterns reflect the overall local tensor information around that voxel. In this work, the local time maps are used as the tensor features $A[]$ in Eq. (2). The detailed implementation will be described in the next section.

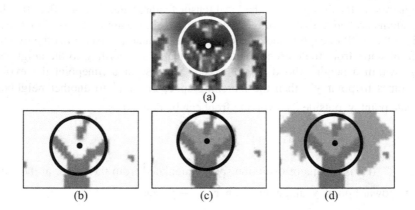

Fig. 2. The local time map calculated around a given voxel (green point). (a) The time map generated from the local fast marching. The color map shows the values of the arrival time at each voxel starting from the green point. The green circle illustrates a neighborhood within which the time map features are selected as the tensor features $A[]$; (b) (c) and (d) illustrate the evolution of the marching front (the boundary of the blue region) at different iterations. It can be seen that the front moves quickly along the fiber directions (brown shows CSF regions).

2.3 Implementation of the FM-Based Simultaneous Registration Algorithm

After fast marching we can obtain the time map around each voxel of interest over the entire brain. It can be seen from Figure 2 that the diffusion speed or arrival time along different directions is very different, which is determined by the DTI image. The front propagates faster along the direction of fiber tracts and slower along other directions. Therefore, the time map calculated from the tensor-based fast marching reflects the diffusion patterns around a voxel.

Back to Eq. (2), The time map obtained from Section 2.2 can be used to calculate the tensor features, thus Eq. (2) is re-written as,

$$
E = \sum_{\mathbf{x} \in \Omega} \left\{ \sum_{\mathbf{y} \in N(\mathbf{x})} \left(t_S(\mathbf{f}(\mathbf{x}) + \mathbf{x}, \mathbf{f}(\mathbf{y}) + \mathbf{y}) - t_{Q(\mathbf{f})D_T Q^T(\mathbf{f}),\mathbf{f}}(\mathbf{x}, \mathbf{y}) \right)^2 \right.
$$
$$
\left. + \mu \left(FA_S(\mathbf{f}(\mathbf{x}) + \mathbf{x}) - FA_T(\mathbf{x}) \right)^2 \right\},
$$

(8)

where $t_S(\mathbf{x}, \mathbf{y})$ stands for the arrival time from voxel $\mathbf{x}$ to voxel $\mathbf{y}$ in the subject image S. $t_{Q(\mathbf{f})D_T Q^T(\mathbf{f}),\mathbf{f}}(\mathbf{x}, \mathbf{y})$ stands for the arrival time map from voxel $\mathbf{x}$ to voxel $\mathbf{y}$ in the deformed template image after considering both tensor reorientation $Q(\mathbf{f})$ and deformation field $\mathbf{f}$. $N(\mathbf{x})$ represents a local neighborhood of voxel $\mathbf{x}$ wherein the local fast marching features are extracted.

However, once the deformation field $\mathbf{f}$ is changed, the time map around each template voxel has to be recalculated based on the deformed and reoriented template image. In fact we cannot simply deform the time maps since the arrival times also change. This is extremely time-consuming, and a fast implementation algorithm should be investigated in order to be able to accomplish the goal. In this work we used an approximation of the time map in the template image.

To simplify the calculation, we seek to only calculate the time map features from the original template image and then correct that time map based on the current deformation, *i.e.*, we calculate the time map around each voxel $\mathbf{x}$, $t_T(\mathbf{x}, \mathbf{y}), \mathbf{y} \in N(\mathbf{x})$ and use it to estimate $t_{QD_T Q^T,\mathbf{f}}(\cdot,\cdot)$ in Eq. (8). As shown in Figure 3, for a smooth deformation field the local angular changes along the fast marching tracks (the pink track in the figure) are relatively small. Thus, we assume that the reorientation of the fast marching track and that of the tensor at a given voxel are similar or the angular difference of the two orientations is small. Thus the projection of the tensor along the marching direction, *i.e.*, $\mathbf{r}^T D_y \mathbf{r}$ in Eq. (4), and the angular differences between vectors $\mathbf{r}_{y'}$ and $\mathbf{r}$ in Eq. (5), are omitted after deforming the template smoothly. The relatively large change will be the distance d in Eq. (7). Thus the time map can be estimated by the distance changes along the marching tracks as,

$$
t_{Q(\mathbf{f})D_T Q^T(\mathbf{f}),\mathbf{f}}(\mathbf{x}, \mathbf{y}) \approx t_T(\mathbf{x}, \mathbf{y})(1 + \frac{|\mathbf{f}(\mathbf{y}) + \mathbf{y} - \mathbf{f}(\mathbf{x}) - \mathbf{x}|_{\mathbf{x} \to \mathbf{y}} - |\mathbf{y} - \mathbf{x}|_{\mathbf{x} \to \mathbf{y}}}{|\mathbf{y} - \mathbf{x}|_{\mathbf{x} \to \mathbf{y}}}),
$$

(9)

where $|\cdot|_{\mathbf{x} \to \mathbf{y}}$ represents the distance along the marching track from $\mathbf{x}$ to $\mathbf{y}$.

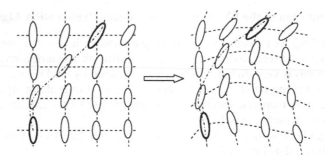

Fig. 3. The local angular changes along the fast marching tracks (*pink or dash-dotted* line) are relatively small for smooth deformation field. For example the fast marching starting from the bottom-left *red* tensor to the top *blue* tensor will follow the same track as shown in *pink* dash-dotted lines before and after deformation. In our simplification, we assume that the angular changes along these tracks are small and thus the time map change can be approximately adjusted by the distance changes due to deformation.

Finally, the simplified the energy function can be defined as,

$$
E = \sum_{x \in \Omega} \left\{ \sum_{y \in N(x)} \left(t_S(\mathbf{f}(\mathbf{x}) + \mathbf{x}, \mathbf{f}(\mathbf{y}) + \mathbf{y}) - t_T(\mathbf{x}, \mathbf{y})(1 + \frac{|\mathbf{f}(\mathbf{y}) + \mathbf{y} - \mathbf{f}(\mathbf{x}) - \mathbf{x}|_{x \to y} - |\mathbf{y} - \mathbf{x}|_{x \to y}}{|\mathbf{y} - \mathbf{x}|_{x \to y}}) \right)^2 \right.
$$
$$
\left. + \mu (FA_S(\mathbf{f}(\mathbf{x}) + \mathbf{x}) - FA_T(\mathbf{x}))^2 \right\}.
$$
(10)

It can be seen that using the simplified version, we only need to calculate the local fast marching feature once for both the template and the subject images. The time map features in the template image are then "deformed" and adjusted in order to calculate the differences between the template image and the subject image.

The algorithm can be summarized as follows:

- Step 1. Select the number of resolutions R and down-sample the input DTI images for multi-resolution registration; set the current resolution $r = R$.
- Step 2. In resolution r, for each voxel whose FA value is greater than a threshold, calculate its local time map using the method described in Section 2.2;
- Step 3. For each control point of the cubic B-Spline $\mathbf{c}$, estimate the gradient of the objective function with respect to the control point, *i.e.*, $\partial E/\partial \mathbf{c}$, update the deformation value of the control point using $\mathbf{v}(\mathbf{c}) = \mathbf{v}(\mathbf{c}) - \varepsilon \partial E/\partial \mathbf{c}$, and update the small portion of the deformation field affected by this control point; All the control points are iterated in this step to update the deformation.
- Step 4. Repeat Step 3 until convergence. After registration in resolution r, if $r = 1$ then go to Step 5 otherwise up-sample the cubic B-Spline model to a higher resolution and calculate its corresponding deformation field. After obtaining the deformation field the template image is reoriented and deformed accordingly using Xu's reorientation method [8]. Finally, we set $r = r - 1$, and go to Step 2 for processing in the next resolution;

- Step 5. Calculate the final deformation field using the resultant cubic B-Spline model and reorient the subject image onto the template space if necessary [8].

Notice the time map on the deformed template image is re-calculated at in each resolution to eliminate large errors due to the simplification.

3 Results

Two sets of experiments are performed in order to evaluate the proposed FM-based simultaneous registration algorithm. In the first set of experiments simulated DTI images are used to evaluate the accuracy of registration by comparing with the known deformations. The FA-based high-dimensional free-form deformation method is also performed for comparison. In the second experiment, we applied the proposed FM-based simultaneous registration algorithm to real diffusion tensor MRI images from normal subjects to demonstrate its performance.

3.1 Experiments on Simulated Datasets

Ten images have been simulated based on the following strategy. First the statistical model-based deformation simulation [21] has been used to simulate the DTI images. More than 100 T1-weighted MR images have been registered onto a template image space, in which both T1-weighted and diffusion tensor images are available, using the high-dimensional registration algorithm [4]. For all the images in this work, the voxel size of the T1-weighted images is $.9375mm \times .9375mm \times 1.5mm$ and that of the DTI images is $2mm \times 2mm \times 2.7mm$. Based on the resultant deformation fields, a statistical model was trained and then used to simulate ten simulated deformations. Finally, we used [8] to warp the DTI image of the template onto ten different subject spaces based on the simulated deformation fields. Thus the tensors of the template DTI image have been undergone both warping and reorientation operations in order to generate the warped DTI images. Since the deformation fields between the template image and the simulated images are known, we used them as our testing images to evaluate the performance of the proposed algorithm. Similarly, the fractional anisotropy images are also calculated from these DTI images and used as one feature of the proposed algorithm. As a comparison, the traditional ways to register DTI image, namely register the FA images using high-dimensional free-form deformable registration has also been tested for comparative purpose. Figure 4 shows the FA maps of the template image and three sample simulated images. It can be seen that the simulated images are different in terms of shape variability and valid anatomical structures (notice the various shapes of the ventricles).

After registering the template image with the simulated images, we calculated the distributions of the deformation errors between the registration results and the ground truth. Suppose the ground truth is f^* and the resultant deformation is f, the difference map Δf is calculated as the voxel-wise Euclidian distance between f and f^*. Figure 5 shows the average histograms for ten images using the proposed FM-based simultaneous registration algorithm and the FA-based free-form deformation algorithm, respectively. It can be seen that the proposed algorithm yields relatively

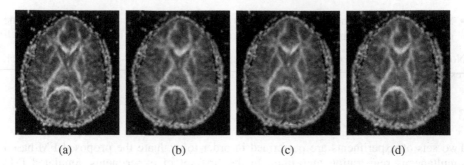

(a)   (b)   (c)   (d)

Fig. 4. The FA maps of the template image and three examples of the simulated images. (a) The template; (b), (c) and (d) the simulated images. Global transformations between template and simulated images have been canceled so that only deformable vector fields are used.

accurate deformation. As the FA is also used in the proposed algorithm as one image feature for registration, the comparative results indicate that by using the neighborhood tensor features the registration can be more robust and accurate. The experiment also shows that the simplification of the energy function works well for DTI image registration.

3.2 Experiments on DTI Images

The second experiment aims to show the application of the proposed algorithm on real DTI images. In order to be able to visually evaluate the performance of the algorithm, we used the proposed algorithm to automatically register a template image with 14 normal adult DTI images provided by S. Mori of Johns Hopkins, under the Human Brain Project and National Research Resource Center grant (1RO1AG20012-01/P41RR15241-01A1). Several specific fiber bundles from the template images are manually selected and the goal was to automatically register the template image with each of the subject images and then label the corresponding fiber bundles in the subject images. On the other hand, these fiber bundles of interest are also manually picked from each subject image, so that we can quantitatively compare the differences between the automatic labeling results and the manual labeling results.

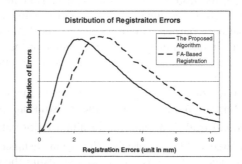

Fig. 5. The distributions of the registration errors of ten simulated images using the FA-based registration and the proposed algorithm

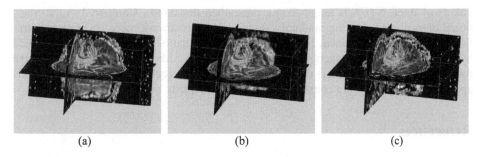

(a)   (b)   (c)

Fig. 6. Example of the fiber labeling of a subject. (a) Fibers of the template image; (b) extracted fiber tracts in the subject image (deformed on to the template image), and (c) the manual selection of the fiber tracts from the subject image.

We used the Hausdorff distances from one fiber in the subject image to all the template fibers of a bundle of interest to classify whether this fiber belongs to the bundle of interest. It is not easy to accurately label the fibers even after image registration due to the complexity of fiber structures. Some fiber classification might need to be combined with image registration in order to precisely extract fiber bundles. For example, after automatic labeling of a region using image registration algorithms, if we simply pick the fibers close to the warped fibers from the atlas, chances are that not all the fibers picked belong to a desired white matter bundle, and on the other hand some fibers belonging to the neuro bundle might not been extracted. Therefore, although in this experiment, we simply use a distance measure for fiber classification, it is worth noting that such distance-based labeling might introduce errors.

Figure 6 shows an example of the results of the selected fiber tracts from corpus callosum using the proposed algorithm. Figure 6 (a) provides the manual selection of the tracts from the template image, and Figure 6 (b) shows the fibers automatically labeled from the subject image (warped on the template image space). Figure 6 (c) displays the manual marked fibers from the subject image. It can be seen that the manual selection and auto-calculated fiber tracts are quite similar.

Finally, it is worth noting that in our experiments, we found that the fiber tracking results from the warped DTI images are not as good as those from the original images. This is because the reorientation algorithms always have some assumptions about how the fibers "should" rotate, which will affect more or less the fiber tracking results. Therefore, as long as the deformable registration provides accurate vector field to define the correspondences among images, fiber tracts and other diffusion characteristics can be first calculated in the original image spaces and then spatially aligned for quantitative intra- and inter-subject analysis.

4   Conclusions

A fast marching-based simultaneous registration algorithm is proposed for DTI brain images. The algorithm not only considers the orientation of tensors but also uses the neighborhood tensor information of each voxel during the registration procedure. The tensor features are extracted by applying a local fast marching algorithm around voxels of interest (FA is larger than a prescribed threshold). Compared to the traditional algorithms using the randomly simulated deformations, more accurate registration results can be obtained. In addition, visual evaluation of the fiber tracts labeled by the FM-based simultaneous registration also shows the promising results. In the future work, we will evaluate the proposed algorithm in real DTI brain image analysis applications such as brain connectivity analysis in Autism or Schizophrenia patients.

References

[1] Alexander, D., Gee, J.C., Bajcsy, R.: Similarity measures for matching diffusion tensor images. In: BMVC, pp. 93–102 (1999)
[2] Corouge, I., Fletcher, P.T., Joshi, S., Gilmore, J.H., Gerig, G.: Fiber tract-oriented statistics for quantitative diffusion tensor MRI analysis. In: Duncan, J.S., Gerig, G. (eds.) MICCAI 2005. LNCS, vol. 3749, pp. 131–139. Springer, Heidelberg (2005)
[3] Assaf, Y., Pasternak, O.: Diffusion tensor imaging (DTI)-based white matter mapping in brain research: a review. J. Mol. Neurosci. 34(1), 51–61 (2008)
[4] Shen, D., Davatzikos, C.: HAMMER: Hierarchical Attribute Matching Mechanism for Elastic Registration. IEEE Trans. on Medical Imaging 21(11), 1421–1439 (2002)
[5] Rueckert, D., Sonoda, L.I., Hayes, D., Hill, D., Leach, M., Hawkes, D.: Nonrigid registration using free-form deformations: application to breast MR images. IEEE Trans. Med. Imaging 18(8), 712–721 (1999)
[6] Pollari, M., Neuvonen, T., Ltjnen, J.: Affine registration of diffusion tensor MR images. In: Larsen, R., Nielsen, M., Sporring, J. (eds.) MICCAI 2006. LNCS, vol. 4191, pp. 629–636. Springer, Heidelberg (2006)
[7] Van Hecke, W., Leemans, A., D'Agostino, E., De Backer, S., Vandervliet, E., Parizel, P.M., Sijbers, J.: Nonrigid coregistration of diffusion tensor images using a viscous fluid model and mutual information. IEEE Trans. Med. Imaging 26(11), 1598–1612 (2007)
[8] Xu, D., Mori, S., Shen, D., van Zijl, P.C.M., Davatzikos, C.: Spatial Normalization of Diffusion Tensor Fields. Magnetic Resonance in Medicine 50, 175–182 (2003)
[9] Yang, J., Shen, D., Davatzikos, C., Verma, R.: Diffusion tensor image registration using tensor geometry and orientation features. In: Metaxas, D., Axel, L., Fichtinger, G., Székely, G. (eds.) MICCAI 2008, Part II. LNCS, vol. 5242, pp. 905–913. Springer, Heidelberg (2008)
[10] Irfanoglu, M.O., Machiraju, R., Sammet, S., Pierpaoli, C., Knopp, M.V.: Automatic deformable diffusion tensor registration for fiber population analysis. In: Metaxas, D., Axel, L., Fichtinger, G., Székely, G. (eds.) MICCAI 2008, Part II. LNCS, vol. 5242, pp. 1014–1022. Springer, Heidelberg (2008)
[11] Ziyan, U., Sabuncu, M.R., O'Donnell, L.J., Westin, C.F.: Nonlinear registration of diffusion MR images based on fiber bundles. In: Ayache, N., Ourselin, S., Maeder, A. (eds.) MICCAI 2007, Part I. LNCS, vol. 4791, pp. 351–358. Springer, Heidelberg (2007)
[12] Chiang, M.C., Leow, A.D., Klunder, A.D., Dutton, R.A., Barysheva, M., Rose, S.E., McMahon, K.L., de Zubicaray, G.I., Toga, A.W., Thompson, P.M.: Fluid Registration of Diffusion Tensor Images Using Information Theory. Med. Img. 27(4), 442–456 (2008)
[13] Hagmann, P., Jonasson, L., Maeder, P., Thiran, J.P., Wedeen, V.J., Meuli, R.: Understanding diffusion MR imaging techniques: from scalar diffusion-weighted imaging to diffusion tensor imaging and beyond. Radiographics, 205–223 (2006)

[14] Jones, D.K., Griffin, L.D., Alexander, D.C., Catani, M., Horsfield, M.A., Howard, R., Williams, S.C.: Spatial normalization and averaging of diffusion tensor MRI data sets. Neuroimage 17(2), 592–617 (2002)
[15] Zhang, H., Yushkevich, P.A., Gee, J.C.: Registration of Diffusion Tensor Images. In: CVPR, pp. 842–847 (2004)
[16] Zhang, H., Yushkevich, P.Z., Alexander, D.C., Gee, J.C.: Deformable registration of diffusion tensor MR images with explicit orientation optimization. Medical Image Analysis 10(5), 764–785 (2006)
[17] Yeo, B.T.T., Vercauteren, T., Fillard, P., Pennec, X., Golland, P., Ayache, N., Clatz, O.: DTI Registration with Finite-Strain Differential. In: ISBI, pp. 700–703 (2008)
[18] Zhang, H., Avants, B.B., Yushkevich, P.A., Woo, J.H., Wang, S., McCluskey, L.F., Elman, L.B., Melhem, E.R., Gee, J.C.: High-dimensional spatial normalization of diffusion tensor images improves the detection of white matter differences: an example study using amyotrophic lateral sclerosis. IEEE Trans. Med. Imaging 26(11), 1585–1597 (2007)
[19] Staempfli, P., Jaermann, T., Crelier, G.R., Kollias, S., Valavanis, A., Boesiger, P.: Resolving fiber crossing using advanced fast marching tractography based on diffusion tensor imaging. Neuroimage 30(1), 110–120 (2006)
[20] Sethian, J.A.: Level Set Methods and Fast Marching Methods. Cambridge Univ. Press, Cambridge (1999)
[21] Xue, Z., Shen, D., Karacali, B., Stern, J., Rottenberg, D., Davatzikos, C.: Simulating Deformations of MR Brain Images for Validation of Atlas-based Segmentation and Registration Algorithms. Neuroimage 33(3), 855–866 (2006)

Discovering Sparse Functional Brain Networks Using Group Replicator Dynamics (GRD)

Bernard Ng[1], Rafeef Abugharbieh[1], and Martin J. McKeown[2]

[1] Biomedical Signal and Image Computing Lab, Department of Electrical Engineering,
[2] Department of Medicine (Neurology), Pacific Parkinson's Research Center,
The University of British Columbia, Vancouver, BC, Canada
`bernardn@ece.ubc.ca, rafeef@ece.ubc.ca,`
`mmckeown@interchange.ubc.ca`

Abstract. Functional magnetic resonance imaging (fMRI) has become increasingly used for studying functional integration of the brain. However, the large inter-subject variability in functional connectivity renders detection of representative group networks very difficult. In this paper, we propose a new iterative method that we refer to as "group replicator dynamics," for detecting sparse functional networks that are common across subjects within a group. The proposed method uses replicator dynamics, which we show to be equivalent to non-negative sparse PCA, and incorporates group information for identifying common networks across subjects with subject-specific weightings of the identified brain regions reflecting individual differences. Finding a separate network for each subject, as opposed to employing traditional averaging approaches, permits statistical testing of group significance. We validated our method on synthetic data, and applying it to real fMRI data detected task-specific group networks that conform well with prior neuroscience knowledge.

Keywords: fMRI, functional connectivity, group analysis, replicator dynamics.

1 Introduction

In recent years, an increasing interest in the functional integration of the brain has emerged for studying higher order cognitive functions [1-3] and neurological diseases [3-7]. Functional integration refers to the interactions between different brain regions and is typically characterized in terms of functional connectivity [8] and effective connectivity [9]. Functional connectivity is defined as the correlations between brain regions, whereas effective connectivity is the influence of a brain region over another brain region. The focus of this paper will be on inferring functional connectivity from functional magnetic resonance imaging (fMRI) data.

The classical approach of analyzing functional connectivity is to pick a seed voxel or region and examine the linear correlations between the seed and all other voxels in the brain [10]. This approach has been widely used for detecting resting-state networks with promising results [10, 11], but suffers from the drawback of neglecting the joint interactions between multiple voxels [12]. To account for such interactions,

J.L. Prince, D.L. Pham, and K.J. Myers (Eds.): IPMI 2009, LNCS 5636, pp. 76–87, 2009.

multivariate techniques such as clustering [13-15], principal component analysis (PCA) [8], and independent component analysis (ICA) [12, 16] have previously been explored. To explicitly exploit the sparse nature of human brain networks [17], we have adopted replicator dynamics [18-21] in this paper, which we show to be a fast solution to the non-negative sparse PCA problem [22, 23] under certain constraints. Enforcing sparsity eases the diffused weighting problem seen in classical PCA [24, 25], where non-zero loadings (i.e. spatial component maps) are often assigned to the majority of voxels within brain, which complicates network identification.

The multivariate methods described above provide effective means of analyzing functional connectivity within a single subject, but the optimal way for performing group analysis is not trivial. The traditional way is to either concatenate [26, 27] or average [27, 28] the voxel time courses across subjects in detecting representative group networks. Alternatively, one can perform connectivity analysis separately on each subject and average the results. For instance, Lohmann and Bohn performed group inference by first estimating the pairwise correlations between voxels for each subject and subsequently applying replicator dynamics on the average correlation matrix [18]. Similarly, van de Heuvel et al. in their study of resting-state networks applied normalized cut to cluster voxels within each subject and used the consistency of the clustermaps to infer group clusters [15]. Provided the functional organization is similar across subjects, the average networks would be reasonable representations of the group. However, if the connection strengths between brain regions vary across subjects, the average group networks may not reflect the features in the individual networks of each subject [29]. Moreover, collapsing the individual networks into a single group network does not permit statistical testing for group significance.

Another challenge associated with group analysis is the need for establishing a correspondence across subjects. Connectivity analysis performed at the voxel level, as often done for most of the aforementioned methods, typically entails spatial normalization, which is prone to mis-registration [30-32] and spatial distortions [33]. An alternative approach to create a subject correspondence without spatial normalization is to define regions of interest (ROIs) in each subject's native space and examine the connectivity between these brain regions. For instance, Marrelec et al. used partial correlation to measure the connectivity between anatomically defined ROIs [34]. Similarly, Ng et al. applied replicator dynamics on anatomically defined ROIs to investigate the effects of task frequency on functional connectivity [21]. To avoid the drawbacks associated with spatial normalization, this ROI-based approach is thus employed in our analysis.

In this paper, we propose a new iterative method for detecting sparse functional networks consistently recruited among a group of subjects. To encourage sparsity, replicator dynamics is used to iteratively update a weight vector that represents the degree to which an ROI belongs to the most coherent network. To facilitate statistical testing of group significance, we propose to learn the dominant network of each subject *individually* (as opposed to applying replicator dynamics to the average correlation matrix of the group [18, 21]) but with group information incorporated within each iteration, so that subject variability can be modeled while ensuring *group* networks are being detected. This iterative scheme, as we will demonstrate with synthetic and real fMRI data, results in functional networks consisting of the same ROIs across subjects yet with different ROI weightings for each subject reflecting the individual differences, thus enabling group significance to be assessed.

2 Materials

After obtaining informed consent, fMRI data were collected from 10 healthy subjects (3 men, 7 women, mean age 57.4 ± 14 years) and 10 Parkinson's disease (PD) patients on and off medication (4 men, 6 women, mean age 66 ± 8 years). Each subject was required to first use their right-hand and then their left hand to squeeze a bulb with sufficient pressure such that a horizontal bar shown on a screen was kept within an undulating pathway. The pathway remained straight during baseline periods, which required a constant pressure to be applied. During the time of stimulus, the pathway became sinusoidal at a frequency of 0.25 Hz (slow), 0.5 Hz (medium) or 0.75 Hz (fast) presented in a pseudo-random order. Each run lasted 260s, alternating between baseline and stimulus of 20 s duration with an extra 20 s baseline period at the beginning and end of each run.

Functional MRI was performed on a Philips Gyroscan Intera 3.0 T scanner (Philips, Best, Netherlands) equipped with a head-coil. T2*-weighted images with blood oxygen level dependent (BOLD) contrast were acquired using an echo-planar (EPI) sequence with an echo time of 3.7 ms, a repetition time of 1985 ms, a flip angle of 90°, an in plane resolution of 128 128 pixels, and a pixel size of 1.9 1.9 mm. Each volume consisted of 36 axial slices of 3 mm thickness with a 1 mm gap. A 3D T1-weighted image consisting of 170 axial slices was further acquired to facilitate anatomical localization of activation.

Each subject's fMRI data was pre-processed using Brain Voyager's (Brain Innovation B.V.) trilinear interpolation for 3D motion correction and sinc interpolation for slice time correction. Further motion correction was performed using motion corrected independent component analysis (MCICA) [35]. The voxel time courses were then high-pass filtered to account for temporal drifts. No spatial warping or smoothing was performed.

Eighteen motor-related ROIs were manually drawn by an expert on each subject's structural scan in their native space based upon anatomical landmarks and guided by a neurological atlas [36] using AMIRA (Mercury Computer Systems, San Diego, USA). ROIs included the bilateral putamen, caudate, globus pallidus, thalamus (THA), cerebellum (CER), primary motor cortex (M1), supplementary motor area (SMA), prefrontal cortex (PFC), and anterior cingulated cortex (ACC). The segmented ROIs were resliced at the fMRI resolution and used to extract the preprocessed voxel time courses within each ROI for subsequent analysis.

3 Methods

We present here a novel iterative method, which we refer to as group replicator dynamics (GRD), for detecting sparse functional networks that are consistent across subjects. Given an initial weight vector for each subject, where the magnitude of the elements represent the degree to which the corresponding ROIs belong to the most coherent network, replicator dynamics is iteratively applied to update these weight vectors, as described in Section 3.1. In each iteration, after all subjects' weight vectors are updated, these updated weight vectors are adjusted based on the group information as described in Section 3.2. These two steps are repeated until convergence.

3.1 Replicator Dynamics

Replicator dynamics is a well-known concept in theoretical biology for modeling the evolution of interacting species [37]. In this model, each species is assigned a fitness value, which is used to determine the fittest species that survives over time. In the context of functional connectivity analysis, each brain region is considered a species, with its fitness measured by the correlation between brain regions. If we let $w^i(0)$ be the initial weight vector of the ith subject as defined above, the most coherent network can be determined by iteratively applying the following replicator equation [37]:

$$w^i(k+1) = \frac{w^i(k).*C^iw^i(k)}{w^i(k)^T C^iw^i(k)} \, , \qquad (1)$$

where .* represents element-wise multiplication, k is the iteration counter, and C^i is the correlation matrix of the ith subject with each element corresponding to the pair-wise correlation between average ROI intensity time courses. To avoid self connections, the main diagonal of C^i is set to zero. Furthermore, to avoid bias during initialization, $w^i(0)$ is set to $1/N_r$, where N_r is the number of brain regions being examined. Using (1), w^i is guaranteed to converge to a local maximum based on the fundamental theorem of natural selection [37], provided C^i is real-value, non-negative, and symmetric. In this paper, positive and negative correlations are assumed to be of equal importance, thus the absolute value of the correlations is used to ensure C^i is non-negative. Nevertheless, networks with positively correlated regions can be separately analyzed by nulling out the negative elements in C^i and vice versa. Upon convergence, only elements corresponding to the most correlated brain regions will be non-zero due to the sparse nature of replicator dynamics as we discuss next.

The objective function that (1) maximizes is in fact the same as PCA, i.e. $w^{iT}C^iw^i$. Thus, one might argue that using PCA will provide similar results as replicator dynamics. However, the results obtained from replicator dynamics can in fact be very different from PCA for the following reason. The first principle component of PCA, w^i, is the solution to the optimization problem:

$$\arg\max_{w^i} w^{i^T}C^iw^i, \quad subject \ to \ \left\|w^i\right\|_2 = 1 \, , \qquad (2)$$

which does not encourage sparsity [24, 25], hence all elements of w^i will likely be non-zero. This problem of diffused weighting complicates network identification, since no clear threshold will necessarily be present for separating out the dominant network from other less correlated brain regions. To impose sparsity, the constraint in (2) needs to be modified to $\|w^i\|_1 \leq K$, where K is a user-defined parameter [38]. The resulting optimization problem is often referred to as sparse PCA:

$$\arg\max_{w^i} w^{i^T}C^iw^i, \quad subject \ to \left\|w^i\right\|_1 \leq K \, . \qquad (3)$$

Various solutions for (3) have been proposed. For instance, d' Aspremont et al. solved (3) using semidefinite programming [25] and Zou et al. solved (3) as a regression problem with lasso (elastic net) constraints [24]. If we further constrain w^i to be non-negative, the resulting problem will be of the form:

$$\arg\max_{w^i} w^{i^T} C^i w^i, \quad subject\ to\ \sum_j w^i_j \leq K, w^i \geq 0 , \tag{4}$$

which is known as non-negative sparse PCA [22, 23]. Examining (1), since all elements of C^i are restricted to be non-negative, w^i will also be non-negative by construction. Moreover, (1) enforces the elements of w^i to sum to one. Thus, replicator dynamics is in fact a solution of the non-negative sparse PCA problem! We note that previous studies [18] have observed an unexplained tendency of the detected networks to comprise of mutually correlated voxels. This observation can actually be explained by our finding of the equivalence between replicator dynamics and non-negative sparse PCA, since imposing sparsity given limited weights (i.e. $\sum w^i_j = 1$) will encourage the weights to be assigned to mutually correlated brain regions.

3.2 Group Replicator Dynamics

If we simply apply (1) separately for each subject until convergence, the detected networks will likely be different across subjects [29]. However, if there exists a core functional network that is common across subjects, we can exploit group information to identify this core network. The underlying assumption is that the majority of subjects use the same core functional network to perform the same task, but in addition, each subject may recruit extra brain regions, which constitutes inter-subject variability. Also, the common core network may not necessarily be the most coherent network for every subject, potentially due to different processing strategies or simply due to different levels of noise [29]. Given $w^i(k)$, to encourage networks consisting of the same brain regions across subjects, one could adjust $w^i(k)$ such that the group entropy is minimized [39, 40]. For analytic simplicity, if we assume $w^i(k)$ are instances of a normal random variable, w, then the entropy of w is given by:

$$\ln\sqrt{(2\pi e)^{N_r}|\Sigma|)} \propto \ln|\Sigma| , \tag{5}$$

where Σ is the covariance of w. To minimize the entropy, a gradient descent approach is used with $w^i(k)$ updated as follows [39, 40]:

$$W(k) = W(k) - \lambda(W_c(k)^T (W_c(k)W_c(k)^T + \alpha I)^{-1}) , \tag{6}$$

where $W(k)$ is a $N_r \times N_s$ matrix with $w^i(k)$ of each subject along the columns and $W_c(k)$ is the same as $W(k)$ but with the subject mean removed from each row. λ governs the learning rate and must be set below α to ensure numerical stability [39]. Since the number of subjects, N_s, will typically be much less than the number of brain regions, N_r, $W_c W_c^T$ will be rank deficient. Hence, αI (with $\alpha = 0.1$) is added to regularize the inversion of $W_c W_c^T$. At each iteration k, after updating all subjects' $w^i(k)$ using (1), (6) is applied to adjust $w^i(k)$ so that elements of $w^i(k)$ that are consistently large across subjects are reinforced, while other elements are suppressed. (1) is then applied to the adjusted $w^i(k)$ at the next iteration, $k+1$, and the same process is repeated until convergence. Since (1) searches for the most coherent network within a subject, while (6) encourages networks to be similar across subjects, the combined effect of (1) and (6) results in highly coherent networks that comprise of the same brain regions across subjects, but with subject-specific ROI weightings reflecting individual differences.

To test if the detected functional network is significantly different from that obtained from random noise, we first approximate the network coherence of each subject, c^i, as $w^{iT}C^iw^i$. A t-test is then applied to the Fisher's Z-transform of the c^i's, which we denote as z^i, to estimate the probability that the z^i's are drawn from a null distribution generated from random noise. To estimate the mean of the null distribution, we temporally permute all the average ROI intensity time courses 10,000 times, calculate the mean z averaged across subjects for each permutation, and take the largest mean z as the null mean. We note that approximating c^i as $w^{iT}C^iw^i$ is legitimate only if the same ROIs are detected as the core functional network across subjects. Otherwise, the estimated c^i's would represent different networks and declaring the presence of a significant common group network under this scenario would be invalid. Also, although applying replicator dynamics to the average correlation matrix [18, 21] may detect a similar group network, collapsing all subjects' networks into a single group network does not permit testing of group significance. We note that subsequent networks can be detected by removing those ROIs detected in the dominant network and reapplying the procedures above [18, 21].

3.3 Empirical Evaluation

To test our proposed connectivity analysis framework, we generated 1,000 synthetic datasets, each consisting of 10 subjects and 20 ROIs for each subject, as summarized in Fig. 1(m). ROIs 1 to 4 were designed to be mutually correlated and form the core functional network. These ROIs were also set to be connected to ROI 10 for the subject 1, ROI 11 for subject 2, etc. to introduce inter-subject variability. Furthermore, we have set ROIs 5 to 9 to be mutually correlated but with lower correlation except for subjects 1 and 2 to test the case where a secondary network is present and the core functional network is not the most coherent network for some of the subjects. The synthetic ROI time courses were generated by convolving a box-car with the hemodynamic response and adding Gaussian noise (Fig. 1(k)) at a level similar to the real data (Fig. 1(l)). The timing of the box-car for ROIs 1 to 4 and the extra subject dependent ROI is set to be exactly the same in our experiments. For ROIs 5 to 9, the stimulus period is shrunk by half to distinguish this secondary network from the core. Also, except for subjects 1 and 2, the noise level is set to be slightly higher than the core to ensure this secondary network is less correlated. For the remaining ROIs, random Gaussian noise is used as the ROI time courses.

The results obtained by applying the proposed group replicator dynamics as well as other related schemes are summarized in Fig. 1(a) to (j), where the average w^i of each subject over 1,000 synthetic datasets are plotted. Applying replicator dynamics separately to each subject (curve with dots) detected ROIs 1 to 4 to be part of the most coherent network for subjects 3 to 10, but not for subjects 1 and 2. This result is expected since ROIs 1 to 4 were designed to have lower mutual correlations than ROIs 5 to 9 for these two subjects. The extra subject-dependent ROI was also assigned roughly equal weights as ROIs 1 to 4. Hence, replicator dynamics alone provides a powerful means of detecting sparse subject-specific networks, but it is not as effective in identifying group networks, where certain heuristics will be required to prune out ROIs 1 to 4 as being the core functional network. We note that computationally estimating the weight vector using (1) took less than a millisecond for each subject.

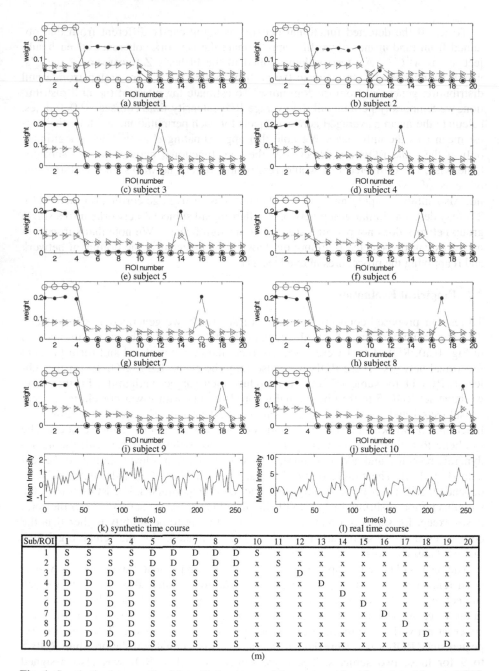

Fig. 1. Synthetic data results. (a) to (j) Average weight vectors of subjects 1 to 10 over 1,000 datasets detected using group replicator dynamics (circle), replicator dynamics (dot), group PCA (triangle), and PCA (cross). (k) Sample synthetic ROI time course with similar noise level as in real data (l). (m) Ground truth. "D" and "S" indicate if an ROI belongs to the dominant or secondary network. "x" implies random noise. Applying group replicator dynamics detected group networks that perfectly matched with the ground truth, but not so for the other methods.

Applying group replicator dynamics (curve with circle) detected ROIs 1 to 4 as the core functional network for all subjects even for subjects 1 and 2. Also, no weight was falsely assigned to the extra subject-dependent ROI for all 1,000 datasets. Furthermore, the p-values obtained for all datasets were well below 0.05. We note that applying replicator dynamics on the average correlation matrix also detected ROIs 1 to 4 as being the core network, but statistical significance could not be assessed since all subjects' information was collapsed in this approach.

For comparison, we also applied PCA to each subject separately (curve with crosses). Weights were assigned to all ROIs even for random noise, although slightly higher weights were on average given to ROIs 1 to 4 and the subject-dependent ROI for subjects 3 to 10, and ROIs 5 to 9 for subjects 1 and 2. However, if we instead examine the weights of each dataset separately, the weights given to ROIs 1 to 9 and the subject-dependent ROI were in fact very similar with weights assigned to ROIs 5 to 9 occasionally being higher than that of ROIs 1 to 4 for subjects 3 to 10, and vice versa for subjects 1 and 2. Thus, defining a subjective threshold to identify the most coherent network would be very difficult and ROIs not belonging to the most coherent network might be falsely detected.

To incorporate group information into PCA, we replaced (1) with $w^i(k+1) = C^i w^i(k)$, $\|w^i(k)\|_2 = 1$ (i.e. estimating the first principal component using the Power method) in our proposed iterative scheme. We refer to this algorithm as group PCA. Using this algorithm resulted in similar networks as obtained by applying PCA to each subject separately. We suspect the reason for this result was that PCA assigned similar weights to every ROI, thus the group entropy of the w^i's would be minute, leading to negligibly small adjustments applied to w^i by (6).

4   Results and Discussion

Fig. 2 summarizes the core functional networks detected by applying group replicator dynamics to our real experimental fMRI data for each combination of subject group and task (e.g. healthy and slow). The correlation matrices for each task were estimated using the corresponding segments of the average ROI intensity time courses. Only the left-handed results are presented due to space limitation.

For healthy subjects, the bilateral cerebellar hemispheres, bilateral SMA, and right M1 were detected as the core network during slow frequency task. At the medium frequency, the bilateral thalami were further detected. Since the thalamus is known to serve as a relay between the cerebellum and the cortex, detecting the thalamus may be a result of increased communication. At the fastest frequency, the left M1 instead of the bilateral thalami were found to be part of the core network. Prior studies suggested that the ipsilateral M1 becomes more involved as task difficulty increases [41], thus detecting the left M1 during a left-handed task at the highest frequency conforms to prior neuroscience findings. For PD patients off medication, the core network detected at the slow frequency was exactly the same as that of the healthy subjects' during the fast frequency. This result suggests that the brain deficits in PD patients made the slow frequency task appeared as difficult as the fast condition, hence the need for the left M1. The same network was detected during medium and fast frequencies. For PD patients on medication, the core network appeared to have normalized to that of healthy subjects at the slow frequency, but with more

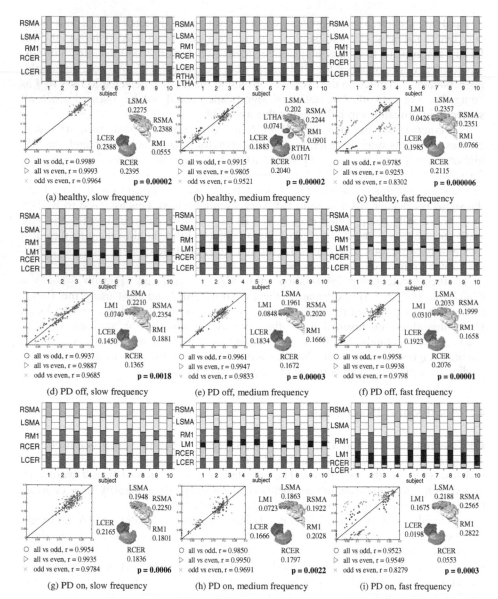

Fig. 2. Real fMRI data results. At the top of each sub-figure is a bar graph of the estimated weight vector of each subject using group replicator dynamics. The ROIs given non-zeros weights are labeled on the side of the bar graph. The bottom left of each sub-figure is a consistency plot. The bottom right of each sub-figure is a 3D rendering of the detected ROIs and the average weights of these ROIs over the subjects. All networks showed high consistency and were detected to be significant at a p-value of 0.05 with Bonferroni correction (i.e. 0.05/18 = 0.0028). Networks detected in PD off medication were similar to those detected in healthy subjects during the fast frequency, demonstrating the effects of brain deficits in PD patients. Upon medication, the network appeared to have normalized back to that of the healthy subjects during slow frequency, but not at medium and fast.

involvement of the right M1, which also matches findings from other prior studies [42]. At the medium frequency, the left M1 again became involved, and at the fast frequency, substantially more involvement of the bilateral M1 and bilateral SMA were found. Increased activity in the SMA upon medication was also observed in prior studies [42]. We note that all detected core networks were significant at a p-value of 0.05 with Bonferroni correction for the number of comparisons (i.e. 0.05/18 = 0.0028). Also, to test for consistency, we divided the time courses into odd and even time points and re-applied our proposed method. The weights obtained by using all time points and only the odd and even time points were very similar with correlations well above 0.9 for most cases. Regarding the constraint of non-negative correlation matrix required for applying replicator dynamics, the correlations of the detected ROIs were all positive. Hence, this constraint was not a major issue for the current experiment. For comparisons, we also applied group PCA to the data, but the results were analogous to the synthetic case, where similar weights were assigned to all ROIs. Thus, no distinct group networks could easily be identified.

5 Conclusions

In this paper, we proposed a new iterative method for detecting common networks within a group of subjects. By exploiting replicator dynamics, which we showed to be equivalent to non-negative sparse PCA, and incorporating group information, our method was able to detect sparse group networks that perfectly matched with the ground truth when applied to synthetic data. In contrast, classical PCA resulted in diffused weightings, which greatly hindered network identification. Applying group replicator dynamics to real fMRI data detected significant task-specific group networks that matched well with prior neuroscience knowledge. Our results thus demonstrated that the combination of sparsity and group information provides an effective means to combat against inter-subject variability in detecting group functional networks.

References

1. Schlosser, R.G., Wagner, G., Sauer, H.: Assessing the Working Memory Network: Studies with Functional Magnetic Resonance Imaging and Structural Equation Modeling. Neurosci. 139, 91–103 (2006)
2. Au Duong, M.V., et al.: Modulation of Effective Connectivity inside the Working Memory Network in Patients at the Earliest Stage of Multiple Sclerosis. NeuroImage 24, 533–538 (2005)
3. Addis, D.R., Moscovitch, M., McAndrews, M.P.: Consequences of Hippocampal Damage across the Autobiographical Memory Network in Left Temporal Lobe Epilepsy. Brain 130(9), 2327–2342 (2007)
4. He, B.J., et al.: The Role of Impaired Neuronal Communication in Neurological Disorders. Curr. Opin. Neurol. 20, 655–660 (2007)
5. Waites, A.B., et al.: Functional Connectivity Networks are Disrupted in Left Temporal Lobe Epilepsy. Ann. Neurol. 59, 335–343 (2006)

6. Au Duong, M.V., et al.: Altered Functional Connectivity Related to White Matter Changes inside the Working Memory Network at the very Early Stage of MS. J. Cereb. Blood Flow Metab. 25, 1245–1253 (2005)
7. Cader, S., et al.: Reduced Brain Functional Reserve and Altered Functional Connectivity in Patients with Multiple Sclerosis. Brain 129(2), 527–537 (2006)
8. Friston, K.J., et al.: Functional Connectivity: The Principal Component Analysis of Large (PET) Data Sets. J. Cereb. Blood Flow Metab. 13, 5–14 (1993)
9. Friston, K.J., Frith, C.D., Frackowiak, R.S.J.: Time-dependent Changes in Effective Connectivity Measured with PET. Hum. Brain Mapp. 1, 69–80 (1993)
10. Biswal, B., et al.: Functional Connectivity in the Motor Cortex of Resting Human Brain using Echo-planar MRI. Magn. Reson. Med. 34, 537–541 (1995)
11. Greicius, M.D., Krasnow, B., Reiss, A.L., Menon, V.: Functional connectivity in the resting brain: a network analysis of the default mode hypothesis. Proc. Natl. Acad. Sci. USA 100, 253–258 (2003)
12. van de Ven, V.G., et al.: Functional Connectivity as Revealed by Spatial Independent Component Analysis of fMRI Measurements during Rest. Hum. Brain. Mapp. 22, 165–178 (2004)
13. Goutte, C., et al.: On Clustering fMRI Time Series. NeuroImage 9(3), 298–310 (2002)
14. Cordes, D., et al.: Hierarchical Clustering to Measure Connectivity in fMRI Resting State Data. Magn. Reson. Imaging. 20, 305–317 (2002)
15. van den Heuvel, M., Mandl, R., Hulshoff Pol, H.: Normalized Cut Group Clustering of Resting-state fMRI Data. PLoS ONE 3(4), e2001 (2008)
16. McKeown, M.J., et al.: Analysis of fMRI Data by Blind Separation into Independent Spatial Components. Hum. Brain. Mapp. 6, 160–188 (1998)
17. Bassett, B.S.: Small-World Brain Networks. The Neuroscientist 12(6), 512–523 (2006)
18. Lohmann, G., Bohn, S.: Using Replicator Dynamics for Analyzing fMRI Data of the Human Brain. Trans. Med. Imaging. 21, 485–492 (2002)
19. Neumann, J., et al.: Meta-analysis of Functional Imaging Data Using Replicator Dynamics. Hum. Brain Mapp. 25, 165–173 (2005)
20. Neumann, J., et al.: The Parcellation of Cortical Areas Using Replicator Dynamics in fMRI. NeuroImage 32, 208–219 (2006)
21. Ng, B., Abugharbieh, R., McKeown, M.J.: Inferring Functional Connectivity using Spatial Modulation Measures of fMRI Signals within Brain Regions of Interest. In: 5th IEEE International Symposium on Biomedical Imaging: From Nano to Marco., pp. 275–572 (2008)
22. Zass, R., Shashua, A.: Nonnegative Sparse PCA. In: Advances in Neural Information Processing Systems, pp. 1561–1568 (2006)
23. Sigg, C.D., Buhmann, J.M.: Expectation Maximization for Sparse and Non-Negative PCA. In: 25th International Conference on Machine Learning, Helsinki, Finland (2008)
24. Zou, H., Hastie, T., Tibshirani, R.: Sparse Principal Component Analysis. J. Computational and Graphical Statistics 15(2), 265–286 (2004)
25. d'Aspremont, A., Bach, F., El Ghaoui, L.: Full Regularization Path for Sparse Principal Component Analysis. In: 24th International Conference on Machine Learning, vol. 227, pp. 177–184. ACM, New York (2007)
26. Calhoun, V.D., et al.: A Method for Making Group Inferences from Functional MRI Data using Independent Component Analysis. Hum. Brain. Mapp. 14, 140–151 (2001)
27. Schmithorst, V.J., Holland, S.K.: Comparison of Three Methods for Generating Group Statistical Inferences from Independent Component Analysis of Functional Magnetic Resonance Imaging Data. J. Magn. Reson. Imaging. 19(3), 365–368 (2004)

28. Bokde, A.L., et al.: Functional Interactions of the Inferior Frontal Cortex during the Processing of Words and Word-like Stimuli. Neuron 30, 609–617 (2001)
29. Goncalves, M.S., et al.: Can Meaningful Effective Connectivities be Obtained between Auditory Cortical Regions. NeuroImage 14, 1353–1360 (2001)
30. Uylings, H.B.M., et al.: Consequences of Large Interindividual Variability for Human Brain Atlases: Converging Macroscopical Imaging and Microscopical Neuroanatomy. Anat. Embryol. 210, 423–431 (2005)
31. Samanez-Larkin, G.R., D'Esposito, M.: Group Comparisons: Imaging the Aging Brain. Soc. Cogn. Affect. Neurosci. 3(3), 290–297 (2008)
32. Wilke, M., Schmithorst, V.J., Holland, S.K.: Assessment of Spatial Normalization of Whole-Brain Magnetic Resonance Images in Children. Hum. Brain Mapp. 17(1), 48–60 (2002)
33. Ng, B., Abugharbieh, R., McKeown, M.J.: Adverse Effects of Template-based Warping on Spatial fMRI Analysis. In: SPIE Conference on Medical Imaging, Orlando, Florida (2009)
34. Marrelece, G., et al.: Partial Correlation for Functional Brain Interactivity Investigation in Functional MRI. NeuroImage 32, 228–237 (2006)
35. Liao, R., Krolik, J.L., McKeown, M.J.: An Information-theoretic Criterion for Intrasubject Alignment of fMRI Time Series: Motion Corrected Independent Component Analysis. Trans. Med. Imaging. 24(1), 29–44 (2005)
36. Talairach, J., Tournoux, P.: Co-Planar Stereotaxic Atlas of the Human Brain: 3-Dimensional Proportional System - an Approach to Cerebral Imaging. Thieme Medical Publishers, New York (1988)
37. Schuster, P., Sigmund, K.: Replicator dynamics. J. Theor. Biol. 100, 533–538 (1983)
38. Tibshirani, R.: Regression Shrinkage and Selection via the LASSO. J. Royal Stat. Soc. series B 58, 267–288 (1996)
39. Cates, J., et al.: Shape Modeling and Analysis with Entropy-Based Particle Systems. In: Karssemeijer, N., Lelieveldt, B. (eds.) IPMI 2007. LNCS, vol. 4584, pp. 333–345. Springer, Heidelberg (2007)
40. Oguz, I., et al.: Cortical Correspondence Using Entropy-based Particle Systems and Local Features. In: 5th IEEE International Symposium on Biomedical Imaging: From Nano to Marco, pp. 1637–1640 (2008)
41. Verstynen, T., et al.: Ipsilateral Motor Cortex Activity during Unimanual Hand Movements Relates to Task Complexity. J. Neurophysiol. 93, 1209–1222 (2005)
42. Haslinger, B., et al.: Event-related Functional Magnetic Resonance Imaging in Parkinson's Disease before and after Levodopa. Brain 124(3), 558–570 (2001)

Multimodal Functional Imaging Using fMRI-Informed Regional EEG/MEG Source Estimation

Wanmei Ou[1], Aapo Nummenmaa[2], Matti Hämäläinen[2], and Polina Golland[1]

[1] Computer Science and Artificial Intelligence Laboratory, MIT, USA
[2] Athinoula A. Martinos Center for Biomedical Imaging, MGH, USA
wanmei@csail.mit.edu

Abstract. We propose a novel method, fMRI-Informed Regional Estimation (FIRE), which utilizes information from fMRI in E/MEG source reconstruction. FIRE takes advantage of the spatial alignment between the neural and the vascular activities, while allowing for substantial differences in their dynamics. Furthermore, with the regional approach, FIRE can be efficiently applied to a dense grid of sources. Inspection of our optimization procedure reveals that FIRE is related to the re-weighted minimum-norm algorithms, the difference being that the weights in the proposed approach are computed from both the current estimates and fMRI data. Analysis of both simulated and human fMRI-MEG data shows that FIRE reduces the ambiguities in source localization present in the minimum-norm estimates. Comparisons with several joint fMRI-E/MEG algorithms demonstrate robustness of FIRE in the presence of sources silent to either fMRI or E/MEG measurements.

Keywords: EEG, MEG, fMRI, Inverse Problem, Expectation-Maximization.

1 Introduction

The principal difficulty in interpreting Electroencephalography (EEG) and magnetoencephalography (MEG) data stems from the ill-posed electromagnetic inverse problem: infinitely many spatial current patterns give rise to identical measurements [10]. Additional assumptions on the spatial current patterns must be incorporated into the reconstruction process to obtain a unique estimate [3].

In addition to the general assumptions about the spatial current patterns such as minimum energy (or ℓ_2-norm), specific prior knowledge about activation locations can be obtained from other imaging modalities. Among them, functional Magnetic Resonance Imaging (fMRI) provides the most relevant information for the reconstruction due to its good spatial resolution. fMRI measures the hemodynamic activity, which indirectly reflects the neural activity measured by E/MEG. Extensive studies of neurovascular coupling have demonstrated similarity in spatial patterns of these two types of activations [13]. However, the timecourses of

J.L. Prince, D.L. Pham, and K.J. Myers (Eds.): IPMI 2009, LNCS 5636, pp. 88–100, 2009.

the neural and the vascular activities differ substantially, and their exact relationship is yet to be characterized in full. In addition to the differences in their physiological origins, E/MEG and fMRI have different sensitivity characteristics. For example, a brief transient neural activity may be difficult to detect in fMRI while sustained weak neural activity may lead to relatively strong fMRI signals but might have a poor signal-to-noise ratio in E/MEG.

The most straightforward way to incorporate fMRI information into E/MEG inverse estimation is the fMRI-weighted Minimum-Norm Estimation (fMNE), [1,12]. This method uses a thresholded Statistical Parametric Map (SPM) from fMRI analysis to construct weights for the standard Minimum-Norm Estimation (MNE), leading to significant improvements when the SPM is accurate. However, the weights depend on arbitrary choices of the threshold and weighting parameters. Moreover, these weights are assumed to be time independent causing excessive bias in the estimated source timecourses. Sato *et al.* [15] combined the Automatic Relevance Determination (ARD) framework and fMNE to achieve more focal estimates. In this method, which we will refer to as fARD, the parameters of a hyperprior are set based on the thresholded SPM. In addition to the arbitrary choice of the threshold similar to that in fMNE, the estimates computed via fARD are often unstable, especially in the regions where the vascular activity is weak.

Here, we propose a novel method, the fMRI-Informed Regional Estimation (FIRE), to improve the accuracy of the E/MEG source estimates. Since the relationship between the dynamics of the evoked neural and the evoked vascular signals is largely unknown, we only model the similarity of spatial patterns in the two processes, as opposed to the Kalman-filter approach in [6]. Furthermore, we expect that the shape of the activation timecourses varies across brain regions, especially for the neural activation timecourses. To account for this fact, FIRE treats the temporal dynamics in different brain regions independently. In other words, there is no constraint imposing similarity of the activation timecourses across regions. We assume the shape of the activation timecourses to be constant within a brain region, modulated by a set of location-specific latent variables. The regions are chosen based on subject-specific cortical parcellation [7]. Handling the temporal dynamics of the two types of activities separately while exploiting their common spatial pattern helps to preserve the temporal resolution of E/MEG and to achieve accurate source localization.

The prior on the latent variables encourages spatially smooth current estimates within a brain region. The prior also encourages the number of activated regions to be small, similar to the ARD approach [17], except that our prior is region-based rather than location-based. Both the activation timecourse model and the choice of brain regions in FIRE are similar to those employed in recent work by Daunizeau *et al.* [4]. However, Daunizeau *et al.* aim to symmetrically infer brain activities visible in either EEG or fMRI data, resulting in an extra random variable to model the vascular activity. The confidence of the estimated brain activities reduces when there are discrepancies between the EEG and the fMRI measurements. Furthermore, due to the complexity of this model, the estimation is limited to a coarse source space. Instead of aiming at a symmetrical inference, we focus on the estimation of current sources. We incorporate the fMRI information to reduce ambiguities in source localization usually present in E/MEG source estimation.

To fit the model to the data, we use the coordinate descent method, alternating between the estimation of current sources and of other model parameters. This iterative update scheme is similar to the re-weighted MNE methods such as FOCal Underdetermined System Solver (FOCUSS) [8]. In contrast to the re-weighted MNE, in our method the weights are jointly determined using both the estimated neural activity and the vascular activity measured by fMRI. Moreover, the estimates at different time points influence each other. The computation of the weights is related to problems arising in continuous Gaussian mixture modeling, which can be efficiently optimized using the Expectation-Maximization (EM) algorithm [5].

In the following, we first discuss the model underlying FIRE, the inference procedure, and the implementation details. We then present the experimental comparisons between FIRE and prior methods for joint E/MEG-fMRI analysis using both simulated and human data, followed by a discussion and conclusions.

2   Methods

2.1   Neurovascular Coupling and Data Models

We assume that the source space comprises N discrete locations on the cortex parcelled into K brain regions. We denote the set indexing the discrete locations in region k by P_k and the cardinality of P_k by N_k.

Fig. 1 illustrates our model. The shape of the source timecourses is identical within a region but varies across regions. Specifically, we let $\mathbf{u}_k$ and $\mathbf{v}_k$ be the

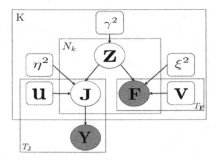

Fig. 1. Graphical interpretation of FIRE. The hidden activity $\mathbf{z}$ models the neurovascular coupling relationship. The hidden current source distribution $\mathbf{J}$ is measured by E/MEG, producing observation $\mathbf{Y}$. $\mathbf{F}$ denotes fMRI measurements. Vectors $\mathbf{u}$ and $\mathbf{v}$ are the unknown neural and vascular waveforms in a certain brain region, respectively. The inner plate represents N_k vertices in region k; the outer plate represents K regions. The bottom left and right plates represent $T_\mathbf{J}$ and $T_\mathbf{F}$ time points in the neural and the vascular measurements, respectively.

unknown waveforms in region k, associated with neural and vascular activities, respectively. We model the neural and the vascular activity strength through a hidden vector variable $\mathbf{z} = [z_1, z_2, \cdots, z_N]^\mathrm{T}$. The continuous scalar z_n indicates the activation strength at location n on the cortical surface. Thus, the probabilistic model for the neural activation timecourse $\mathbf{j}_n$ and the vascular activation timecourse $\mathbf{f}_n$ at location n in region k can be expressed as

$$p\left(\mathbf{j}_n, \mathbf{f}_n | z_n; \mathbf{u}_k, \mathbf{v}_k, \eta_k^2, \xi_k^2\right) = \mathcal{N}\left(\mathbf{j}_n; z_n \mathbf{u}_k, \eta_k^2 \mathbf{I}\right) \mathcal{N}\left(\mathbf{f}_n; z_n \mathbf{v}_k, \xi_k^2 \mathbf{I}\right), \quad (1)$$

where η_k^2 and ξ_k^2 are noise variances. We construct all matrices such that each row represents a location or a sensor and each column represents a particular time point. Thus, we let $N \times T_\mathbf{J}$ matrix $\mathbf{J} = [\mathbf{j}_1, \mathbf{j}_2, \cdots, \mathbf{j}_N]^\mathrm{T}$ be the neural current on the cortex for all $T_\mathbf{J}$ time points. We assume that the vascular signal $\mathbf{f}_n$ at location n is directly observable through fMRI. We let $N \times T_\mathbf{F}$ matrix $\mathbf{F} = [\mathbf{f}_1, \mathbf{f}_2, \cdots, \mathbf{f}_N]^\mathrm{T}$ be the fMRI measurements on the cortex over $T_\mathbf{F}$ time points. Note that our neurovascular coupling model captures only the spatial alignment between the two types of activities; it does not impose temporal similarity between the signals.

The neural currents $\mathbf{j}_n$ are detected with E/MEG described by the standard observation model. We let $M \times T_\mathbf{J}$ matrix $\mathbf{Y} = [\mathbf{y}(1), \mathbf{y}(2), \cdots, \mathbf{y}(T_\mathbf{J})]$ be the E/MEG measurements at all $T_\mathbf{J}$ time points. Column t of matrix $\mathbf{J}$, $\mathbf{j}(t)$, denotes the neural current distribution at time t. The quasi-static Maxwell's equations imply that E/MEG signals at time t are instantaneous linear combinations of the currents at different locations:

$$\mathbf{y}(t) = \mathbf{A}\mathbf{j}(t) + \mathbf{e}(t) \qquad \forall\, t = 1, 2, \cdots, T_\mathbf{J}, \quad (2)$$

where $\mathbf{e}(t)$ is the measurement noise. The $M \times N$ forward matrix $\mathbf{A}$ is determined by the electromagnetic properties of the head, the geometry of the sensors, and the locations of the sources. With spatial whitening in the sensor space, $\mathbf{e}(t) \sim \mathcal{N}(0, \mathbf{I})$. The number of sources N ($\sim 10^3 - 10^4$) is much larger than the number of measurements M ($\sim 10^2$), leading to an infinite number of solutions satisfying Eq. (2) even for $\mathbf{e}(t) = \mathbf{0}$. In general, $\mathbf{j}_n$ should be modeled as three timecourses corresponding to the three Cartesian components of the current. However, due to the columnar organization of the cortex, we can further constrain the current orientation to be perpendicular to the cortical surface and consider a scalar timecourse at each location.

2.2   Priors and Parameter Settings

To encourage the activation patterns to be smooth within a region, we impose a prior on the modulating variables. Specifically, we define $\mathbf{z}_k = \{z_n\}_{n \in P_k}$ and assume $\mathbf{z}_k \sim \mathcal{N}(\mathbf{0}, \gamma_k^2 \boldsymbol{\Phi}_k)$, where the variance γ_k^2 indicates the activation strength in region k, and $\boldsymbol{\Phi}_k$ is a fixed matrix that acts as a regularizer by penalizing the sum of squared differences between neighboring locations. This spatial prior is particularly important for the brain regions where vascular activity is too weak to measure, but the neural activity can be detected by E/MEG.

Our $\mathbf{\Phi}_k$ is similar to the regularizer used in the Low Resolution Brain Electromagnetic Tomography (LORETA) [14], except that we apply $\mathbf{\Phi}_k$ to individual brain regions while LORETA's spatial regularizer is applied to the whole brain. We assume separate variance γ_k^2 for different brain regions since the strength of current is expected to vary significantly between regions with and without active sources. This choice is similar to the recent work in the application of ARD to E/MEG reconstruction [15,17], except that their work assumes independent γ^2 for each location in the brain.

Since the forward model $\mathbf{A}$ is underdetermined, the current distribution $\mathbf{J}$, produced by our neurovascular coupling model, can fully explain the E/MEG data. In other words, without the noise term η_k^2 (i.e., $\mathbf{j}_n = z_n \mathbf{u}_k$), the fMRI data can exert too much influence on the reconstruction results. Although we can estimate the noise variance of the current source timecourses η_k^2 by extending the inference procedure, we find the corresponding estimate unstable without a prior. Based on preliminary empirical testing, we fix $\eta_k^2 = 1$. With proper temporal whitening of the fMRI data, we can also assume that $\xi_k^2 = \eta_k^2$. Fixing $\eta_k^2 = \xi_k^2$ helps to significantly reduce the computational burden of the estimation.

To summarize, our model can be mathematically expressed as

$$p(\mathbf{Y}, \mathbf{J}, \mathbf{F}, \mathbf{z}; \mathbf{\Theta}) = p(\mathbf{Y}|\mathbf{J})p(\mathbf{J}, \mathbf{F}|\mathbf{z}; \mathbf{\Theta})p(\mathbf{z}; \mathbf{\Theta}), \tag{3}$$

where $\mathbf{\Theta} = [\theta_1, \theta_2, \cdots, \theta_K]$ is the combined set of parameters, and $\theta_k = \{\mathbf{u}_k, \mathbf{v}_k, \gamma_k^2\}$. $p(\mathbf{Y}|\mathbf{J})$ is the E/MEG data model in Eq. (2). $p(\mathbf{J}, \mathbf{F}|\mathbf{z}; \mathbf{\Theta})$ is our neurovascular coupling model in Eq. (1), and $p(\mathbf{z}; \mathbf{\Theta})$ is the prior on $\mathbf{z}$. Therefore,

$$\log p(\mathbf{Y}, \mathbf{J}, \mathbf{F}, \mathbf{z}; \mathbf{\Theta}) = \sum_{t=1}^{T_J} \log \mathcal{N}(\mathbf{y}(t); \mathbf{Aj}(t), \mathbf{I}) +$$
$$\sum_{k=1}^{K} \sum_{n=1}^{N_k} \log \left[\mathcal{N}(\mathbf{j}_n; z_n \mathbf{u}_k, \eta_k^2 \mathbf{I}) \mathcal{N}(\mathbf{f}_n; z_n \mathbf{v}_k, \xi_k^2 \mathbf{I}) \right] + \sum_{k=1}^{K} \log \mathcal{N}(\mathbf{z}_k; 0, \gamma_k^2 \mathbf{\Phi}_k).$$

2.3   Inference

Our goal is to estimate the current source $\mathbf{J}$ and the timecourses $\mathbf{u}$ and $\mathbf{v}$. We treat the activation strength $\mathbf{z}$ as an auxiliary variable, and marginalize it out in the analysis. We formulate the inference as

$$\{\mathbf{J}^*, \ \mathbf{\Theta}^*\} = \underset{\mathbf{J}, \ \mathbf{\Theta}}{\arg\max} \log p(\mathbf{Y}, \mathbf{J}, \mathbf{F}; \mathbf{\Theta})$$

$$= \underset{\mathbf{J}, \ \mathbf{\Theta}}{\arg\max} \log \int_{\mathbf{z}} p(\mathbf{Y}, \mathbf{J}, \mathbf{F}, \mathbf{z}; \mathbf{\Theta}) d\mathbf{z} = \underset{\mathbf{J}, \ \mathbf{\Theta}}{\arg\max} \log \left(p(\mathbf{Y}|\mathbf{J})p(\mathbf{J}, \mathbf{F}; \mathbf{\Theta}) \right).$$

$$\tag{4}$$

With marginalization of $\mathbf{z}$, $p(\mathbf{J}, \mathbf{F}; \mathbf{\Theta})$ acts as the prior for $\mathbf{J}$. Since both $\mathbf{J}$ and $\mathbf{F}$ are linear functions of $\mathbf{z}$, $p(\mathbf{J}, \mathbf{F}; \mathbf{\Theta})$ is a continuous Gaussian mixture model.

The difficulty in inference with the proposed model is caused by the intertwining between space and time, reflected by the intersection of the temporal plates and the spatial plates in Fig. 1. That is because the output of a given E/MEG sensor is a mixture of signals from the entire source space. Hence, the inference must be performed for all time points and all locations simultaneously. FIRE is thus substantially more computationally demanding compared to standard temporally independent E/MEG estimation and voxel-wise fMRI analysis.

Due to the special structure in our model when one set of variables is fixed, we can derive an efficient gradient descent method with two alternating steps. In the first step, we fix Θ and derive a closed-form solution for $\mathbf{J}$. In the second step, we fix $\mathbf{J}$ and show that Θ can be efficiently estimated through the EM algorithm. Section 5 discusses an alternative approach to this inference problem.

For a fixed $\Theta = \widehat{\Theta}$, $p(\mathbf{Y}, \mathbf{J}, \mathbf{F}; \widehat{\Theta})$ is a jointly-Gaussian distribution. Thus, the estimate of $\mathbf{J}$ is the conditional mean:

$$\widehat{\mathbf{J}} = \arg\max_{\mathbf{J}} \log p(\mathbf{Y}, \mathbf{J}, \mathbf{F}; \widehat{\Theta}) = E\left[\mathbf{J} | \mathbf{Y}, \mathbf{F}; \widehat{\Theta}\right] = \mathbf{\Gamma}_{\mathbf{w},\mathbf{J}}^{\mathrm{T}} \mathbf{\Gamma}_{\mathbf{w}}^{-1} \mathbf{w}, \tag{5}$$

where $\mathbf{w}^{\mathrm{T}} = \left[(\mathrm{vec}(\mathbf{Y}))^{\mathrm{T}} (\mathrm{vec}(\mathbf{F}))^{\mathrm{T}}\right]$ includes both E/MEG and fMRI measurements. Operator $\mathrm{vec}(\cdot)$ concatenates adjacent columns of a matrix. $\mathbf{\Gamma}_{\mathbf{w}}$ is the covariance matrix of $\mathbf{w}$, and $\mathbf{\Gamma}_{\mathbf{w},\mathbf{J}}$ is the cross-covariance matrix between $\mathbf{w}$ and $\mathrm{vec}(\mathbf{J})$. Thus, E/MEG and fMRI measurements jointly determine the estimate of the neural activity. Eq. (5) is similar to the standard MNE solution [10], but it also includes the correlation between $\mathbf{Y}$ and $\mathbf{F}$ and the correlation among different time points of $\mathbf{J}$.

For a fixed $\mathbf{J} = \widehat{\mathbf{J}}$, we optimize the parameters Θ:

$$\widehat{\Theta} = \arg\max_{\Theta} \log p(\widehat{\mathbf{J}}, \mathbf{F}; \Theta). \tag{6}$$

As shown in Fig. 1, when the current distribution $\mathbf{J}$ is fixed, the E/MEG measurement $\mathbf{Y}$ does not provide additional information for the parameter estimation. Since the parameters for different regions are independent for a fixed $\widehat{\mathbf{J}}$, the estimates for different regions can be obtained independently. Furthermore, parameter Θ can be efficiently estimated using the EM algorithm by re-introducing the latent variable $\mathbf{z}$, which is the auxiliary variable describing activation strength. This method can be thought of as an extension of the EM algorithm for probabilistic PCA [16] to two sets of data [2]. For region k, the parameter estimates $\widehat{\theta}_k$ can be obtained by optimizing the lower bound of the log-probability:

$$\log p\left(\{\widehat{\mathbf{j}}_n, \mathbf{f}_n\}_{n \in P_k}; \theta_k\right) \geq \int_{\mathbf{z}_k} q(\mathbf{z}_k) \log p\left(\{\widehat{\mathbf{j}}_n, \mathbf{f}_n\}_{n \in P_k}, \mathbf{z}_k; \theta_k\right) d\mathbf{z}_k, \tag{7}$$

where $q(\mathbf{z}_k) = p\left(\mathbf{z}_k | \{\widehat{\mathbf{j}}_n, \mathbf{f}_n\}_{n \in P_k}; \widehat{\theta}_k\right)$ is the posterior probability computed in the E-step. Since $\{\widehat{\mathbf{j}}_n, \mathbf{f}_n\}_{n \in P_k}$ and $\mathbf{z}_k$ are jointly-Gaussian distributed for a fixed $\widehat{\theta}_k$, $q(\mathbf{z}_k)$ is also a Gaussian distribution. We use $\langle \cdot \rangle_q$ to denote the expectation with respect to the posterior distribution $q(\mathbf{z}_k)$, i.e., $\langle \cdot \rangle_q \triangleq \left[\cdot | \{\widehat{\mathbf{j}}_n, \mathbf{f}_n\}_{n \in P_k}; \widehat{\theta}_k\right]$. Since the M-step depends only on quantities related to the first- and the second-order statistics of $\mathbf{z}_k$, we only need to update those quantities in the E-step:

$$\langle \mathbf{z}_k \mathbf{z}_k^{\mathrm{T}} \rangle_q \leftarrow \left[\frac{1}{\gamma_k^2} \mathbf{\Phi}_k^{-1} + \left(\frac{\mathbf{u}_k^{\mathrm{T}} \mathbf{u}_k + \mathbf{v}_k^{\mathrm{T}} \mathbf{v}_k}{\eta_k^2} \right) \mathbf{I} \right]^{-1}$$

$$\langle \mathbf{z}_k \rangle_q \leftarrow \frac{\langle \mathbf{z}_k \mathbf{z}_k^{\mathrm{T}} \rangle_q}{\eta_k^2} \left[\left(\mathbf{u}_k^{\mathrm{T}} \widehat{\mathbf{j}}_1 + \mathbf{v}_k^{\mathrm{T}} \mathbf{f}_1 \right), \cdots, \left(\mathbf{u}_k^{\mathrm{T}} \widehat{\mathbf{j}}_{N_k} + \mathbf{v}_k^{\mathrm{T}} \mathbf{f}_{N_k} \right) \right]^{\mathrm{T}}$$

$$\langle \mathbf{z}_k^{\mathrm{T}} \mathbf{\Phi}_k^{-1} \mathbf{z}_k \rangle_q \leftarrow \langle \mathbf{z}_k \rangle_q^{\mathrm{T}} \mathbf{\Phi}_k^{-1} \langle \mathbf{z}_k \rangle_q + \mathrm{tr} \left(\mathbf{\Phi}_k^{-1} \langle \mathbf{z}_k \mathbf{z}_k^{\mathrm{T}} \rangle_q \right).$$

In the M-step, we fix $q(\mathbf{z}_k)$ and optimize Eq. (7). With some algebra, we arrive at the update equations for the model parameters:

$$\widehat{\mathbf{u}}_k \leftarrow \frac{\sum_{n \in P_k} \langle z_n \rangle_q \widehat{\mathbf{j}}_n}{\mathrm{tr}(\langle \mathbf{z}_k \mathbf{z}_k^{\mathrm{T}} \rangle_q)}, \quad \widehat{\mathbf{v}}_k \leftarrow \frac{\sum_{n \in P_k} \langle z_n \rangle_q \mathbf{f}_n}{\mathrm{tr}(\langle \mathbf{z}_k \mathbf{z}_k^{\mathrm{T}} \rangle_q)}, \quad \text{and} \quad \widehat{\gamma_k^2} \leftarrow \frac{\langle \mathbf{z}_k^{\mathrm{T}} \mathbf{\Phi}_k^{-1} \mathbf{z}_k \rangle_q}{N_k}. \tag{8}$$

We iterate the EM algorithm until convergence which usually takes less than ten iterations. We then re-estimate $\mathbf{J}$ according to Eq. (5).

To summarize, the algorithm proceeds as follows:

(i) Initialize $\widehat{\mathbf{J}}$ as the MNE estimate.
(ii) Until convergence:
   1. Compute $\widehat{\mathbf{\Theta}}$ using the EM algorithm: E-step for the hidden variable $\mathbf{z}$ followed by M-step for the model parameters $\mathbf{\Theta}$.
   2. Update $\widehat{\mathbf{J}}$ according to Eq. (5) for $\mathbf{\Theta} = \widehat{\mathbf{\Theta}}$.

3   Implementation

For the computation of the forward matrix $\mathbf{A}$, we need to specify the E/MEG forward model and the source space. We employ the single-compartment boundary-element model for the MEG forward computations [9]. The source space is confined to a mesh on the cortical surface with approximately 5-mm resolution, corresponding to about 5000 vertices per hemisphere.

The functional regions are defined by parceling the cortical folding pattern using the FreeSurfer software, resulting in 35 parcels per hemisphere [7]. The boundaries of adjacent parcels are defined along sulci. We merge adjacent parcels that contain fewer than 30 vertices. Our neurovascular coupling model requires an orientation reference for each brain region. Here, we set the orientation reference to be the largest left singular vector of the matrix formed by the outward cortical normals within a region.

We apply the standard preprocessing to fMRI data, then estimate the hemodynamic response function (HRF) at each voxel with a 15-bin finite impulse response regressor covering a 20-s time window using the FS-FAST software (MGH, Boston, MA). The estimated HRF is used as $\mathbf{f}_n$ in our model. For a source space of $N \sim 10^4$ vertices and timecourses of $T_\mathbf{J} \sim 10^2$ and $T_\mathbf{F} \sim 10^1$ samples, FIRE takes less than 20 iterations until the energy function reduces less than 0.1% from the energy of the previous iteration. In each iteration of the coordinate descent algorithm, the estimate of Θ takes 30 seconds, while the estimate of $\mathbf{J}$ takes 4 minutes on a standard PC (2.8 GHz CPU and 8 GB RAM), leading to the total run time of approximately 1.5 hours. Estimating $\mathbf{J}$ involves an inversion of an $(MT_\mathbf{J} + NT_\mathbf{F}) \times (MT_\mathbf{J} + NT_\mathbf{F})$ dense symmetric matrix $\mathbf{\Gamma_w}$, which is too large to store in memory. Instead, we employ the conjugate gradient descent method to solve the corresponding system of linear equations. It usually takes 100 iterations until convergence.

4 Results

We first compare FIRE to MNE, fMNE, and fARD using simulated data. We then extend the comparison to human MEG and fMRI data from a somatosensory study.

4.1 Simulation Studies

To simulate MEG measurements, we created two patches on the cortical sheet, with current source orientation along the outward normal to the cortical surface. Shown in the lateral-occipital view of the right hemisphere (Fig. 2), Patch A contains 20 vertices and is located in the inferior parietal region. Patch B contains 32 vertices and is located in the superior parietal region. We simulated neural and vascular timecourses in these two patches for three different scenarios: no silent activity, silent vascular activity, and silent neural activity. In the two cases with silent activities, we kept the activity of patch B unchanged while silencing neural or vascular activity in patch A. The simulated neural signals are shown as solid black lines in the rightmost column of Fig. 2. The activation maps corresponding to the peaks of the two simulated neural signals are shown in the first column.

For the forward calculations, we employed the sensor configuration of the 306-channel Neuromag VectorView MEG system used in our human studies and added Gaussian noise to the signals. The resulting signals have a SNR of 3 dB, within the typical SNR range of real MEG data. Since the two patches are close in the highly folded cortex and they exhibit neural activity during overlapping time intervals, it is particularly difficult to obtain accurate current source estimates.

Columns two to five in Fig. 2 depict the current estimates using different methods. Following [12], the fMNE weighting parameters are set to 1 and 0.1 for active and inactive fMRI locations, respectively. Since the estimates from different methods are not directly comparable in amplitude, the threshold for each method is chosen to be $1/6$ of the maximum absolute value of the corresponding current estimates $\mathbf{J}^*$. The rightmost column in Fig. 2 presents the estimated timecourses (dashed) of the most active vertex, in terms of energy, in both patches.

No Silent Activity. As shown in Fig. 2(a), the MNEs extend across adjacent gyri. fMNE, fARD, and FIRE correctly localize the two patches at the peak activation, but FIRE provides a better estimate of the spatial extent of the activations. The fARD estimate is unstable, as reflected by the large fluctuations in the estimated timecourses in patch B (green).

Silent Vascular Activity. When the vascular activity in patch A is silent, fMNE shows excessive bias towards patch B. Without a large weight, the amplitude of the estimated timecourses (blue) in patch A is significantly lower than the corresponding estimates in patch B. It would be therefore easy to miss neural activation in patch A when interpreting the results (column three in Fig. 2(b)). In contrast, by combining neural and vascular information in the re-weighted scheme, FIRE avoids such a bias. Its estimate in patch A (column five) is similar to that obtained from MNE (column one). As the weights for patch B increase and the weights for patch A decrease in the fARD update, the estimate in patch B explains the activation in patch A. As shown in the timecourse panel, the estimated timecourse in patch B (green) is similar in shape to the simulated timecourse in patch A (black solid). The change of sign is due to the fact that the outward normals for patch A and patch B are in approximately opposite directions.

Silent Neural Activity. As shown in Fig. 2(c), all methods can correctly localize the neural activity in patch B, except for the small false positive in patch A for fARD. By assigning identical weights to patches A and B, fMNE estimates a timecourse for patch A (blue) that is noisier than the corresponding one produced by FIRE (red). FIRE suppresses the weights for patch A since the current estimates in that patch are close to zero; its results are closer to the simulations.

4.2   Median-Nerve Experiments

We also tested the method using human experimental data. The median nerve at the right wrist was stimulated according to an event-related protocol, with a random inter-stimulus-interval ranging from 3 to 14 s. This stimulus activates a complex cortical network [11], including the contralateral primary somatosensory cortex (cSI) and bilateral secondary somatosensory cortices (cSII and iSII).

MEG and fMRI data were acquired in separate sessions. The MEG measurements were acquired using a 306-channel Neuromag VectorView MEG system. A 200-ms baseline before the stimulus was used to estimate the noise covariance matrix of the MEG sensors. An average signal, computed from approximately 100 trials, was used as the input to each method. The fMRI images were acquired using a Siemens 3T machine (TR=1.5 s, $64 \times 64 \times 24$, $3 \times 3 \times 6 \, \text{mm}^3$, single channel head coil). Anatomical images, from a 3T scanner, were used to construct the source space and the forward model.

In the leftmost column in Fig. 3, approximate locations for cSI (solid), cSII (dashed), and iSII (dashed) are highlighted on the fMRI activation maps ($p \leq 0.005$). Given the expected activations, we partitioned the post-central region into two regions, separately covering cSI and cSII. Note that in the noisy SPM, the sites of fMRI activations do not exactly agree with the locations of the expected current sources.

Columns two to five in Fig. 3 present the estimates at 75 ms after stimulus onset, during which cSI, cSII, and iSII should be activated. The threshold was set separately for each hemisphere since the activation in iSII is much weaker

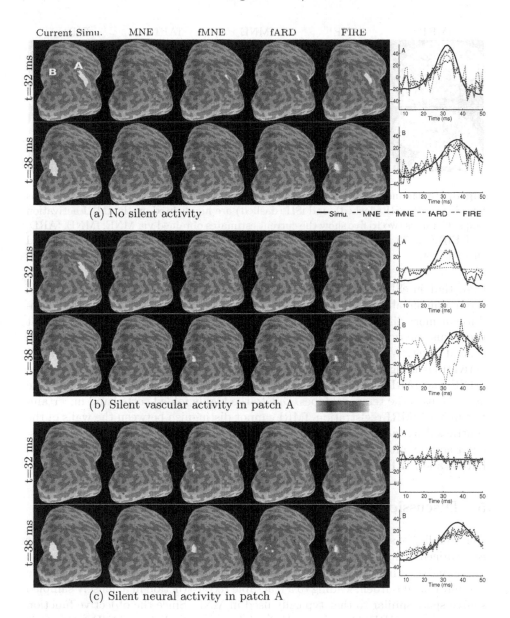

Fig. 2. Current source estimates in three scenarios. Lateral-occipital view of the right hemisphere is shown. Patch A and patch B are highlighted in the top left panel; the rest of the figures follow the same convention. (a) Neither neural nor vascular activity is silent. (b) Vascular activity in patch A is silent. (c) Neural activity in patch A is silent. The first column illustrates the simulated current distributions with a selected threshold at the peak activations. The next four columns show the estimates from MNE, fMNE, fARD, and FIRE. Hot/cold colors correspond to outward/inward current flow. The rightmost column shows the simulated (black solid) and the estimated (dashed) timecourses from the most active vertices in patch A (top) and B (bottom) for the corresponding methods.

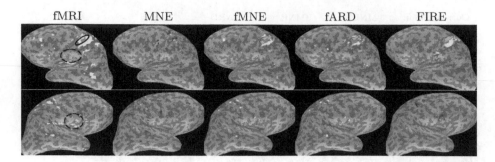

Fig. 3. Human median-nerve experiments. In the first column, approximate locations for cSI (solid), cSII (dashed), and iSII (dashed) are highlighted on the fMRI activation maps. Columns two to five show the current estimates obtained via MNE, fMNE, fARD, and FIRE at 75 ms after stimulus onset. Hot/cold colors indicate outward/inward current flow.

than that in cSI and cSII. For each method, the threshold is set to be 1/6 of the maximum absolute value of the corresponding current estimates. MNE produces a more diffuse estimate, including physiologically unlikely activations at the gyrus anterior to the cSI area. In contrast, FIRE pinpoints cSI on the post-central gyrus. With the prior knowledge from fMRI, the detected cSII and iSII activations using fMNE, fARD, and FIRE are within the expected areas. The fMNE and fARD show stronger weighting towards the fMRI, reflected by the activations in the temporal lobes. Due to the highly folded cortex and uncertainties in MRI-fMRI registration, fMRI cannot distinguish between the walls of the central sulcus and the post-central sulcus, causing both walls to show strong vascular activity after mapping of the fMRI volume onto the cortex. Hence, fMNE, fARD, and FIRE estimates extend to both sulcal walls mentioned above.

5   Discussion

The coupling of spatial and temporal domains in the joint fMRI-E/MEG analysis constrained many previous models to operate on a coarse source space. The use of region-based neurovascular coupling model proposed in this paper reduces the computational burden, leading to a tractable reconstruction in a densely sampled source space similar to that typically used in MNE. Since the objective function is not convex, FIRE depends on the initialization. We believe MNE estimate is a reasonable choice for initialization since it is unbiased.

As an alternative to the coordinate descent inference procedure proposed in this work, one could treat both $\mathbf{J}$ and $\mathbf{z}$ as latent variables in the EM framework. Since $\mathbf{J}$, $\mathbf{z}$, and the measurements are jointly Gaussian, the posterior distribution of the latent variables is also Gaussian, leading to a closed-form update. Similar to the derivations in Eq. (8), the M-step updates depend on the second order statistics of the latent variables. Since $\mathbf{J}$ is not fixed in this EM procedure, the estimate at each location depends on the estimate at all other locations in the source space, as opposed to the region-independent estimation when $\mathbf{J}$ is fixed. Therefore, the computation of the second-order statistics is infeasible except for an extremely coarse discretization of the source space.

The estimation of $\mathbf{u}_k$ and $\mathbf{v}_k$ is closely related to the canonical correlation analysis (CCA). CCA seeks vectors to project two high dimensional data sets ($\{\hat{\mathbf{j}}_n\}_{n \in P_k}$ and $\{\mathbf{f}_n\}_{n \in P_k}$ in our case) to a low dimensional space so as to maximize the correlation coefficient. The probabilistic interpretation of CCA has been established in [2].

Our neurovascular coupling model is designed for fixed-orientation current estimates, since the latent-variable model assumes that the spatial concordance of neural and vascular activities is characterized by a scalar. For free-orientation current estimates, the neurovascular coupling model would have to be adjusted to handle the correspondence between the current flow in three directions and a single vascular activation timecourse at a certain location. Moreover, FIRE assumes a single activation waveform pair, $\mathbf{u}$ and $\mathbf{v}$, in a region. The validity of this assumption depends on the size of the region and the distance between two activation sources. We cannot directly extend FIRE to multiple activation waveform pairs per region, since such an extension does not capture the fact that the shape of the vascular activation timecourses from two distinct sources is often highly similar but the neural processes are different. In the situation where there are two distinct current sources in one region, our preliminary results demonstrate that FIRE can localize the two current sources, but the estimated timecourses are combinations of the true timecourses. We defer the extension for free-orientation estimate and the extension for multiple activation sources per region to future work.

6 Conclusions

In contrast to most joint fMRI-E/MEG models, FIRE explicitly takes into account the inherent differences in the data measured by E/MEG and fMRI. The corresponding estimates can be efficiently computed with an iterative procedure which bears similarity with re-weighted MNE methods, except that the weights are based on both the current estimates in the last iteration and the fMRI data via the proposed neurovascular coupling model. This construction of the weights reduces the excessive sensitivity to fMRI present in many joint fMRI-E/MEG analysis methods, leading to more accurate current estimates as demonstrated by analysis of both simulated and human data.

Acknowledgments. We thank Dr. Raij and Dr. Siracusa for stimulating discussion. This work was supported in part by NIH NIBIB NAMIC U54-EB005149, NIH NCRR NAC P41-RR13218, NIH NCRR P41-RR14075 grants, and the NSF CAREER Award 0642971. Wanmei Ou is partially supported by the PHS training grant DA022759-03.

References

1. Ahlfors, S., Simpson, G.: Geometrical interpretation of fMRI-guided MEG/EEG inverse estimates. NeuroImage 22, 323–332 (2004)
2. Bach, F., Jordan, M.: A probabilistic interpretation of canonical correlation analysis. Technical Report 688, UC Berkeley (2005)
3. Baillet, S., et al.: Electromagnetic brain mapping. IEEE Sig. Proc. Mag. (2001)
4. Daunizeau, J., et al.: Symmetrical event-related EEG/fMRI information fusion in a variational Bayesian framework. NeuroImage 36, 69–87 (2007)
5. Dempster, A., et al.: Maximum likelihood from incomplete data via the EM algorithm. J. of Roy. Stat. Soc. B 39, 1–38 (1977)
6. Deneux, T., Faugeras, O.: EEG-fMRI fusion of non-triggered data using Kalman filtering. In: ISBI, pp. 1068–1071 (2006)
7. Fischl, B., et al.: Whole brain segmentation: automated labeling of neuroanatomical structures in the human brain. Neuron 33, 341–355 (2002)
8. Gorodnitsky, I., Rao, B.: Sparse signal reconstruction from limited data using FOCUSS: a re-weighted MNE algorithm. IEEE Trans. Sig. Proc. 45, 600–616 (1997)
9. Hämäläinen, M., Sarvas, J.: Realistic conductivity geometry model of the human head for interpretation of neuromagnetic data. IEEE Biomed. Eng. 36, 165–171 (1989)
10. Hämäläinen, M., et al.: Magnetoencephalography - theory, instrumentation, and applications to noninvasive studies of the working human brain. Rev. Mod. Phys. 65, 413–497 (1993)
11. Hari, R., Forss, N.: Magnetoencephalography in the study of human somatosensory cortical processing. Philos. Trans. R. Soc. Lond. B 354, 1145–1154 (1999)
12. Liu, A., et al.: Spatiotemporal imaging of human brain activity using functional MRI constrained magnetoencephalography data: Monte Carlo simulations. PNAS 95, 8945–8950 (1998)
13. Logothetis, N., Wandell, B.: Interpreting the BOLD signal. Annu. Rev. Physiol. 66, 735–769 (2004)
14. Pascual-Marqui, R., et al.: Low resolution electromagnetic tomography: a new method for localizing electrical activity in the brain. Int. J. Psychophysiol. 18, 49–65 (1994)
15. Sato, M., et al.: Hierarchical Bayesian estimation for MEG inverse problem. NeuroImage 23, 806–826 (2004)
16. Tipping, M., Bishop, C.: Probabilistic principal component analysis. J. Royl. Stat. Soc. B 61, 611–622 (1999)
17. Wipf, D., Nagarajan, S.: A unified Bayesian framework for MEG/EEG source imaging. NeuroImage 44, 947–966 (2009)

Tractography Segmentation Using a Hierarchical Dirichlet Processes Mixture Model

Xiaogang Wang[1], W. Eric L. Grimson[1], and Carl-Fredrik Westin[2]

[1] Computer Science and Artificial Intelligence Lab,
Massachusetts Institute of Technology, Cambridge, MA, 02139, USA
[2] Computational Research Laboratory, Childrens Hospital,
Harvard Medical School, Boston, MA 02115, USA
{xgwang,welg}@csail.mit.edu, westin@bwh.harvard.edu

Abstract. In this paper, we propose a new nonparametric Bayesian framework to cluster white matter fiber tracts into bundles using a hierarchical Dirichlet processes mixture (HDPM) model. The number of clusters is automatically learnt from data with a Dirichlet process (DP) prior instead of being manually specified. After the models of bundles have been learnt from training data without supervision, they can be used as priors to cluster/classify fibers of new subjects. When clustering fibers of new subjects, new clusters can be created for structures not observed in the training data. Our approach does not require computing pairwise distances between fibers and can cluster a huge set of fibers across multiple subjects without subsampling. We present results on multiple data sets, the largest of which has more than 120,000 fibers.

1   Introduction

Diffusion Magnetic Resonance Imaging (dMRI) is an MRI modality that has gained tremendous popularity over the past five years and is one of the first methods that made it possible to visualize and quantify the organization of white matter in the human brain in vivo. Extracting connectivity information from dMRI, termed "tractography", is an especially active area of research, as it promises to model the pathways of white matter tracts in the brain, by connecting local diffusion measurements into global trace-lines. In neurological studies of white matter using tractography it is often important to identify anatomically meaningful fiber bundles. Similar fibers form clusters of points, where each cluster is identified as a "fiber bundle".

In this paper, we propose a nonparametric Bayesian framework to cluster fibers into bundles. The 3D space of the brain is quantized into voxels. A bundle is modeled as a multinomial distribution over voxels and orientations. This probabilistically models the spatial variation of the pathways of fibers. The models of bundles are learnt from how voxels are connected by fibers instead of comparing distances between fibers. If two voxels are connected by many fibers, both of the voxels have large weights in the model of the same bundle, which means that they are on the same pathway of white matter tracts. Many existing approaches

J.L. Prince, D.L. Pham, and K.J. Myers (Eds.): IPMI 2009, LNCS 5636, pp. 101–113, 2009.

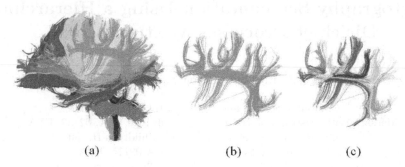

$$(a) \qquad\qquad\qquad (b) \qquad\qquad\qquad (c)$$

Fig. 1. An example of multiscale clustering. The spatial range of the whole brain is $200 \times 200 \times 200$. (a): The clustering result when the space is quantized into voxels of size $11 \times 11 \times 11$. The bundles correspond to structures at a large scale. (b): One bundle from (a). (c): The space is quantized into voxels of size $3 \times 3 \times 3$ and the bundle in (b) is further clustered into smaller bundles corresponding to structures at a finer scale.

have difficulty in determining the number of clusters and in clustering a very large set of fibers. Our approach automatically learns the number of clusters from data with a Dirichlet process (DP) prior [1]. While the space and time complexities of existing distance-based fiber clustering approaches are at least $O(M^2)$, where M is the number of fibers, the space complexity of our approach is $O(M)$ since it does not compute and store pairwise distances between fibers.

After the models of bundles have been learnt from training data without supervision, they are used as priors to cluster/classify new fibers. When clustering fibers of new subjects, our approach adapts the models of bundles to new data and creates new clusters for structures which are not observed in training data, instead of fixing the number of clusters as current methods do. Our framework can be extended to multiscale clustering. First cluster fibers using a large size of voxels and bundles correspond to structures at a large scale. Then each bundle can be further clustered using a smaller size of voxels, leading to structures at a finer scale. An example is shown in Figure 1. Multiscale clustering makes it easier for experts to identify white matter structures across different scales.

1.1   Related Work

Automatically clustering fibers has drawn a lot of attention in recent years. A typical framework is to first define a pairwise similarity/distance between fibers and to input the similarity matrix to standard clustering algorithms. Brun et al. [2] computed the Euclidean distances between 9-D fiber shape descriptors. Jonasson et al. [3] measured the similarity between two fibers by counting the number of points sharing the same voxel. Gerig et al. [4] proposed three measures related to Hausdorff distance: closest point distance, mean of closest distances and Hausdorff distance. Various clustering algorithms, such as hierarchical clustering (single-link and complete-link) [4,5], fuzzy c-means [6], k-nearest neighbors [7], normalized cuts [2] and spectral clustering [3,8] were used. Mean of closest distances and spectral clustering were popular among possible choices [8,9].

These clustering algorithms required manually specifying the number of clusters or a threshold for deciding when to stop merging/splitting clusters, both of which are difficult to know especially when the data sets are complicated and noisy. Moberts et al. [9] showed that the performance of clustering varied dramatically when different numbers of clusters were chosen. To avoid this difficulty, O'Donnell and Westin [8] first chose a large cluster number for spectral clustering and then manually merged clusters to obtain models for white matter structures.

Another drawback of this framework is the high space and time complexities of computing pairwise distances between fibers when the data set is large. Whole brain tractography produces between $10,000$ and $100,000$ fibers per subject. It is difficult to compute a $100,000 \times 100,000$ similarity matrix or even to store it in memory. Some clustering algorithms, such as spectral clustering, need to compute the eigenvectors of this huge similarity matrix. This problem becomes more serious when clustering fibers of multiple subjects. The current solutions are to cluster only a small portion of the whole data set after subsampling or to do some numerical approximation based on the sampled subset [8]. However, important information from the full data set may be lost after subsampling.

Maddah et al. [10] proposed a probabilistic approach to cluster fibers without computing pairwise distances. They used a Dirichlet distribution[1] as a prior to incorporate anatomical information. This approach is different from ours. It used a parametric model, assuming that the number of clusters is known and required manual initialization of cluster centers. [10] required establishing point correspondence which was difficult, while our approach does not.

Dirichlet process mixtures (DPM) models were applied to medical image analysis in recent years because of their capability to learn the number of clusters and their flexibility to adapt to a wide variety of data. Adelino [11] used a DPM model for brain MRI tissue classification. In [12,13] DPM models were used to model spatial brain activation patterns in functional magnetic resonance imaging. In [14], Jbabdi et al. modeled the connectivity profiles of a brain region as an infinite mixture of multivariate Gaussian distributions with a DP prior. To the best of our knowledge, our work is the first to use HDPM for tractography segmentation to automatically learn the number of clusters from data. Our approach is related to the work [15] where HDPM models were used for word-document analysis. HDPM was also used for trajectory analysis in visual surveillance [16].

2 Method

We begin by introducing DP in Section 2.1. In Section 2.2 and 2.3 we propose our HDPM model for clustering fibers and use Gibbs sampling for inference. In

---

[1] Dirichlet distribution is used as a prior of finite mixture models. These models can only well adapt to data from particular distributions. Dirichlet process in our approach is used as a prior in infinite mixture models. These models can well adapt to a wide variety of data.

Section 2.3, we explain how to use the learned models of bundles as a prior to cluster new data.

2.1   Dirichlet Process

DP [1] is used as a prior to sample probability measures. It is defined by a concentration parameter α, which is a positive scalar, and a base probability measure H. A probability measure G randomly drawn from $DP(\alpha, H)$ is always a discrete distribution,

$$G = \sum_{k=1}^{\infty} \pi_k \delta_{\phi_k}, \tag{1}$$

which can be obtained from a stick-breaking construction [17]. In Eq (1), ϕ_k is a parameter vector sampled from H, δ_{ϕ_k} is a Dirac delta function centered at ϕ_k, and π_k ($\sum_{k=1}^{\infty} \pi_k = 1$) is a non-negative scalar constructed by $\pi_k = \pi_k' \prod_{l=1}^{k-1} (1 - \pi_l')$, $\pi_k' \sim Beta(1, \alpha)$.

G can be used as a prior for infinite mixture models. Let $\{w_i\}$ be a set of observed data points. w_i is sampled from a density function $p(\cdot|\theta_i)$ parameterized by θ_i, and θ_i (which is one of the ϕ_ks in Eq (1)) is sampled from G. Data points sharing the same parameter vector ϕ_k are clustered together under this mixture model. Given parameter vectors $\theta_1, \ldots, \theta_N$ of N data points, the parameter vector θ_{N+1} of data point w_{N+1} can be sampled from a prior by integrating out G,

$$\theta_{N+1}|\theta_1, \ldots, \theta_N, \alpha, H \sim \sum_{k=1}^{K} \frac{n_k}{N + \alpha} \delta_{\theta_k^*} + \frac{\alpha}{N + \alpha} H. \tag{2}$$

There are K distinct parameter vectors $\{\theta_k^*\}_{k=1}^K$ (identifying K components) among $\theta_1, \ldots, \theta_N$. n_k is the number of points with parameter vector θ_k^*. θ_{N+1} can be assigned as one of the existing components (w_{N+1} is assigned to one of the existing clusters) or can sample a new component from H (a new cluster is created for w_{N+1}). The posterior of θ_{N+1} is

$$p(\theta_{N+1}|w_{N+1}, \theta_1, \ldots, \theta_N, \alpha, H) \propto p(w_{N+1}|\theta_{N+1})p(\theta_{N+1}|\theta_1, \ldots, \theta_N, \alpha, H). \tag{3}$$

It is likely for the Dirichlet process mixture (DPM) model to create a new component if existing components cannot well explain the data. There is no limit to the number of components. These properties make DP ideal for modeling data clustering problems when the number of clusters is not well-defined in advance.

2.2   Hierarchical Dirichlet Process Mixture Model

In probability theory, statistics, and machine learning, a graphical model is a graph that represents independences among random variables. The graphical model of our HDPM model is shown in Figure 2. There are M fibers and each fiber j has N_j points which are ordered sequentially. $o_{ji} = (u_{ji}, \Delta u_{ji})$ is the observed 3D coordinate $u_{ji} = (x_{ji}, y_{ji}, z_{ji})$ and shift $\Delta u_{ji} = u_{ji+1} - u_{ji}$ of point i on fiber j. The 3D space of the brain is uniformly quantized into voxels and

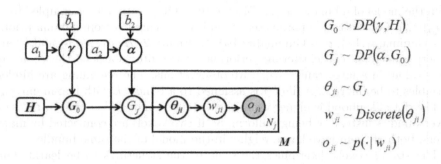

$$G_0 \sim DP(\gamma, H)$$

$$G_j \sim DP(\alpha, G_0)$$

$$\theta_{ji} \sim G_j$$

$$w_{ji} \sim Discrete(\theta_{ji})$$

$$o_{ji} \sim p(\cdot \,|\, w_{ji})$$

Fig. 2. The graphical model of our HDPM model. The right side list the distributions where the random variables are sampled from. G_0 is a prior on the whole data set. G_j is a prior on fiber j. Both G_0 and G_j are sampled from DP. θ_{ji} is the model of a bundle sampled for a point. w_{ji} and o_{ji} are the code and observation of a point.

shifts are quantized into three orientations $\Delta u_1 = (1,0,0)^T$, $\Delta u_2 = (0,1,0)^T$ and $\Delta u_3 = (0,0,1)^T$. A codebook is built, in which codes (entries of the codebook) are indices of voxels and orientations. Let u_w be the centroid of the voxel and d_w be the index of the orientation vector corresponding to code w. Quantization is done in a probabilistic way,

$$p(o_{ji}|w) = p(u_{ji}|u_w)p(\Delta u_{ji}|d_w), \qquad (4)$$

$$p(u_{ji}|u_w) \propto \begin{cases} \cos^2\left(\frac{\|u_{ji}-u_w\|^2}{2R^2}\pi\right), & \|u_{ji}-u_w\| \leq R \\ 0, & \|u_{ji}-u_w\| > R \end{cases}, \qquad (5)$$

$$p(\Delta u_{ji}|d_w) \propto \begin{cases} 1, & d_w = \arg\max_d \frac{|\Delta u_{ji}\cdot\Delta u_d|}{\|\Delta u_{ji}\|\cdot\|\Delta u_d\|} \\ 0, & \text{otherwise} \end{cases}. \qquad (6)$$

Since we do not distinguish the starting and ending points of a fiber, the sign of the correlation between Δu_{ji} and Δu_d is ignored in Eq (6). The statistical model ϕ_k of a bundle is a multinomial distribution over voxels and orientations. Optionally, if the symmetry across hemispheres is considered, we can do bilateral clustering as in [8]. Assuming that the brain is aligned and $x = 0$ is the midsagittal plane, we modify observed 3D coordinates as $u_{ji} = (|x_{ji}|, y_{ji}, z_{ji})$ ignoring the signs of x coordinates. Thus, learnt models of bundles are symmetric to the midsagittal reflection.

A prior G_0 on the whole data set is sampled from a DP, $G_0 \sim DP(\gamma, H)$, where the base measure H is a Dirichlet distribution. $G_0 = \sum_{k=1}^{\infty} \pi_{0k}\delta_{\phi_k}$ is a infinite mixture in which components $\{\phi_k\}$ are models of bundles. For a fiber j, a prior G_j is sampled from a DP, $G_j = DP(\alpha, G_0)$. It was shown that in HDPM all the G_j share the same set of components $\{\phi_k\}$ as G_0, however, they have different weights π_j over $\{\phi_k\}$, i.e. $G_j = \sum_{k=1}^{\infty} \pi_{jk}\delta_{\phi_k}$ [15]. Thus the models of bundles are learnt from all the fibers, and fibers have different distributions over bundles. For a point i on fiber j, the model θ_{ji} ($\theta_{ji} \in \{\phi_k\}$) of a bundle is sampled from G_j, $\theta_{ji} \sim G_j$. Its index of voxel and orientation w_{ji} is sampled from the model of a bundle, $w_{ji} \sim$ Discrete(θ_{ji}). Observation o_{ji} is sampled from $p(o_{ji}|w_{ji})$. Concentration parameters γ and α are sampled from gamma priors, $\gamma \sim$ Gamma(a_1, b_1), $\alpha \sim$ Gamma(a_2, b_2). In Figure 2, H, a_1, a_2, b_2 and b_2 are hyperparameters. The clustering performance is quite robust to the choice of their values in a large range. $\{o_{ji}\}$ are observations. The remaining are hidden variables to be inferred. A fiber j is assigned to a bundle k with maximum π_{jk}.

The data likelihood is higher when the distribution of a fiber concentrates on fewer bundles instead of being uniform. So if two voxels are connected by many fibers, both of them have large weights in the model of the same bundle.

The size of voxels determines the scale of the structures to be learnt. Our framework can be extended to multiscale clustering. First cluster fibers using a large size of voxels and bundles correspond to structures at a large scale. Then each bundle can be further clustered using a smaller size of voxels, showing structures at a finer scale. Multiscale clustering makes it easier for experts to identify white mater structures across different scales.

2.3   Inference

We use the Gibbs sampling inference proposed in [15], which is based on Chinese restaurant franchise. First we introduce some notations. c_{ji} is the index of the bundle assigned to point i on fiber j. n_{jk} is number of points assigned to bundle k on fiber j. n_j is the number of point on fiber j. m_{kw} is the number of points with code w and being assigned to bundle k. m_k is the total number of points assigned to bundle k. n_{jk}^{-ji}, m_{kw}^{-ji} and m_k^{-ji} mean that they are statistics without counting c_{ji}. $H = $ Dir($h, \ldots, h$) is a flat Dirichlet prior. L is the size of the codebook.

During the sampling procedure, suppose that K models of bundles (clusters) have been created and assigned to data. Then,

$$G_0 = \sum_{k=1}^{K} \pi_{0k} \delta_{\phi_k} + \pi_{0u} G_u, \qquad G_u \sim DP(\gamma, H) \qquad (7)$$

The Gibbs sampling scheme proposed in [15] integrated out $\{\pi_{jk}\}$ and $\{\phi_k\}$ without sampling them. The posterior of c_{ji} is given by

$$p(c_{ji}|\{c_{j'i'}\}_{j'i' \neq ji}, \{w_{ji}\}, \{\pi_{0k}\}, \alpha) \propto \begin{cases} (n_{jk}^{-ji} + \alpha \pi_{0k}) \cdot \frac{n_{kw_{ji}}^{-ji} + h}{n_k^{-ji} + Lh}, & k \in \{1, \ldots, K\} \\ \alpha \pi_{0u} \cdot \frac{1}{L}, & k \text{ is new} \end{cases}$$
$$(8)$$

This posterior is the product of two terms which explain how many points on fiber j are assigned to bundle k $(n_{jk}^{-ji} + \alpha \pi_{0k})$, and how well the code w_{ji} fits the model of an existing bundle $((n_{kw_{ji}}^{-ji} + h)/(n_k^{-ji} + Lh))$ or a flat distribution $(1/L)$ to create a new bundle. This shows that points on the same fiber tend to choose the same bundle. The posteriors of $\{\pi_{0k}\}$, γ and α involve more details of the Chinese restaurant franchise. They can be found in [15]. We need one more step to sample w_{ji} which is not observed in our model but observed in [15],

$$p(w_{ji}|o_{ji}, \{w_{j'i'}\}_{j'i' \neq ji}, \{c_{j'i'}\}) \qquad (9)$$

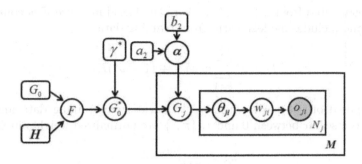

Fig. 3. The graphical model of our HDPM model for clustering testing data. F is used as the base measure to sample the prior G_0^* on the new data set. F includes the models of bundles in G_0 learnt from training data.

$$\propto p(o_{ji}|w_{ji})p(w_{ji}|\{w_{j'i'}\}_{j'i'\neq ji},\{c_{j'i'}\}) \propto p(o_{ji}|w_{ji})\frac{n_{c_{ji}w_{ji}}^{-ji}+h}{n_{c_{ji}}^{-ji}+Lh}. \qquad (10)$$

where $p(o_{ji}|w_{ji})$ is given by Eq (4).

Although $\{\phi_k\}$ and $\{\pi_{jk}\}$ are not explicitly sampled during the Gibbs sampling procedure, they can be estimated from any single sample,

$$\hat{\phi}_{kw} = \frac{m_{kw}+h}{m_k+Lh}, \quad \hat{\pi}_{jk} = \frac{n_{jk}+\alpha\pi_{0k}}{n_j+\alpha}.$$

The space complexity of our approach is $O(M)$. The time complexity of each Gibbs sampling iteration is $O(M)$. It is difficult to provide theoretical analysis on the convergence of Gibbs sampling. In practice, we stop burn-in when the data likelihood converges. From our empirical observation, the time complexity of our approach is much lower than $O(M^2)$. Recently some more efficient inference approaches, such as variational inference [18], and parallel sampling [19], have been proposed and applied to DPM and HDPM models. In future work, we will study how to improve the inference of our model using these schemes.

2.4   Clustering New Data

After the models of bundles have been learnt from training data without supervision, we can fix G_0 and the number of clusters to classify new fibers. Thus our model is converted to a parametric model.

Optionally, we can use the models learnt from training data as priors to cluster instead of classifying new data. The pre-learnt models can adapt to new data, and new clusters can be created for structures not observed in the training data. Our HDPM model for clustering testing data is shown in Figure 3. Suppose that G_0 represented in Eq (7) has been learnt from training data and K clusters are created. A prior G_0^* on testing data is to be learnt. Different from the model shown in Figure 2, where G_0 is generated from a DP with a flat base measure

H, G_0^* is generated from $DP(\gamma^*, F)$, where the based measure F is constructed from G_0 and includes models learnt from training data.

$$F = \omega^* \sum_{k=1}^{K} \hat{\pi}_{0k} \delta_{\phi_k^*} + (1 - \omega^*) H \qquad (11)$$

F is composed of two parts: the models learnt from training data and a flat prior. ω^* is a scalar between 0 and 1. $\{\hat{\pi}_{0k}\}$ are normalized weights in G_0,

$$\hat{\pi}_{0k} = \frac{\pi_{0k}}{\sum_{k'=1}^{K} \pi_{0k'}}.$$

This assumes that before observing any testing data, there already exist K models of bundles $\{\phi_k^*\}_{k=1}^K$. However, instead of letting ϕ_k^* be equal to ϕ_k in Eq (7), we sample ϕ_k^* from a Dirichlet distribution choosing ϕ_k as prior,

$$\phi_k^* \sim Dir(\xi_k^* \cdot \phi_k + H),$$

where ξ_k^* is a positive scalar. Thus the models of bundles can adapt to testing data instead of being fixed.

The choice of γ^*, ω^* and ξ_k^* controls how much the models learnt from the training data affect the clustering of testing data. The two extreme cases are that the pre-learnt models have no effect on clustering new data ($\omega^* = 0$, $\xi_k^* = 0$) and that the models learnt from new data are exactly the same as those learnt from training data ($\gamma^* = \infty$, $\omega = 1$, $\xi_k^* = \infty$).

Suppose there are K^* models of bundles assigned to testing data. Then an explicit construction of G_0^* is given by

$$G_0^* = \sum_{k=1}^{K} \pi_{0k}^* \delta_{\phi_k^*} + \sum_{k=K+1}^{K^*} \pi_{0k}^* \delta_{\phi_k^*} + \pi_{0u}^* G_{0u}^*. \qquad (12)$$

Models $\{\phi_k^*\}_{k=1}^K$ have been seen in training data. They are sampled from priors $Dir(\xi_k^* \cdot \phi_k + H)$ and are updated using testing data. $\{\phi_k^*\}_{k=K+1}^{K^*}$ are new models not found in training data. They are sampled from a flat prior $Dir(H)$. The remaining parts are the same as described in Section 2.2.

3   Results

We evaluate our approach on multiple data sets. The spatial range of the whole brain is roughly $200 \times 200 \times 200$. The size of voxels is $11 \times 11 \times 11$. We choose the hyperparameters in Figure 2 as $a_1 = a_2 = b_1 = b_2 = 1$, $h = 0.3$. We do bilateral clustering. Running on a computer with 3GHz CPU, it takes around one minute to cluster $1,000$ fibers and around four hours to cluster $60,000$ fibers.

The first data set has $3,152$ fibers with ground truth. They are manually labeled to six anatomical structures. Figure 4 (a)-(d) plots the clustering results of our approach and a spectral clustering approach, compared with the ground

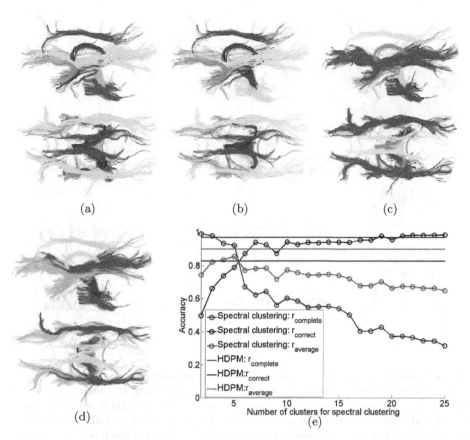

(a)   (b)   (c)

(d)   (e)

Fig. 4. Compare the results of two clustering approaches with the ground truth on a data set with 3, 152 fibers. Two views are plotted for each result. (a) Ground truth. (b) Our approach. (c) Spectral clustering when the number of clusters is 6. (d) Spectral clustering when number of clusters is 7. (e) The accuracies of completeness and correctness of spectral clustering and our approach (HDPM).

truth. Colors are used to distinguish clusters. Since clusters may be permuted in different results, the meaning of colors is not consistent across different results. The spectral clustering approach uses the mean of closest distances as the distance measure, which was found the most effective in previous studies [9,8]. The clustering result of our approach is close to the ground truth. Although the correct number of clusters has been set, two anatomical structures are merged in the result of the spectral clustering approach. A few outlier fibers form a small cluster. As the number of clusters increases to 7, the two anatomical structures still cannot be separated, instead, another structure splits into two clusters.

There are two important aspects, called *correctness* and *completeness*, to be considered when comparing a clustering result with the ground truth [9]. Correctness implies that fibers of different anatomical structures are not clustered together. Completeness means that fibers of the same anatomical structures are

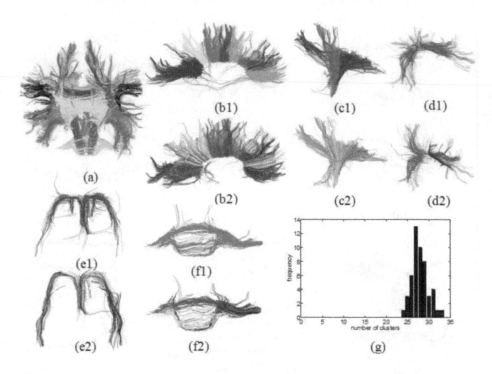

Fig. 5. Compare results of our approach and the approach proposed in [8], in which experts manually merged the clusters from spectral clustering to obtain anatomical structures. (a) Clustering all the fibers using our approach. (b1)-(f1) show the obtained anatomical structures by merging clusters from our approach (totally 27 clusters). (b2)-(f2) show the obtained anatomical structures by merging clusters from spectral clustering (totally 200 clusters). Colors are used to distinguish clusters. (g) plots the frequency of the numbers of clusters learnt by our approach when running 50 trials of Gibbs sampling with random initializations.

clustered together. Putting all the fibers into the same cluster results in 100% completeness and 0% correctness. Putting every fiber into a singleton cluster results in 100% correctness and 0% completeness. To measure correctness, we randomly sample 5,000 pairs of fibers which are in different anatomical structures according to the ground truth and calculate the accuracy ($r_{correct}$) of they are also in different clusters according to the clustering result. To measure completeness, we randomly sample 5,000 pairs of fibers which are in the same anatomical structures and calculate the accuracy ($r_{correct}$) of they are also in the same clusters. $r_{average} = (r_{correct} + r_{complete})/2$ is also computed. The accuracies of our approach and spectral clustering are plotted in Figure 4 (e). As we increase the number of clusters from 2 to 25, the correctness of spectral clustering increases and its completeness decreases. Its best $r_{average}$ is found when the number of clusters is five, which is close to the ground truth, and it is lower than $r_{average}$ of our approach. The correctness of our approach is almost consistently better than spectral clustering until spectral clustering chooses more than 20

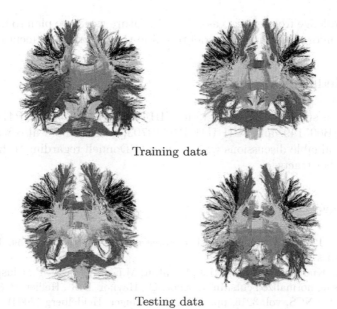

Training data

Testing data

Fig. 6. Cluster fibers across multiple subjects

clusters. The completeness of our approach is significantly better than spectral clustering when the number of clusters of spectral clustering is larger than 5.

We compare our approach with the approach proposed in [8] on a larger data set with 12, 420 fibers. In [8], fibers were first grouped into a large number of clusters (200) and then experts merged these clusters to obtain anatomical structures. In this data set there are 10 anatomical structures. Our approach clusters these fibers to 27 clusters. We also manually merge them to these 10 anatomical structures, however its takes much less effort than [8] since the number of clusters is smaller. Figure 5 shows some of the anatomical structures obtained by the two approaches. 83.2% fibers have consistent anatomical labels according to the two results. To evaluate how our approach is sensitive to initialization, we run 50 trials of Gibbs sampling with random initializations. Figure 5 (g) plots the frequency of the numbers of clusters learnt from data.

Figure 6 shows the results of clustering fibers across multiple subjects. The training data has 63, 751 fibers of two subjects. The models of bundles are learnt from all these fibers. The testing data has 61, 572 fibers of two subjects.

4   Conclusion

We propose a nonparametric Bayesian framework for tractography segmentation. The number of clusters is automatically learnt from data through DP. This method has much lower space complexity than distance-based clustering methods can cluster a very large set of fibers. Our Bayesian model is very flexible to include knowledge from experts as priors. In future work, we plan to incorporate anatomical information in the model to guide tractography segmentation.

Acknowledgments

This work was supported by NIH grants NIH R01 MH074794, NIH P41 RR13218, NIH U54 EB005149, and NIH U41 RR019703. The authors also want to acknowledge valuable discussions with Lauren O'Donnell regarding techniques for clustering fiber tracts.

References

1. Ferguson, T.S.: A bayesian analysis of some nonparametric problems. The Annals of Statistics 1, 209–230 (1973)
2. Brun, A., Knutsson, H., Park, H.J., Shenton, M.E., Westin, C.-F.: Clustering fiber traces using normalized cuts. In: Barillot, C., Haynor, D.R., Hellier, P. (eds.) MICCAI 2004. LNCS, vol. 3216, pp. 368–375. Springer, Heidelberg (2004)
3. Jonasson, L., Hagmann, P., Thiran, J.P., Wedeen, V.J.: Fiber tracts of high angular resolution diffusion mri are easily segmented with spectral clustering. In: International Society for Magnetic Resonance in Medicine, p. 1310 (2005)
4. Gerig, G., Gouttard, S., Corouge, S.: Analysis of brain white matter via fiber tract modeling. In: Proc. of IEEE Engineering in Medicine and Biology, pp. 4421–4424 (2004)
5. Xia, Y., Turken, A.U., Whitfield-Gabrieli, S.L., Gabrieli, J.D.: Knowledge-based classification of neuronal fibers in entire brain. In: Duncan, J.S., Gerig, G. (eds.) MICCAI 2005. LNCS, vol. 3749, pp. 205–212. Springer, Heidelberg (2005)
6. Maddah, M., Grimson, W.E.L., Warfield, S.K., Wells, W.M.: A unified framework for clustering and quantitative analysis of white matter fiber tracts. Medical Image Analysis 12, 191–202 (2008)
7. Ding, Z., Gore, J.C., Anderson, A.W.: Classification amd quantification of neuronal fiber pathways using diffusion tensor MRI. Magnetic Resonance in Medicine 49, 716–721 (2003)
8. O'Donnell, L.J., Westin, C.F.: Automatic tractography segmentation using a high-dimensional white matter atlas. IEEE Trans. on Medical Imaging 26, 1562–1575 (2007)
9. Moberts, B., Vilanova, A., Jake, J.W.: Evaluation of fiber clustering methods for diffusion tensor imaging. In: Proc. of IEEE Visualization, pp. 65–72 (2005)
10. Maddah, M., Zollei, L., Grimson, W.E.L., Wells III, W.M.: Modeling of anatomical information in clustering of white matter fiber trajectories using dirichlet distribution. In: MMBIA, pp. 1–7 (2008)
11. Adelino, R., Ferreira, S.: A dirichlet process mixture model for brain MRI tissue classification. Medical Image Analysis 11, 169–182 (2006)
12. Kim, S., Smyth, P.: Hierarchical dirichlet processes with random effects. In: Proc. of NIPS, pp. 697–704 (2006)
13. Thirion, B., Tucholka, A., Keller, M., Pinel, P.: High level group analysis of FMRI data based on dirichlet process mixture models. In: Karssemeijer, N., Lelieveldt, B. (eds.) IPMI 2007. LNCS, vol. 4584, pp. 482–494. Springer, Heidelberg (2007)

14. Jbabdi, S., Woolrich, M.W., Behrens, T.: Multiple-subjects connectivity-based parcellation using hierarchical dirichlet process mixture models. NeuroImage 44, 373–384 (2009)
15. Teh, Y.W., Jordan, M.I., Beal, M.J., Blei, D.M.: Hierarchical dirichlet processes. Journal of the American Statistical Association 101, 1566–1581 (2006)
16. Wang, X., Ma, K.T., Ng, G.W., Grimson, W.E.L.: Trajectory analysis and semantic region modeling using a nonparametric Bayesian model. In: Proc. of CVPR, pp. 1–8 (2008)
17. Sethuraman, J.: A constructive definition of dirichlet priors. Statistica Sinica 4, 639–650 (1994)
18. Blei, D.M., Jordan, M.I.: Variational inference for dirichlet process mixtures. Bayesain Analysis 1, 121–144 (2006)
19. Asuncion, A., Smyth, P., Welling, M.: Asynchronous distributed learning of topic models. In: Proc. of NIPS (2008)

A Statistical Model of White Matter Fiber Bundles Based on Currents

Stanley Durrleman[1,2], Pierre Fillard[3], Xavier Pennec[1], Alain Trouvé[2],
and Nicholas Ayache[1]

[1] Asclepios Team-Project, INRIA - Sophia Antipolis-Méditerranée, France
[2] Centre de Mathématiques et Leurs Applications (CMLA), ENS-Cachan, France
[3] Lab. de Neuroimagerie Assistée par Ordinateur - CEA/Neurospin, Saclay, France

Abstract. The purpose of this paper is to measure the variability of a
population of white matter fiber bundles without imposing unrealistic
geometrical priors. In this respect, modeling fiber bundles as currents
seems particularly relevant, as it gives a metric between bundles which
relies neither on point nor on fiber correspondences and which is robust
to fiber interruption. First, this metric is included in a diffeomorphic
registration scheme which consistently aligns sets of fiber bundles. In
particular, we show that aligning directly fiber bundles may solve the
aperture problem which appears when fiber mappings are constrained by
tensors only. Second, the measure of variability of a population of fiber
bundles is based on a statistical model which considers every bundle as a
random diffeomorphic deformation of a common template plus a random
non-diffeomorphic perturbation. Thus, the variability is decomposed into
a geometrical part and a "texture" part. Our results on real data show
that both parts may contain interesting anatomical features.

1 Introduction

The primary goal of Computational Anatomy is to study the variability of
anatomical structures in populations. This analysis can be used to classify
populations (e.g. pathologic versus control), or to drive the segmentation of
anatomical structures in new images. Variability measures usually rely on correspondences determined by registration. More generally, shape differences can be
captured by the geometrical deformation of one structure onto another. These
deformations are used to learn how a prototype structure (called also atlas or
template) deform within a population. This requires to define a proper registration method and to infer a statistical model on the deformations between an
atlas (to be estimated) and each subject in the population.

While such statistical analysis have already been proposed for sulcal lines [1,2],
and subcortical structures [3,4], much fewer tools are available for white matter
fiber bundles obtained in diffusion MRI. These structures are of great importance
as they may contribute to map brain connections between functional areas, or
to understand effects of neurological pathologies (like Alzheimer's disease) onto
the brain white matter. Most recent approaches are based on the nonlinear

J.L. Prince, D.L. Pham, and K.J. Myers (Eds.): IPMI 2009, LNCS 5636, pp. 114–125, 2009.

registration of fractional anisotropy (FA) maps [5,6] or tensor images [7,8]. The deformation resulting from this image registration is then applied to fibers. In these methods, one may question if the fiber bundles are correctly aligned since the bundling information is not visible in FA or tensor images. Fibers which belong to the same bundle connect specific brain regions together and should therefore be preserved during registration. For this reason, we propose here to use directly fiber bundles as constraints to drive the registration.

Recent approaches measuring variability of fiber bundles rely on point or fiber correspondences between bundles [9,10,11]. However, tractography algorithms were never shown to produce stable and reproducible results. Thus, the comparison of bundles should not rely on individual fibers or points but rather on the global shape of the bundles. Furthermore, tractography might be valid only locally: the true neuronal pathway may correspond to the union of several pieces of fibers and one should not blindly consider sets of connected points produced by tractography as true fibers. The solution of considering a bundle as an unconnected cloud of points is not satisfactory either, since it does not take into account the local orientation of the bundles encoded by the tangents of the fibers. Therefore, an ideal framework for fiber bundles should be robust to *curve connectivity and sampling*, and should take into account the *local orientation* of the bundle. Similarly, a distance between bundles (used as a dissimilarity measure during registration) should rely *neither on point nor on fiber correspondences*. In this paper, we propose to use the framework based on currents, that precisely models curves as a set of unconnected oriented points. This framework is robust to fiber interruption and provides a dissimilarity metric on curve sets that does not assume any kind of correspondences. Conversely, it is sensitive to the local fiber orientation and to the point density: a single fiber will be unlikely to influence registration, which makes currents naturally robust to outliers. Finally, currents are compatible with the diffeomorphic registration method in [12], and therefore can be used for pairwise registration of fiber bundles.

Once a registration framework of fiber bundles modeled as currents is defined, it can be used to define a statistical model of variability. From the perspective of the deformable models, we consider the bundles of different subjects as random diffeomorphic deformations of an unknown template perturbed by non-diffeomorphic variations (called residues in the sequel). Following the work of [4], we jointly estimate this prototype bundle along with its deformations onto each subject's anatomy. In a second time, statistical analysis of bundles is achieved by a principal component analysis (PCA) of the diffeomorphic deformations and the residues to extract their principal modes of variations. The former accounts for the smooth variations of the template within the population: stretching, shrinking, dilation or torsion, while the later accounts for all variations that cannot be captured by regular diffeomorphisms, called *texture* in the sequel: fiber creation or topology changes. This model is not based on strong assumptions and can therefore retrieve a large range of geometrical variations.

The paper is organized as follows. Sec. 2 shows how currents are used to model fiber bundles and how they are interfaced with a diffeomorphic registration scheme. The statistical model is developed in Sec. 3. In Sec. 4, we evaluate the method on real data. We compare pairwise registrations of 5 fiber bundles with the alignment obtained from FA and tensors images. Finally, we build the atlas from 6 subjects and analyze the variability of the corticobulbar tract.

2   Fiber Bundles Registration Based on Currents

2.1   Fiber Bundles Modeled as Currents

Currents are geometrical objects originally introduced in medical image analysis to model curves and surfaces [12]. In this section, we recall the properties which are relevant for our topic and refer the reader to [12,13,4] for more details.

In the framework of currents, a set of fibers is characterized by the way it integrates vector fields. Given ω a square integrable $3D$ vector field, a bundle B made of several fibers F_i integrates ω thanks to:

$$B(\omega) = \sum_{F_i \in B} \int_{F_i} \omega(x)^t \tau_i(x) dx, \tag{1}$$

where $\tau_i(x)$ is the oriented tangent vector of the fiber F_i at point x. A fiber bundle may be seen as a set of wires sending information in one direction at a constant rate. Eq. 1 computes the total rate of information that goes through the orthogonal sections (i.e. equipotential surfaces) of ω. To characterize a fiber bundle, we measure how this quantity varies while the equipotentials of ω varies. For this purpose, we define the test space W, in which ω varies, as the set of the convolutions between any square integrable vector fields and a smoothing kernel. This excludes from W the vector fields with too high spatial frequencies. Formally, W is the reproducing kernel Hilbert space (r.k.h.s.) whose kernel K^W is Gaussian: $K^W(x, y) = \exp(- \|x - y\|^2 / \lambda_W^2) I_3$ for any points $(x, y)^1$. The standard deviation, λ_W, is the typical scale at which the vector fields ω varies spatially. In this setting, any set of smooth curves is a continuous linear mapping from W to $\mathbb{R}$. The space of currents W^* is the space containing such objects.

W^* is a vector space. The addition of two pieces of curves is simply the union of them. In Eq. 1, each fiber F_i or each piece of these fibers can be seen as a current individually: the union of them (their addition) is still a current. For instance, Eq. 1 would not change if each F_i were split into a collection of small segments. *It does not depend on the connectivity of the fibers within the bundle.*

Any current in W^* may be decomposed into an *infinite* sum of delta Dirac currents, which play the role of basis vectors. A Dirac current δ_x^τ is defined by: $\delta_x^\tau(\omega) = \tau^t \omega(x)$. It models an oriented point and encodes the direction τ of the fiber bundle at point x. Each segment of the polygonal lines returned by tractography is approximated by a Dirac current δ_x^τ where x is the center of the segment and τ its direction. This approximation converges in the space of

---

[1] K^W is the Green's function of $L^t L$ for some differential operator L. The inner product in W is defined then by $\langle \omega, \omega' \rangle_W = \langle L(\omega), L(\omega) \rangle_{L^2}$. See [14] for more details.

currents as the sampling of the curves becomes finer. In this sense, the modeling is *weakly sensitive to the sampling* of the fibers. As a consequence, a bundle B is approximated by a *finite* sum over all segments within the bundle: $\sum_i \delta_{x_i}^{\tau_i}$.

In addition, the space of currents W^* is provided with a norm and an inner product, which define a distance between two bundles B and B' as: $\|B - B'\|_{W^*} = \sup_{\|\omega\|_W \leq 1} |B(\omega) - B'(\omega)|$. Following our analogy, this measures the rate of information along the wires of B and the wires of B' that goes through the orthogonal sections of the same ω. We look for the regular ω ($\|\omega\|_W \leq 1$) which makes this difference the largest possible, i.e. that captures the more differences between the two structures. This geometric distance compares bundles globally, *without assuming any kind of fiber or point correspondences between them*. The smaller the standard deviation λ_W, the smaller the scale at which ω varies, the finer the geometrical details captured by this distance.

This distance has a closed form. On the Dirac currents, the inner product is given by $\langle \delta_x^\alpha, \delta_y^\beta \rangle_{W^*} = \alpha^t K^W(x,y)\beta$. By linearity, the inner product between two bundles $B = \sum_{i=1}^n \delta_{c_i}^{\tau_i}$ and $B' = \sum_{j=1}^m \delta_{c'_j}^{\tau'_j}$ is given by:

$$\langle B, B' \rangle_{W^*} = \sum_{i=1}^n \sum_{j=1}^m \tau_i^t K^W(c_i, c'_j)\tau'_j \tag{2}$$

This inner product (and hence the distance $\|B - B'\|_{W^*}$) does not require any condition on the curves sampling (n may not equal m, for instance). It compares all pairs of tangents (τ_i, τ'_j) weighted by a function of their distance $\|c_i - c'_j\|$.

Since the space of currents is a vector space provided with an inner product, we can directly compute the mean and the covariance matrix of a population of fiber bundles. However, this statistical analysis would not be relevant with unregistered fiber bundles. This will be used, instead, to perform PCA on the residuals that remain after registration.

2.2 Spatially Consistent Registration of Fiber Bundles

Our goal is to align two sets of fiber bundles segmented in images of two different subjects. The algorithm introduced in [12] finds precisely a *consistent deformation of the underlying 3D space* that best matches two sets of labeled currents. The deformations are chosen as $3D$ diffeomorphisms (smooth deformations with smooth inverses), solution at time $t = 1$ of the flow equation: $\frac{\partial \phi_t(x)}{\partial t} = v_t(\phi_t(x))$, with initial condition $\phi_0 = \text{Id}$ (no deformation). The time-varying vector field $(v_t)_{t \in [0,1]}$ is the speed vector field of the deformation, which is supposed to belong to a r.k.h.s. V with Gaussian kernel K^V. The standard deviation of K^V, λ_V, determines the typical scale of the deformation: the greater, the smoother the deformation. The regularity of the final deformation ϕ_1^v is measured by integrating the norm of the speed vector field over time: $d_V^2(\text{Id}, \phi_1^v) = \int_0^1 \|v_t\|_V^2 dt$. The registration consists therefore in minimizing:

$$J(v) = \sum_{i=1}^N \|\phi_1^v \star B_i - B'_j\|_{W^*}^2 + \gamma d_V^2(\text{Id}, \phi_1^v) \tag{3}$$

where γ is the usual trade-off between fidelity to data and regularity. $\phi \star B$ denotes the geometrical transportation of the fiber bundle B by the diffeomorphism ϕ: each point x moves to $\phi(x)$ and each tangent τ is transformed into $d_x\phi(\tau)$, where $d_x\phi$ is the Jacobian matrix of ϕ. This geometrical transportation is conveyed in the space of currents thanks to $(\phi \star B)(\omega) = B((d\phi)^t \omega \circ \phi)$, which results simply from a change of variable in Eq. 1. On Dirac currents, we have $\phi \star \delta_x^\tau = \delta_{\phi(x)}^{d_x\phi(\tau)}$.

It is proved that the speed vector field minimizing Eq. 3 *is parametrized* by momenta $\alpha_k(t)$ at the points $x_k(t)$ of the moving bundle B: $v_t(x) = \sum_k K^V(x, x_k(t)) \alpha_k(t)$ [12,15]. Once time is discretized, Eq. 3 is therefore minimized via a gradient descent on the parameters: $(\alpha_k(t_p))$. Moreover, the resulting diffeomorphisms are geodesic. Thanks to Euler-Lagrange equations [15], they are entirely determined by their initial momenta $\alpha_k(0)$: *the tangent-space representation* of the diffeomorphism. The metric on this tangent space is given by $\|\alpha(0)\|^2 = \|v_0\|_V^2 = \alpha(0)^t k^V \alpha(0)$ where k^V is the matrix $(K^V(x_i, x_j))_{i,j}$. From now on, we denote ϕ^α the diffeomorphism ϕ_1^v with initial momenta α.

Applying this registration framework directly to fiber bundles, which may have up to 10^5 segments, raises computational issues. The computation of the data fidelity term in Eq. 3 ($\|\phi_1^v \star B - B'\|_{W^*}$) requires to compare every segments of B with every segments of B', as shown in Eq. 2. Hopefully, this complexity is reduced thanks to the approximation scheme of [13].

3 A Statistical Model of Fiber Bundles

In this section, we show how to use the modeling based on currents and the previous registration tool to define a statistical model on fiber bundles. Following [16,4], we model our observations as deformations of an unknown prototype bundle (also called template or atlas) perturbed by non-diffeomorphic variations (the residues). Formally, we consider the bundles $(B_i)_{i=1...N}$ (the same bundle for N different subjects) as instances of the following process:

$$B_i = \phi_i \star \bar{B} + \varepsilon_i \tag{4}$$

where the bundles B_i are seen as currents, ϕ_i are diffeomorphisms that deform the unknown template $\bar{B}$ supposed to be a current as well. ε_i are the residual perturbations which account for everything that cannot be captured by a regular deformation. The ε_i's are supposed to be i.i.d. zero-mean Gaussian random variables in the space of currents. To infer a random model on the deformations ϕ_i, we use their tangent-space representation: an instance ϕ^α is simulated by shooting geodesically an instance of the momenta α (vector of finite dimension).

We estimate the template $\bar{B}$, the deformations ϕ_i and the residues ε_i with a Maximum A Posteriori approach with an approximation, as in [4]. As a result, we minimize:

$$\min_{\bar{B}, \alpha_i} \left\{ \sum_{i=1}^N \left\| \phi^{\alpha_i} \star \bar{B} - B_i \right\|_{W^*}^2 + \gamma d_V^2 (\mathrm{Id}, \phi^{\alpha_i}) \right\} \tag{5}$$

We start by setting $\phi_i = \mathrm{Id}$ (i.e. $\alpha_i = 0$, no deformation) and $\bar{B} = \sum_{i=1}^{N} B_i/N$, the empirical mean in the space of currents. Then, we minimize the functional by considering that $\bar{B}$ and the α_i's are fixed alternatively. The first step consists in registering $\bar{B}$ to each B_i, leading to initial momenta (α_i). The second step consists in updating $\bar{B}$ by minimizing $J(\bar{B}) = \sum_{i=1}^{N} \left\| \phi^{\alpha_i} \star \bar{B} - B_i \right\|_{W*}^2$. This last minimization benefits from the approximation scheme of [13,4].

Eventually, the algorithm returns an unbiased template $\bar{B} = \sum_{k=1}^{n_B} \delta_{x_k}^{\tau_k}$ and the deformations ϕ^{α_i} of $\bar{B}$ to each B_i. We perform a PCA on the momenta (α_i), and another PCA on the residual perturbations $\varepsilon_i = \phi^{\alpha_i} \star \bar{B} - B_i$. We shoot geodesically in the direction (resp. in the opposite direction) of the first mode of momenta, m_α (resp. $-m_\alpha$), to give the first mode of deformation at $+\sigma$ (resp. $-\sigma$): $\phi^{\pm m_\alpha}$. The PCA on residues is performed in the space of currents. This leads to the mean $\bar{\varepsilon} = \sum_i \varepsilon_i/N$ and the first mode at $\pm\sigma$: $m_\varepsilon = \bar{\varepsilon} \pm \sum_i E_i(\varepsilon_i - \bar{\varepsilon})$, where E is the first eigenvector of the covariance matrix $(\langle \varepsilon_i - \bar{\varepsilon}, \varepsilon_j - \bar{\varepsilon} \rangle_{W*})_{i,j}$. As linear combinations of the input currents, the mean and the first mode can be approximated using the scheme of [13] for a better visualization.

This joint statistical modeling accounts for both diffeomorphic and non-diffeomorphic variability. It is not biased by arbitrary point or fiber correspondences between different subjects. It does not impose strong prior on the nature of the variability. For instance, it does not assume that fibers of a bundle come from a mean line whose samples have been randomly moved, as in [9]. The major prior of our model consists in where to put the separation between the geometrical part (captured by the diffeomorphisms) and the texture part (contained in the residues). This separation is determined by the regularity parameters: λ_V, λ_W and the trade-off γ. In this paper, we set these parameters manually, whereas they could be set automatically along the lines of [16] for instance.

4   Experiments

Six brain DTI data sets acquired on a 1.5T GE scanner on healthy volunteers were used in this study. Image dimensions are $128 \times 128 \times 30$, and resolution is $1.8 \times 1.8 \times 4$mm. 25 non-collinear diffusion gradients and a b-value of $1000 s.mm^{-2}$ were used. Fiber tractography was performed using MedINRIA [2], which includes a robust tensor estimation and a streamline tractography algorithm using log-Euclidean tensor interpolation [17]. Manual segmentation of five fiber bundles was done: the entire corpus callosum, the corticospinal and the corticobulbar tracts, and the left and right arcuate fasciculi (Fig. 4-a).

First, we evaluate the methodology developed in Sec. 2 by registering the bundles of two subjects and comparing the result with FA and tensor registration (Sec. 4.1). Second, our framework for atlas construction is evaluated with the construction of a diffeomorphic atlas of the five bundles of our data set (Sec. 4.2) and the statistical analysis of the corticobulbar tract (Sec. 4.3).

---

[2] http://www-sop.inria.fr/asclepios/software/MedINRIA/

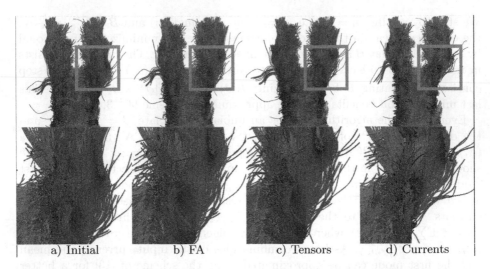

| a) Initial | b) FA | c) Tensors | d) Currents |

Fig. 1. Diffeomorphic registration of two corpus callosum fibers. Bottom images are a closeup on the green squared region. Initial tracts (a) and registered tracts using FA (b), tensors (c) or bundles (d) as constraints. Overlap of blue and red fibers is greater using currents, especially in the left and right parts of the genu of the corpus callosum.

4.1   Fiber Bundle Registration

Diffeomorphic registration of fiber bundles using currents is compared to non-linear registration of FA [18] and tensor [8] images. Pairwise registrations of 5 fiber bundles segmented in 2 subjects are conducted. For FA and tensor-based bundle registration, deformation fields were computed between images and applied to bundles afterwards: bundles were not tracked again after registration. Note that the three methods produce diffeomorphic transformations and can be compared. The parameters were adjusted to produce deformations of about the same smoothness. Concerning our registration scheme, we set the regularity of the deformation $\lambda_V = 20$mm, the spatial scale of the currents $\lambda_W = 5$mm and the trade-off between regularity and fidelity-to-data: $\gamma = 10^{-4}$. For clarity purpose, we present registration results of two bundles only: the corpus callosum (CC) (Fig. 1) and the corticospinal tract (CST) (Fig. 2), since they highlight the most striking differences between methods.

Fig. 1 a) shows two misaligned CC. Fig. 1 b) and c) present the registration of those bundles computed using respectively FA and tensor images. The registration of the fiber bundles with our method (Fig. 1 d) shows a greater overlap, synonym of a better alignment. Local improvements are noticeable in the left and right parts of the genu. This result shows that *the bundle information acts as a stronger prior* to align fiber tracts than the tensor image. Moreover, one can still notice few red fibers not aligned with the blue bundle in the exterior of the tract, which illustrates *the robustness of our methodology to outliers*.

Registration of two CST shows similar effects, especially in the anterior part expanded in a green square in Fig. 2. In those regions, multiple bundles may

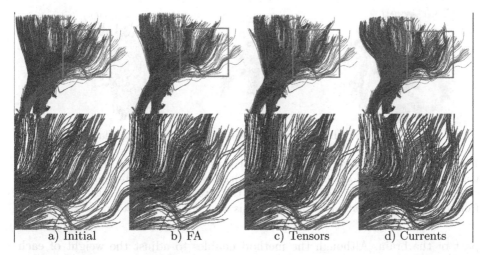

| a) Initial | b) FA | c) Tensors | d) Currents |

Fig. 2. Registration of two corticospinal tracts. Bottom images are a closeup on the green squared region. Initial tracts (a) and registered tract using FA (b), tensors (c) or bundles (d) as constraints. Currents better warp the red fibers in the anterior part of the tract, highlighting the aperture problem inherent to FA and tensor-based approaches. Registration in the posterior part is mainly constrained by the corpus callosum which strongly pushes the fibers toward the posterior part of the brain.

coexist whereas FA and tensor images are uniform, as shown in Fig. 3. Therefore, image-based registration is unable to correctly align the bundles, since bundle boundaries are not visible in images. This is an *aperture problem* inherent to FA and tensor-based methods. The bundling information is an extra information brought either by experts or by automatic bundling methods with anatomical priors. During our global registration, the CC acts as a stronger constraint than CST since it has much more fibers. This impacts the registration of the posterior part of the CST in Fig 2, whose fibers are pushed by the CC toward the posterior

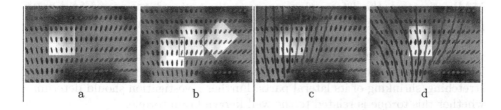

| a | b | c | d |

Fig. 3. Illustration of the aperture problem in FA and tensor registration. **a and b:** Tensor fields of two subjects overlapped with FA images are shown (sagittal slice, inside the corona radiata). Without any prior, it is impossible to determine whether the rectangle in image **a** matches with any in image **b**: this is the aperture problem. **c and d:** two schematic fiber bundles in red and blue were added. It becomes clearer that the rectangle of image **c** has a unique correspondence in image **d**. The aperture problem is partly solved using the bundles as priors.

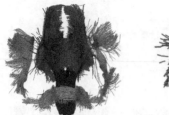 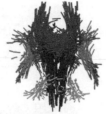 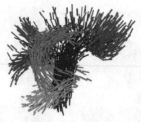

(a) One subject   (b) template (occipital view) (c) template (lateral view)

Fig. 4. Template of five bundles: the corticospinal tract (blue), the corticobulbar tract (yellow), the callosal fibers (red), the left and right arcuates (green). (a): one subject among the six of the data set. (b,c) the estimated unbiased atlas. Data result from a random deformation on the atlas, plus a random perturbation.

part of the brain. Although the method enables to adjust the weight of each bundle during registration, the choice of such weights still remain arbitrary.

4.2 Fiber Atlas Construction

As explained in Sec. 3, we estimate a template such that the input data result from random deformations of this template added with random perturbations in the space of currents. As emphasized in Section 2.2, there is only one global deformation acting on all 5 bundles together, and 5 independent perturbations for each bundle. The template consists of five prototype bundles shown in Fig. 4. It has been computed by fixing the parameters of currents $\lambda_W = 5$mm, of deformations $\lambda_V = 20$mm and the trade-off $\gamma = 10^{-4}$.

4.3 Variability Analysis of the Corticobulbar Tract

We show here how the first mode of deformations and the first mode of residues describe the variability of the corticobulbar tract within the studied population. The "geometrical" variability is captured by the deformations. As a result of the MAP estimation, the deformations appear to be centered: the norm of the mean parameters is 0.42 times the standard deviation, not significantly different from 0. The first mode of the deformations at $\pm\sigma$ is shown in Fig. 5, first row. It shows the variability of the template which was captured by the regular diffeomorphisms. The main variations are a torque of the frontal part of the bundle, as well as a stretching/shrinking of its lateral parts. Further investigation should determine whether this torque is related to the well-known brain torque.

The variability in terms of "texture" is captured by the residual perturbations. The residues are centered: the mean current is 0.36 times its standard deviation. The first residual mode m_ε is shown in Fig. 5, second row. It shows an asymmetry in the number of fibers in each lateral part of the bundle. This result shows, undoubtedly, that the variability left aside from the diffeomorphisms is not pure noise, *but still contains some interesting anatomical features*. In our case, further investigation is needed to determine whether this fiber creation/deletion effect is

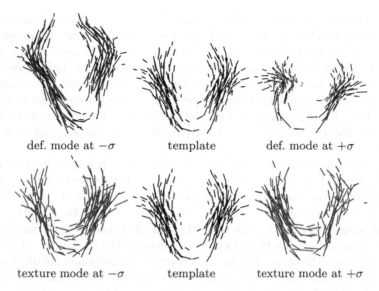

def. mode at $-\sigma$ template   def. mode at $+\sigma$

texture mode at $-\sigma$ template   texture mode at $+\sigma$

Fig. 5. Variability of the corticobulbar bundle (view from top) **Row 1: First deformation mode at** $\pm\sigma$. The diffeomorphic variability of the population around the prototype bundle (middle) is mainly a torque at the basis of the bundle and a stretching/shrinking effect of the left and right parts of the bundle. **Row 2: First "texture" mode at** $\pm\sigma$. The texture mode (what remains once the diffeomorphic variability is discounted) at $+\sigma$ (resp. $-\sigma$) shows that the left (resp. right) part of the bundle becomes thicker, while its right (resp. left) part becomes thinner.

due to a true anatomical variability or to an artifact of the tracking algorithm. In any case, this shows how our modeling analyzes all the geometrical information without imposing strong priors on the kind of the variations we are looking for.

5   Discussion and Conclusion

In this paper, we proposed a novel framework for the statistical analysis of fiber bundles using currents. Our methodology does not impose point-to-point or fiber-to-fiber correspondences, a crucial feature in regards to the variability of tractography algorithms outputs. It is also robust to outliers and weakly dependent of the fiber sampling. Diffeomorphic registrations produce smooth and invertible deformation fields which match consistently a set of fiber bundles of one subject onto another. This registration scheme is further extended by a statistical model of fiber bundles, which estimates a template and its variability in a population. The variability is, in turn, decomposed into a geometrical part accounting for smooth deformations and a texture part which accounts for non-diffeomorphic changes in a population.

Pairwise registration shows that FA and tensor-based registration are less adapted than currents for fiber bundles registration, as bundle boundaries are not visible in those images (aperture problem). A misalignment of bundles may result in a loss of statistical power in group comparisons since contributions of several unrelated fiber bundles may be confounded. The method presented here optimally uses the strong prior that fibers belong to consistent bundles and ensure a proper alignment of those for statistical comparisons. This statistical analysis was evaluated on five fiber bundles extracted in six subjects. It shows consistent results with known anatomical variability (brain torque), which is put in evidence for the first time on fibers. Even with such a small dataset, our analysis managed to decompose the variability into two parts that are likely to describe relevant anatomical features.

The method, however, raises several questions. First, it is sensitive to the total number of fibers of a bundle, or fiber density, that may vary between two subjects. These variations may be caused by the tractography algorithm itself, as fiber density is generally an arbitrary parameter set by the method. One solution would consist in normalizing this density by relying the fiber density to physical properties of the neural fibers, like the neural flux transported by the bundle. Second, our method requires all fibers in a bundle, and by extension all bundles of different subjects, to have a consistent orientation: all fibers should start at the same cortical region and end in the same region. We cannot reasonably assume that tractography algorithms produce consistently oriented fibers. In this work, reorientation was performed with an empirical procedure. For larger datasets, an automatic reorientation procedure has to be included, or the modeling based on currents has to be adapted to account for non-oriented curves.

Future work will focus on evaluating the method on much larger dataset to strengthen the interpretation of our results. Automatic bundling can be used to produce a complete set of anatomically relevant fiber bundles, as in [19,20]. Then, our measure of variability could be used to segment fiber bundles in new images. It could be used also to classify patients according to pathologies, to find consistent sub-groups within populations, to detect abnormalities via deviations from the normal variability. One can imagine to extend this framework to automatically mine geometrical dataset.

Acknowlegments. We would like to thank Denis Ducreux, MD, Bicêtre Hospital, Paris, for providing the brain datasets. This work was partially supported by European IP project Health-e-child (IST-2004-027749) and Microsoft Research.

References

1. Durrleman, S., Pennec, X., Trouvé, A., Thompson, P., Ayache, N.: Inferring brain variability from diffeomorphic deformations of currents: an integrative approach. Medical Image Analysis 12(5), 626–637 (2008)
2. Fillard, P., Arsigny, V., Pennec, X., Hayashi, K., Thompson, P., Ayache, N.: Measuring brain variability by extrapolating sparse tensor fields measured on sulcal lines. NeuroImage 34(2), 639–650 (2007)
3. Vaillant, M., Miller, M., Younes, L., Trouvé, A.: Statistics on diffeomorphisms via tangent space representations. NeuroImage 23, 161–169 (2004)
4. Durrleman, S., Pennec, X., Trouvé, A., Ayache, N.: A forward model to build unbiased atlases from curves and surfaces. In: Proc. of MFCA 2008 (2008)

5. Goodlett, C., Fletcher, P., Gilmore, J., Gerig, G.: Group statistics of DTI fiber bundles using spatial functions of tensor measures. In: Metaxas, D., Axel, L., Fichtinger, G., Székely, G. (eds.) MICCAI 2008, Part II. LNCS, vol. 5242, pp. 1068–1075. Springer, Heidelberg (2008)
6. Smith, S., Jenkinson, M., Johansen-Berg, H., Rueckert, D., Nichols, T., Mackay, C., Watkins, K., Ciccarelli, O., Cader, M., Matthews, P., Behrens, T.: Tract-based spatial statistics: Voxelwise analysis of multi-subject diffusion data. NeuroImage 31, 1487–1505 (2006)
7. Zhang, H., Yushkevich, P.A., Rueckert, D., Gee, J.C.: Unbiased white matter atlas construction using diffusion tensor images. In: Ayache, N., Ourselin, S., Maeder, A. (eds.) MICCAI 2007, Part II. LNCS, vol. 4792, pp. 211–218. Springer, Heidelberg (2007)
8. Yeo, B., Vercauteren, T., Fillard, P., Pennec, X., Golland, P., Ayache, N., Clatz, O.: DTI registration with exact finite-strain differential. In: ISBI 2008, pp. 700–703 (2008)
9. Corouge, I., Fletcher, P., Joshi, S., Gouttard, S., Gerig, G.: Fiber tract-oriented statistics for quantitative diffusion tensor MRI analysis. Medical Image Analysis (10), 786–798 (2006)
10. Ziyan, U., Sabuncu, M.R., O'Donnell, L.J., Westin, C.-F.: Nonlinear Registration of Diffusion MR Images Based on Fiber Bundles. In: Ayache, N., Ourselin, S., Maeder, A. (eds.) MICCAI 2007, Part I. LNCS, vol. 4791, pp. 351–358. Springer, Heidelberg (2007)
11. Batchelor, P.G., Calamante, F., Tournier, J.D., Atkinson, D., Hill, D.L.G., Connelly, A.: Quantification of the shape of fiber tracts. MRM 55(4), 894–903 (2006)
12. Vaillant, M., Glaunès, J.: Surface matching via currents. In: Christensen, G.E., Sonka, M. (eds.) IPMI 2005. LNCS, vol. 3565, pp. 381–392. Springer, Heidelberg (2005)
13. Durrleman, S., Pennec, X., Trouvé, A., Ayache, N.: Sparse approximation of currents for statistics on curves and surfaces. In: Metaxas, D., Axel, L., Fichtinger, G., Székely, G. (eds.) MICCAI 2008, Part II. LNCS, vol. 5242, pp. 390–398. Springer, Heidelberg (2008)
14. Saitoh, S.: Theory of Reproducing Kernels and Its Applications. Pitman Research Notes in Mathematics Series, vol. 189. Wiley, Chichester (1988)
15. Miller, M.I., Trouvé, A., Younes, L.: On the metrics and Euler-Lagrange equations of computational anatomy. Annual Review of Biomed. Eng. 4, 375–405 (2002)
16. Allassonnière, S., Amit, Y., Trouvé, A.: Towards a coherent statistical framework for dense deformable template estimation. J. Roy. Stat. Soc. B 69(1), 3–29 (2007)
17. Fillard, P., Arsigny, V., Pennec, X., Ayache, N.: Clinical DT-MRI estimation, smoothing and fiber tracking with log-Euclidean metrics. IEEE Trans. on Medical Imaging 26(11), 1472–1482 (2007)
18. Vercauteren, T., Pennec, X., Malis, E., Perchant, A., Ayache, N.: Insight into efficient image registration techniques and the demons algorithm. In: Karssemeijer, N., Lelieveldt, B. (eds.) IPMI 2007. LNCS, vol. 4584, pp. 495–506. Springer, Heidelberg (2007)
19. Maddah, M., Wells, W.M., Warfield, S.K., Westin, C.F., Grimson, W.E.L.: Probabilistic clustering and quantitative analysis of white matter fiber tracts. In: Karssemeijer, N., Lelieveldt, B. (eds.) IPMI 2007. LNCS, vol. 4584, pp. 372–383. Springer, Heidelberg (2007)
20. El Kouby, V., Cointepas, Y., Poupon, C., Rivière, D., Golestani, N., Pallier, C., Poline, J.B., Bihan, D.L., Mangin, J.F.: MR diffusion-based inference of a fiber bundle model from a population of subjects. In: Duncan, J.S., Gerig, G. (eds.) MICCAI 2005. LNCS, vol. 3749, pp. 196–204. Springer, Heidelberg (2005)

Neural Tractography Using
an Unscented Kalman Filter

James G. Malcolm[1], Martha E. Shenton[1,2], and Yogesh Rathi[1]

[1] Psychiatry Neuroimaging Laboratory, Harvard Medical School, Boston, MA
malcolm@bwh.harvard.edu
[2] VA Boston Healthcare System, Brockton Division, Brockton, MA

Abstract. We describe a technique to simultaneously estimate a local neural fiber model and trace out its path. Existing techniques estimate the local fiber orientation at each voxel independently so there is no running knowledge of confidence in the estimated fiber model. We formulate fiber tracking as recursive estimation: at each step of tracing the fiber, the current estimate is guided by the previous. To do this we model the signal as a mixture of Gaussian tensors and perform tractography within a filter framework. Starting from a seed point, each fiber is traced to its termination using an unscented Kalman filter to simultaneously fit the local model and propagate in the most consistent direction. Despite the presence of noise and uncertainty, this provides a causal estimate of the local structure at each point along the fiber. Synthetic experiments demonstrate that this approach reduces signal reconstruction error and significantly improves the angular resolution at crossings and branchings. *In vivo* experiments confirm the ability to trace out fibers in areas known to contain such crossing and branching while providing inherent path regularization.

1   Introduction

The advent of diffusion weighted magnetic resonance imaging has provided the opportunity for non-invasive investigation of neural architecture. Using this imaging technique, neuroscientists want to ask how neurons originating from one region connect to other regions, or how strong those connections may be. For such studies, the quality of the results relies heavily on the chosen fiber representation and the method of reconstructing pathways.

To begin studying the microstructure of fibers, we need a model to interpret the diffusion weighted signal. Such models fall broadly into two categories: parametric and nonparametric. One of the simplest parametric models is the diffusion tensor which describes a Gaussian estimate of the diffusion orientation and strength at each voxel [1, 2]. While robust, this model can be inadequate in cases of mixed fiber presence or more complex orientations [3, 4]. To handle more complex diffusion patterns, various parametric models have been introduced: weighted mixtures [5, 6, 7, 8], higher order tensors [9], directional functions [10, 11, 12], and diffusion oriented transforms [13].

Nonparametric models often provide more information about the diffusion pattern. Instead of estimating a discrete number of fibers as in parametric models, nonparametric techniques estimate an oriented distribution function (ODF) describing an arbitrary

J.L. Prince, D.L. Pham, and K.J. Myers (Eds.): IPMI 2009, LNCS 5636, pp. 126–138, 2009.
© Springer-Verlag Berlin Heidelberg 2009

configuration of fibers. For this estimation, Tuch [14] introduced Q-ball imaging to numerically compute the ODF using the Funk-Radon transform. The use of spherical harmonics simplified the computation with an analytic form [15, 16, 17] and spherical ridgelets further reduced the coefficients required [18]. Recently, Poupon et al. [19] demonstrated online direct estimation of single-tensor and harmonic coefficients using a linear Kalman filter. Another approach to producing an ODF is to assume a model for the signal response of a single-fiber and use spherical deconvolution [20, 21, 22, 11, 23]. A good review of both parametric and nonparametric models can be found in [24, 25].

Based on these models, several techniques attempt to reconstruct pathways. Deterministic tractography involves directly following the diffusion pathways. In the single tensor model, this means simply following the principal diffusion direction [26], while multi-tensor models often include techniques for determining the number of fibers present or when pathways branch [27, 7, 28, 29]. Kalman and particle filters have been used with single tensor streamline tractography [30, 31, 32], but these are used for path regularization and not to estimate the underlying fiber model. Another approach to regularizing single tensor tractography uses a moving least squares estimate weighted with the previous tensor [33]. While this present study focuses on deterministic techniques, probabilistic methods have been developed to form connections by diffusing out a connectivity map according to the ODF [34, 35, 36, 37].

While parametric methods directly describe the principal diffusion directions, interpreting the ODFs from model independent representations typically involves determining the number and orientation of principal diffusion directions present [38, 39, 20]. For example, Bloy et al. [40] find them as maxima on the surface of a high-order tensor; Descoteaux et al. [25] deconvolve with a sharpening kernel before extracting maxima; and Schultz et al. [41] decompose a high-order tensor into a mixture of rank-1 tensors. Ramirez et al. [42] provide a quantitative comparison of several such techniques.

1.1 Our Contributions

Of the approaches listed above, almost all fit the model at each voxel independent of other voxels. In this paper, we describe a method to estimate the model parameters and perform tractography simultaneously within a causal filter. In this way, the estimation at each position builds upon the previous estimates along the fiber.

To begin estimating within a finite dimensional filter, we model the diffusion signal using a simple weighted mixture of two Gaussian tensors [5, 6, 43]. This enables estimation directly from the raw signal data without separate preprocessing or regularization steps. Because the signal reconstruction is nonlinear, we use the unscented Kalman filter to perform model estimation and then propagate in the most consistent direction. Using causal estimation in this way yields inherent path regularization, low signal reconstruction error, and accurate fiber resolution at crossing angles not found with independent optimization. We further note that the approach presented here generalizes to arbitrary fiber model with finite dimensional parameter space, and since the estimation is inherently smooth, it does not require arbitrary termination criteria such as curvature.

2 Approach

The main idea of our approach is to trace the local fiber orientations using the estimation at previous positions to guide estimation at the current position. In a loop, the Kalman filter estimates the model at the current position, moves a step in that direction, and then begins estimation again. Recursive estimation in this manner greatly improves the accuracy of resolving individual orientations and yields inherently smooth tracts despite the presence of noise and uncertainty.

Section 2.1 provides the necessary background on modeling the measurement signal using tensors and defines the specific two-fiber model employed in this study. Then, Section 2.2 describes how this model can be estimated using an unscented Kalman filter.

2.1 Modeling Local Fiber Orientations

In diffusion weighted imaging, image contrast is related to the strength of water diffusion, and our goal is to accurately relate these signals to an underlying model of fiber orientation. At each image voxel, diffusion is measured along a set of distinct gradients, $\mathbf{u}_1, ..., \mathbf{u}_n \in \mathbb{S}^3$ (on the unit sphere), producing the corresponding signal, $\mathbf{s} = [\, s_1, ..., s_n \,]^T \in \mathbb{R}^n$. For voxels containing a mixed diffusion pattern, a general weighted formulation is written as,

$$s_i = s_0 \sum_j w_j e^{-b\mathbf{u}_i^T D_j \mathbf{u}_i}, \tag{1}$$

where s_0 is a baseline signal intensity, b is an acquisition-specific constant, w_j are convex weights, and D_j is a tensor representing a diffusion pattern [6, 7].

From that general mixture model, we choose a restricted form with two equally-weighted tensors. This choice is guided by several previous studies. Behrens et al. [37] showed that at a b-value of 1000 the maximum number of detectable fibers is two. Several other studies have also found two tensors to be sufficient [6, 7, 38, 8]. Using this as a practical guideline, we chose a mixture of two Gaussians for a fiber model. Also, we assume the shape of each tensor to be ellipsoidal, $i.e.$ there is one dominant principal diffusion direction $\mathbf{m}$ with eigenvalue λ_1 and the remaining orthonormal directions have equal eigenvalues $\lambda_2 = \lambda_3$ (as in [44, 43, 8, 11]). Last, following the study of [38], we assume an equal combination (50%-50%) of the two tensors. While the effect of this second choice appears to have little to no effect on experiments, we have yet to quantify any potential loss in accuracy. These assumptions leave us with the following model used in this study:

$$s_i = \tfrac{s_0}{2} \left(e^{-b\mathbf{u}_i^T D_1 \mathbf{u}_i} + e^{-b\mathbf{u}_i^T D_2 \mathbf{u}_i} \right), \tag{2}$$

where D_1, D_2 are each expressible as, $D = \lambda_1 \mathbf{m}\mathbf{m}^T + \lambda_2 \left(\mathbf{p}\mathbf{p}^T + \mathbf{q}\mathbf{q}^T \right)$, with $\mathbf{m}, \mathbf{p}, \mathbf{q} \in \mathbb{S}^3$ forming an orthonormal basis aligned to the principal diffusion direction $\mathbf{m}$. The free model parameters are then $\mathbf{m}_1, \lambda_{11}, \lambda_{21}, \mathbf{m}_2, \lambda_{12}$, and λ_{22}.

2.2 Estimating the Fiber Model

Given the measured signal at a particular voxel, we want to estimate the underlying model parameters that explain this signal. As in streamline tractography, we treat the fiber as the trajectory of a particle which we trace out. At each step, we examine the measured signal at that position, estimate the underlying model parameters, and propagate forward in the most consistent direction.

To use a state-space filter for estimating the model parameters, we need the application-specific definition of four filter components:

1. The system state ($\mathbf{x}$): the model parameters
2. The state transition ($f[\cdot]$): how the model changes as we trace the fiber
3. The observation ($h[\cdot]$): how the signal appears given a particular state
4. The measurement ($\mathbf{y}$): the actual signal obtained from the scanner

For our state, we directly use the model parameters for the two-tensor model in Eq. 2:

$$\mathbf{x} = [\,\mathbf{m}_1 \ \lambda_{11} \ \lambda_{21} \ \mathbf{m}_2 \ \lambda_{12} \ \lambda_{22}\,]^T, \tag{3}$$

where $\mathbf{m} \in \mathbb{S}^2$ and $\lambda \in \mathbb{R}^+$. For the state transition we assume identity dynamics; the local fiber configuration does not undergo drastic change from one position to the next. Our observation is the signal reconstruction, $\mathbf{y} = \mathbf{s} = [\,s_1, ..., s_n\,]^T$ using s_i from Eq. 2, and our measurement is the actual signal interpolated at the current position.

Since the signal reconstruction using tensors is a nonlinear processes, we employ an unscented Kalman filter to perform estimation. Similar to classical linear Kalman filtering, the unscented version seeks to reconcile the predicted state of the system with the measured state and addresses the fact that those two processes–prediction and measurement–may be nonlinear or unknown. It does this in two phases: first it uses the system transition model to predict the next state and observation, and then it uses the new measurement to correct this state estimate. In what follows, we present the algorithmic application of the filter. For more thorough treatments, see [45, 46].

Suppose the system of interest is at time t and we have a Gaussian estimate of its current state with mean, $\mathbf{x}_t \in \mathbb{R}^n$, and covariance, $P_t \in \mathbb{R}^{n \times n}$. Prediction begins with the formation of a set $\mathbf{X}_t = \{\chi_i\} \subset \mathbb{R}^n$ of $(2n + 1)$ sample states with associated convex weights, $w_i \in \mathbb{R}$, spread around the current state. We use the covariance, P_t, to distribute this set deterministically:

$$\chi_0 = \mathbf{x}_t \qquad w_0 = \kappa/(n + \kappa) \qquad w_i = w_{i+n} = \frac{1}{2(n+\kappa)}$$

$$\chi_i = \mathbf{x}_t + \left[\sqrt{(n + \kappa)P_t}\right]_i \qquad \chi_{i+n} = \mathbf{x}_t - \left[\sqrt{(n + \kappa)P_t}\right]_i \tag{4}$$

where $[A]_i$ denotes the ith column of matrix A and κ is an adjustable scaling parameter. Next, this set is propagated through the state transition function, $\hat{\chi} = f[\chi] \in \mathbb{R}^n$, to obtain a new predicted sample set: $\mathbf{X}_{t+1|t} = \{f[\chi_i]\} = \{\hat{\chi}_i\}$. Since in this study we assume the fiber configuration does not change, we may write this as, $\mathbf{x}_{t+1|t} = f[\mathbf{x}_t] = \mathbf{x}_t$. These are then used to calculate the predicted system mean state, $\hat{\mathbf{x}}_{t+1|t} = \sum_i w_i \hat{\chi}_i$, and covariance, $P_{xx} = \sum_i w_i \left(\hat{\chi}_i - \hat{\mathbf{x}}_{t+1|t}\right)\left(\hat{\chi}_i - \hat{\mathbf{x}}_{t+1|t}\right)^T + Q$, where Q is the injected process noise bias. This procedure comprises the *unscented transform* used to estimate the behavior of a nonlinear function: spread sample points based on your current uncertainty, propagate those samples using your transform function, and measure the spread of those transformed samples.

To obtain the predicted observation, we again apply the unscented transform this time using the predicted states, $\mathbf{X}_{t+1|t}$, to estimate what we expect observe from the measurement of each state: $\gamma = h[\hat{\chi}] \in \mathbb{R}^m$. Keep in mind that for this study, our observation is the signal reconstruction from Eq. 2, and the measurement itself is looking at the diffusion-weighted signal, $\mathbf{s}$, interpolated at the current position. From these, we obtain the predicted set of observations, $\mathbf{Y}_{t+1|t} = \{h[\hat{\chi}_i]\} = \{\gamma_i\}$, and may calculate its mean, $\hat{\mathbf{y}}_{t+1|t} = \sum_i w_i \, \hat{\gamma}_i$, and covariance, $P_{yy} = \sum_i w_i \left(\hat{\gamma}_i - \hat{\mathbf{y}}_{t+1|t}\right)\left(\hat{\gamma}_i - \hat{\mathbf{y}}_{t+1|t}\right)^T +$ R, where R is the injected measurement noise bias. The cross correlation between the state and observation is given as: $P_{xy} = \sum_i w_i \left(\hat{\chi}_i - \hat{\mathbf{x}}_{t+1|t}\right)\left(\hat{\gamma}_i - \hat{\mathbf{y}}_{t+1|t}\right)^T$.

As is done in the classic linear Kalman filter, the final step is to use the Kalman gain, $K = P_{xy}P_{yy}^{-1}$, to correct our prediction and provide us with the final estimated system mean and covariance,

$$\mathbf{x}_{t+1} = \hat{\mathbf{x}}_{t+1|t} + K(\mathbf{y}_t - \hat{\mathbf{y}}_{t+1|t}) \tag{5}$$

$$P_{t+1} = P_{xx} - KP_{yy}K^T, \tag{6}$$

where $\mathbf{y}_t \in \mathbb{R}^m$ is the actual signal measurement taken at this time.

To summarize the proposed technique, we are using the unscented Kalman filter to estimate the two-tensor model parameters. Tractography involves maintaining for each fiber its model parameter state, covariance, and position. At each iteration of the algorithm, we predict the new state which in this case is simply identity: $\mathbf{x}_{t+1|t} = \mathbf{x}_t$. Our actual measurement $\mathbf{y}_t$ in Eq. 5 is to look at the diffusion-weighted signal, $\mathbf{s}$, recorded by the scanner at this position. At subvoxel positions we interpolate directly on the diffusion-weighted images. With these, we step through the equations above to find the new estimated model parameters, $\mathbf{x}_{t+1}$. Last, we move a small step in the most consistent principal diffusion direction, either $\mathbf{m}_1$ or $\mathbf{m}_2$, and then repeat the process from that new location.

3 Experiments

We first use experiments with synthetic data to validate our technique against ground truth. We confirm that our approach accurately estimates the true underlying signal and reliably recognizes crossing fibers over a broad range of angles. Comparing against two alternative multi-fiber optimization techniques, we find the filtered approach gives consistently superior results (Section 3.1). Next, we perform tractography through crossing fiber fields and qualitatively examine the underlying orientations and branchings (Section 3.2). Lastly, we examine a real dataset to demonstrate how causal estimation is able to pick up fibers and branchings known to exist *in vivo* yet absent using other techniques (Section 3.3).

Following the experimental method of generating synthetic data found in [22, 25, 41], we used the average eigenvalues of the 300 voxels with highest fractional anisotropy (FA) in our real data set: $\{1200, 100, 100\}\mu m^2$/msec (FA=0.91). We generated synthetic MR signals according to Eq. 2 using these eigenvalues to form an anisotropic tensor at both $b = 1000$ and $b = 3000$ using 81 gradient directions uniformly spread on the hemisphere. Two levels of Rician noise was introduced: relatively

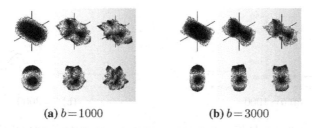

(a) $b = 1000$ (b) $b = 3000$

Fig. 1. Synthetic two-fiber voxel signal at a 60° angle *(black wires indicate axes)* showing the qualitative level of noise introduced. Each column shows the same signal from two viewpoints. Noise levels are pure (ground truth, no noise), "clean" (minimal noise), and "dirty" (heavy noise) *(left to right in each group).*

little noise which we call "clean" ($\sigma = 0.1$, SNR≈ 5 dB) and significant noise which we call "dirty" ($\sigma = 0.2$, SNR≈ 10 dB). To get an idea of this level of noise, Fig. 1 visualizes a sample voxel with two fibers at a 60° angle.

Throughout the experiments, we make comparisons against three alternative techniques. First, we use the same two-tensor model from Section 2.1 with a variant matching pursuit for brute force, dictionary-based optimization [47]. In our implementation, we simply project against a dictionary populated with the same pure two-tensor signals used to generate the synthetic data only oriented at 341 directions on the hemisphere, thus any error is due to the method's sensitivity to noise and discretization. Further, this is in effect the theoretical limit on performance for independent optimization techniques. This approach highlights the effect of using the same model but changing the optimization technique to one that treats each voxel independently. Second, we use spherical harmonics for modeling [22] and fiber-ODF sharpening for peak detection as described in [25] (order $l = 8$, regularization $L = 0.006$). This provides a comparison with an independently estimated, model-free representation. Note that this technique is very similar to spherical deconvolution. We will often refer to this method as "sharpened spherical harmonics". Last, when performing tractography on real data, we use single-tensor streamline tractography as a baseline[1].

3.1 Signal Reconstruction and Angular Resolution

While the independent optimization techniques can be run on individually generated voxels, care must be taken in constructing reasonable scenarios to test the causal filter. For this purpose, we constructed a 2D field through which to navigate (see Fig. 4a). In the middle is one long fiber pathway where the filter begins estimating a single tensor but then runs into a field of voxels with two crossed fibers at a fixed angle. In this crossing region we calculated error statistics. Similarly, we computed the angular error over this region using both sharpened spherical harmonics and matching pursuit. We generated several similar fields, each at a different fixed angle. By varying the size of the crossing region or the number of fibers run, we ensured that each technique performed at least 500 estimations.

---

[1] Using the freely available Slicer 2.7 (http://www.slicer.org).

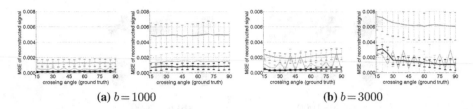

(a) $b = 1000$ (b) $b = 3000$

Fig. 2. Mean squared error (MSE) between reconstructed signal and ground truth signal at various crossing angles. Notice how the increased noise has little effect on the filter *(black)* compared to using matching pursuit *(light gray)* or spherical harmonics *(dark gray)*. Each subfigure shows both the clean and dirty experiments *(left, right)*.

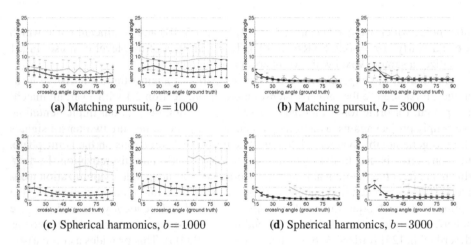

(a) Matching pursuit, $b = 1000$ (b) Matching pursuit, $b = 3000$

(c) Spherical harmonics, $b = 1000$ (d) Spherical harmonics, $b = 3000$

Fig. 3. Average angle error at various crossing angles comparing all three techniques: matching pursuit, sharpened spherical harmonics, and the proposed filter *(black)*. The filter provides stable and consistent estimation compared to either alternative technique. Each subfigure shows both the clean and dirty experiments *(left, right)*.

In the first experiment, we look at signal reconstruction error. We calculate the mean squared error of the reconstructed signal, s, against the ground truth signal, $\hat{s}$ (pure, no noise): $\|s - \hat{s}\|^2 / \|\hat{s}\|^2$. Fig. 2 shows the results of using the proposed filter, matching pursuit, and spherical harmonics. Over each technique's 500+ estimations, the trendlines indicate the mean error while the bars indicate one standard deviation. Spherical harmonics appear to produce a smooth fit to the given noisy data. Matching pursuit, despite having a dictionary filled only with the correct eigenvalues, shows the effect of discretization and sensitivity to noise. This experiment demonstrates that the proposed filter accurately and reliably estimates the true underlying signal.

In the second experiment, we looked at the error in angular resolution by comparing the filtered approach to matching pursuit and sharpened spherical harmonics. Matching pursuit again shows the effects of noise and discretization. Consistent with the results reported in [25, 17], spherical harmonics are generally unable to detect and resolve angles below 50° for $b = 1000$ or below 40° for $b = 3000$. Fig. 3c and Fig. 3d confirm this, respectively. This experiment demonstrates that for $b = 1000$, the filtered approach consistently resolves angles down to 20-30° with 5° error compared to independent optimization which fails to reliably resolve below 60° with as much as 15° error. For $b = 3000$, the filtered approach consistently resolves down to 20-30° with 2-3° error compared to independent optimization which cannot resolve below 50° with 5° error.

3.2 Synthetic Tractography

Having verified the technique's accuracy, we now turn to the resulting tractography. Fig. 4a shows a synthetic crossing fiber field at three fixed angles: 40°, 50°, 60° ($b = 3000$, noisy). From the bottom, we start several fibers that propagate upward where they encounter the crossing region. In Fig. 4b, we take a closer look at several neighboring sample voxels estimated within that crossing region, and we show the ODFs reconstructed using sharpened spherical harmonics and the proposed filter. As expected, at 40°, using spherical harmonics often only reports a single angle *(circled)*. Further, a closer examination of the reported axes shows the bias toward a single averaged axis as reported in [38, 41]. In contrast, the filtered results are consistent and accurate. For illustration, the 40° and 50° fields in Fig. 4a show how detected branchings may be followed.

3.3 Tractography on Real Data

We tested our approach on a real human brain scan of 51 diffusion weighted images with voxel size of $1.66 \times 1.66 \times 1.7 \, \text{mm}^3$ and $b = 900 \, \text{s/mm}^2$.

In this study, we focus on fibers originating in the corpus callosum. Specifically, we trace out the lateral transcallosal fibers that run through the corpus callosum out to the lateral gyri. It is known that single-tensor streamline tractography only traces out the dominant pathways forming the U-shaped callosal radiation (Fig. 5a and Fig. 6a). Several studies document this phenomena, among them the works of Descoteaux et

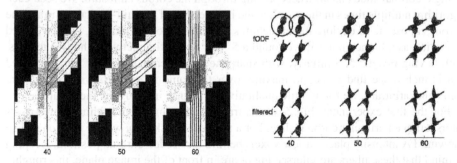

(a) Single fiber producing branches; several fibers maintaining parallel tracts.

(b) Estimated ODFs: spherical harmonics (top) and filtered two-tensor (bottom).

Fig. 4. Closeup of the estimated ODFs of several neighboring voxels estimated within the crossing region at fixed angles: 40°, 50°, 60°. Notice that spherical harmonics *(top row)* show an angular bias and have trouble finding both axes at 40° *(circled)*.

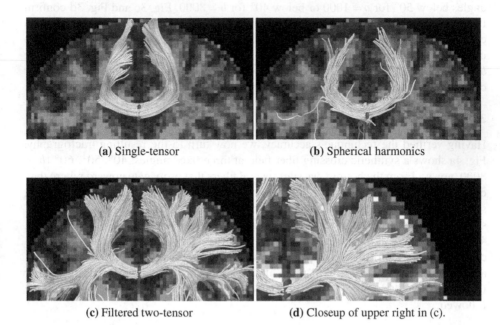

     (a) Single-tensor   (b) Spherical harmonics

    (c) Filtered two-tensor   (d) Closeup of upper right in (c).

Fig. 5. Filtered tractography (c),(d) picks up many fiber paths consistent with the underlying structures. Both single-tensor streamline (a) and sharpened spherical harmonics (b) are unable to find the majority of these pathways. Seed region indicated in gray.

al. [25] and Schultz et al. [41] have side-by-side comparisons. These fibers have been reported in using diffusion spectrum imaging [27], probabilistic tractography [11, 48, 25] and more recently with tensor decomposition [41].

    In this study, we focus on two basic experiments: looking at the tracts surrounding a single coronal slice and all tracts passing through the corpus callosum. We seed each algorithm multiple times in the voxels at the intersection of the mid-sagital plane and the corpus callosum. To explore the branchings found using our technique, we considered a position as a branch point if we found a 5°-40° separation between the two tensors, both having FA$\geq$0.15. Similarly, with sharpened spherical harmonics, we considered it a branch if we find a second maxima over the same range. While thresholds are somewhat arbitrary, we found little qualitative difference in adjusting these values.

    For the first experiment, Fig. 5 shows tracts originating from within a few voxels intersecting a particular coronal slice. For a reference backdrop, we use a coronal slice showing FA intensity placed a few voxels behind the seeded coronal position. Keeping in mind that these fibers are intersecting or are in front of the image plane, this roughly shows how the fibers navigate the areas of high anisotropy (bright regions). Similar to the results in [25, 41], Fig. 5b shows that spherical harmonics only pick up a few fibers intersecting the U-shaped callosal radiata. In contrast, our proposed algorithm traces out many pathways consistent with the apparent anatomy. To emphasize transcallosal

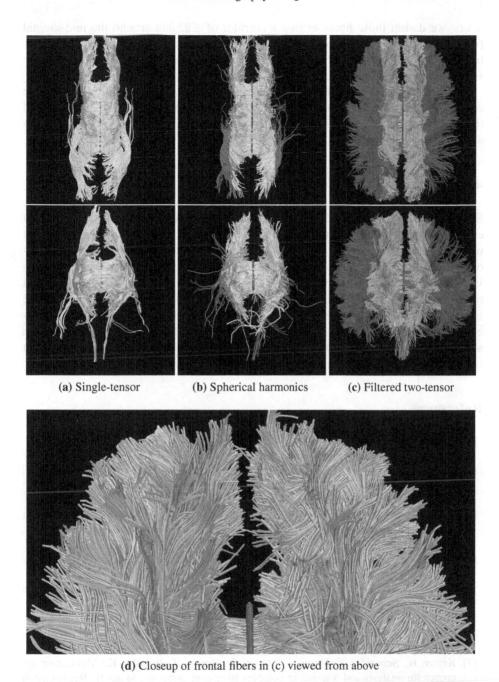

(a) Single-tensor   **(b)** Spherical harmonics   **(c)** Filtered two-tensor

(d) Closeup of frontal fibers in (c) viewed from above

Fig. 6. Tracing fibers originating from the center of the entire corpus callosum with views from above *(top row)* and front-to-back *(bottom)*. The proposed filtered tractography (c) is able to find many of the lateral projections *(darkened)* while single-tensor (a) is unable to find any and few are found with sharpened spherical harmonics (b). Seed region indicated in gray.

tracts, we darken those fibers exiting a corridor of ± 22 mm around the mid-sagittal plane. Fig. 5d provides a closer inspection of Fig. 5c where, to emphasize the underlying anatomy influencing the fibers, we use the actual coronal slice passing through the voxels used to seed this run.

For the second experiment, Fig. 6 shows a view of the whole brain to highlight the overall difference between the three methods. Here again we darken the transcallosal fibers found using the proposed filter. Fig. 6d provides a closeup of the frontal lobe from above to show the various pathways infiltrating the gyri.

4   Conclusions

Studies involving deterministic tractography rely on the underlying model estimated at each voxel as well as the reconstructed pathways. In this work, we demonstrated that using a causal filter provides robust estimates of much higher accuracy than independent estimation techniques. While the model we employed has been used previously in various forms, we primarily focused on the optimization technique used to estimate that model. Framing that estimation within a recursive filter allowed us to apply a standard technique for nonlinear estimation. We believe that exploring both alternative models and filtering techniques will provide more accurate and comprehensive information about neural pathways and ultimately enhance non-invasive diagnosis and treatment of brain disease.

References

[1] Basser, P., Jones, D.: Diffusion-tensor MRI: theory, experimental design and data analysis - A technical review. NMR in Biomedicine 25, 456–467 (2002)

[2] Behrens, T., Woolrich, M., Jenkinson, M., Johansen-Berg, H., Nunes, R., Clare, S., Matthews, P., Brady, J., Smith, S.: Characterization and propagation of uncertainty in diffusion-weighted MR imaging. Magnetic Resonance in Medicine 50, 1077–1088 (2003)

[3] Alexander, D., Barker, G., Arridge, S.: Detection and modeling of non-Gaussian apparent diffusion coefficient profiles in human brain data. Magnetic Resonance in Medicine 48, 331–340 (2002)

[4] Frank, L.: Characterization of anisotropy in high angular resolution diffusion-weighted MRI. Magnetic Resonance in Medicine 47, 1083–1099 (2002)

[5] Alexander, A., Hasan, K., Tsuruda, J., Parker, D.: Analysis of partial volume effects in diffusion-tensor MRI. Magnetic Resonance in Medicine 45, 770–780 (2001)

[6] Tuch, D., Reese, T., Wiegell, M., Makris, N., Belliveau, J., Wedeen, V.: High angular resolution diffusion imaging reveals intravoxel white matter fiber heterogeneity. Magnetic Resonance in Medicine 48, 577–582 (2002)

[7] Kreher, B., Schneider, J., Mader, I., Martin, E., Hennig, J., Il'yasov, K.: Multitensor approach for analysis and tracking of complex fiber configurations. Magnetic Resonance in Medicine 54, 1216–1225 (2005)

[8] Peled, S., Friman, O., Jolesz, F., Westin, C.F.: Geometrically constrained two-tensor model for crossing tracts in DWI. Magnetic Resonance in Medicine 24(9), 1263–1270 (2006)

[9] Hlawitschka, M., Scheuermann, G.: HOT-lines: Tracking lines in higher order tensor fields. In: Visualization, pp. 27–34 (2005)

[10] McGraw, T., Vemuri, B., Yezierski, B., Mareci, T.: Von Mises-Fisher mixture model of the diffusion ODF. In: Int. Symp. on Biomedical Imaging, pp. 65–68 (2006)

[11] Kaden, E., Knøsche, T., Anwander, A.: Parametric spherical deconvolution: Inferring anatomical connectivity using diffusion MR imaging. NeuroImage 37, 474–488 (2007)

[12] Rathi, Y., Michailovich, O., Shenton, M., Bouix, S.: Directional functions for orientation distribution estimation. Medical Image Analysis (in press, 2009)

[13] Özarslan, E., Shepherd, T., Vemuri, B., Blackband, S., Mareci, T.: Resolution of complex tissue microarchitecture using the diffusion orientation transform. NeuroImage 31(3) (2006)

[14] Tuch, D.: Q-ball imaging. Magnetic Resonance in Medicine 52, 1358–1372 (2004)

[15] Anderson, A.: Measurement of fiber orientation distributions using high angular resolution diffusion imaging. Magnetic Resonance in Medicine 54(5), 1194–1206 (2005)

[16] Hess, C., Mukherjee, P., Han, E., Xu, D., Vigneron, D.: Q-ball reconstruction of multimodal fiber orientations using the spherical harmonic basis. Magnetic Resonance in Medicine 56, 104–117 (2006)

[17] Descoteaux, M., Angelino, E., Fitzgibbons, S., Deriche, R.: Regularized, fast, and robust analytical Q-ball imaging. Magnetic Resonance in Medicine 58, 497–510 (2007)

[18] Michailovich, O., Rathi, Y.: On approximation of orientation distributions by means of spherical ridgelets. In: Int. Symp. on Biomedical Imaging, pp. 939–942 (2008)

[19] Poupon, C., Roche, A., Dubois, J., Mangin, J.F., Poupon, F.: Real-time MR diffusion tensor and Q-ball imaging using Kalman filtering. Medical Image Analysis 12(5), 527–534 (2008)

[20] Jian, B., Vemuri, B.: A unified computational framework for deconvolution to reconstruct multiple fibers from diffusion weighted MRI. Trans. on Medical Imaging 26(11), 1464–1471 (2007)

[21] Jansons, K., Alexander, D.: Persistent angular structure: New insights from diffusion MRI data. Inverse Problems 19, 1031–1046 (2003)

[22] Tournier, J.D., Calamante, F., Gadian, D., Connelly, A.: Direct estimation of the fiber orientation density function from diffusion-weighted MRI data using spherical deconvolution. NeuroImage 23, 1176–1185 (2004)

[23] Kumar, R., Barmpoutis, A., Vemuri, B., Carney, P., Mareci, T.: Multi-fiber reconstruction from DW-MRI using a continuous mixture of von Mises-Fisher distributions. In: Mathematical Methods in Biomedical Image Analysis (MMBIA), pp. 1–8 (2008)

[24] Alexander, D.: Multiple-fiber reconstruction algorithms for diffusion MRI. Annals of the New York Academy of Sciences 1046 (2005)

[25] Descoteaux, M., Deriche, R., Anwander, A.: Deterministic and probabilistic Q-ball tractography: from diffusion to sharp fiber distributions. Technical Report 6273, INRIA (2007)

[26] Basser, P., Pajevic, S., Pierpaoli, C., Duda, J., Aldroubi, A.: In vivo fiber tractography using DT-MRI data. Magnetic Resonance in Medicine 44, 625–632 (2000)

[27] Hagmann, P., Reese, T., Tseng, W.Y., Meuli, R., Thiran, J.P., Wedeen, V.: Diffusion spectrum imaging tractography in complex cerebral white matter: An investigation of the centrum semiovale. In: Int. Symp. on Magnetic Resonance in Medicine (ISMRM), p. 623 (2004)

[28] Guo, W., Zeng, Q., Chen, Y., Liu, Y.: Using multiple tensor deflection to reconstruct white matter fiber traces with branching. In: Int. Symp. on Biomedical Imaging, pp. 69–72 (2006)

[29] Qazi, A., Radmanesh, A., O'Donnell, L., Kindlmann, G., Peled, S., Whalen, S., Westin, C.F., Golby, A.: Resolving crossings in the corticospinal tract by two-tensor streamline tractography: Method and clinical assessment using fMRI. NeuroImage (2008)

[30] Gössl, C., Fahrmeir, L., Putz, B., Auer, L., Auer, D.: Fiber tracking from DTI using linear state space models: Detectability of the pyramidal tract. NeuroImage 16, 378–388 (2002)

[31] Björnemo, M., Brun, A., Kikinis, R., Westin, C.F.: Regularized stochastic white matter tractography using diffusion tensor MRI. In: Dohi, T., Kikinis, R. (eds.) MICCAI 2002. LNCS, vol. 2488, pp. 435–442. Springer, Heidelberg (2002)

[32] Zhang, F., Goodlett, C., Hancock, E., Gerig, G.: Probabilistic fiber tracking using particle filtering. In: Ayache, N., Ourselin, S., Maeder, A. (eds.) MICCAI 2007, Part II. LNCS, vol. 4792, pp. 144–152. Springer, Heidelberg (2007)

[33] Zhukov, L., Barr, A.: Oriented tensor reconstruction: Tracing neural pathways from diffusion tensor MRI. In: Visualization, pp. 387–394 (2002)

[34] Parker, G., Alexander, D.: Probabilistic Monte Carlo based mapping of cerebral connections utilizing whole-brain crossing fiber information. In: Taylor, C.J., Noble, J.A. (eds.) IPMI 2003. LNCS, vol. 2732, pp. 684–696. Springer, Heidelberg (2003)

[35] Campbell, J.W., Siddiqi, K., Rymar, V., Sadikot, A., Pike, G.: Flow-based fiber tracking with diffusion tensor and Q-ball data: Validation and comparison to principal diffusion direction techniques. NeuroImage 27(4), 725–736 (2005)

[36] Hosey, T., Williams, G., Ansorge, R.: Inference of multiple fiber orientations in high angular resolution diffusion imaging. Magnetic Resonance in Medicine 54, 1480–1489 (2005)

[37] Behrens, T., Johansen-Berg, H., Jbabdi, S., Rushworth, M., Woolrich, M.: Probabilistic diffusion tractography with multiple fibre orientations: What can we gain? NeuroImage 34, 144–155 (2007)

[38] Zhan, W., Yang, Y.: How accurately can the diffusion profiles indicate multiple fiber orientations? A study on general fiber crossings in diffusion MRI. J. of Magnetic Resonance 183, 193–202 (2006)

[39] Seunarine, K., Cook, P., Hall, M., Embleton, K., Parker, G., Alexander, D.: Exploiting peak anisotropy for tracking through complex structures. In: Mathematical Methods in Biomedical Image Analysis (MMBIA), pp. 1–8 (2007)

[40] Bloy, L., Verma, R.: On computing the underlying fiber directions from the diffusion orientation distribution function. In: Metaxas, D., Axel, L., Fichtinger, G., Székely, G. (eds.) MICCAI 2008, Part I. LNCS, vol. 5241, pp. 1–8. Springer, Heidelberg (2008)

[41] Schultz, T., Seidel, H.: Estimating crossing fibers: A tensor decomposition approach. Trans. on Visualization and Computer Graphics 14(6), 1635–1642 (2008)

[42] Ramirez-Manzanares, A., Cook, P., Gee, J.: A comparison of methods for recovering intravoxel white matter fiber architecture from clinical diffusion imaging scans. In: Metaxas, D., Axel, L., Fichtinger, G., Székely, G. (eds.) MICCAI 2008, Part I. LNCS, vol. 5241, pp. 305–312. Springer, Heidelberg (2008)

[43] Friman, O., Farnebäck, G., Westin, C.F.: A Bayesian approach for stochastic white matter tractography. Trans. on Medical Imaging 25(8), 965–978 (2006)

[44] Parker, G., Alexander, D.: Probabilistic anatomical connectivity derived from the microscopic persistent angular structure of cerebral tissue. Phil. Trans. R. Soc. B 360, 893–902 (2005)

[45] Julier, S., Uhlmann, J.: Unscented filtering and nonlinear estimation. IEEE 92(3), 401–422 (2004)

[46] van der Merwe, R., Wan, E.: Sigma-point Kalman filters for probabilistic inference in dynamic state-space models. In: Workshop on Advances in Machine Learning (2003)

[47] Mallat, S., Zhang, Z.: Matching pursuits with time-frequency dictionaries. Trans. on Signal Processing 41, 3397–3415 (1993)

[48] Anwander, A., Descoteaux, M., Deriche, R.: Probabilistic Q-Ball tractography solves crossings of the callosal fibers. In: Human Brain Mapping, p. 342 (2007)

Multi-fiber Reconstruction from DW-MRI Using a Continuous Mixture of Hyperspherical von Mises-Fisher Distributions*

Ritwik Kumar[1], Baba C. Vemuri[1], Fei Wang[2], Tanveer Syeda-Mahmood[2], Paul R. Carney[3], and Thomas H. Mareci[4]

[1] Dept. of CISE, University of Florida, Gainesville, FL, USA
[2] IBM Almaden Research Center, San Jose, CA, USA
[3] Dept. of Pediatrics, University of Florida, Gainesville, FL, USA
[4] Dept. and Molecular Biology, University of Florida, Gainesville, FL, USA

Abstract. Multi-fiber reconstruction has attracted immense attention lately in the field of diffusion weighted MRI analysis. Several mathematical models have been proposed in literature but there is still scope for improvement. The key issues of importance in multi-fiber reconstruction are, fiber detection accuracy, robustness to noise and computational efficiency. To this end, we propose a novel mathematical model for representing the MR signal attenuation in the presence of multiple fibers at a single voxel and estimate the parameters of this model given the diffusion weighted MRI data. Our model for the diffusion MR signal consists of a continuous mixture of Hyperspherical von Mises-Fisher distributions. Being a continuous mixture, our model does not require the specification of the number of mixture components. We present a closed form expression for this continuous mixture that leads to a computationally efficient implementation. To validate our model we present extensive results on both synthetic and real data (human and rat brain) and demonstrate that even in presence of noise, our model clearly outperforms the state-of-the-art methods in fiber orientation estimation while maintaining a substantial computational advantage.

1   Introduction

Diffusion Weighted Magnetic Resonance Imaging (DW-MRI), arguably one of the most important imaging inventions of the twentieth century, is the only existing non-invasive and in-vivo imaging method that allows examination of neural tissue architecture at a microscopic scale. By quantitatively capturing the diffusion of water molecules in the brain tissues one can determine the white matter fiber tracts even in the presence of complex local geometries such as fiber crossings ([21,17,6]) and connectivity of different brain regions ([8]).

DW-MRI works by measuring the loss of precession synchronization of hydrogen molecules when a pair of directional magnetic gradient pulses with opposing

---

* This research was in part supported by UF Alumni Fellowship to RK, NIH EB007082 to BCV and NIH EB004752 to PC and TM.

J.L. Prince, D.L. Pham, and K.J. Myers (Eds.): IPMI 2009, LNCS 5636, pp. 139–150, 2009.

polarity are applied. This is quantitatively captured in the DW-MR image as the loss of signal required to pull the precession back in synchronization, defined for each gradient direction. From this raw data, water displacement probabilities (PDF) at each voxel can be obtained by computing the fourier transform of the corresponding signal attenuation function, reconstructed from its directional samples. The local fiber orientation can then be inferred by computing the maxima of the displacement probability function or the orientation distribution function (ODF), which can be obtained by radially integrating or by taking the radial iso-surface of the PDF. Further processing of this information, for instance, via tractography can reveal connections between different regions of the brain.

From the above description it readily follows that the accurate reconstruction of the signal attenuation from its directional, often noisy, samples is of fundamental importance to the success of subsequent steps. In this paper we present a novel technique to accomplish this, which provides superior accuracy for fiber orientation detection while maintaining computational efficiency advantage over the state-of-the-art techniques. Our method captures the inherent antipodal symmetry of the DW-MR signal using the Knutsson mapping [16] and models the signal attenuation function using a continuous mixture of Hyperspherical von Mises-Fisher distributions, for which we have derived a closed form expression.

Over the last two decades, various methods have been suggested for MR signal attenuation and ODF modeling. Pioneering work in this field was presented in [7] which modeled diffusion by rank 2 tensors (DTI). Though effective in characterizing the diffusivity function in most of white matter, DTI could not explain complex fiber geometry such as crossings. To address this, techniques using spherical harmonics [13] and higher order tensors [22], [4] were proposed using high resolution data (HARDI), but these produced diffusivity functions whose peaks are known not to correspond to the fiber orientations [21]. Bypassing the signal reconstruction, direct ODF modeling was proposed in [10] and [14] using Q-Ball imaging but this produced a displacement probability function which was corrupted via convolution with a zeroth order Bessel function. Diffusion Spectrum imaging [12] was proposed as an alternate to Q-Ball but it suffers from time intensive sampling requirements. Diffusion Orientation Transform, proposed in [21], analytically evaluated the radial component of the fourier integral but it yields a displacement probability that is also corrupted via convolution with a function that can not be specified in analytic form.

In contrast to the above methods are the multi-compartmental models (e.g. [25,3,20,9]) that use a discrete mixture of basis functions to approximate the MR signal attenuation. Though effective, these methods face the model selection problem of fixing the number of mixture components a priori, and this was addressed by the deconvolution based approaches ([24,1,2]), which assume a distribution of fibers at each voxel. More recently, continuous mixture models have been proposed in [15] and [17] which model MR signal attenuation as a continuous mixture of some appropriately chosen bases and recover model parameter by solving linear systems.

Of all the methods presented above, multi-compartmental models and continuous mixture models are most closely related to our technique presented here. In particular, it is related to the work presented by McGraw et al. [20], Bhalerao et al. [9], Jian et al. [15] and Kumar et al. [17].

McGraw et al. [20] and Bhalerao et al. [9] present multi-compartmental models for MR signal attenuation modeling using discrete mixtures of von Mises-Fisher and Hyperspherical von Mises-Fisher distributions respectively. Both of these techniques require computationally intensive non-linear optimizations to recover the model parameters at each voxel. Furthermore, [20] suffers from the well known model selection problem, where the number of mixture components are arbitrarily set. Though the method in [9] tries to avoid this problem using Akaike information criterion, it however results in choosing between one or two components by exhaustively comparing the two choices, which puts this technique only on a slightly better footing than the one in [20].

Jian et al. [15] and Kumar et al. [17] formulate their models in the continuous mixture framework, which allows them to overcome the model selection problems associated with discrete mixtures mentioned above. Though Jian et al. [15] define the current state-of-the-art in terms of fiber orientation detection accuracy, their technique requires eigenvalues of the diffusion tensors in the continuous mixture to be fixed, in order to translate its discretization problem from $\mathcal{P}_3$, space of symmetric positive definite matrices, to that of discretizing $\mathcal{S}^2$, the sphere. Moreover, since it seeks non negative weights, it requires the use of the Non-Negative Least Squares [18] algorithm at each voxel of the DW-MRI data, which can be computationally intensive. The model proposed by Kumar et al. [17] avoids these problems at the expense of being less accurate than the method in [15].

Our method addresses all of of the above mentioned pitfalls by providing more accurate fiber orientation detection results than [15] while maintaining the computational advantage similar to [17].

2 Theory

2.1 Knutsson Mapping

DW-MR data is inherently antipodally symmetric. If a mixture model for its estimation uses basis functions which are not inherently antipodally symmetric, it would need additional constraints to enforce antipodal symmetry of the estimation. Existing mixture models like those described in [20] and [17] handle antipodal symmetry by combining pairs of basis functions with antipodal orientations into one basis function. Here we use a much more seamless method that uses higher dimensional mapping called Knutsson mapping [16] to account for antipodal symmetry.

Knutsson [16] proposed a mapping $\nu : \mathcal{S}_2 \to \mathcal{S}_4$ which was agnostic to directions, $\nu(\overrightarrow{x}) = \nu(-\overrightarrow{x})$, locally preserved angular metric for constant magnitude vectors, $|\delta\nu(\overrightarrow{x})| = \alpha \cdot |\delta\overrightarrow{x}|$ with α being some constant and lead to direction independent magnitude in the mapped space, $|\nu(\overrightarrow{x})| = \beta$ for some constant β. This mapping is defined as

$$\nu([r,\theta,\phi]) = [\sin^2(\theta)\cos 2\phi, \sin^2(\theta)\sin 2\phi, \sin 2\theta \cos \phi, \sin 2\theta \sin \phi, \sqrt{3}(\cos^2 \theta - \frac{1}{3})],$$
(1)

where $[r,\theta,\phi]$ is the spherical parameterization of a vector in $\mathcal{S}_2$.

Knutsson mapping proves to be a handy tool for dealing with data which only depends on axes and not directions, like DW-MR data. In the context of continuous mixture model, this mapping alleviates the need to pair antipodal bases into one. But as a result of this mapping, the problem now is no longer defined in $\mathcal{S}_2$ and would require analysis in $\mathcal{S}_4$. It was employed in the past by [9] in context of processing MR signals.

2.2 Continuous Mixture of Hyperspherical von Mises-Fisher Distributions

A continuous mixture model defined on the spherical domain $\mathcal{S}_{p-1}$ can be represented as

$$f(\mathbf{x}) = \int_{\mathcal{S}_{p-1}} D(\boldsymbol{\mu})K(\mathbf{x},\boldsymbol{\mu})d\boldsymbol{\mu},$$
(2)

where $K(\mathbf{x},\boldsymbol{\mu})$ is called the basis function or the kernel and $D(\boldsymbol{\mu})$ is called the mixing density. Here x and $\boldsymbol{\mu}$ are vectors in $\mathcal{S}_{p-1}$. This formulation can be looked at as a generalization of the discrete mixture of basis functions where the continuous mixing density has replaced the discrete mixing weights.

Here, we seek a continuous mixture of Hyperspherical von Mises-Fisher distributions [19], which for the most general case (defined on $\mathcal{S}_{p-1}$), is given as

$$M_p(\mathbf{x};\boldsymbol{\mu},\kappa) = (\frac{\kappa}{2})^{p/2-1}\frac{\exp(\kappa\boldsymbol{\mu}^T\mathbf{x})}{\Gamma(p/2)I_{p/2-1}(\kappa)}.$$
(3)

where $\boldsymbol{\mu}$, (with $\| \boldsymbol{\mu} \| = 1$) is the mean direction along which the distribution is oriented with a concentration given by parameter $\kappa \geq 0$. I_ν is the Bessel function of the first kind and order ν.

As mentioned in the previous section, in order to handle antipodal symmetry we project the vectors from $\mathcal{S}_2$ to $\mathcal{S}_4$, and thus, the kernel function for our continuous mixture model should also be defined in $\mathcal{S}_4$, hence it has the form

$$M_5(\mathbf{x};\boldsymbol{\mu},\kappa) = \frac{1}{3}\sqrt{\frac{2}{\pi}}\frac{\kappa^{3/2}}{I_{3/2}(\kappa)}\exp(\kappa\boldsymbol{\mu}^T\mathbf{x}).$$
(4)

Note that in this expression $\mathbf{x}$ and $\boldsymbol{\mu}$ are defined as vectors in $\mathcal{S}^4$ and not $\mathcal{S}^2$.

It can be noted in Eq. 2 that the mixing density is a density defined on the domain of integration. In our case, it needs to be defined on $\mathcal{S}_4$. As the spherical analog of the Gaussian distribution, Hyperspherical von Mises-Fisher density again presents itself as a natural choice. But since the formulation in Eq. 2 is convolutional in nature, if both the mixing density and the kernel are chosen to be single lobed functions, so would be the continuous mixture. In order to provide our model flexibility to accommodate intra-voxel orientation heterogeneity (IVOH), we use a discrete mixture of hyperspherical von Mises-Fisher distributions as the mixing density, given as

$$D_5(\boldsymbol{\mu}; \{\boldsymbol{\gamma}_i\}, \kappa') = \sum_{i=1}^{N} w_i \frac{1}{3} \sqrt{\frac{2}{\pi}} \frac{\kappa'^{3/2}}{I_{3/2}(\kappa')} \exp\left(\kappa' \boldsymbol{\gamma}_i^T \boldsymbol{\mu}\right). \tag{5}$$

This density is parameterized by a discrete collection of N directions $\{\boldsymbol{\gamma}_i\}$, and constant concentration κ'. We must point out that N here decides the resolution of spherical discretization and is in no way related to the number of expected fiber bundles. This kind of discretization is often used in continuous mixtures ([15], [17]) and should be looked at as the number of basis functions to be used while reconstructing the MR signal attenuation. Generally the quality of reconstruction improves as this resolution increases. For our method we obtain the set of direction $\{\boldsymbol{\gamma}_i\}$ by a 4th order subdivision of the icosahedral tessellation of the unit hemisphere. Note that we have not discretized the space for parameter κ' as we will set it later based on numerical considerations.

Substituting the expressions for the kernel and the mixing density in Eq .2 leads to the following expression for the MR signal attenuation $S(\mathbf{q})/S_0$

$$\frac{S(\mathbf{q})}{S_0} = \int_{S_P} \sum_{i=1}^{N} w_i \frac{2(\kappa'\kappa)^{\frac{3}{2}}}{9\pi I_{\frac{3}{2}}(\kappa') I_{\frac{3}{2}}(\kappa)} \exp\left(\kappa' \boldsymbol{\gamma}_i^T \boldsymbol{\mu}\right) \exp\left(\kappa \boldsymbol{\mu}^T \mathbf{q}\right) d\boldsymbol{\mu}, \tag{6}$$

where $S(\mathbf{q})$ is the DW-MRI signal value associated with reciprocal space vector $\mathbf{q}$, S_0 the zero gradient signal. Here we make the important observation that if κ is set to unity, this expression can be looked at as a Laplace transform of the Hyperspherical von Mises-Fisher distribution in $\mathcal{S}_4$, which we have analytically evaluated to be

$$\frac{S(\mathbf{q})}{S_0} = \sum_{i=1}^{N} w_i \frac{\sqrt{2}\kappa'^{\frac{3}{2}}/(3\sqrt{\pi} I_{\frac{3}{2}}(1) I_{\frac{3}{2}}(\kappa'))}{(\kappa' \cosh(\kappa') - \sinh(\kappa'))} \left[\frac{\cosh(\|\kappa'\mu_i + \mathbf{q}\|)}{\|\kappa'\mu_i + \mathbf{q}\|^2} - \frac{\sinh(\|\kappa'\mu_i + \mathbf{q}\|)}{\|\kappa'\mu_i + \mathbf{q}\|^3}\right]. \tag{7}$$

This expression provides the value of signal attenuation when the magnetic gradient is applied in the direction $\mathbf{q}$. Since the MR data is obtained for multiple such directions, unknown weights w_i can be obtained by solving a linear system using the method described subsequently.

2.3   Numerical Solution

When the data is available for various gradient directions $\mathbf{q}_j$, unknown weights from the expression in Eq. 7 can be obtained by solving a system of linear equations $Aw = S$, where w is the vector of N unknown weights, S is the vector that contains the M acquired MR signal samples $S(\mathbf{q}_j)/S_0$, and A is the $M \times N$ matrix where the entry A_{ji} in the jth row and the ith column is given by

$$A_{ji} = \frac{\sqrt{2}\kappa'^{\frac{3}{2}}/(3\sqrt{\pi} I_{\frac{3}{2}}(1) I_{\frac{3}{2}}(\kappa'))}{(\kappa \cosh(\kappa') - \sinh(\kappa'))} \left[\frac{\cosh(\|\kappa'\mu_i + \mathbf{q}_j\|)}{\|\kappa'\mu_i + \mathbf{q}_j\|^2} - \frac{\sinh(\|\kappa'\mu_i + \mathbf{q}_j\|)}{\|\kappa'\mu_i + \mathbf{q}_j\|^3}\right]. \tag{8}$$

Since the data can be noisy and the number of fibers (bundles) at a voxel are sparse (as compared to N), we obtain the unknown weights by using a regularized least squares formulation leading to the minimization of the following expression

$$w = \underset{w'}{\operatorname{argmin}} ||Aw' - S||^2 + \lambda ||w'||^2 \qquad (9)$$

which leads to the following closed form solution for the unknown w

$$w = A^T (AA^T + \lambda I)^{-1} S. \qquad (10)$$

This expression can be evaluated without inverting any matrix. This constrained least squares is also called Damped Least Squares and has been employed in the past in [15].

At this stage we set the parameters κ' and λ so as to ensure better conditioning of the process in Eq. 10. We must point out that these parameters need to be set only once, as the matrix A remains the same even if the actual MR data changes from voxel to voxel.

2.4   Fiber Orientation Recovery

The water molecule displacement probability function can be obtained from the signal attenuation function via a Fourier transform given as

$$P(\mathbf{r}) = \int \frac{S(\mathbf{q})}{S_0} e^{-2\pi i \mathbf{q}^T \mathbf{r}} d\mathbf{q}, \qquad (11)$$

where $\mathbf{q}$ is the reciprocal space vector, $S(\mathbf{q})$ is the DW-MRI signal value associated with vector $\mathbf{q}$, S_0 the zero gradient signal and $\mathbf{r}$ is the displacement vector. Through there are various methods available in literature for obtaining the water displacement probability, in our implementation we use the method proposed in [5] for its effectiveness. Once the water displacement probability has been obtained, fiber orientations can be recovered by finding the maxima of either a radial iso-surface of $P(\mathbf{r})$ or the radial integral of $P(\mathbf{r})$. We use the former of these techniques to evaluate the fiber orientation primarily on account of its simplicity and good accuracy.

3   Experimental Results and Discussion

First, we try to quantitatively capture the performance of our technique relative to various state-of-the-art methods. Towards this, in Fig. 1(A) we present fiber orientation detection errors for Mixture of Wisharts (MoW) [15], continuous mixture of von Mises-Fisher distributions (MovMF) [17], Q-Ball Orientation Distribution Function [10], Diffusion Orientation Transform (DOT) [21] and the proposed method for various noise levels in the signal. For this experiment we simulated a 2-fiber crossing using the so called Söderman's model proposed in [23] which captures the MR signal attenuation from particles diffusing inside a cylindrical boundary.

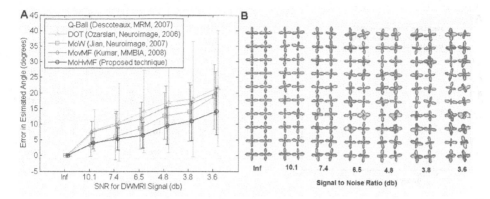

Fig. 1. (A). Fiber orientation detection accuracy comparison with DOT [21], MoW [15], Q-Ball ODF [10] and MovMF [17]. **(B).** Probability profiles for 2 fibers crossing at 90° as the amount of noise increases from left to right.

The signal was simulated for 81 gradient directions with a b value of $1250\,s/mm^2$. We added Rician noise to the data with increasing variance and obtained signal with the signal to noise ratio (SNR) ranging from ∞ (for no noise) to 3.6 (large noise). It can be readily noted from Fig. 1(A) that the proposed method provides noise robust performance and achieves higher accuracy as compared to MoW, Q-Ball ODF, MovMF and DOT.

Next in Fig. 1(B) we visualize the probability profiles generated by our method for the various noise levels used in Fig. 1(A). We have presented 2 column of water displacement probability profiles for each case with the corresponding SNR mentioned below it. It can be noted that as the SNR decreases the computed probability profiles starts showing deviations from the expected 90° crossings with near perfect detection in the first column (noiseless case).

We used the same 2-fiber crossing testbench to evaluate the computational efficiency of the proposed method. For this experiment we implemented MoW [15] and MovMF [17] and our method in MATLAB 7.4. Then we noted the time taken by each technique for 2 fiber crossing reconstruction for scan volumes of varying sizes. The experiment was conducted on an Intel Centrino 2.4 GHz machine with 3 GB memory and the obtained run times are reported in Fig. 2(A). It can be noted that our method maintains the same computational efficiency as MovMF and is substantially faster than MoW. The primary reason for this is that for MoW, the linear system is solved using non-negative least squares method while our method uses a simpler linear system solver.

In Fig. 2(B) we present more comprehensive quantitative results for our method as both the number of fibers in the crossings and the intra-fiber angles are varied. For this experiment, we simulated MR signal attenuation with various different fiber crossing angles and with varying amount of noise. The angles in the second column are the maximum inter-fiber angle for the cases with multiple fibers. In the next eight columns fiber orientation detection errors (in degrees) are presented with the corresponding SNR mentioned in the column headings. Following observations

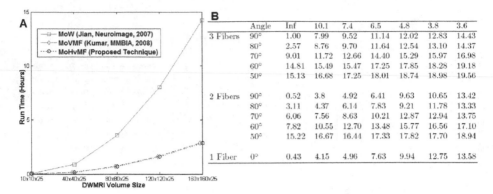

Fig. 2. (A) Computational efficiency comparison as the scan volume size increases. It can be noted that our technique provides better performance than competing methods (MoW[15] and MovMF [17]). **(B)** Fiber orientation detection errors (in degrees) for 1, 2 and 3 fiber crossings. The second column indicates the maximum inter-fiber angular separation when multiple fibers are present. Column headings for next eight columns indicate the SNR in db.

can be made from these results. Firstly, as the number of fibers crossing at each voxel increases, so does the ambiguity in detection of fiber orientation and thus results for single fiber are better than 2 or 3 fibers. Secondly, for all the cases (1, 2 or 3 fibers), as the noise level increases, so does the orientation detection error rates. Thirdly, as the angle between the intersection fibers decreases, the error rates go up. Note that as long as the error rates are not larger than half the fiber separation angle, number of fibers can still be accurately detected and thus for all the cases presented, correct number of fibers can be resolved irrespective of the error.

Thus far we presented results on simulated data for quantitative comparison of various methods, next we present comprehensive results of our method on real human and rat brain data. In these results we have shown water molecule displacement probability iso-surfaces estimated from the reconstructed signal using the proposed method. Each probability profiles is colored according to the dominant fiber direction and the color map is provided in the top left corner of both Fig. 3 and Fig. 4 respectively. The peaks of the probability profile indicate the fiber orientation.

We present results on human brain data in Fig. 3. This data was acquired using 46 gradient directions with repetition time of 8.5 sec and b value of 800 s/mm^2 on a 3 Tesla Phillips scanner. The matrix size was 128 × 128 × 60 and the data was acquired at 2 mm × 2 mm × 2 mm resolution. In Fig. 3, images (A) and (C) show the coming together of the corpus callosum splenium and corpus callosum genu bundles with the inferior fronto-occipital tract respectively. At the join of these two bundles, fiber crossings can be seen and the plotted spherical functions depict the multiple lobes whose peaks point to the direction of the fibers, using which we can track fibers ([8]) as shown in Fig. 3(A)(iv) and Fig. 3(C)(iv). Fig. 3(B) shows another slice with single fiber bundles as well as fiber crossings.

In Fig. 4 we present results obtained on rat brain data acquired using a 17.6 Tesla Bruker scanner. The data used in Fig. 4(A) and 4(C) was obtained from an ex-

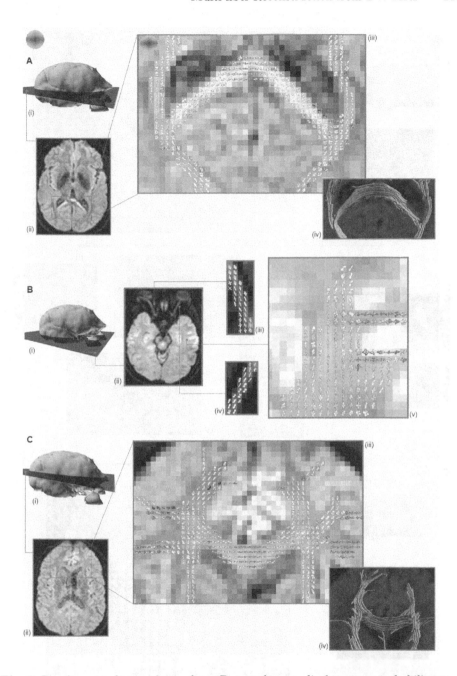

Fig. 3. Results using human brain data. Detected water displacement probability profiles for various human brain regions including regions showing merging of the **A**. corpus callosum splenium and the inferior fronto-occipital tract and **C**. corpus callosum genu and the inferior fronto-occipital tract are presented. Part **B** shows single fiber bundles as well as fiber crossings.

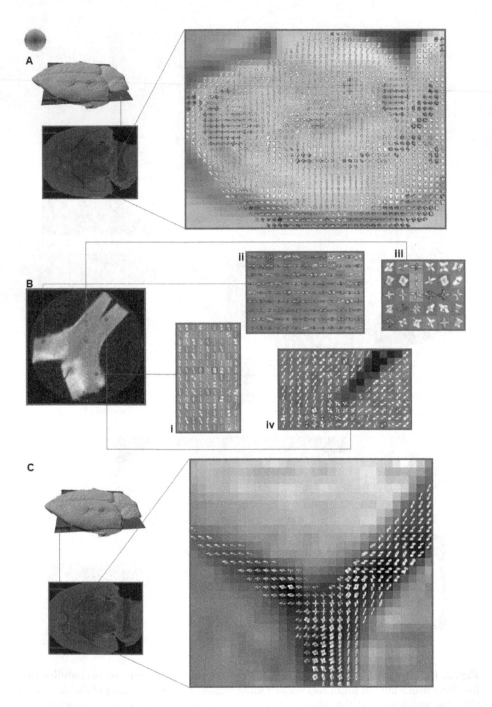

Fig. 4. Results using rat brain data. Detected fiber orientations in – **A**. Rat brain hippocampus, **B**. Optic chiasm from a rat brain and **C**. Cingulum and corpus callosum crossing.

cised perfusion-fixed rat brain. Thirty-two images were acquired using a spin-echo, pulsed-field-gradient sequence with repetition time 1.4 s, echo time 28 ms, field of view 30 mm $\times$ 15 mm, matrix 200 $\times$ 100 with 32 continuous 0.3 mm thick slices measured (oriented parallel to the long-axis of the brain). 46 diffusion weighted images were collected with 5 signal averages with approximate b values of 1250 s/mm^2, whose orientations were determined by the tessellation on a hemisphere. The data used in Fig. 4(B) was obtained from excised, perfusion-fixed rat optic chiasm in 46 gradient directions with the b value as 1250 s/mm^2.

Fig. 4(A) shows fiber orientations in the hippocampus region of the rat brain. The zoomed-in region of interest shows fiber crossings and single fiber structures consistent with already published reports on hippocampal structure [11]. In Fig. 4(B) we present estimated fiber orientations from various regions of myelinated axons from the two optic nerve bundles crossing each other to reach their respective contra-lateral optic tracts. Inset images (i) and (ii) show the optic tract where voxels are composed of single fibers. Inset (iii) shows the crossing fibers while the inset (iv) shows the fibers going their separate ways after the crossing. Fig. 4(C) shows fibers of cingulum and corpus callosum (upper right) intersecting each other. Single fibers and fiber crossings can be seen to be correctly rendered using our method.

4   Conclusion

In this paper we introduced a novel mathematical model for modeling the MR signal attenuation leading to high fiber orientation detection accuracy and computational efficiency. We have experimentally demonstrated that our method is particularly robust to the presence of noise and outperforms existing methods in terms of fiber orientation detection accuracy. Further, since our techniques leads to a linear system which we solve using damped least squares, it is more computationally efficient, as compared to existing methods that employ non-linear techniques and constrained linear least-squares techniques. Through extensive experiments on rat and human brain data, we showed that the proposed technique can provide excellent fiber detection results for real data as well.

References

1. Alexander, D.C.: Maximum entropy spherical deconvolution for diffusion MRI. In: Christensen, G.E., Sonka, M. (eds.) IPMI 2005. LNCS, vol. 3565, pp. 76–87. Springer, Heidelberg (2005)
2. Adam, W., Anderson, A.W.: Measurement of fiber orientation distributions using high angular resolution diffusion imaging. MRM 54(5) (2005)
3. Assaf, Y., Freidlin, R.Z., Rohde, G.K., Basser, P.J.: New modeling and experimental framework to characterize hindered and restricted water diffusion in brain white matter. MRM (2004)
4. Barmpoutis, A., Jian, B., Vemuri, B.C., Shepherd, T.M.: Symmetric positive 4th order tensors and their estimation from diffusion weighted MRI. In: Karssemeijer, N., Lelieveldt, B. (eds.) IPMI 2007. LNCS, vol. 4584, pp. 308–319. Springer, Heidelberg (2007)

5. Barmpoutis, A., Vemuri, B.C., Forder, J.R.: Fast displacement probability profile approximation from hardi using 4th-order tensors. In: ISBI (2008)
6. Barmpoutis, A., Vemuri, B.C., Howland, D., Forder, J.R.: Extracting tractosemas from a displacement probability field for tractography in dw-MRI. In: Metaxas, D., Axel, L., Fichtinger, G., Székely, G. (eds.) MICCAI 2008, Part I. LNCS, vol. 5241, pp. 9–16. Springer, Heidelberg (2008)
7. Basser, P.J., Mattiello, J., Lebihan, D.: Estimation of the Effective Self-Diffusion Tensor from the NMR Spin Echo. J. Magn. Reson. B 103 (1994)
8. Basser, P.J., Pajevic, S., Pierpaoli, C., Duda, J., Aldroubi, A.: In vivo fiber tractography using dt-MRI data. Magnetic Resonance in Medicine 44(4) (2000)
9. Bhalerao, A., Westin, C.-F.: Hyperspherical von mises fisher mixture (hvmf) modelling of high angular resolution diffusion MRI. In: Ayache, N., Ourselin, S., Maeder, A. (eds.) MICCAI 2007, Part I. LNCS, vol. 4791, pp. 236–243. Springer, Heidelberg (2007)
10. Descoteaux, M., Angelino, E., Fitzgibbons, S., Deriche, R.: Regularized, fast and robust analytical q-ball imaging. Magnetic Resonance in Medicine 58 (2007)
11. Shepherd, T.M., et al.: Structural insights from high-resolution diffusion tensor imaging and tractography of the isolated rat hippocampus. NeuroImage (2006)
12. Wedeen, V.J., et al.: Mapping complex tissue architecture with diffusion spectrum magnetic resonance imaging. MRM 54(6) (2005)
13. Frank, L.R.: Characterization of anisotropy in high angular resolution diffusion-weighted MRI. MRM 47(6) (2002)
14. Hess, C.P., Mukherjee, P., Han, E.T., Xu, D., Vigneron, D.B.: Q-ball reconstruction of multimodal fiber orientations using the spherical harmonic basis. MRM (2006)
15. Jian, B., Vemuri, B.C., Özarslan, E., Carney, P.R., Mareci, T.H.: A novel tensor distribution model for the diffusion weighted mr signal. NeuroImage (2007)
16. Knutsson, H.: Producing a continuous and distance preserving 5-d vector repesentation of 3-d orientation. In: IEEE Computer Society Workshop on Computer Architecture for Pattern Analysis and Image Database Management (1985)
17. Kumar, R., Barmpoutis, A., Vemuri, B.C., Carney, P.R., Mareci, T.H.: Multi-fiber reconstruction from dw-MRI using a continuous mixture of von mises-fisher distributions. MMBIA (2008)
18. Lawson, C., Hanson, R.J.: Solving Least Squares Problems. Prentice-Hall, Englewood Cliffs (1974)
19. Mardia, K.V., Jupp, P.: Directional Statistics, 2nd edn. John Wiley, New York (2000)
20. McGraw, T.E., Vemuri, B.C., Yezierski, R., Mareci, T.H.: Von Mises-Fisher mixture model of the diffusion ODF. In: ISBI (2006)
21. Özarslan, E., Shepherd, T.M., Vemuri, B.C., Blackband, S.J., Mareci, T.H.: Resolution of complex tissue microarchitecture using the diffusion orientation transform (DOT). NeuroImage 31, 1086–1103 (2006)
22. Özarslan, E., Mareci, T.H.: Generalized diffusion tensor imaging and analytical relationships between diffusion tensor imaging and high angular resolution diffusion imaging. MRM 50(5) (2003)
23. Söderman, O., Jönsson, B.: Restricted diffusion in cylindirical geometry. J. Magn. Reson. B 117(1) (1995)
24. Tournier, J.-D., Calamante, F., Gadian, D.G., Connelly, A.: Direct estimation of the fiber orientation density function from diffusion-weighted MRI data using spherical deconvolution. NeuroImage (2004)
25. Tuch, D.S., Reese, T.G., Wiegell, M.R., Makris, N., Belliveau, J.W., Wedeen, V.J.: High angular resolution diffusion imaging reveals intravoxel white matter fiber heterogeneity. MRM (2002)

Regression Models of Atlas Appearance

Torsten Rohlfing[1], Edith V. Sullivan[2], and Adolf Pfefferbaum[1,2]

[1] Neuroscience Program, SRI International, Menlo Park, CA, USA
torsten@synapse.sri.com, dolf@synapse.sri.com
[2] Department of Psychiatry and Behavioral Sciences, Stanford University, Stanford CA, USA
edie@stanford.edu

Abstract. Models of object appearance based on principal components analysis provide powerful and versatile tools in computer vision and medical image analysis. A major shortcoming is that they rely entirely on the training data to extract principal modes of appearance variation and ignore underlying variables (e.g., subject age, gender). This paper introduces an appearance modeling framework based instead on generalized multi-linear regression. The training of regression appearance models is controlled by independent variables. This makes it straightforward to create model instances for specific values of these variables, which is akin to model interpolation. We demonstrate the new framework by creating an appearance model of the human brain from MR images of 36 subjects. Instances of the model created for different ages are compared with average shape atlases created from age-matched sub-populations. Relative tissue volumes vs. age in models are also compared with tissue volumes vs. subject age in the original images. In both experiments, we found excellent agreement between the regression models and the comparison data. We conclude that regression appearance models are a promising new technique for image analysis, with one potential application being the representation of a continuum of mutually consistent, age-specific atlases of the human brain.

1 Introduction

This paper describes framework for creating models of object appearance. Whereas principal component analysis (PCA) drives the common active shape model (ASM) pioneered by Cootes *et al.* [1], our framework is instead based on a generalized linear regression model (GLRM). On a high level of abstracting, one can think of the difference between these two approaches as supervised (GLRM) vs. unsupervised (PCA) learning of the model. While regression has been used for non-linear refinement of PCA-based ASMs [2] and for shape regression [3], we believe that this is the first application of regression to generate appearance models.

The immediate benefit of using regression instead of PCA is that it explicitly models the changes of appearance in response to independent variables, such as subject age or sex (see schematic comparison of PCA-based vs. regression shape model in Fig. 1). Such a model is, therefore, able to generate instances linked to specific sets of independent variable values, which we demonstrate herein by creating an appearance regression model of the human brain. Using this model, we are able to generate atlases of the brain for specific ages, sexes, or, in future work, disease conditions.

J.L. Prince, D.L. Pham, and K.J. Myers (Eds.): IPMI 2009, LNCS 5636, pp. 151–162, 2009.

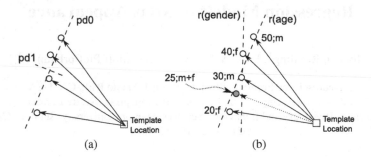

Fig. 1. Schematic comparison of shape models based on PCA and regression, each using the same mapping of one template point location to four corresponding data point locations. *(a)* The PCA-based model provides two orthogonal principal directions based entirely on the data point locations. *(b)* The regression-based model (here, multi-linear model) provides one regression line per independent variable (here, age and sex). The regression lines are not necessarily orthogonal. Unlike the PCA-based model, the regression model can be instantiated for specific independent variable values (here, marked by the solid circle, 25 years of age, half male/half female).

Atlases of human brain anatomy have an important role in studies of brain anatomy and function. They serve as standard reference coordinate systems, to which data from all subjects in typical imaging-based studies are registered for statistical analysis. They can also be used to outline regions of interest, which can then be propagated via registration to images from individual subjects (i.e., atlas-based segmentation [4])

When based on a single individual [5], an atlas represents an anatomy associated with a well-determined set of subject independent variable values (e.g., that person's age and sex). When an entire group of subjects is used to construct a population atlas [6], on the other hand, then the atlas is representative for an entire range of independent variable values, but it is no longer specific.

For the study of the human brain, the regression-based modeling framework bridges the gap between these two concepts: the atlas regression model covers an entire range of independent variable values, according to the individual images, from which it was created, yet every instance we create from the model corresponds to a specific set of independent variable values. From the same input population we can thus create many different atlases, each specific, but *all related to one another* by dense mutual coordinate correspondences. Regions of interest outlined on one atlas instance transfer immediately to all other instances from the same model, which enables comparable studies of different subject populations, each of them using a study-appropriate atlas.

The remainder of this paper is organized as follows. Section 2 describes the general mathematical framework behind the regression appearance model. Section 3 describes the application of the regression appearance model to generate atlases from multi-modality MR image data acquired from 36 subjects. Section 4 presents atlases resulting from this population, analyzed in terms of how well they model effects (e.g., age) in the input data. Section 5 discusses of the benefits of regression appearance models and differences between them and PCA-based models.

2   Regression Appearance Model

In this section, we introduce the mathematical framework of the regression appearance model. The purpose of this model is to determine the correspondence between subject independent variables and image appearance based on co-registered images. The principal idea is illustrated by a data flow diagram in Fig. 2. A regression shape model [3] is first constructed from spatial correspondences between the input images via regression over the independent variables associated with them. Correspondences are determined herein via image registrations (see Section 3.3 for details), which relates our model to the statistical deformation model [7], but landmark-based point correspondences are an equally valid input.

When the shape model is instantiated for a particular set of atlas independent variables, all input images can be separately reformatted into the model coordinate space. In this space, we then perform a second regression on the reformatted image intensities at each pixel. The result of instantiating the second regression model is then the final atlas, which combines the two models for shape and intensity appearance.

2.1   Definitions

For $k = 1, \ldots, K$, let I_k be images from K subjects. For each k, let $\vec{p}_k$ be a vector of length P, which contains the values of P independent variables for subject k. Numerical independent variables, such as age, are used directly, whereas discrete independent variables, such as sex and diagnosis, are binary dummy-coded as 0 and 1.[1]

Furthermore, let $\Omega = \{\vec{x}_n | 0 < n \leq N\}$ be the voxel coordinates of a template grid to which all K images are registered. For each input image I_k, the template space thus relates to the space of I_k via the deformation field $U_k = \{\vec{u}_{k,n} \in \mathbb{R}^3 | 0 < n \leq N\}$ such that

$$\vec{x}_n \mapsto \vec{x}_n \mid \vec{u}_{k,n}. \tag{1}$$

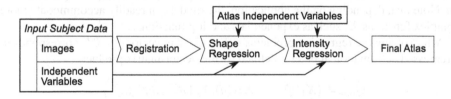

Fig. 2. Data flow diagram. Coordinate transformations are determined between the input images via image registration. The resulting transformations are then used to create a shape regression model based on the subjects' independent variable values. The latter are then also used to obtain local regression models of pixel intensities. The combined shape and intensity models are instantiated for selected atlas independent variables to create the final atlas.

---

[1] As an example, with independent variables age, sex, and Alzheimer's disease, a 56 year-old control man could be represented by $\vec{p} = (56, 1, 0)$, whereas a 65 year-old woman with Alzheimer's disease would analogously be represented by $\vec{p} = (65, 0, 1)$.

To account for differences in pose, orientation, and scale [7], the pure deformation (excluding affine) component is determined for each pixel n as

$$(d_{k,n}^x, d_{k,n}^y, d_{k,n}^z)^T = \mathbf{J}_k^{-1} \vec{u}_{k,n},$$ (2)

where $\mathbf{J}_k$ is the Jacobian of the global affine transformation T_k that maps from the template space to the space of image I_k.

2.2 Shape Regression

Shape regression is performed by constructing, via a GLRM [8], a deformation field that maps the original template space into a space corresponding to a given set of subject independent variables. To this end, one needs to solve (via singular value decomposition, see [9], Chapter 15.4) the three regression problems

$$\vec{b}_n^x = \mathbf{G}\vec{a}_n^x, \vec{b}_n^y = \mathbf{G}\vec{a}_n^y, \text{ and } \vec{b}_n^z = \mathbf{G}\vec{a}_n^z$$ (3)

for $\vec{a}_n^x, \vec{y}_n^z, \vec{a}_n^z$ at each pixel n. Here,

$$\vec{b}_n^x = (d_{1,n}^x, \ldots, d_{K,n}^x)^T, \vec{b}_n^y = (d_{1,n}^y, \ldots, d_{K,n}^y)^T, \text{ and } \vec{b}_n^z = (d_{1,n}^z, \ldots, d_{K,n}^z)^T$$ (4)

are the observed deformation vector components for the K inputs. The design matrix

$$\mathbf{G} = \begin{pmatrix} X_1(\vec{p}_1) & \cdots & X_M(\vec{p}_1) & 1 \\ \vdots & \ddots & \vdots & \vdots \\ X_1(\vec{p}_K) & \cdots & X_M(\vec{p}_K) & 1 \end{pmatrix}$$ (5)

is composed of M functions applied to each of the subject independent variables for $k = 1, \ldots K$. Later in this paper, we use two particular models: a first-order (linear) and a second-order (quadratic) model. For the linear model, $M = P$ and $X_m(\vec{p}) \equiv p_m$. The second-order model contains all functions of the linear model and incorporates as additional functions X all second-order monomials of the elements in $\vec{p}$. For example, the first two additional functions could be $X_{P+1}(\vec{p}) \equiv p_1^2$, $X_{P+2}(\vec{p}) \equiv p_1 p_2$, and so on. Note that, depending on the application, the model can readily accommodate more complex functions X, such as exponentials and log functions.

After solving the regression problems in Eq. (3), any vector $\vec{q} \in \mathbb{R}^P$ corresponds to a regressed deformation at pixel n defined by the vector-matrix product

$$\vec{Q}_{\vec{q},n} = (X_1(\vec{q}), \ldots, X_M(\vec{q}), 1) \left(\vec{a}_n^{(x)}, \vec{a}_n^{(y)}, \vec{a}_n^{(z)} \right).$$ (6)

Taken over all n, these deformation vectors define a deformation field, $\mathbf{Q}_{\vec{q}}$, that maps coordinates from the original template space to the regression space corresponding to $\vec{q}$ via

$$\vec{x}_n \mapsto \vec{x}_n + \vec{Q}_{\vec{q},n}.$$ (7)

In the simplest application of $\mathbf{Q}_{\vec{q}}$, its inversion[2] can be used to reformat the non-regression template into the new coordinate space.

---

[2] See Noblet et al. [10] for a survey of numerical deformation field inversion techniques.

2.3 Intensity Regression

Once the regression-based deformation $\mathbf{Q}_{\vec{p}}$ has been determined for a given indepen-dent variable vector $\vec{q}$, all K input images can be reformatted directly into the corresponding space by concatenating the numerical inversion of $\mathbf{Q}_{\vec{q}}$ with the template-to-subject transformation U_k.

The resulting K reformatted images, now all in the same space with pixel-by-pixel correspondence, can be combined into the final atlas image. Instead of using the usual intensity averaging, however, we use the same regression model already used to construct the regression template coordinate space.

For that, the design matrix, $\mathbf{G}$, is identical to the one used for deformation field regression, $\vec{b}_n$ contains the intensities of the K corresponding intensities in the refor-matted images at pixel n, and the final image intensity is given by scalar multiplication of instantiation variable values $\vec{q}$ and fitted parameters $\vec{a}_n$.

3 Application to Atlas Generation

3.1 Subjects and Imaging

Images were acquired from 36 subjects, 18 men and 18 women. The average age of the men was 51.3 years (range=20 to 83), that of the women 53.2 years (range=20 to 85). These subjects were subdivided in three distinct age groups: young (25.5 ± 4.3, range = 20 to 33 years), middle-aged (52.4 ± 4.4, range = 46 to 58), and elderly (77.7 ± 4.9, range = 67 to 85 years). Each age group comprised six men and six women. All subjects were right-handed, non-smoking, and healthy, recruited from the local community for ongoing studies in our group.

Four imaging sequences were collected on a 3.0T GE scanner. For T_1-weighted structural images, acquisition parameters were: 3D axial IR-prep SPoiled Gradient Recalled (SPGR), TR=6.5 ms, TE=1.54 ms, thick=1.25 mm, skip=0, locations=124. For T_2-weighted and proton density-weighted imaging: 2D axial dual-echo fast spin echo (FSE), TR=10,000 ms, TE=14/98 ms, thick=2.5 mm, skip=0, locations=62. Acquisi-tion parameters for diffusion tensor imaging were: 2D echo-planar diffusion-weighted images (DWI), TR=7500 ms, TE=97.6 ms, thick=2.5 mm, skip=0, locations=62, b=0 (5 NEX), plus 15 non-collinear diffusion directions b=860 s/mm² (2 NEX), plus 15 op-posite polarity non-collinear diffusion directions b=860 s/mm² (2 NEX) FOV=240 mm, x-dim=96, y-dim=96, reconstructed to 128×128 pixels. For field map computation to spatially unwarp DWI: 2D axial dual-echo gradient echo (GRE)TR=460 ms, TE=3/5 ms, thick=2.5 mm, skip=0, locations=62.

3.2 Image Pre-processing

The SPGR and FSE images were corrected for B_1-induced intensity bias fields by applying a second-order polynomial multiplicative bias field, computed using an in-house implementation of a model-free entropy-minimization algorithm [11]. A brain mask was extracted from the late-echo FSE image using the FSL Brain Extraction Tool, BET [12], which was propagated to the SPGR and early-echo FSE images via co-registration. The skull-stripped SPGR images were then segmented using FAST [13] into probability maps for gray matter (GM), white matter (WM), and cerebrospinal fluid (CSF).

In the DWI, eddy-current distortions were minimized on a slice-by-slice basis by within-slice registration that takes advantage of the symmetry of the opposing polarity acquisition [14]. The individual repeat acquisitions for each diffusion direction were averaged, eliminating the need to account for the cross terms between imaging and diffusion gradients producing 15 images per location for tensor computation. A field map was constructed from the complex difference image between two echoes (3 and 5 ms) of the GRE after unwrapping with FSL's PRELUDE tool. B_0 inhomogeneity distortion was corrected with FUGUE, the FSL Utility for Geometrically Unwarping EPIs [15]. Tensor fields were then reconstructed, and maps of fractional anisotropy (FA) and mean diffusivity (MD) computed, using Camino [16].

3.3   Groupwise Alignment

The entire intersubject registration procedure is applied to bias-corrected SPGR images. It is described in detail in an earlier paper and is, therefore, only summarized here. An empty template coordinate space, which is defined independently of the N input images, is mapped to each of these images spaces via a coordinate transformation, $\mathbf{T}_n$, for $0 < n \leq N$.

The initial, linear alignments are 9-parameter affine transformations (shift, rotation, anisotropic scale). These were computed using a multi-image generalization of mutual information based on a continuous approximation of joint and marginal image entropies [17]. The nonrigid transformations are represented by free-form deformations based on third-order B-splines [18]. These were computed using a stack entropy image similarity measure [19]. Both registration stages employed a simple but effective multi-level, multi-resolution gradient descent scheme. Both stages also enforced zero sums over all images for each of the transformation parameters, which is a hard constraint based on the regularization term proposed by Studholme & Cardenas [20].

4   Results

Nonrigid shape (i.e., excluding scale) differences between male and female atlases, while clearly present, were small compared with aging effects (see Fig. 3). All regression atlases shown below are, therefore, mixed-sex atlases with equal male and female contributions. In Fig. 4, representative axial slices are shown from the SPGR, tissue classification, FA, and MD channels of regression atlases created in age increments of 10 years. The regressed tissue classifications were generated by mapping the individual tissue classifications into regressed atlas space, followed by label voting. The typical aging effects (increasing CSF volume, decreasing FA, increasing MD) are readily apparent from these images.

4.1   First vs. Second Order Models: Comparison with Sub-population Atlases

One way to assess whether the regression appearance model is effective at modeling the effect of independent variables on brain structure is to compare an atlas generated by

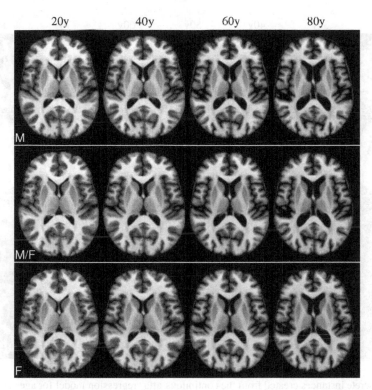

Fig. 3. Comparison of sex vs. age effects in atlases instantiated from the same 36-subject regression model. *Top row:* all-male atlases, *middle row:* male/female mixed-sex atlases, *bottom row:* all-female atlases. Note that affine differences including scale were eliminated from the model (see text).

the model with one generated from a parameter-matched population of subjects. More precisely, for each of the three 12-subject age groups in our input population, we create a separate brain atlas using the same registration technique outlined in Section 3.3. We then compare the resulting atlas with one generated by the 36-subject regression model for the age defined by the mean age of the 12-subject subgroup.

The atlases created by both a first-order and a second-order model are shown with corresponding slices of the respective subgroup atlases in Fig. 5. There are some differences in the cortical folding patterns, which is not surprising given the distinct sets of input individuals. In general, however, and in particular for subcortical structures, all atlases are highly consistent with each other. The second-order model appears to capture the accelerating increase in lateral ventricle volume better than the first-order model, which is particularly evident by comparing difference images between the middle-aged and older atlas images (Fig. 5, second and third row).

4.2 Age Effects: Regression Atlases vs. Subjects

For each subject and for each atlas shown in Fig. 4, we computed the relative volumes of cerebrospinal fluid (CSF), gray matter (GM), and white matter (WM) in percent of

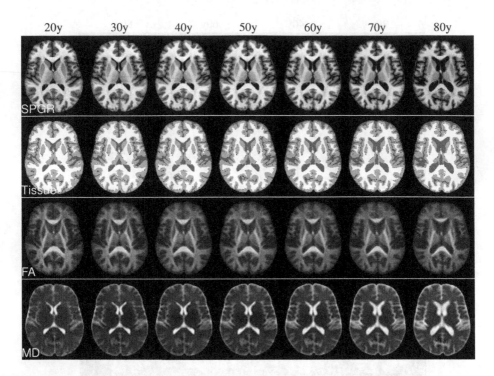

Fig. 4. Discrete instances created from the continuous atlas regression model for ages 20 through 80 years in 10 year increments. *Rows from top to bottom:* SPGR, maximum-likelihood tissue segmentation, DTI-FA, and DTI-MD.

intra-cranial volume (ICV). For each of the three "tissue" types, these relative volumes are plotted against age in Fig. 6. There is excellent agreement between the relative volumes in subjects and regression atlases for all three tissue types, albeit with slight overestimation of WM volume and underestimation of CSF volume. Note that the overall effects of increasing CSF volume, decreasing GM volume, but constant WM volume are perfectly consistent with well-established aging effects in the brain [21].

Well-known aging effects of decreasing FA and increasing MD with age are also shown by our subject population and modeled by the regression atlases, as is shown in Fig. 7. We note here that the slope of the age effects is modeled quite accurately, as is (in the second-order regression atlases at least) the well-established increasing speedup of both effects with age.

The regression models that we created are consistently over-estimating FA and under-estimating MD compared with the individual input images. We note, however, that simply averaging over all WM pixels is quite crude and ignores effects such as anterior-posterior gradients in aging effects on the brain. More importantly perhaps, the tissue classification in the regression atlases in some sense represents a combination of multiple classifications (one from each input image), which has been shown in other contexts to be more accurate than the individual classifications [22]. Applying more accurate WM maps (i.e., one that includes fewer non-WM pixels) in the regression atlases than in the individual images would certainly explain a bias towards higher FA and lower MD as observed here.

5 Discussion

This paper has described a method for modeling atlas appearance, based on regression rather than PCA. The effectiveness of the framework was demonstrated by applying it to generate models of human brain atlas appearance that depended on subject age and sex. Atlases instantiated from these models showed excellent agreement with three subgroup atlases created from young, middle-aged, and older subjects separately via groupwise registration. The regression atlases also accurately modeled aging effects on tissue volumes and DTI measures observed in the input data, and consistent with the neuroscience literature [21].

It is important to emphasize that the regression model of appearance is not intended, nor able, to replace PCA-based models for every application. Indeed, both methods complement each other: in applications where there are no meaningful independent variables, the PCA-based model is the only one applicable. This is, for example, the case with one standard example of shape models, the training of hand outlines [1]. In cases where controlled independent variables determine the data, however, the regression-based model can make use of this *a priori* knowledge.

From a theoretical point of view, there are also some relevant differences between the PCA-based and regression-based model: whereas the PCA uses explicit coupling, for example over all pixels in an image or deformation field, via the joint covariance matrix, the regression model uses an implicit coupling via the use of the same regression design matrix at every pixel. The regression model furthermore imposes more intuitive bounds on instantiated values of independent variables, i.e., it is intuitive from the training data, at what point the model instantiation turns from an interpolation into an extrapolation.

As with other regression methods, problems in our framework can arise from cor-related independent variables, for example when all diseased subjects are men, and all controls are women. In such cases, the method can be extended to partial least squares regression [23] by first performing PCA on the original independent variables, and then performing regression with respect to the dominant principal components. While this would remedy numerical problems, the model created from such a pathological subject population would suffer from the inability to separate the effects of correlated variables, a problem remedied by study design rather than post-acquisition analysis.

One important application of immediate interest for our work are the popular "op-timized VBM" [24] studies, which commonly use *study-specific templates* for spatial normalization. These templates are generated from the data to be analyzed (or a "nor-mal" subgroup thereof), and thus the results represented within their coordinate systems are not comparable with one another as every study uses its own specific template. Also, quality assurance must be repeated for every study-specific template used. Instead of study-specific templates, our work enables the instantiation of *study-appropriate tem-plates* from a regression model. All templates instantiated from the same model are guaranteed to be spatially compatible with one another and they have high certainty to be of identical quality.

First-order Model Instantiation   Second-order Model Instantiation   Subgroup Atlas

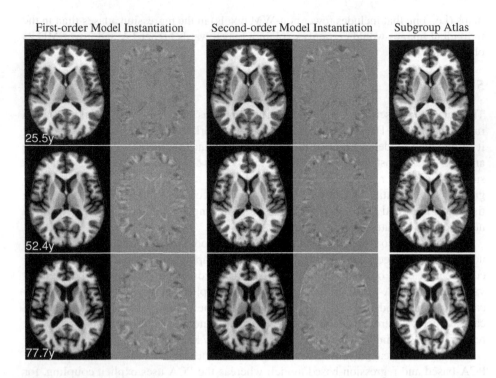

Fig. 5. Comparison of regression atlases instantiated for the mean subject age in each group of the three age groups with atlases computed independently from each group. *Top to bottom:* young, middle-aged, elderly group. *Left column:* SPGR for first-order model regression atlas and difference with subgroup atlas. *Middle column:* SPGR for second-order model regression atlas and difference with subgroup atlas. *Right column:* subgroup atlas. All difference image are shown using the same gray level scale, centered at zero.

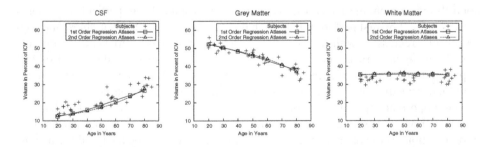

Fig. 6. Comparison of tissue volume vs. age in subjects and regression atlases. *Left to right:* CSF, gray matter, white matter. All tissue volumes are relative to the ICV to account for head size differences. Measurements for first-order and second-order regression atlases are connected by line segments. There are no regression lines in these figures, i.e., the lines representing the regression atlases are measurements in their own right and not fits of the subject measurements.

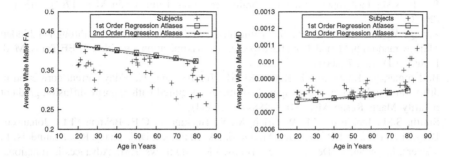

Fig. 7. FA and MD vs age effects in regression atlases compared with individual subjects. *Left:* mean FA, averaged over all pixels classified as white matter in each subject and each atlas. *Right:* mean MD, averaged over all white matter pixels.

Acknowledgments

This work was supported by grants AG017919, AA005965, and AA12388.

References

1. Cootes, T.F., Taylor, C.J., Cooper, D.H., Graham, J.: Active shape models – Their training and application. Comput. Vision Image Understanding 61(1), 38–59 (1995)
2. Sozou, P., Cootes, T., Taylor, C., Di-Mauro, E.: A non-linear generalisation of PDMs using polynomial regression. In: Proceedings of the Conference on British Machine Vision, Surrey, UK, vol. 2, pp. 397–406. BMVA Press (1994)
3. Davis, B.C., Fletcher, P.T., Bullitt, E., Joshi, S.: Population shape regression from random design data. In: IEEE 11th International Conference on Computer Vision, ICCV, October 2007, pp. 1–7 (2007)
4. Miller, M.I., Christensen, G.E., Amit, Y., Grenander, U.: Mathematical textbook of deformable neuroanatomies. Proc. Natl. Acad. Sci. USA 90(24), 11944–11948 (1993)
5. Holmes, C.J., Hoge, R., Collins, L., Woods, R., Toga, A.W., Evans, A.C.: Enhancement of MR images using registration for signal averaging. J. Comput. Assist. Tomogr. 22(2), 324–333 (1998)
6. Evans, A.C., Collins, D.L.: A 305-member MRI-based stereotactic atlas for CBF activation studies. In: Proc. of the 40th Annual Meeting of the Society for Nuclear Medicine (1993)
7. Rueckert, D., Frangi, A.F., Schnabel, J.A.: Automatic construction of 3-D statistical deformation models of the brain using nonrigid registration. IEEE Trans. Med. Imag. 22(8), 1014–1025 (2003)
8. Friston, K.J., Holmes, A.P., Worsley, K.J., Poline, J.B., Frith, C., Frackowiak, R.S.J.: Statistical parametric maps in functional imaging: A general linear approach. Hum. Brain Map. 2, 189–210 (1995)
9. Press, W.H., Teukolsky, S.A., Vetterling, W.T., Flannery, B.P.: Numerical Recipes in C: The Art of Scientific Computing, 2nd edn. Cambridge University Press, Cambridge (1992)
10. Noblet, V., Heinrich, C., Heitz, F., Armspach, J.P.: Accurate inversion of 3-D transformation fields. IEEE Trans. Image Processing 17(10), 1963–1968 (2008)
11. Likar, B., Viergever, M.A., Pernus, F.: Retrospective correction of MR intensity inhomogeneity by information minimization. IEEE Trans. Med. Imag. 20(12), 1398–1410 (2001)

12. Smith, S.M.: Fast robust automated brain extraction. Hum. Brain Map. 17(3), 143–155 (2002)
13. Zhang, Y., Brady, M., Smith, S.: Segmentation of brain MR images through a hidden Markov random field model and the expectation-maximization algorithm. IEEE Trans. Med. Imag. 20(1), 45–57 (2001)
14. Bodammer, N., Kaufmann, J., Kanowski, M., Tempelmann, C.: Eddy current correction in diffusion-weighted imaging using pairs of images acquired with opposite diffusion gradient polarity. Magn. Reson. Med. 51(1), 188–193 (2004)
15. Smith, S.M., Jenkinson, M., Woolrich, M.W., Beckmann, C.F., Behrens, T.E., Johansen-Berg, H., Bannister, P.R., De Luca, M., Drobnjak, I., Flitney, D.E., Niazy, R.K., Saunders, J., Vickers, J., Zhang, Y., De Stefano, N., Brady, J.M., Matthews, P.M.: Advances in functional and structural MR image analysis and implementation as FSL. NeuroImage 24(S1), 208–219 (2004)
16. Cook, P.A., Bai, Y., Nedjati-Gilani, S., Seunarine, K.K., Hall, M.G., Parker, G.J., Alexander, D.C.: Camino: Open-source diffusion-MRI reconstruction and processing. In: 14th Scientific Meeting of the International Society for Magnetic Resonance in Medicine, Seattle, WA, USA, May 2006, p. 2759 (2006)
17. Russakoff, D.B., Tomasi, C., Rohlfing, T., Maurer Jr., C.R.: Image similarity using mutual information of regions. In: Pajdla, T., Matas, J.(G.) (eds.) ECCV 2004. LNCS, vol. 3023, pp. 596–607. Springer, Heidelberg (2004)
18. Rueckert, D., Sonoda, L.I., Hayes, C., Hill, D.L.G., Leach, M.O., Hawkes, D.J.: Nonrigid registration using free-form deformations: Application to breast MR images. IEEE Trans. Med. Imag. 18(8), 712–721 (1999)
19. Learned-Miller, E.G.: Data driven image models through continuous joint alignment. IEEE Trans. Pattern Anal. Machine Intell. 28(2), 236–250 (2006)
20. Studholme, C., Cardenas, V.: A template free approach to volumetric spatial normalization of brain anatomy. Pattern Recogn. Lett. 25(10), 1191–1202 (2004)
21. Pfefferbaum, A., Mathalon, D.H., Sullivan, E.V., Rawles, J.M., Zipursky, R.B., Lim, K.O.: A quantitative magnetic resonance imaging study of changes in brain morphology from infancy to late adulthood. Arch. Neurol. 51(9), 874–887 (1994)
22. Rohlfing, T., Brandt, R., Menzel, R., Maurer Jr., C.R.: Evaluation of atlas selection strategies for atlas-based image segmentation with application to confocal microscopy images of bee brains. NeuroImage 21(4), 1428–1442 (2004)
23. Wold, S., Ruhe, A., Would, H., Dunn, W.: The collinearity problem in linear regression. The partial least squares (PLS) approach to generalized inverses. SIAM J. Sci. Stat. Comput. 5(3), 735–743 (1984)
24. Good, C.D., Johnsrude, I.S., Ashburner, J., Henson, R.N.A., Friston, K.J., Frackowiak, R.S.J.: A voxel-based morphometric study of ageing in 465 normal adult human brains. NeuroImage 14(1), 21–36 (2001)

Non-rigid Image Registration with Uniform Spherical Structure Patterns

Shu Liao and Albert C.S. Chung

Lo Kwee-Seong Medical Image Analysis Laboratory,
Department of Computer Science and Engineering,
The Hong Kong University of Science and Technology, Hong Kong
liaoshu@cse.ust.hk, achung@cse.ust.hk

Abstract. Non-rigid image registration is a challenging task in medical image analysis. In recent years, there are two essential issues. First, intensity similarity is not necessarily equivalent to anatomical similarity when the anatomical correspondences between subject and template images are established. Second, the registration algorithm should be robust against monotonic gray-level transformation when aligning anatomical structures in the presence of bias fields. In this paper, a new feature based non-rigid registration method is proposed to deal with these two problems. The proposed method is based on a new type of image feature, called Uniform Spherical Structure Pattern (USSP). USSP encodes voxel-wise interaction information and geometric properties of anatomical structures. It is computationally efficient, rotation invariant and theoretically monotonic gray-level transformation invariant. The USSP feature is integrated with the Markov random field (MRF) discrete labeling framework to define energy function for registration in this paper. If the segmentation results are available, explicit anatomical correspondence can be established as an additional energy term. The energy function is optimized via the *alpha*-expansion algorithms. The proposed method is compared with three widely used non-rigid registration methods on both simulated and real databases obtained from BrainWeb and IBSR. Experimental results demonstrate that the proposed method achieves the highest registration accuracy among all the compared methods.

1 Introduction

Non-rigid image registration plays an important role in medical image analysis. Its clinical applications include, but not limited to, anatomical analysis and statistical parametric mapping. Many novel methods have been proposed during the last decade. They can be broadly classified into three categories: landmark based, intensity based and feature based registration methods. Landmark based registration methods extract anatomical features from manually located landmark points. Transformations are estimated based on such anatomical features [1,2]. Landmark based registration methods use prior knowledge obtained from manually placed landmark points and thus they are usually computationally efficient.

J.L. Prince, D.L. Pham, and K.J. Myers (Eds.): IPMI 2009, LNCS 5636, pp. 163–175, 2009.
© Springer-Verlag Berlin Heidelberg 2009

However, to produce accurate registration results, these methods need sufficient number of landmark points and therefore require additional burdens. Intensity based registration methods define a similarity measure metric evaluated from voxel intensity distributions to guide the registration process [3,4]. An essential issue related to intensity based registration methods is intensity similarity is not necessarily equivalent to anatomical similarity. Feature based registration methods use feature vectors as signatures for each voxel. Then the registration process is formulated as a feature matching and optimization problem.

Despite the fact that many aforementioned methods have been proposed to tackle the non-rigid registration problem, two challenges arise in recent years. First, the goal of non-rigid image registration is to establish anatomical correspondence between the template and the subject images. Using absolute voxel intensity values alone to characterize anatomical properties may be insufficient, as pointed out in [5], and can make the similarity measure function stuck at local minima. As such, effective anatomical region descriptor is needed. Second, the registration algorithm should be robust against monotonic gray-level bias fields, which commonly exist during the imaging process. Otherwise, the registration algorithm may prefer to align the bias fields instead of aligning anatomical structures, as discussed in [6].

Therefore, we are motivated to propose a new feature based non-rigid registration method which can accurately capture the geometric properties of the anatomical structures and theoretically robust against the monotonic gray-level bias fields. There are three main contributions in this paper. (i) A new anatomical region descriptor, called uniform spherical structure pattern (USSP) is designed to capture the anatomical geometry of the input images. (ii) The USSP descriptor is theoretically invariant to monotonic gray-level bias fields and image rotation. (iii) If the segmentation results of input images are available, an explicit anatomical energy term based on the Fisher's separation criteria (FSC) is proposed to measure the distance of different tissue classes between the subject and the template images. Markov random field (MRF) discrete labeling has been shown to be a robust framework to model the non-rigid registration process in recent years [7,8]. In this paper, the USSP feature is integrated with the MRF labeling framework to define the energy function which guides the registration process. The α-expansion algorithm is used to minimize the MRF energy function. The proposed method is evaluated on both the simulated and real 3D databases obtained from BrainWeb and IBSR and compared with three widely used registration algorithms. It is observed that the proposed method achieves the highest registration accuracy among all the compared methods.

2   Feature Extraction with Uniform Spherical Structure Patterns

In this section, we describe the design details of the uniform spherical structure pattern (USSP) region descriptor, analyze its properties, and show how to use USSP to extract anatomical features from input images.

2.1 Basic Spherical Structure Patterns

Suppose for a given input image G, for each voxel $v \in G$, we define a sphere S_v, which is centered at v with radius R. N_v samples are uniformly taken on the surface of S_v using the sampling method proposed in [9]. Samples which do not fall exactly into the image grid are interpolated by using the trilinear interpolation method. Then, for each voxel i on the surface of S_v, it is thresholded to binary numbers "0" or "1" by using the Equation 1:

$$B_i = \begin{cases} 0, \text{if } I_i < I_v, \\ 1, \text{if } I_i \geq I_v, \end{cases} \tag{1}$$

where I_i is the intensity of voxel i, and I_v is the intensity of the center voxel v.

The thresholded surface represents the geometric features surrounding the voxel v as the binary values reflect the voxel-wise interactions between the neighboring voxels and the center voxel. The thresholded surface is called the basic spherical structure pattern (BSSP). Local binary pattern [10] is a special case of BSSP in the 2D case. The formal definition of BSSP is given as follows:

Definition 1: *Basic spherical structure pattern (BSSP) is the thresholded spherical surface obtained from the original spherical neighborhood centered at the reference voxel by using the Equation 1.*

BSSP is monotonic gray-level transformation invariant because the neighboring voxels are converted to the binary digits by comparing their intensity values with the center voxel intensity. As long as the relative difference between two voxel intensity values does not change, the thresholded surface remains the same.

2.2 Uniform Spherical Structure Patterns

Though the BSSP proposed in Section 2.1 is monotonic gray-level transformation invariant, there are many types of BSSP which are too sparse to reliably reflect the anatomical features of input images. In this section, we define the uniform spherical structure pattern (USSP) which is a subset of BSSP and represents fundamental image structures. USSP is defined as follows:

Definition 2: *Uniform spherical structure patterns (USSP) are basic spherical structure patterns (BSSP), which have AT MOST two continuous regions of "0"s and "1"s.*

For example, Figures 1 (a) and (b) are USSPs, while Figure 1 (c) is not a USSP. The pseudo code of determining whether a BSSP is a USSP or not is presented in the Algorithm 1. The time complexity of the Algorithm 1 is analyzed as follows. Finding the largest connected component by using the BFS algorithm needs $O(N)$ time. Operation 3 also needs $O(N)$ time in the worst case. Other operations take constant computation time. Therefore, the Algorithm 1 takes $O(N)$ time, which is a linear time algorithm.

Algorithm 1. Determining whether a BSSP is a USSP

Input: A BSSP with radius R and N neighboring voxels on the surface.

Output: true or false (whether the input is a USSP or not).

1. Randomly select a neighboring voxel i on the surface of the input BSSP
2. Find the largest connected component starting from i based on its binary digit B_i using the Breadth First Search (BFS), set a flag for each voxel belonging to that largest connected component
3. FOR each unflagged neighboring voxel $t \in BSSP$ with binary digit B_t
4.   IF ($B_t == B_i$)
5.   Return false
6.   END IF
7. END FOR
8. Return true

USSP contains important physical meanings regarding the fundamental image structures. For example, Figure 1 (a) represents a dark spot as all the surrounding voxels' intensity values are higher than or equal to the intensity of the center voxel. Figure 1 (b) reflects that there is an edge along the center voxel as half of the neighboring voxels' intensity values are lower than the intensity of the center voxel and lie on the same continuous region, while the other half of the neighboring voxels just act as the opposite. All the non-uniform spherical structure patterns are considered as a single type of image structure in this paper.

To further illustrate that USSP encodes dominant information and represents the fundamental image structures, Figures 2 (a) to (c) plot the proportions of USSPs among all the BSSPs with different parameters for 20 image volumes

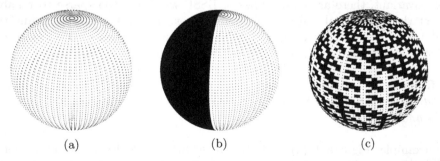

(a)   (b)   (c)

Fig. 1. (a) An example of USSP, with all "1"s (white region) on the surface. There is only one continuous region of all "1"s on the surface; (b) An example of USSP, with half the surface of "0"s (black region) and half the surface of "1"s (white region). There are two continuous regions (i.e., one with "0"s, the other with "1"s); (c) An example of non-uniform SSP. There are more than two continuous regions with "0"s and "1"s on the surface.

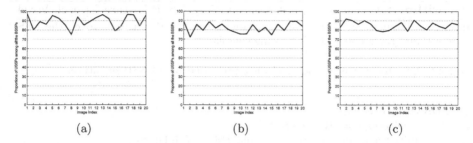

(a)   (b)   (c)

Fig. 2. Proportions (in %) of USSPs among all the BSSPs of 20 image volumes obtained from IBSR, with parameters: (a) Radius = 1, Number of Neighboring Samples = 25; (b) Radius = 2, Number of Neighboring Samples = 36; (c) Radius = 3, Number of Neighboring Samples = 49

obtained from IBSR[1]. It is observed from Figure 2 that USSPs have dominant proportions among all the BSSPs (i.e., mostly over 80%) with different parameters. Therefore, USSP can reliably capture the anatomical properties of the input image volumes. In the rest of the paper, we will only focus on extracting USSP features from the input images.

2.3   Feature Extraction of Rotation Invariant USSPs

Though USSP contains dominant information and represents fundamental images structures, it is still not rotation invariant up to the current stage. When the image rotates, the positions of the binary digits on the surface of USSP will be shifted accordingly. As pointed out in [11], rotation invariance is a desired property for feature based non-rigid registration methods.

Therefore, we design an algorithm to extract rotation invariant USSP features. It is observed that no matter how the image rotates, the region areas of "0"s and "1"s (i.e., the number of voxels belonging to "0"s and "1"s) of a USSP pattern do not change. Therefore, the number of voxels belonging to "0" or "1" binary digits can be used to denote the types of USSP, which should be invariant to rotation. In this paper, the type ID of the USSP is determined by the number of "0"s in the USSP. All the non-uniform BSSPs are treated as a single type pattern. Algorithm 2 presents the procedure for calculating rotation invariant USSP signatures for each voxel v from a local cubic square window W centered at v, assuming that the radius R and number of neighboring samples N are given. The time complexity of the Algorithm 2 is $O(|G| \times |W| \times N)$, where $|G|$ is the number of voxels of the input image G, $|W|$ is the window size and N is the number of neighboring samples used for USSP.

It should be noted that Algorithm 2 only takes care of the area of "0" region to determine the USSP type. A more detailed USSP type classification can be

---

[1] http://www.cma.mgh.harvard.edu/ibsr/

Algorithm 2. Calculate the Rotation Invariant USSP Feature for each Voxel

---

Input: An input image G, a local cubic square window W for each voxel, the USSP radius R and the number of neighboring samples N.

Output: A vector image K, each voxel is represented by a USSP signature.

1. FOR each voxel $v \in G$
2. $SubVolume = (W$ center at $v)$
3.   Initialize a new feature histogram, $H[0...(N+1)] = 0$
4.   FOR each voxel $t \in SubVolume$
5.   Calculate its corresponding BSSP Q_t with parameters R and N
6.   Determine whether Q_t is a USSP or not using Algorithm 1
7.   IF Q_t is a USSP
8. $PatternID = $ Number of "0"s in Q_t
9. $H[PatternID] = H[PatternID] + 1$
10.   ELSE
11. $H[N+1] = H[N+1] + 1$
12.   END IF
13.   END FOR
14.   Normalize $H[0...(N+1)]$ such that $\sum_{i=0}^{N+1} H[i] = 1$
15. $K(v) = H[0...(N+1)]$
16. END FOR
17. Return K

---

achieved if we also take care of the shape of the "0" region. However, there are too many possible shape combinations and will result in unstable anatomical feature description as some of the USSP occurrences are too small. This makes the USSP feature histogram too sparse to reliably mirror the anatomical properties of the input images. Radius R in the Algorithm 2 affects the scale of interest to extract the anatomical structures. In this paper, the radius R is determined by adopting the best scale selection principle proposed in [12].

The rotation invariant USSP feature also preserves the monotonic gray-level transformation invariant property of BSSP. Figure 3 shows an example. Figure 3 (a) is an image slice obtained from BrainWeb with no bias field distortion. Figure 3 (b) is a type-A bias field obtained from BrainWeb with 40% inhomogeneity. Figure 3 (c) is the resulting bias field distorted image. The region inside the green rectangle is the region of interest (ROI). The rotation invariant USSP feature vectors with 49 neighboring samples are extracted from the ROI by treating the ROI as the $SubVolume$ in the Algorithm 2. Figures 3 (f) and (g) are the rotation invariant USSP feature vectors extracted from the ROI before and after bias field distortion respectively. For comparison purpose, the intensity histograms of the ROI before and after bias field distortion are also shown in Figures 3 (d) and (e). It is observed that the intensity histograms of ROI before and after bias field distortion have large variations. The rotation invariant

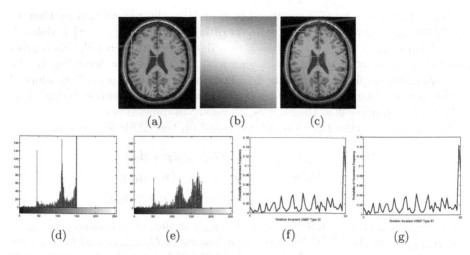

(a)   (b)   (c)

(d)   (e)   (f)   (g)

Fig. 3. (a) The original image; (b) The bias field of 40% inhomogeneity; (c) Resulting image after applying the bias field in (b) to the original image in (a); (d) Intensity histogram of ROI (green rectangle region in (a)) in the original image; (e) Intensity histogram of ROI (green rectangle region in (c)) in the bias field distorted image; (f) Rotation invariant USSP feature of ROI in the original image; (g) Rotation invariant USSP feature of ROI in the bias field distorted image

USSP feature vectors extracted from ROI before and after bias field distortion are almost the same (i.e., just with slight variations). Therefore, the robustness of the USSP features against bias field distortion is implied.

3   MRF Labeling Formulation for Registration

Recently, the MRF discrete labeling framework is shown to be able to robustly model the non-rigid registration process [7,8]. In this paper, the USSP feature is integrated with the MRF discrete labeling framework to define the energy function. An explicit anatomical correspondence energy term is also proposed based on the Fisher's separation criteria (FSC) [13,14] if the segmentation results of the input images are available.

The general form of the MRF energy function by considering clique size order up to two is expressed as:

$$E_f = E_{data} + E_{smoothness}$$
$$= \sum_{p \in \Omega} D_p(l_p) + \sum_{(p,q) \in N} V_{p,q}(l_p, l_q), \qquad (2)$$

where Ω is the set of voxels, N is the neighborhood system defined in Ω. In this paper, the 4-connected neighborhood system is used. $D_p(l_p)$ is the energy function, which penalizes the cost of assigning label l_p to voxel p, and $V_{p,q}(l_p, l_q)$ penalizes the cost of label discrepancy between two neighboring voxels.

The deformation space is quantized to transform the registration problem to the MRF labeling problem. A discrete set of labels $L \in \{l^1, l^2, ..., l^n\}$ is defined. Each label l^i $(1 \leq i \leq n)$ corresponds to a displacement vector $\boldsymbol{d_i}$. Each label assignment l_p to voxel p denotes moving p to a new position according to the corresponding displacement vector $\boldsymbol{d_{l_p}}$. The quantization step in [7] is adopted in this paper. Each voxel can be displaced off the original position bounded by a discretized window $\Psi = \{0, \pm s, \pm 2s, ..., \pm ws\}^d$ of dimension d.

The energy function $D_p(l_p)$ is defined based on the USSP features as:

$$
\begin{aligned}
D_p(l_p) &= D_p(G_{template}(\boldsymbol{p}), G_{subject}(\boldsymbol{p} + \boldsymbol{d_{l_p}}) \\
&= D_p(K_{template}(\boldsymbol{p}), K_{subject}(\boldsymbol{p} + \boldsymbol{d_{l_p}})) \\
&= JSD(K_{template}(\boldsymbol{p}) \| K_{subject}(\boldsymbol{p} + \boldsymbol{d_{l_p}})),
\end{aligned}
\tag{3}
$$

where $G_{template}$ is the template image, $G_{subject}$ is the subject image, $K_{template}$ and $K_{subject}$ are the USSP feature vector images of $G_{template}$ and $G_{subject}$ respectively obtained via the Algorithm 2. $JSD(\cdot)$ denotes the Jensen-Shannon divergence. Therefore, based on the Equation 3, the data term E_{data} at iteration t is defined as:

$$
E_{data}^t = \sum_{p \in \Omega} JSD(K_{template}(\boldsymbol{p}) \| K_{subject}^{t-1}(\boldsymbol{p} + \boldsymbol{d_{l_p}})),
\tag{4}
$$

where $K_{subject}^{t-1}$ denotes the USSP feature vector image of the subject image resulting from the previous transformation prior to iteration t.

The piece-wise truncated absolute distance is adopted as the smoothness potential function:

$$
V_{p,q}(l_p, l_q) = \min(\lambda, |\boldsymbol{d_{l_p}} - \boldsymbol{d_{l_q}}|),
\tag{5}
$$

where λ is a constant represents the maximum penalty. The truncated absolute distance is a metric as stated in [15].

If the segmentations of the template image and the subject image are available, an explicit anatomical energy term can be established as an additional energy term based on FSC. Suppose that the input images are segmented into c classes of tissues. Let $V_i^T (1 \leq i \leq c)$ and $V_i^S (1 \leq i \leq c)$ denote the volumes of voxels belonging to tissue class i of the template and the subject images, N_i^T and N_i^S denote the numbers of voxels in V_i^T and V_i^S. $\boldsymbol{F_{i,j}^T}$ and $\boldsymbol{F_{i,j}^S}$ denote the USSP feature vectors from the jth voxel of the ith class tissue of the template and the subject images at current iteration. We first calculate the mean of the ith class tissue of the template and the subject images as: $\boldsymbol{m_i^T} = \frac{1}{N_i^T} \sum_{k=1}^{N_i^T} \boldsymbol{F_{i,k}^T}$, $\boldsymbol{m_i^S} = \frac{1}{N_i^S} \sum_{k=1}^{N_i^S} \boldsymbol{F_{i,k}^S}$.

Then, according to the principles of FSC [13], the 1-D space of the projected feature vector which can maximize the separability of the feature vector cluster of V_i^T and V_i^S is given by:

$$
y_z = (\boldsymbol{m_i^T} - \boldsymbol{m_i^S})^T \mathbf{S}^{-1} \boldsymbol{F_z},
\tag{6}
$$

where $\mathbf{S}^{-1}$ is the inverse of the pooled covariance matrix, $\boldsymbol{F_z}$ is the USSP feature vector of voxel z belonging to the ith class tissue of either the template image or the subject image. Therefore, the 1-D projections of $\boldsymbol{m_i^T}$ and $\boldsymbol{m_i^S}$ according to the Equation 6 are:

$$K_i^T = (\boldsymbol{m_i^T} - \boldsymbol{m_i^S})^T \mathbf{S}^{-1} \boldsymbol{m_i^T}, \tag{7}$$

$$K_i^S = (\boldsymbol{m_i^T} - \boldsymbol{m_i^S})^T \mathbf{S}^{-1} \boldsymbol{m_i^S}. \tag{8}$$

This 1-D projection maximizes the following FSC measure function [13] of tissue class i of the template image and the subject image:

$$f_i = \frac{|K_i^T - K_i^S|}{\sqrt{(\sigma_i^T)^2 + (\sigma_i^S)^2}}, \tag{9}$$

where σ_i^T and σ_i^S are the standard deviations of the projected USSP feature vector belonging to the ith tissue class of the template image and the subject image.

When the FSC measure function in Equation 9 is minimized, the anatomical similarity of tissue class i is maximized. The explicit anatomical energy term is defined by summing up the FSC measure functions defined in the Equation 9 of all the tissue classes. Therefore, now the total energy function becomes:

$$E_f = E_{data} + E_{smoothness} + E_{anatomy}$$

$$= \sum_{p \in \Omega} D_p(l_p) + \sum_{(p,q) \in N} V_{p,q}(l_p, l_q) + \sum_{i=1}^{c} f_i. \tag{10}$$

In order to minimize the energy function defined in Equations 2 and 10, the $alpha$-expansion algorithm [15] is adopted.

4   Experimental Results

The proposed method is evaluated by performing non-rigid registration experiments on both the simulated and real 3D datasets obtained from BrainWeb[2] and IBSR[3] respectively. It is also compared with three state-of-the-art algorithms: FFD [3], Demons [4] and HAMMER [11]. In all the experiments, the local cubic square window W in the Algorithm 2 was set to $16 \times 16 \times 16$, and number of neighboring samples N of each USSP was 49. The 3D displacement window for the proposed method was $\Psi = \{0, \pm 1, \pm 2, ..., \pm 12\}^3$. The maximum penalty parameter λ defined in Equation 5 was set to 20.

---

[2] http://www.bic.mni.mcgill.ca/brainweb/
[3] http://www.cma.mgh.harvard.edu/ibsr/

Table 1. The mean values of P and SDs of GM, WM and CSF with different methods. BR denotes before registration, USSP (WOE) denotes using USSP features without the explicit anatomical energy term, USSP (WE) denotes using USSP features with the explicit anatomical energy term.

Tissue	BR	FFD	Demons	HAMMER	USSP (WOE)	USSP (WE)
Gray	0.41923±0.07	0.73816±0.06	0.77416±0.05	0.79563±0.06	0.84281±0.05	0.86725±0.04
White	0.48344±0.03	0.77825±0.04	0.78024±0.06	0.81093±0.02	0.83527±0.08	0.86103±0.07
CSF	0.37025±0.06	0.73072±0.06	0.74281±0.03	0.75682±0.02	0.79093±0.06	0.84774±0.03

4.1   Experiments with Simulated Data

In this section, the proposed method is evaluated on the simulated 3D T1 image data obtained from BrainWeb. 20 image volumes from different subjects were used. One of the image volumes was served as the template image, and the others were used as the subject images. Each image has resolution of $256 \times 256 \times 181$ voxels. The segmentation results are provided by BrainWeb. Before registration, the skull stripping process was performed on each image as it is a required step for HAMMER [11] to be compared in this paper. The software Brain Suite version 2 obtained from USC[4] was used to accomplish the skull removing process.

Figures 4 (b) to (e) show the reconstructed average brain images after the registration using FFD [3], Demons [4], HAMMER [11] and the proposed method (without explicit anatomical energy term). Figure 4 (a) is the template image for reference. The control point spacing of FFD is $2.5mm$, as suggested in [16]. It is visually observed that the proposed method achieves the best registration accuracy as the average brain images obtained via the proposed method preserve most of the details of the template image and are sharper than those obtained by the other compared methods. The tissue overlap of gray matter (GM), white matter (WM) and cerebrospinal fluid (CSF) between the template and the transformed subject images is also adopted as the evaluation measure [16] to analyze the registration accuracy. It is defined as $P = \frac{N(A \cap B)}{N(A \cup B)}$, where A and B denote the regions of a specific tissue in two images. The average values of P and the standard deviations of GM, WM and CSF before registration, registration after using FFD [3], Demons [4], HAMMER [11] and the proposed method with and without the explicit anatomical energy term are listed in Table 1. As observed in the Table 1, the proposed method achieves the highest value of P among all the compared methods for the simulated 3D data sets. If the explicit anatomical energy term is used, the registration accuracy can be further improved.

4.2   Experiments with Real Data

In this section, the proposed method is further evaluated by performing registration experiments on the 3D real datasets obtained from IBSR. 20 skull-stripped image volumes with segmentation results are obtained. Each of them has resolution around $256 \times 256 \times 64$ voxels. The experimental settings are similar to

---

[4] http://brainsuite.usc.edu/

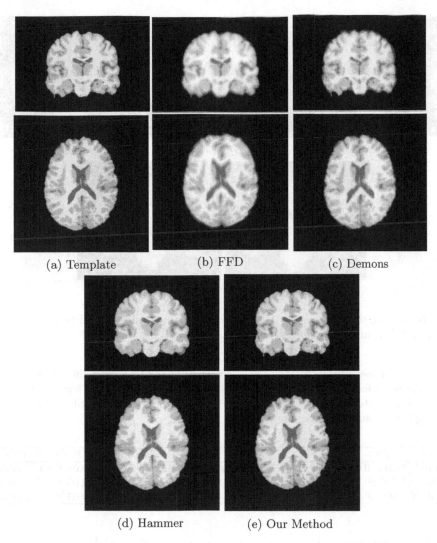

(a) Template   (b) FFD   (c) Demons

(d) Hammer   (e) Our Method

Fig. 4. (a) The template image; Average brain obtained using: (b) FFD, (c) Demons, (d) HAMMER and (e) the proposed method

the settings described in Section 4.1. The same cross section of the template image, the resulting average brain images obtained via various methods are shown in Figure 5. The control point spacing of FFD was again set to $2.5mm$. It is visually observed from Figure 5 that the proposed method has the highest registration accuracy among all the compared methods, especially in the region of gyral crowns, sulcal roots and ventricles, which are important and salient regions of the brain anatomical structures. The tissue overlap measure values P of different approaches are listed in Table 2. It is shown that USSP has the highest value of P, which echoes the visual results shown in Figure 5. FFD [3], Demons

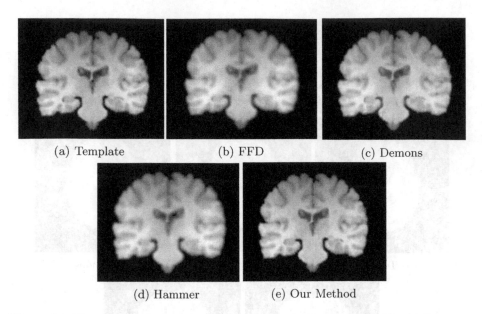

(a) Template   (b) FFD   (c) Demons

(d) Hammer   (e) Our Method

Fig. 5. (a) The template image; Average brain obtained using: (b) FFD, (c) Demons, (d) HAMMER and (e) the proposed method

Table 2. The mean values of P and SDs of GM, WM and CSF with different methods. BR denotes before registration, USSP (WOE) denotes using USSP features without the explicit anatomical energy term, USSP (WE) denotes using USSP features with the explicit anatomical energy term.

Tissue	BR	FFD	Demons	HAMMER	USSP (WOE)	USSP (WE)
Gray	0.54082±0.06	0.74034±0.04	0.76477±0.03	0.78174±0.05	0.82073±0.04	0.84624±0.05
White	0.52147±0.05	0.76285±0.06	0.77830±0.04	0.80627±0.05	0.83816±0.06	0.86216±0.06
CSF	0.33094±0.07	0.72192±0.04	0.76693±0.04	0.75906±0.04	0.79631±0.03	0.83772±0.04

[4], HAMMER [11] and the proposed method took about 7, 5, 10 and 11 hours respectively to register one image pair on a 3.2GHz P4 CPU with 2GB RAM.

5   Conclusion

In this paper, a new feature extraction method for non-rigid image registration is proposed. The uniform spherical structure pattern (USSP) feature is designed to extract monotonic gray-level transformation invariant and rotation invariant anatomical features from the input image volumes. The proposed feature can be extracted efficiently as the extraction process only requires several voxel-wise comparison operations. The registration problem is formulated as a Markov random field (MRF) labeling and energy minimization problem based on the USSP features. If the segmentation results of the input images are available, an explicit anatomical energy term can also be established easily based on the Fisher's separation criteria (FSC) measure function. From the experimental results on both the simulated and real 3D datasets, it is demonstrated that the proposed method gives the highest registration accuracy among all the compared methods.

References

1. Rohr, K.: Image registration based on thin plate splines and local estimates of anisotropic landmark localization uncertainties. In: Wells, W.M., Colchester, A.C.F., Delp, S.L. (eds.) MICCAI 1998. LNCS, vol. 1496, pp. 1174–1183. Springer, Heidelberg (1998)
2. Thompson, P., Toga, A.: A surface-based technique for warping three-dimensional images of the brain. TMI 15, 402–417 (1996)
3. Rueckert, D., Sonoda, L., et al.: Nonrigid registration using free-form deformations: Application to breast MR images. TMI 18, 712–721 (1999)
4. Thirion, J.: Image matching as a diffusion process: an analogy with maxwell's demons. MedI. A 2, 243–260 (1998)
5. Tu, Z., Narr, K., et al.: Brain anatomical structure segmentation by hybrid discriminative/generative models. TMI 27, 495–508 (2007)
6. Dirk, L., et al.: Nonrigid image registration using conditional mutual information. In: Karssemeijer, N., Lelieveldt, B. (eds.) IPMI 2007. LNCS, vol. 4584, pp. 725–737. Springer, Heidelberg (2007)
7. Tang, W., Chung, A.: Non-rigid image registration using graph-cuts. In: Ayache, N., Ourselin, S., Maeder, A. (eds.) MICCAI 2007, Part I. LNCS, vol. 4791, pp. 916–924. Springer, Heidelberg (2007)
8. Glocker, B., et al.: Inter and intra-modal deformable registration: Continuous deformations meet efficient optimal linear programming. In: Karssemeijer, N., Lelieveldt, B. (eds.) IPMI 2007. LNCS, vol. 4584, pp. 408–420. Springer, Heidelberg (2007)
9. Yershova, A., LaValle, S.: Deterministic sampling methods for spheres and so(3). In: ICRA, pp. 3974–3980 (2004)
10. Ojala, T., Pietikainen, M., Maenpaa, T.: Multiresolution gray-scale and rotation invariant texture classification with local binary patterns. PAMI 24, 971–987 (2002)
11. Shen, D., Davatzikos, C.: HAMMER: Hierarchical attribute matching mechanism for elastic registration. TMI 21, 1421–1439 (2002)
12. Wu, G., Qi, F., Shen, D.: Learning-based deformable registration of mr brain images. TMI 25, 1145–1157 (2006)
13. Fisher, A.: The Mathematical Theory of Probabilities. Macmillan, Basingstoke (1923)
14. Kruizinga, P., Petkov, N.: Nonlinear operator for oriented texture. TIP 8, 1395–1407 (1999)
15. Yuri, B., Olga, V., Ramin, Z.: Fast approximate energy minimization via graph cuts. PAMI 23, 1222–1239 (2001)
16. Crum, W., Rueckert, D., et al.: A framework for detailed objective comparison of non-rigid registration algorithms in neuroimaging. In: Barillot, C., Haynor, D.R., Hellier, P. (eds.) MICCAI 2004. LNCS, vol. 3216, pp. 679–686. Springer, Heidelberg (2004)

Joint Bayesian Cortical Sulci Recognition and Spatial Normalization

Matthieu Perrot[1,2,4], Denis Rivière[1,4], Alan Tucholka[1,3,4], and Jean-François Mangin[1,2,4]

[1] CEA, Neurospin, LNAO, Saclay, France
[2] INSERM U.797, Orsay, France
[3] INRIA Saclay-île-de-France, Parietal, Saclay, France
[4] IFR 49, Paris, France
matthieu.perrot@cea.fr
http://www.lnao.fr

Abstract. In this paper, we study the recognition of about 60 sulcal structures over a new T1 MRI database of 62 subjects. It continues our previous work [7] and more specifically extends the localization model of sulci (SPAM). This model is sensitive to the chosen common space during the group study. Thus, we focus the current work on refining this space using registration techniques. Nevertheless, we also benefit from the sulcuswise localization variability knowledge to constrain the normalization. So, we propose a consistent Bayesian framework to jointly identify and register sulci, with two complementary normalization techniques and their detailed integration in the model: a global rigid transformation followed by a piecewise rigid-one, sulcus after sulcus. Thereby, we have improved the sulci labeling quality to a global recognition rate of 86%, and moreover obtained a basic but robust registration technique.

Keywords: cortical folds labeling, sulci, registration, SPAM, EM.

1 Introduction

Group studies involve one of the most intriguing and challenging problem of brain imaging. Indeed, the human cortex is highly convoluted by series of intricated folds and vary strongly from one individual to another. Cortical anatomy, fibers of white matter and functional activity are known to be interwoven in some way still to be defined. Therefore, matching of anatomical structures is fundamental to hugely reduce the intersubject anatomo-functional variability.

Fortunately, some of the largest sulci are relatively stable either in their localization, their shape or according to their neighbouring folds [7]. Moreover, the deepest part of the main sulci are rather well-localized and organized [16,2]. Therefore, the major sulci are often used either to assess the quality of a normalization or as landmarks for co-registration. Indeed, sulci labels and brain normalization are interrelated. Most of the time, normalization and sulci labeling are two well-separated sequential steps. Either the first step [17] provides a

J.L. Prince, D.L. Pham, and K.J. Myers (Eds.): IPMI 2009, LNCS 5636, pp. 176–187, 2009.

common space to the second [7,6,15], or the second yields constraints to the first one [8]. We face here a kind of chicken-egg dilemma. Thus, most methods choose to break the loop and use a weaker approach to replace one of the two steps. They either use a normalization process based only on MRI intensities or geometrical features which can not disambiguate some folds, or use a poor common space to estimate sulci variability for labeling purpose. Nevertheless, we can go further and use the best of the two steps. In fact, iterative answers [19] can be build to overcome the dilemma to some extent. In the following, we propose such a method in a full Bayesian framework (close to the model proposed in [20]) to jointly find sulci labels and a robust registration to a well-defined common space.

This paper extends the sulcuswise localization models and the Bayesian framework introduced in our previous works [7]. Here, we kept aside the structural aspect of our works (in particular the study of neighbouring sulci relations [6]) to focus on the specific topic of joint sulci recognition and registration.

2 Database

The number of subjects in the learning database and the quality of the sulcal delineation across them is a crucial component to correctly guide the model design and enhance the performance of the recognition system. Beyond the largest folds, no ground truth exists. Indeed, the definition of the secondary and tertiary folds is a research subject in its own right. For that reason, many incoherences remained in the labeling of the database used previously [7]. Thus, an in-depth study of the cortical folds has been carried out. As a result, a difficult work, several months long, has been done in this direction to carefully question and correct our previous database, and extend it up to 62 subjects (all with left and right hemispheres). The first and third authors of this paper have jointly labeled the whole database and compared their opinions to justify their choices. Hence, manual sulci identification has been made as homogeneous and consistent as possible, based only on anatomical information extracted from T1 MRI. To that end, a set of 63 labels is used on the left hemisphere and 62 on the right one. The rules used to specify the labeling are based on the sulcal roots theory [2].

Several heterogeneous databases (our former database, a diffusion-dedicated database [3], a twins database [4] and some subjects from the ICBM database) were grouped from several sites: SHFJ, CHU La Pitié Salpêtrière, CHU La Timone, McGill (4 different 1.5T scanners with various spatial resolution). Most of the subjects are right-handed men, between 25 and 35 years old.

A collection of tools (released in the Brainvisa software [1]) has been developed to help the manual labeling, speed up the process and quickly compare many brains together.

We briefly remind here what we mean by sulcus. We used the Brainvisa [1] anatomical segmentation pipeline [5] to extract the cortical folds. We get a raw brain negative mold which is skeletonized and over-segmented according to depth, curvature and topological criteria. Thereby, we obtained a collection of elementary sulcal pieces to be labeled. Lastly, a sulcus is a set of such sulcal

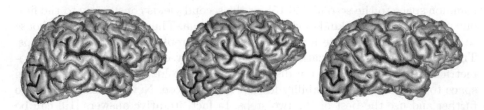

Fig. 1. Sulcal patterns variability: 3 manually labeled brains from our new database

pieces with the same label. Remember that the challenging part of sulci labeling is to stick the sulcal pieces together to give one sulcus, or to find the boundaries between sulci.

3   Models and Methods

Previously, we introduced a model to automatically identify sulci from localization information [7]. This labeling method and the model estimation are based on the strong assumption that all subjects (from training and testing databases) live in a common space. Hence, the more accurate the chosen data normalization process, the more efficient this model. We had used the well-known Talairach coordinate system [12]. This system is based on the alignement of the anterior and posterior commissures (AC-PC) and the interhemispheric plane, followed by the scaling of the brain boundaries along the three cardinal axes with the Talairach atlas.

In this paper, our main goal is still to infer a full labeling $L = \{L_i\}_{i \in \mathcal{E}}$ of brain folds. Namely, we have to find the label L_i of each elementary anatomical structure i to be labeled (in our application sulcal pieces: see section 2 for details). Here, $\mathcal{E}$ denotes the whole set of these structures. The labeling is based on localization information $D = \{D_i\}_{i \in \mathcal{E}}$ (in our case, D_i is the set of the 3D coordinates of the voxels of the structure i from the MRI data, but other information could be considered). These data are expressed in a common referential space (for instance the Talairach one) thanks to a transformation from the subject space and defined by the parameter Θ (equal to θ_{Tal} in the case of the Talairach space). Hence, the MAP (Maximum A Posteriori) formulation of labeling from our previous model can be rewriten as follows:

$$P(\textbf{Labeling}|\textbf{Data}) = P(L|D\Theta = \theta_{Tal}) \propto P(D|L\Theta = \theta_{Tal})P(L|\Theta = \theta_{Tal}) \quad (1)$$

In the same way, we can reconsider the formulation of the estimation of the localization model $\mathcal{M}$ (in this paper we use SPAM models, see section 3.4 for details) from a training database $\mathcal{A}$, by the introduction of normalization parameters (from subject space to the Talairach one): $\theta_{a,tal}$ for each subject $a \in \mathcal{A}$:

$$P(\textbf{Model}|\textbf{Training Set}) = P(\mathcal{M}|\{D_a L_a; \Theta_a = \theta_{a,tal}\}_{a \in \mathcal{A}}) \quad (2)$$

where each subscript a stands for data specific to the subject a.

In the following, we first introduce the general principles of a natural extension of this model which considers the re-estimation of normalization parameters (for global and sulcuswise rigid registration techniques). Then, the method details are given for the joint registration and labeling, and for the joint registration and model estimation. Finally, the method is derived for a specific sulcuswise localization model used in our experiments : the SPAM model.

3.1   Normalization and Registration

The Talairach coordinate system is really reliable only for the deepest anatomical structures (thalamus, putamen, caudate nucleus...) and quite inaccurate for the cortical folds. Besides, in the considered database (see section 2), AC-PC alignements have been done manually. In this paper, we propose to automatically define a better common space by transforming each subject using registration techniques with respect to our localization models. The pratical application of this idea is not straightforward and depends on the chosen normalization, since the registration is done between a subject and a probabilistic model rather than a mean subject or an atlas. In the following sections, we will state how to introduce the normalization step in a meaningful way to extend our previous model, estimate it from a training database, and use it to help the labeling process on a new unlabeled subject.

In this context, we choose to further study two specific complementary registration methods. The first one is rigid and defined by global parameters $\theta_g = (R_g, t_g)$, where R_g is a rotation matrix and t_g a translation vector. It will provide a refined version of the Talairach space. Its optimization does not need any specific prior thanks to the strong constraints defined by the labelwise localization models. It also provides a good initialization for any second step non-linear registration.

To this end, many methods could be used and integrated in the considered model of this paper. Nevertheless, state of the art diffeomorphic registration techniques are extremely time consuming. Do not forget that our first goal is not to provide a perfect registration but to infer sulci labels. So we can afford the use of simpler methods if it is done with enough care.

As a second step, we suggest a simple non-linear registration method that extends naturally the global approach to a sulcuswise one. It is defined by a set of parameters $\theta_s = \{\theta_{s,l}\}_{l \in \mathcal{L}} = \{(R_{s,l}, t_{s,l})\}_{l \in \mathcal{L}}$ with one rigid registration for each label l. Obviously, without constraints, some counterintuitive phenomena can occur because this registration is non-diffeomorphic. In fact, various structures could cross each other after registration and result in a poor local labeling. Besides, some neighbouring sulci have similar shapes and could be easily confused without strong enough constraints. This method has severe drawbacks that can be hugely reduced and controled with the use of a well chosen referential space for initialization and strong priors to control the range of available local transformations. To that end, we used independent priors for each label. The translations are estimated by a full-covariance 3D-Gaussian. For the rotations, we split their prior in 2 components based on the standard vector-rotation parametrization. We have chosen generalizations of multivariate Gaussian distributions: Von Mises distribution for the rotation angle, Kent or Bingham distributions for the direction of the rotation (see [11] for an overview). The local rigid transformations of a point x depends on the chosen reference point g. Indeed, $R \cdot x + t = R \cdot (x - g) + (t - R \cdot g - g) + g = R \cdot x_g + t_g + g$ with x_g and t_g expressed in the local coordinate system defined by g. The case $g = 0$ corresponds to the global arbitrary coordinates. To be as sharp as possible, the translation prior needs to be estimated from t_g with a well chosen reference g. A natural choice, for a given label, is to use the gravity center of all sulci with this label over the database, with coordinates expressed in the normalized space of the model.

These approaches are quite well integrated in the following models and lead to drastic simplifications of the optimization scheme. They allow the use of a simplified model without any statistical dependency, which results in a fast and efficient optimization method (see eq. 9).

3.2   Joint Registration and Labeling

Here we suppose that the model $\mathcal{M}$ is known. Either, it may has been learned with (according to the method suggested in the section 3.3) or without (according to our previous work [7]) normalization refinement. Thereby, in this section, all probabilities $P(\cdot)$ are defined implicitely given $\mathcal{M}$. The following formula extends the equation 1 to find jointly the labels l and the registration parameters θ:

$$l^*, \theta^* = \underset{l,\theta}{\operatorname{argmax}}\, P(L = l\Theta = \theta | D) \tag{3}$$

Direct optimization of this quantity is difficult and time consuming. However, we can consider other quantities of interest as the marginal probabilities over Θ and L: $P(L|D)$ and $P(\Theta|D)$ respectively. According to our model design (independence assumptions and registration methods), it induces simplifications. Thus, we choose to first optimize the registration θ regarding L as hidden labels, and then optimize labels under the best θ^* previously obtained:

$$\begin{cases} \theta^* = \underset{\theta}{\operatorname{argmax}}\, P(\Theta=\theta|D) = \underset{\theta}{\operatorname{argmax}}\, P(\theta) \sum_{L=l} P(L = l|\theta) P(D|L = l; \theta) \\ l^* = \underset{l}{\operatorname{argmax}}\, P(L=l|D; \Theta=\theta^*) = \underset{l}{\operatorname{argmax}}\, P(D|L = l; \Theta = \theta^*) P(L = l|\Theta=\theta^*) \end{cases}$$
$$\tag{4}$$

θ^* can be estimated by the iterative Expectation Maximization (EM) algorithm [9] which reaches a local optimum from a well-chosen initialization $\theta^{(0)}$:

$$\theta^{(n+1)} = \underset{\theta}{\operatorname{argmax}}\, Q\left(\theta \middle| \theta^{(n)}\right) \tag{5}$$

with

$$\begin{aligned} Q\left(\theta \middle| \theta^{(n)}\right) &= \mathbb{E}_L\left[log(P(DL\theta)) \middle| D\theta^{(n)}\right] \\ &= \sum_{L=l} P\left(L = l \middle| D\theta^{(n)}\right) log\left[P(D|L = l\theta) P(L = l|\theta) P(\theta)\right] \end{aligned} \tag{6}$$

where $\mathbb{E}_L[\cdot]$ stands for the expectation over L.

Currently, we will consider a widely spread assumption of conditional independence of all $\{D_i\}_{i\in\mathcal{E}}$ given L. Besides, the labels prior $P(L)$ does not depend on the transformation θ, and so we derive the above expression for global rigid registration:

$$Q_g\left(\theta_g\middle|\theta_g^{(n)}\right) = \sum_{l\in\mathcal{L}}\sum_{i\in\mathcal{E}} P\left(L_i = l_i\middle|D_i\theta_g^{(n)}\right) log\left[P(D_i|L_i\theta_g)P(L_i = l_i)P(\theta_g)\right]$$
(7)

The optimization of θ is now regarded as a standard parameter optimization within the framework of mixture models. Indeed, $P(L_i = l_i|\theta)$ is the prior of the model l_i defined by the likelihood $P(D_i|L_i = l_i\theta)$ (in our case these generative models are SPAM: see section 3.4). Finally, the $\{D_i\}_{i\in\mathcal{E}}$ are realizations of the mixture model.

For local registration, we supposed $P(\theta_s) = \prod_{l\in\mathcal{L}} P(\theta_{s,l})$, where each $\theta_{s,l}$ stands for sulcuswise local registration parameters.

$$Q_s\left(\theta_s\middle|\theta_s^{(n)}\right) = \sum_{l\in\mathcal{L}}\sum_{i\in\mathcal{E}} P\left(L_i = l\middle|D_i\theta_{s,l}^{(n)}\right) log\left[P(D_i|L_i\theta_{s,l})P(L_i)P(\theta_{s,l})\right] \quad (8)$$

$$\theta_s^* = \left\{\underset{\theta_{s,l}}{argmax} \sum_{i\in\mathcal{E}} P\left(L_i = l\middle|D_i\theta_{s,l}^{(n)}\right) log\left[P(D_i|L_i\theta_{s,l})P(\theta_{s,l})\right]\right\}_{l\in\mathcal{L}} \quad (9)$$

Hence, the optimization of θ follows repeated sequences of local marginal posteriors $P(L_i|D_i\theta)$ estimations (E-step) which yields weights for the registrations optimizations (M-step). The weights can be read into links between structures to be labeled and the mixture model components. For the sulcuswise case, thanks to the independence assumption of the $\{\theta_{s,l}\}_{l\in\mathcal{L}}$, the registration optimization is done independently for each label l.

Lastly, a full labeling l^* is obtained by MAP as in our previous works [7] but after applying the transformation induced by the parameter θ^*:

$$l^* = \{l_i^*\}_{i\in\mathcal{E}} = \left\{\underset{l_i}{argmax}\, P(D_i|L_i = l_i; \Theta = \theta^*)P(L_i = l_i|\Theta = \theta^*)\right\}_{i\in\mathcal{E}} \quad (10)$$

3.3   Joint Registration and Model Estimation

We are interested here by the supervised estimation of our model parameters $\mathcal{M}$. We supposed a training database $\mathcal{A}$ is avalaible (in this work, we use the database described in section 2) with one known label $L_{a,i}$ for each sulcal piece i and each subject $a \in \mathcal{A}$. Previously, the model estimation was built from the Talairach space. Now, we supposed that the registration parameters θ_a (that move each subject $a \in \mathcal{A}$ from the Talairach space to a new refined common space) are unknown and have to be computed at the same time as the model $\mathcal{M}$. To generalize the previous formulation (see equation 2), the ideal measure to optimize is then expressed as below:

$$m^*, \{\theta_a^*\}_{a\in\mathcal{A}} = \underset{m,\{\theta_a\}_{a\in\mathcal{A}}}{argmax}\, P(\mathcal{M} = m\{\Theta_a = \theta_a\}_{a\in\mathcal{A}}|\{D_aL_a\}_{a\in\mathcal{A}}) \quad (11)$$

One way to approximate the maximization of this quantity is to alternate the optimization of the model parameters and that of the registration parameters:

$$
\begin{cases}
m^{(n)} & = \underset{m}{\operatorname{argmax}} \; P\left(\mathcal{M} = m \middle| \{D_a L_a\}_{a \in \mathcal{A}}; \left\{\Theta_a = \theta_a^{(n)}\right\}_{a \in \mathcal{A}}\right) \\
\left\{\theta_a^{(n+1)}\right\}_{a \in \mathcal{A}} & = \underset{\{\theta_a\}_{a \in \mathcal{A}}}{\operatorname{argmax}} \; P\left(\{\Theta_a = \theta_a\}_{a \in \mathcal{A}} \middle| \{D_a L_a\}_{a \in \mathcal{A}}; \mathcal{M} = m^{(n)}\right)
\end{cases}
\tag{12}
$$

Under the independence assumption of subjectwise registration parameters $\{\theta_a\}$ and those of sulcal pieces, the optimization becomes:

$$
\begin{cases}
m_l^{(n)} = \underset{m_l}{\operatorname{argmax}} \quad P\left(\mathcal{M}_l = m_l \middle| \{D_{a,i} L_{a,i} = l\}_{\substack{a \in \mathcal{A} \\ i \in \mathcal{E}_{a,l}}} ; \left\{\Theta_a = \theta_a^{(n)}\right\}_{a \in \mathcal{A}}\right) \\
\theta_a^{(n+1)} = \underset{\theta_a}{\operatorname{argmax}} \; P\left(D_a | L_a; \Theta_a = \theta_a \mathcal{M} = m^{(n)}\right) P\left(\Theta_a = \theta_a | L_a; \mathcal{M} = m^{(n)}\right)
\end{cases}
\tag{13}
$$

with $\mathcal{M} = \{\mathcal{M}_l\}_{l \in \mathcal{L}}$, where $\mathcal{M}_l$ is the set of parameters monitoring the generative model of sulcus l, and $\mathcal{E}_{a,l}$ the set of sulcal pieces of subject a restricted to those with the label l.

The optimization of $\mathcal{M}$ reduces to normalizing each subject a based on their respective transformation θ_a and compute a standard model estimation in this reference space (see section 3.4 for SPAM estimation). For its part, the optimisation of the registration parameters θ_a boils down to find the best transformation to fit the data to the given model $\mathcal{M} = m^{(n)}$ constrainted by the prior $P\left(\Theta_a = \theta_a | L_a; \mathcal{M} = m^{(n)}\right)$.

3.4　SPAM and Registration

The model presented in this paper is based on a mixture of sulcuswise generative models based on localization data. So far, no assumption has been made on these models. In this section, we will show how to use a specific model to represent this information: the SPAM model (Statistical Probabilistic Anatomy Map [13]) already used in our previous work [7] and extending older sulci analysis of [14]. This model gives voxelwise probabilities. In our current context, the likelihood is defined through a transformation θ and for a given label l, the probability of finding one structure at the spatial position x is given by:

$$
P_{SPAM}(x | L = l\theta\mathcal{M}) = \frac{(K_\sigma * f_l)(\Phi_\theta(x))}{\sum_{x \in \Omega}(K_\sigma * f_l)(\Phi_\theta(x))}
\tag{14}
$$

with $K_\sigma * f$ standing for the convolution of f and K_σ which is a 3-dimensional spherical Gaussian kernel of covariance $\sigma^2 Id$, $f_l(x)$ is the frequency of appearance of label L at position x over the database (with $\{\{f_l(x)\}_{x \in \Omega}, \sigma\} \in \mathcal{M}$) and Φ_θ is a transformation function to transform x spatial coordinates from an initial reference space through the registration parameterized by θ. For a given sulcal piece i, its set of voxel coordinates $\mathcal{V}_i$, with voxelwise indepence assumption, the joint likelihood writes:

$$
P_{SPAM}(\mathcal{V}_i | l\theta) = \prod_{x \in \mathcal{V}_i} P_{SPAM}(x | l\theta)^{\frac{1}{|\mathcal{V}_i|}}
\tag{15}
$$

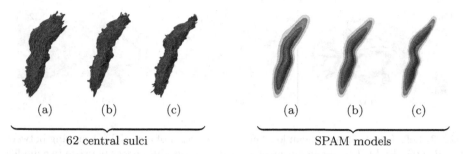

(a)	(b)	(c)	(a)	(b)	(c)

62 central sulci   SPAM models

Fig. 2. Effects of constrained registration on SPAM model estimation: localization uncertainties are reduced from (a) to (c). Models are estimated from (a) Talairach space, (b) with global registration, (c) with local registration. SPAM models are represented conveniently by 3 nested isosurfaces of the probability corresponding to 30, 60 and 80% of the whole probability mass.

with $|\mathcal{V}_i|$ the number of voxels of the sulci which behaves like a normalization factor. Indeed, during the segmentation stage of folds, sulcal pieces of various size are obtained. Hence, this quantity erases size effects and gives comparable posteriors (used to weight the registration during the EM).

In this paper we consider only rigid transformations: a global one with $\varPhi_{g\theta}(\boldsymbol{x})$ $= R_g \cdot \boldsymbol{x} + \boldsymbol{t_g}$ and local ones with $\varPhi_{s,l\theta}(\boldsymbol{x}) = R_{s,l} \cdot \boldsymbol{x} + \boldsymbol{t}_{s,l}$, for each label l. During the registration stage, we have to optimize the parameter set θ. A SPAM model is non-parametric and currently represented as a 3D-volume of probabilities. Thus, analytical optimization is not easy. In this paper, we choose to use the well-known Powell's method [10] to cover the 6-parameter space made up of $\boldsymbol{w}$ (vector-rotation parametrization of R) and the translation $\boldsymbol{t}$ to maximize the matching. See figure 2 to notice the refinement of the raw SPAM model (fig. 2 (a)) by the use of registration techniques.

Lastly, the SPAM model is introduced in our joint labeling and registration framework, replacing $P(D_i = d_i | L_i = l_i; \theta)$ by $P_{SPAM}(\mathcal{V}_i | L = l_i; \theta)$ with $\mathcal{V}_i = d_i$.

4   Results and Discussion

The following results are based on the new database of 62 subjects: left and right hemispheres (versus only 26 right hemispheres before) presented in section 2. All estimations are obtained from a leave-one-out scheme. Namely, for each subject a full model estimation (SPAM, variability estimation of registration parameters: rotations and translations, label priors) is computed from all subjects but the tested one. Then, the unseen subject is labeled from its related model. Thereby, the following results are much more reliable than our previous ones [7].

In the following, we consider three error rates (see equation 16) ranging between 0 and 100%. The two first rates are global error measures where each sulcuswise contribution is weighted by its size. The first E_{mass} is kept here for comparison purposes with our old results [7]. The second one E_{SI} draws inspiration from the measure called similarity index (SI [18]). It is more comprehensive

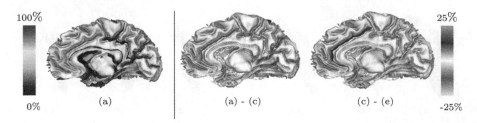

Fig. 3. Left: Leave-one-out mean local error rates E_{local} of a model (a) ranging between 0 and 100%. Right: Leave-one-out mean local error rates differences between two models named by a letter (begining of section 4) to highlight the enhancements. (a) - (c) shows improvements due to a full use of global registration with labeling according to model (a). (c) - (e) shows improvements of the best local registration with labeling according to model (c).

than the first one only based on false positive errors. It also removes errors shared by several sulci (extra or missing sulcal pieces) by counting them only once. Quite on the contrary, the last $E_{local}(l)$ is local and rather draconian. It takes all errors involving a given label l into account (false positive and true negative) without redundancy correction:

$$E_{mass} = \frac{\sum\limits_{l \in \mathcal{L}} FP(l)}{\sum\limits_{l \in \mathcal{L}} FP(l) + TP(l)} \quad E_{SI} = \sum\limits_{l \in \mathcal{L}} w_l \frac{FP(l) + FN(l)}{FP(l) + FN(l) + 2*TP(l)} \quad E_{local}(l) = \frac{FP(l) + FN(l)}{FP(l) + FN(l) + TP(l)}$$

(16)

where w_l is the true size of the sulcus l normalized by the sum of the sizes of all sulci, $FP(l)$, $FN(l)$ and $TP(l)$ stands respectively for false postive, false negative and true positive errors of label l. Each of these measures is computed comparing the manual labels to the automatic ones, and weighted so that each sulcal piece counts as much as its size.

In the following, five models will be discussed and named by letters for a better understanding. (a) basic SPAM model estimated from Talairach, with independent labeling from Talairach (eq. 2). (b) basic SPAM model estimated from Talairach, with joint labeling and global rigid registration from Talairach (eq. 7). (c) globally refined SPAM model (eq. 13) from Talairach, with joint labeling and global rigid registration from Talairach (eq. 7). (d) locally refined SPAM model (eq. 13) from Talairach, with joint labeling and local rigid registration from Talairach (eq. 9). (e) is like (d) but the reference space is not Talairach but the one estimated by a first model estimation or labeling with model (c) (see section 3.1).

The basic SPAM model (a) already gives low error rates. Since, the labeling is done for each sulcal piece independently, severe errors remain (huge sulci parts missing, double outlines). We have tested previously [7] and with some success the use of a Markov field [6] to fix these issues, but this is beyond the scope of the current paper. We suggest here that some of these errors can be considered as registration errors or referential inadequacy between the subject and the model.

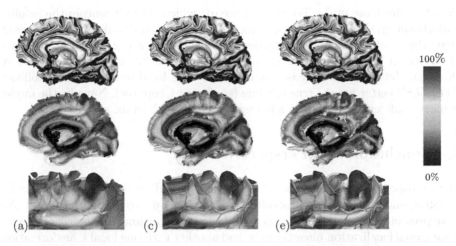

Fig. 4. Some effects of joint labeling and registration on an arbitrary subject which gives bad recognition of the posterior cingulate fissure label (post.C.F) with model (a). Top: local posterior probabilities of the post.C.F mapped on each sulcal piece of the subject. Middle: estimated SPAM models mixed with their respective automatic and registred sulci of the considered subject: look at the enhancement on the post.C.F (yellow color). Bottom: zoomed and cropped version of the previous row. Letters denote models fully described at the begining of section 4: (a) basic SPAM models, (c) with global registration and (e) with local registration. Note that the labeling are almost the same between (c) and (e), but with model (e) the matching is better.

In fact, global error rates are significantly reduced by using the joint labeling and global registration (see table 1 (b)). Moreover, the errors decrease again, with the use of the globally refined SPAM models (c). The enhancements are quite uniformly distributed over the brain (see figure 3). Thus, the two joint approaches at learning and testing stages are effective. In the case of the non-linear transformation, each local registration is constrainted independently. So the more the referential space is reliable, the stronger the constraints are. As expected, initializing the local methods (model estimation and labeling) with the registration result of the global one (e) gives sharper and stronger constraints

Table 1. Leave-one-out mean (over 62 subjects) percentage of global SI and mass error rates (and their standard deviations between parenthesis) for all models listed at the begining of section 4

		No registration	Global registration		local registration	
		(a)	(b)	(c)	(d)	(e)
E_{SI}	Left	17.55 (5.93)	15.27 (2.74)	14.59 (2.88)	16.79 (4.35)	14.22 (2.96)
	Right	16.83 (3.77)	14.70 (3.09)	13.97 (2.91)	15.61 (3.72)	13.48 (3.13)
E_{mass}	Left	16.64 (3.69)	14.56 (2.54)	14.01 (2.62)	16.61 (4.17)	14.11 (2.79)
	Right	15.96 (3.66)	13.95 (2.98)	13.37 (2.82)	15.29 (3.51)	13.30 (2.99)

than the direct use of the Talairach space (d) which actually worsen the results. Unfortunately, this step does not bring about any global significant improvement (see table 1 (c) versus (e)), but rather some local ones at the medial frontal part of the brain for instance (see figure 3). Indeed, the labeling quality is nearly the same, but its reliability is enhanced since the local posteriors probabilities $P(L_i|D_i\Theta)$ better fits the true labeling (see figure 4, top row). Namely, the model is more confident in the given labeling (see figure 4, bottom row).

5   Conclusion and Perspectives

In this paper, we have proposed new models extending our previous works [7] coupling sulci labeling and constrainted registration in a common framework. We have presented two complementary rigid-based registration techniques: one to reduce global localization uncertainties, and another with one local transformation per sulcus. The proposed methods give significant improvements. Their resulting labelings are almost the same but the local approach yields more reliable posterior probabilities which may be helpful for further processings (morphometry studies for instance). Originally, we were interested in the labeling enhancement. Finally, our models also provide a registration method constrainted by reliable anatomical landmarks: the sulci. On the contrary of most landmark-based normalization methods, in our case no labeling is needed to set the constraints: the process is fully automatic. It would be interesting to compare the registration capacities of these methods with standard ones.

Many statistical independence assumptions have been made during the model design, so there is still room for improvement. In fact, the labeling of a sulcal piece should be done in relation with its neighbourhood: a Markov field can do the job (as in our previous work [7] [6], but registration has now to be included). We can also consider registration methods constrainted so that the local anatomical organization of folds are preserved in some way. Nevertheless, more complicated models may need adapted approximations to run properly. These extensions are partially complementary and may benefit from each other.

Acknowledgements. We are indebted to Cyril Poupon and Philippe Pinel for the access to their databases.

References

1. http://brainvisa.info
2. Régis, J., Mangin, J.-F., Ochiai, T., Frouin, V., Rivière, D., Cachia, A., Tamura, M., Samson, Y.: Sulcal root generic model: a hypothesis to overcome the variability of the human cortex folding patterns. Neurol. Med. Chir. 45, 1–17 (2005)
3. Poupon, C., Poupon, F., Allirol, L., Mangin, J.-F.: A database dedicated to anatomo-functional study of human brain connectivity. In: 12th Ann. Meet. Org. Human Brain Mapping (2006)

4. Pinel, P., Thirion, B., Meriaux, S., Jobert, A., Serres, J., Bihan, D.L., Poline, J.-B., Dehaene, S.: Fast reproducible identification and large-scale databasing of individual functional cognitive networks. BMC Neurosci. 8, 91 (2007)
5. Mangin, J.-F., Frouin, V., Bloch, I., Régis, J., Lopez-Krahe, J.: From 3D Magnetic Resonance Images to Structural Representations of the Cortex Topography Using Topology Preserving Deformations. Journal of Mathematical Imaging and Vision 5, 297–318 (1995)
6. Rivière, D., Mangin, J.-F., Papadopoulos-Orfanos, D., Martinez, J.-M., Frouin, V., Régis, J.: Automatic Recognition of Cortical Sulci Using a Congregation of Neural Networks. MIA 6, 77–92 (2002)
7. Perrot, M., Rivière, D., Mangin, J.-F.: Identifying cortical sulci from localization, shape and local organization. In: ISBI, pp. 420–423 (2008)
8. Cathier, P., Mangin, J.-F., Pennec, X., Rivière, D., Papadopoulos-Orfanos, D., Régis, J., Ayache, N.: Multisubject non-rigid registration of brain MRI using intensity and geometric features. In: Niessen, W.J., Viergever, M.A. (eds.) MICCAI 2001. LNCS, vol. 2208, pp. 734–742. Springer, Heidelberg (2001)
9. Dempster, A., Laird, N., Rubin, D.: Maximum likelihood from incomplete data via the em algorithm. Journal of the Royal Statistical Society, Series B 39(1), 1–38 (1977)
10. Powell, M.J.D.: An Efficient Method for Finding the Minimum of a Function of Several Variables Without Calculating Derivatives. Computer Journal 7, 155–162 (1964)
11. Mardia, K.V., Jupp, P.: Directional Statistics, 2nd edn. John Wiley and Sons Ltd., Chichester (2000)
12. Talairach, J., Tournoux, P.: Co-planar Stereotaxic Atlas of the Human Brain. Georg Thieme Verlag, Stuttgart (1988)
13. Evans, A.C., Collins, D.L., Neelin, P., MacDonald, D., Kamber, M., Marrett, T.S.: Three-Dimensional Correlative Imaging: Applications in Human Brain Mapping. Functional Neuroimaging 14, 145–161 (1994)
14. Le Goualher, G., Collins, D.L., Barillot, C., Evans, A.C.: Automatic Identification of Cortical Sulci Using a 3D Probabilistic Atlas. In: Wells, W.M., Colchester, A.C.F., Delp, S.L. (eds.) MICCAI 1998. LNCS, vol. 1496, pp. 509–518. Springer, Heidelberg (1998)
15. Lohmann, G., von Cramon, D.Y.: Automatic labelling of the human cortical surface using sulcal basins. Medical image analysis 4(3), 179–188 (2000)
16. Lohmann, G., von Cramon, D.Y., Colchester, A.C.F.: Deep Sulcal Landmarks Provide an Organizing Framework for Human Cortical Folding. Cerebral Cortex 18(6), 1415–1420 (2008)
17. Tosun, D., Prince, J.L.: A Geometry-Driven Optical Flow Warping for Spatial Normalization of Cortical Surfaces. TMI 27(12), 1739–1753 (2008)
18. Yang, F., Kruggel, F.: Optimization Algorithms for Labeling Brain Sulci Based on Graph Matching. In: ICCV, pp. 1–7 (2007)
19. Vaillant, M., Davatzikos, C.: Hierarchical Matching of Cortical Features for Deformable Brain Image Registration. In: Kuba, A., Sámal, M., Todd-Pokropek, A. (eds.) IPMI 1999. LNCS, vol. 1613, pp. 182–195. Springer, Heidelberg (1999)
20. Yeo, B., Sabuncu, M., Desikan, R., Fischl, B., Golland, P.: Effects of registration regularization and atlas sharpness on segmentation accuracy. Med. Image Anal. 12(5), 603–615 (2008)

Image-to-Physical Registration for Image-Guided Interventions Using 3-D Ultrasound and an Ultrasound Imaging Model

Andrew P. King, Ying-Liang Ma, Cheng Yao, Christian Jansen, Reza Razavi, Kawal S. Rhode, and Graeme P. Penney

Division of Imaging Sciences, King's College London, U.K.
andrew.king@kcl.ac.uk

Abstract. We present a technique for automatic intensity-based image-to-physical registration of a 3-D segmentation for image-guided interventions. The registration aligns the segmentation with tracked and calibrated 3-D ultrasound (US) images of the target region. The technique uses a probabilistic framework and explicitly incorporates a model of the US image acquisition process. The rigid body registration parameters are varied to maximise the likelihood that the real US image(s) were formed using the US imaging model from the probe transducer position. The proposed technique is validated on images segmented from cardiac magnetic resonance imaging (MRI) data and 3-D US images acquired from 3 volunteers and 1 patient. We show that the accuracy of the algorithm is 2.6-4.2mm and the capture range is 9-18mm. The proposed technique has the potential to provide accurate image-to-physical registrations for a range of image guidance applications.

1 Introduction

Image-guidance systems make preprocedure images available during interventions to aid in navigation and to improve the confidence of clinicians. Often the preprocedure image is segmented to delineate structures of interest, and this information is used to form a 'roadmap' for the intervention. An important feature of image-guidance technologies is the alignment of the preprocedure image with the physical space of the clinical environment. In minimally invasive interventions, because of the lack of access to the target structures, many previously proposed solutions have used external markers or features whose corresponding locations are identified in both the preprocedure image and the physical coordinate system. However, because the features are external they are sometimes far from the structures of interest, which introduces possible errors into the alignment. Furthermore, markers attached to the skin are likely to move, making the resulting registration unreliable. In this paper we propose a technique to register a 3-D preprocedure segmented image with physical space using intraprocedure 3-D US images that allows us to register directly using images of the target region.

J.L. Prince, D.L. Pham, and K.J. Myers (Eds.): IPMI 2009, LNCS 5636, pp. 188–201, 2009.
© Springer-Verlag Berlin Heidelberg 2009

Registration between US images and preprocedure images (or segmented images) such as magnetic resonance imaging (MRI) or computed tomography (CT) is a difficult problem because of the low signal-to-noise ratio of US images, their limited field of view and the fact that different image features can be produced in US and CT/MRI by the same underlying anatomy. Furthermore, image quality is highly dependent on the subject and the experience of the sonographer. Previous examples of registration between 3-D US and 3-D preprocedure images include Roche et al [1], who used a similarity measure that incorporated both intensity and MRI gradient information; Leroy et al [2], who registered CT to freehand 3-D US images by preprocessing both modalities to increase the common features between them; Penney et al [3], who registered MRI and freehand 3-D US liver images by remapping both to an intermediate vessel probability representation; Huang et al [4], who proposed a technique in which both 3-D US and CT images were preprocessed prior to registration using mutual information and normalised cross correlation as similarity measures; and Wein et al [5], who registered CT to freehand 3-D US images by simulating US images from CT images.

Most of these examples implicitly introduce knowledge of an imaging process by preprocessing one or both modalities before registration. For example, US images can produce high intensities at tissue boundaries, so a MRI or CT gradient image is often used to highlight such boundaries. We propose a technique that explicitly incorporates knowledge of an imaging process into the registration. We use an US imaging model similar to that previously proposed in US image segmentation [6] and simulation [7]. Our technique involves automatically segmenting a preprocedure MRI image and then augmenting the segmentation with knowledge of the acoustic properties of the tissue types. The registration attempts to maximise the likelihood that a real 3-D US image was formed by the known imaging model by varying the rigid body motion parameters. We demonstrate our technique on cardiac MRI and 3-D US images.

2   Method and Materials

Figure 1 gives an overview of the proposed technique. The preprocedure MRI image is segmented, and each voxel is assigned a label indicating its anatomical region. Each voxel in the segmentation is augmented with knowledge of the acoustic properties of its tissue type. Next, the segmented image is transformed by the starting estimate for the registration (which we denote by the matrix transformation R in Figure 1). The current alignment and the acoustic properties are used to produce a probability density map based on an US imaging model. The map consists of a probability density function at each location in the preprocedure image indicating which US intensities are most likely to occur at that location, based on the US imaging model we will describe in Section 2.2. The probability density map is compared with the real US image to determine an overall likelihood that the US image was produced using the current registration. Finally, the rigid body registration parameters are varied to maximise the

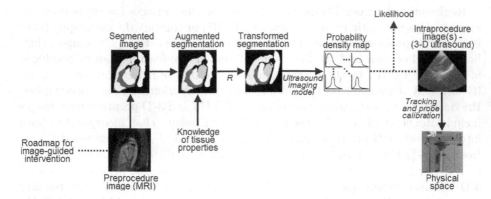

Fig. 1. An overview of the proposed technique to register a segmented preprocedure image to physical space using tracked and calibrated 3-D US images. The preprocedure MRI image is segmented and augmented with knowledge of the acoustic properties of the tissue types. This augmented segmentation, together with an US imaging model, is used to form a probability density map. This map defines how likely it is that any given US image was formed from the imaging model and the current registration, R. R is varied to optimise the likelihood. The 3-D US to physical space transformation is known through a combination of probe calibration and tracking.

likelihood. Calibration and tracking of the US probe allows the registration to be used to compute the overall image to physical transformation for the intervention. Our technique is designed to work with multiple US images. However, for simplicity, in the following Method sections we describe its operation for a single US image.

2.1 Segmentation

For the segmentation we used the automatic atlas-based cardiac segmentation technique described in [8]. This segments the heart into the blood pools of the four chambers, the myocardium, the ascending and descending aorta and the pulmonary artery. We also precompute a gradient image and a Euclidean distance map [9] of the segmented image for use in forming the probability density map.

2.2 The 3-D US Imaging Model

The US imaging model defines a probability density function for any given location in the preprocedure image. Images acquired by state-of-the-art US machines undergo a range of postprocessing operations to make them more easily interpreted by the human visual system, such as time-gain compensation, log compression and low-pass filtering [10]. It is important that any US imaging model should match as closely as possible the true processes that produce the final image intensities. However, the parameters of this processing are normally unknown. Techniques have been proposed for determining some of the parameters (e.g. [11] for the log compression parameters) but to determine the precise parameters of all postprocessing operations would be very difficult. It is sometimes possible to switch off some or all of these processes to simplify the acquisition (e.g. [12]), but this is not routine clinical practice and may make acquisition more difficult for the sonographer. Therefore we chose to leave the processing in place and propose a simplified US imaging model that captures the important elements of the combined US image acquisition and postprocessing operations.

To enable the US image acquisition process to be modelled we augment the segmented image with two extra pieces of information about the acoustic properties of anatomical regions: the characteristic acoustic impedance, Z, which is a tissue property that is analogous to electrical impedance; and the scattering strength, α, which indicates the expected reflection strength due to scatterers in a homogeneous tissue region [10]. We will discuss how these parameter values were set later in this section. The US imaging model defines a probability for each intensity for each voxel, given an augmented segmentation, a current registration and the US probe transducer position (which is known and constant in the US image coordinate system). Before describing the model in detail we first define some terms:

- $f_U(\boldsymbol{x})$: the 3-D US image intensity at coordinate $\boldsymbol{x}$.
- $f_L(\cdot)$: the segmented image of region labels.
- Ω_L: the set of region labels in the segmented image f_L.
- $\boldsymbol{n}_L(\cdot)$: the unit normal vector computed by normalising the gradient of $f_L(\cdot)$.
- $d(\cdot)$: the Euclidean distance transform of the segmented image, $f_L(\cdot)$, i.e. it indicates a distance (in mm) to the nearest region boundary for each voxel.
- R: the current registration from the segmented image to the 3-D US image.

In our proposed model we define probabilities separately for boundaries and homogeneous regions. The overall probability density at US voxel location $\boldsymbol{x}$ given a current registration R is defined as:

$$p(\boldsymbol{x}, R) = \max\left(p_r(\boldsymbol{x}, R), p_b(\boldsymbol{x}, R)\right) \tag{1}$$

where $p_r(\cdot)$ and $p_b(\cdot)$ are the region and boundary probability densities respectively. These densities define a probability for the occurrence of each intensity value at the given coordinate location. The US image coordinate $\boldsymbol{x}$ is transformed to preprocedure image coordinates using the transformation R^{-1}. All probability densities, $p_r(\boldsymbol{x}, R)$ and $p_b(\boldsymbol{x}, R)$, are normalised so that they sum to 1 in the range $[0 \ldots N_U]$, where N_U is the maximum intensity value for the US images (255 in our experiments).

The region probability p_r is a function of the scattering strength α_l of the voxels' tissue types,

$$p_r(\boldsymbol{x}, R) = \begin{cases} G\left(f_U(\boldsymbol{x}), \alpha_l, \sigma_U\right) & \text{if } l \in \Omega_L, \\ \frac{1}{N_U+1} & \text{otherwise} \end{cases} \tag{2}$$
$$\text{where } l = f_L\left(R^{-1} \cdot \boldsymbol{x}\right)$$

In (2), α_l is the scattering strength for tissue region l and $G\left(f_U(\boldsymbol{x}), \alpha_l, \sigma_U\right)$ is the value at $f_U(\boldsymbol{x})$ of a normal distribution centred on α_l with standard deviation σ_U, i.e. $G(x, \alpha, \sigma) = \frac{1}{\sigma\sqrt{2\pi}}\exp\left(\frac{-(x-\alpha)^2}{2\sigma^2}\right)$. The value of σ_U represents the spread of US image intensities due to scatter. We used a value of 30 for the experiments presented in this paper, which means that the normal distribution falls to half of its peak value at a difference of 35 in intensity value. This value was chosen based on observations of this spread in a single sample image. The formulation in (2) defines the expected US intensities of known tissue types. If the tissue type is not known the probability is uniform. Previously in the literature the Rayleigh distribution has been commonly used to represent the variation of intensity values in 'raw' (i.e. unprocessed) US images (e.g. [6][12]). The K distribution and the family of Gamma distributions (of which the Rayleigh distribution is one) [13] have also been proposed. However, log-compression and low-pass filtering alter the distribution of intensity values. Based on our observations, we believe that a normal distribution better captures the true variation of postprocessed US image intensities. Other distributions that have been proposed for postprocessed US images include the Weibull distribution and the family of Gamma distributions [14].

Boundary probabilities are assigned only for voxels within 5mm of a boundary, i.e. $d(\cdot) \leq 5$. For the boundary probability we use a simple model based on a scaled maximum intensity,

$$p_b = G\left(f_U(\boldsymbol{x}), \beta_{bt}\beta_{inc}\beta_{ac}N_U, \sigma_U\right) \tag{3}$$

β_{bt} represents the effect of beam thickness artefacts, β_{inc} the effect of the angle of incidence of the beam with the surface normal and β_{ac} the effect of acoustic impedance differences between two adjacent regions [10].

Beam Thickness Effect. Beam thickness artefacts [15] are the result of the finite thickness of the US image plane and cause a blurring effect in the US image along the beam direction. In unprocessed US images, this effect has been modelled using a triangular windowing function [7], but log compression postprocessing causes a nonlinear drop-off in intensity away from the true boundary. Therefore we chose to model the beam thickness effect using a normal distribution,

$$\beta_{bt} = G\left(d\left(R^{-1}\cdot\boldsymbol{x}\right), 0, \sigma_{bt}\right) \tag{4}$$

where σ_{bt} is the standard deviation of the normal distribution. We used a value of 2.7 for σ_{bt}, which means that the normal distribution falls to half of its peak value at a distance of 3.2mm from the boundary. Recall that $d(\cdot)$ represents the distance to the nearest boundary.

Angle of Incidence. When an US beam hits a surface the strength of the reflection is dependant on the angle of incidence between the beam and the surface normal. The reflection is strongest when the beam hits the surface perpendicularly (i.e. the angle of incidence is 0°) and falls to zero at an angle of incidence of 90°.

The US probe transducer position is known and fixed in the US image coordinate system. In the segmented image it can be determined by transforming it by the inverse of the current registration estimate, R. Therefore for each voxel in the segmented image a vector from the probe to the voxel can be computed. The surface normal at any voxel in the segmented image is known from the gradient image, $n_L(\cdot)$. The angle between these two vectors is the angle of incidence. The angle of incidence factor β_{inc} is computed as

$$\beta_{inc} = \cos\left(\|n_L(R^{-1} \cdot x) \cdot \left(R_\theta^{-1} \cdot \gamma(x)\right)\|\right)^n \tag{5}$$

where $\gamma(x)$ is the probe direction unit vector to voxel x in the US image and R_θ is the rotational component of R. Normally the reflection intensity would be modelled as the cosine of the angle of incidence (i.e. $n = 1$), but log-compression of the US image causes stronger reflections at a wider range of angles. Therefore in our experiments we used a value of $n = 0.5$.

Acoustic Impedance Difference. Finally, the *reflection coefficient*, β_{ac}, indicates the reflection strength between the region at x and the nearest adjacent region based on their relative acoustic impedances, Z_1 and Z_2, [10]

$$\beta_{ac} = \left(\frac{Z_2 - Z_1}{Z_2 + Z_1}\right)^2 \tag{6}$$

Z_1 and Z_2 are known from the augmented segmentation (see Figure 1).

Knowledge of Tissue Properties. The segmented image is augmented with two pieces of information about the acoustic properties of the tissue: the characteristic acoustic impedance and the scattering strength for each tissue type. Estimated values for the characteristic acoustic impedance of human tissue are available in the literature. We used the values from [16], i.e. 1.61 for blood, 1.7 for muscle and 0.0004 for air ($kg\ m^{-2}\ s^{-1} \times 10^6$). Voxels in the segmented image that did not have a region label were assumed to be air. This is valid in our application of cardiac image registration because the heart is mostly surrounded by the lungs. Values for the scattering strength (i.e. the expected intensity of a homogeneous region) are dependent on the postprocessing settings of the US machine. Therefore we estimated values for muscle, blood pool and aorta from a single sample image (acquired from a different subject not used in the experiments presented in this paper). All test images were preprocessed to simulate the settings of the sample image (see Section 2.4).

2.3   Registration

The registration between the segmented image and the US image(s) was performed by varying the rigid body motion parameters, ϕ, to maximise the sum of log probabilities over the image domains of the US images being used in the registration. For multiple US images the log probabilities for all images are summed.

$$\tilde{\phi} = \underset{\phi}{\operatorname{argmax}} \sum_{u} \sum_{x \in \Omega_u} \log p(x, R(\phi)) \qquad (7)$$

where $\phi = (T_x, T_y, T_z, \theta_x, \theta_y, \theta_z)$ is a vector containing the six rigid-body motion parameters, $R(\phi)$ is the matrix transformation produced from these motion parameters, $\tilde{\phi}$ is the final motion estimate and Ω_u is the image domain of US image u. The optimisation was performed using a simple hill-climbing strategy.

2.4   Materials

All MRI images were acquired using a 1.5 Tesla cylindrical bore Philips Achieva MRI scanner. High resolution cardiac volumes were acquired using a 3-D balanced TFE sequence, which was gated at end-exhale and cardiac triggered and gated at late diastole (typically: reconstructed voxel size $1.37 \times 1.37 \times 1.37\text{mm}^3$, 110 sagittal slices, 256×256 matrix, scan time approximately 5 minutes).

All 3-D US images were acquired by an experienced sonographer using an iE33 3-D real-time echocardiography system with a X3-1 3 to 1 MHz broadband matrix array transducer (Philips Healthcare). Infrared light emitting diodes (LEDs) were attached to the US probe to enable it to be tracked using an Optotrak tracking system (Northern Digital Inc.). The probe was calibrated using the method described in [17]. Images were acquired from modified parasternal or apical views, depending on the available acoustic windows for each subject.

Data were acquired from 3 volunteers and 1 patient. The volunteers were all male and aged between 20-23. The patient was male, aged 52, and underwent a pulmonary vein ablation catheterisation to treat atrial fibrillation. All subjects gave informed consent. For volunteer C and patient A optical tracking information was not available. In these cases the relative positions of the US images were automatically computed by coregistering them using the technique described in [18].

All MRI images were acquired with the subjects in a supine position. For volunteer B and patient A the US images were acquired in a supine position. Volunteer C was on their side for US image acquisition. For volunteer A US images were acquired in both the supine position and on their side. Because of the relative movement of the heart and the descending aorta when a subject moves onto their side the descending aorta was excluded from the segmentation for the experiments in which US images were acquired on the subjects' side. Two 3-D US images were acquired for each experiment. Prior to registration, each US image was preprocessed as follows (see Figure 2).

- *Intensity rescaling*: The images were rescaled to ensure that the intensities in the blood pool matched those in the sample image from which the scattering strengths were estimated. First, a rectangular region of the left ventricle was manually delineated in each US image and the mean intensity within the region computed. Next, the US image intensities were linearly scaled so

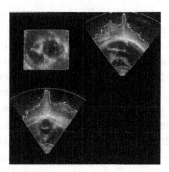

Fig. 2. Filtering a 3-D US image to remove artefacts. The figure shows three orthogonal slices through the 3-D volume centred on the cursor. The white lines outline the area filtered out by the artefact filtering algorithm. The image shown is the parasternal image for volunteer C.

that the mean intensity within the left ventricle region matched the mean intensity in the left ventricle of the sample image whilst maintaining the same maximum intensity in the image. This process is similar to the linear scaling process applied by most US machines to improve visualisation of the images.

– *Artefact filtering*: A simple 3-D artefact removal algorithm was employed which is similar to that employed in 2-D in [3][2]. The algorithm works by tracing a series of lines which represent US beam paths, i.e. radial lines from the transducer face. For each line, starting at the furthest point in the image from the probe position, the algorithm moves towards the probe and labels all voxels as artefacts until a threshold value is reached. Beyond this all voxels are labelled as non-artefact. In addition, a region within 30mm of the probe was labelled as artefact to remove artefacts close to the transducer face. See Figure 2.

2.5 Experiments

We performed experiments to test the accuracy, robustness and precision of the proposed registration technique. In the absence of a gold standard transformation between the MRI and US images, we defined an error measure based on features identified in both the MRI and US images. For each subject, the surfaces of the four chambers of the heart and the myocardium, the centre line of the descending aorta and one point at the lateral extreme of the papillary muscle in the left ventricle were extracted from the segmented MRI image. Next, a number of features were manually identified in both US images. The features used depended on the field of view of each US image, including points on the boundaries of the four chambers and myocardium, points in the centre line of the descending aorta and the papillary muscle, where visible. The overall error measure for each subject was defined as the root mean square (RMS) distance from all US image feature points to their corresponding MRI features.

To test the proposed registration technique, a number of random starting positions were generated. First, an approximate registration between the MRI and US coordinate systems was determined manually. From this initial registration, we executed our registration algorithm to register the images. From this registration, random noise was added to the 6 rigid body motion parameters to produce a series of random starting positions. The error measure was computed for each starting position. A subset of the starting positions was selected to ensure a good spread of initial error values (30 starting positions were chosen with error measures between 3mm and 32mm). Finally, the proposed registration technique was executed from each selected starting position. The registration was performed using only a single US image and also using both US images. The final error measure was computed for each registration result and each result was visually assessed and classified as either a success or a failure. To determine the precision of the proposed technique, for all successful registrations, the mean and standard deviation of the final locations of the US feature points were computed.

3   Results

Overlaid US and segmented MRI images for a sample successful registration are shown in Figure 3. Registration results for all subjects are presented in Figure 4. The accuracy, precision and robustness results for these datasets are given in Table 1. The results show that accuracy of the technique is 2.6-4.2mm. Generally using two US images instead of one in the registration leads to improved robustness, particularly if the images are acquired from different acoustic windows (i.e. apical and parasternal). Better results are also obtained if the subject is on their side during US image acquisition.

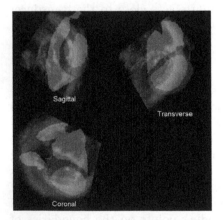 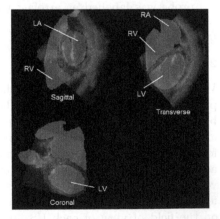

Fig. 3. Three orthogonal slices through a MRI segmentation and a 3-D US image overlaid to illustrate a sample registration result: left: starting position; right: after registration. Annotations show the positions of the left ventricle (LV), right ventricle (RV), left atrium (LA) and right atrium (RA) in the three slices.

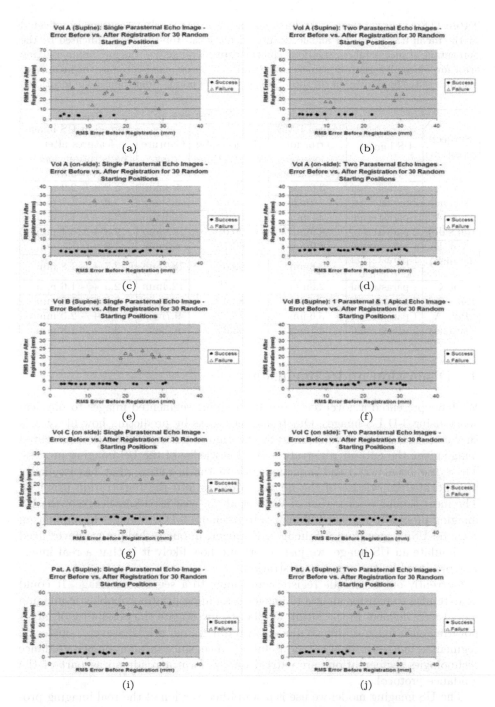

Fig. 4. Registration results: left column results are for a single US image and right column results are for two US images. (a), (b) vol. A, supine; (c), (d) vol. A, on side; (e), (f) vol. B, supine; (g), (h) vol. C, on side; (i), (j) pat. A, supine.

Table 1. Summary of accuracy, robustness and precision results. Accuracy is indicated by the mean RMS error for all successful registrations. Robustness is indicated by the percentage of successful registrations and the capture range (i.e. the maximum starting error for which all registrations were successful). Precision is indicated by the mean/s.d. distance of the final locations of the US image feature points from their mean locations.

Subject (position)	US images	Accuracy Mean RMS error for successful registrations	Robustness % successful registrations	Capture range	Precision Spread of US image features after registration, mean +/- s.d.
Vol. A (supine)	1 parasternal	3.6mm	23.3%	4.9mm	5.2 +/- 2.9 mm
	2 parasternal	4.2mm	40.0%	9.5mm	3.0 +/- 1.7 mm
Vol. A (on side)	1 parasternal	2.7mm	83.3%	10.9mm	2.9 +/- 1.6 mm
	2 parasternal	3.5mm	90.0%	10.9mm	2.8 +/- 1.4 mm
Vol. B (supine)	1 parasternal	3.0mm	66.7%	9.3mm	1.6 +/- 1.5 mm
	1 parasternal & 1 apical	2.8mm	90.0%	18.7mm	2.7 +/- 1.8 mm
Vol. C (on side)	1 parasternal	2.8mm	76.7%	12.4mm	2.5 +/- 1.6 mm
	2 parasternal	2.6mm	83.3%	13.0mm	2.0 +/- 1.5 mm
Pat. A (supine)	1 parasternal	3.6mm	56.7%	9.7mm	3.5 +/- 2.0 mm
	2 parasternal	4.1mm	63.3%	9.7mm	3.3 +/- 1.8 mm

4   Discussion and Conclusions

We have presented a novel technique for aligning segmented images to physical space using 3-D US images. Our technique works by predicting how likely it is that a real US image was produced by the anatomy described by the segmented image given the current registration and knowledge of the US imaging process. There has been very little previous work in the literature that has explicitly incorporated knowledge of the imaging process into the registration problem. The most similar work is that of Wein et al [5], who used knowledge of the US imaging process to register CT images to freehand 3-D US images by simulating B-mode US images from CT images. However, in our technique we never need to simulate an US image, we just determine how likely it is that a real image was produced by the current registration.

Currently our technique registers an image to a segmented image. It could be extended to register images to images if an appropriate probabilistic imaging model were defined. In the future we plan to investigate the possibility of incorporating such image-to-image models into our framework. However, registering segmented images to images is a useful advance, since in many image-guidance technologies segmentations are carried out to form a roadmap as part of the guidance protocol.

The US imaging model we use is a simplified version of the real imaging process. For example, we have ignored the effect of attenuation of the US signal beyond highly reflecting boundaries and we have used a generalised model of the postprocessing operations performed by the US machine. We used a normal distribution to model the variation of intensity values within homogeneous regions. However, Tao et al [14] have suggested that Gamma and Weibull distributions may better model this variation. In future work we plan to investigate the impact of these models on our technique. There is an inherent trade-off between the realism/accuracy of the model and its computational complexity. We have attempted to incorporate the most important elements of the US imaging process whilst preserving its simplicity and avoiding impacting on the work of the sonographer. The execution time of the current implementation of the algorithm is currently about 7 minutes for a $224 \times 208 \times 201$ US image, run on a 2.16 GHz Pentium 4 PC. However, because the step size is successively reduced during the optimisation to refine the registration an approximate alignment is normally available after about 1 minute. The execution time could be further reduced by subsampling the US images. Our main clinical application is the registration of a preprocedure roadmap to physical space for cardiac catheterisations [19]. In such procedures preparation of the patient and gaining intravascular access typically takes at least 15 minutes so we believe that the algorithm is fast enough to fit into our clinical protocol with minimal inconvenience.

The results we have presented are encouraging, and have also provided some useful insight into what type of image acquisition protocol would be required if the technique were to be incorporated into the clinical workflow. The best result occurred when it was possible to acquire US images from two different acoustic windows (parasternal and apical). This is because the two images are more likely to highlight different anatomical features, increasing the amount of information available to the registration algorithm. Also, results seem to be better when the subject was on their side (which is common practice for US image acquisition), although this may not be possible for some image guidance applications. For supine subjects it seems to be important to get good coverage of the descending aorta in the US images (there was good aorta coverage for volunteer B but not so good for volunteer A and patient A). If the aorta is not clearly visible in the US images then there can be rotational errors in the registration due to the ball-like shape of the left ventricle. The capture range of the proposed technique is 9-18mm when using more than 1 US image. It is feasible that a manual registration or simple feature based registration [20] could align MRI and US images to within this margin. The accuracy of the technique is 2.6-4.2mm which is within the clinical accuracy requirement for many image guidance applications. For example, for image-guided cardiac catheterisations we estimate the accuracy requirement to be 5mm.

Acknowledgements

This work was co-funded by the Technology Strategy Boards Collaborative Research and Development programme, following an open competition (grant no. 17352), Philips Healthcare, Best, Netherlands, EPSRC grant EP/D061474/1 and EPSRC fellowship GR/T02799/03. We thank the anonymous reviewers for their constructive suggestions.

References

1. Roche, A., Pennec, X., Malandain, G., Ayache, N.: Rigid registration of 3D ultrasound with MR images: A new approach combining intensity and gradient information. IEEE Transactions on Medical Imaging 20, 1038–1049 (2001)
2. Leroy, A., Mozer, P., Payan, Y., Troccaz, J.: Rigid registration of freehand 3D ultrasound and CT-scan kidney images. In: Barillot, C., Haynor, D.R., Hellier, P. (eds.) MICCAI 2004. LNCS, vol. 3216, pp. 837–844. Springer, Heidelberg (2004)
3. Penney, G.P., Blackall, J.M., Hamady, M.S., Sabharwal, T., Adam, A., Hawkes, D.J.: Registration of freehand 3D ultrasound and magnetic resonance liver images. Medical Image Analysis 8, 81–91 (2004)
4. Huang, X., Hill, N.A., Ren, J., Peters, T.M.: Rapid registration of multimodal images using a reduced number of voxels. In: Proceedings SPIE Medical Imaging, vol. 6141 (2006)
5. Wein, W., Brunke, S., Khamene, A., Callstrom, M.R., Navab, N.: Automatic CT-ultrasound registration for diagnostic imaging and image-guided intervention. Medical Image Analysis 12, 577–585 (2008)
6. Cardinal, M.R., Meunier, J., Soulez, G., Maurice, R.L., Therasse, E., Cloutier, G.: Intravascular ultrasound image segmentation: A three-dimensional fast-marching method based on gray level distributions. IEEE Transactions on Medical Imaging 25(5), 590–601 (2006)
7. Shams, R., Hartley, R., Navab, N.: Real-time simulation of medical ultrasound from CT images. In: Metaxas, D., Axel, L., Fichtinger, G., Székely, G. (eds.) MICCAI 2008, Part II. LNCS, vol. 5242, pp. 734–741. Springer, Heidelberg (2008)
8. Zhuang, X., Hawkes, D.J., Crum, W.R., Boubertakh, R., Uribe, S., Atkinson, D., Batchelor, P., Schaeffter, T., Razavi, R., Hill, D.L.G.: Robust registration between cardiac MRI images and atlas for segmentation propagation. In: Proceedings SPIE Medical Imaging (2008)
9. Maurer Jr., C., Qi, R., Raghavan, V.: A linear time algorithm for computing exact Euclidean distance transforms of binary images in arbitrary dimensions. IEEE Transactions on Pattern Analysis and Machine Intelligence 25(2), 265–269 (2003)
10. Webb, S. (ed.): The Physics of Medical Imaging. Institute of Physics Publishing (1988)
11. Sanches, J.M., Marques, J.S.: Compensation of log-compressed images for 3-d ultrasound. Ultrasound in Medicine and Biology 29(2), 239–253 (2003)
12. Dias, J.M.B., Leitão, J.M.N.: Wall position and thickness estimation from sequences of echocardiographic images. IEEE Transactions on Medical Imaging 15(1), 25–38 (1996)
13. Nillesen, M.M., Lopata, R.G.P., Gerrits, I.H., Kapusta, L., Thussen, J.M., de Korte, C.L.: Modeling envelope statistics of blood and myocardium for segmentation of echocardiographic images. Ultrasound in Medicine and Biology 34(4), 674–680 (2008)
14. Tao, Z., Tagare, H.D., Beaty, J.D.: Evaluation of four probability distribution models for speckle in clinical cardiac ultrasound images. IEEE Transactions on Medical Imaging 25(11), 1483–1492 (2006)
15. Goldstein, A., Madrazo, B.: Slice-thickness artifacts in gray-scale ultrasound. J. Clin. Ultrasound 9, 365–375 (1981)
16. Feng, D.D.: Biomedical Information Technology. Academic Press, London (2008)

17. Ma, Y.L., Rhode, K.S., Gao, G., King, A.P., Chinchapatnam, P., Schaeffter, T., Hawkes, D.J., Razavi, R., Penney, G.P.: Ultrasound calibration using intensity-based image registration: For application in cardiac catheterization procedures. In: Proceedings SPIE Medical Imaging (2008)
18. Grau, V., Becher, H., Noble, A.: Registration of multiview real-time 3-D echocardiographic sequences. IEEE Transactions on Medical Imaging 26(9), 1154–1165 (2007)
19. Rhode, K.S., Hill, D.L.G., Edwards, P.J., Hipwell, J., Rueckert, D., Sanchez-Ortiz, G., Hegde, S., Rahunathan, V., Razavi, R.: Registration and tracking to integrate X-ray and MR images in an XMR facility. IEEE Transactions on Medical Imaging 22(11), 1369–1378 (2003)
20. Ma, Y.L., Rhode, K.S., King, A.P., Cauldfield, D., Cooklin, M., Razavi, R., Penney, G.P.: Echocardiography to magnetic resonance image registration for use in image-guided electrophysiology procedures. In: Proceedings SPIE Medical Imaging (2009)

Automatic Cortical Sulcal Parcellation Based on Surface Principal Direction Flow Field Tracking

Gang Li[1], Lei Guo[1], Jingxin Nie[1], and Tianming Liu[2]

[1] School of Automation, Northwestern Polytechnical University, Xi'an, China
[2] Department of Computer Science and Bioimaging Research Center,
The University of Georgia, Athens, GA, USA

Abstract. Automatic parcellation of cortical surfaces into sulcal based regions is of great importance in structural and functional mapping of human brain. In this paper, a novel method is proposed for automatic cortical sulcal parcellation based on the geometric characteristics of the cortical surface including its principal curvatures and principal directions. This method is composed of two major steps: 1) employing the hidden Markov random field model (HMRF) and the expectation maximization (EM) algorithm on the maximum principal curvatures of the cortical surface for sulcal region segmentation, and 2) using a principal direction flow field tracking method on the cortical surface for sulcal basin segmentation. The flow field is obtained by diffusing the principal direction field on the cortical surface. The method has been successfully applied to the inner cortical surfaces of twelve healthy human brain MR images. Both quantitative and qualitative evaluation results demonstrate the validity and efficiency of the proposed method.

Keywords: Sulcal region segmentation, sulcal basin segmentation.

1 Introduction

The human cerebral cortex is a highly convoluted and complex anatomical structure composed of sulci and gyri, corresponding to the valleys and ridges of the cortical surface representation respectively. Major cortical sulci and gyri are common macroscopic anatomical landmarks in human brains, even though the precise pattern of sulci and gyri geometry could vary considerably across individuals [1]. Thus, major cortical sulci and gyri have been extensively used for assisting deformable registration of brain MR images [2, 3], analyzing the variation of healthy human brain [4], as well as differentiating between normal brain and diseased ones [5]. Since it is very time consuming to manually annotate sulci, automatic sulci extraction has received attention as a research goal in recent years. Therefore, a wide variety of automatic or semi-automatic methods have been proposed for extraction of sulci [6, 7, 8, 9, 10] or sulcal fundi [11, 12, 13, 14, 15].

In this paper, we present an original method for parcellation of the cortical surface into sulcal regions and corresponding sulcal basins based on the geometric characteristics of principal curvatures and principal directions. By definitions, sulcal regions

J.L. Prince, D.L. Pham, and K.J. Myers (Eds.): IPMI 2009, LNCS 5636, pp. 202–214, 2009.

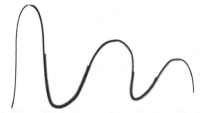

Fig. 1. A 2D schematic illustration of sulcal regions and sulcal basins. The red color parts indicate two sulcal regions. The blue and green parts represent two adjacent sulcal basins.

are the buried regions surrounding sulcal space on cortical surfaces [9], while sulcal basins are the regions bounded by gyral crest lines which separate different basins [8]. Thus, adjacent sulcal basins meet at the gyral crest lines on the cortical surface and partition of the cortical surface into sulcal basins produces a complete parcellation of the cortical surface [8]. Figure 1 shows a 2D schematic illustration of sulcal regions and sulcal basins. The basic ideas of our method are twofold. Firstly, since the maximum principal curvatures are negative at sulcal regions and positive at gyral regions, we model the histogram distribution of maximum principal curvatures using finite mixture Gaussian model and employ the hidden Markov random field model (HMRF) and the expectation maximization (EM) algorithm [16] based on the maximum principal curvatures of the cortical surface for sulcal region segmentation. Secondly, as the principal directions corresponding to the maximum principal curvatures point either towards or away from sulcal regions at a surface vertex, we follow the principal directions or the opposite directions of principal directions to reach sulcal bottom regions. The set of vertices that flow to the same sulcal bottom region are naturally grouped together as a sulcal basin. Thus, partition of the cortical surface into different sulcal basins is naturally achieved. Notably, the estimated principal direction might be noisy and unreliable at flat cortical areas. To deal with this issue, we design a novel principal direction field diffusion method on the triangularized cortical surface by minimization an energy function, in order to generate a smooth flow field from the noisy principal direction field.

The major contributions of this paper are threefold. Firstly, we extended the hidden Markov random field model and the expectation maximization (HMRF-EM) algorithm to triangular cortical surfaces for sulcal region segmentation based on maximum principal curvatures. Secondly, we designed a novel principal direction field diffusion method on the cortical surface to produce a smooth principal direction flow field from the noisy principal direction field. Finally, we developed a new method called flow field tracking for sulcal basin segmentation using the generated flow field. It should be noted that the methods of principal direction field diffusion and flow field tracking are not limited to the work on cortical surfaces only, but could be potentially generalized for surface mesh segmentation in many other applications.

2 Methods

Given a triangular cortical surface, our method for cortical sulcal parcellation performs following steps, as shown in figure 2. Firstly, the principal curvatures and

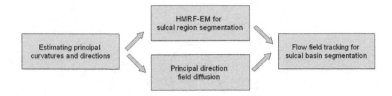

Fig. 2. The flow chart of the proposed cortical sulcal parcellation method

principal directions of each vertex on the cortical surface are estimated. Then, the HMRF-EM framework is adopted to achieve sulcal region segmentation on the cortical surface based on maximum principal curvatures. Afterwards, the principal direction field is diffused to produce a smooth flow field on the cortical surface by minimization an energy function. Finally, the flow field tracking method is performed in the produced flow field to partition the cortical surface into different sulcal basins. In subsequent sections, each step will be explained in detail.

2.1 Estimating Principal Curvatures and Principal Directions

We adopt a robust finite differences method to estimate the principal curvatures, the principal directions and the principal curvature derivatives along with the principal directions as described in [17]. For sulcal region and sulcal basin segmentation, we are interested both in the maximum principal curvature, which is the principal curvature with the largest absolute value in the two principal curvatures, and in its corresponding principal direction (maximum principal direction). The maximum principal curvature and maximum principal direction measure the maximum strength and direction of the normal direction variation respectively. However, the opposite direction of the maximum principal direction can also be considered as the maximum principal direction. To force the maximum principal directions uniformly point toward sulcal bottom regions, which are the regions with large negative maximum principal curvatures, if the directional derivative of maximum principal curvature along maximum principal direction is positive, we flip maximum principal direction to the opposite direction. As a result, the maximum principal directions uniformly point toward the

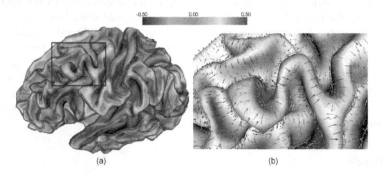

(a)   (b)

Fig. 3. An example of the estimated maximum principal curvatures and maximum principal directions on a cortical inner surface. (a) The maximum principal curvature. (b) The maximum principal direction of the bounded rectangular cortical region in (a). Color bar is on the top.

steep decreasing direction of maximum principal curvature. Figure 3 shows an example of the estimated maximum principal curvature and maximum principal direction on a cortical inner surface of a hemisphere.

2.2 Sulcal Region Segmentation Based on the HMRF-EM

As mentioned before, e.g. in figure 3, the maximum principal curvatures are negative at sulcal regions and positive at gyral regions. Therefore, we model the histogram distribution of maximum principal curvatures using finite mixture Gaussian model. Herein we employ the maximum principal curvature as a feature for sulcal region segmentation, rather than previously used mean curvature [10, 12, 13, 15] or sulcal depth [9, 10, 14]. Because mean curvature is calculated as the average of the maximum and minimum principal curvatures. However, the minimum principal curvatures might be very small values at both sulcal and gyral regions. Therefore, minimum principal curvatures are not good features for distinguishing between them. In comparison, the maximum principal curvatures are more discriminative than mean curvature for sulcal region segmentation. To demonstrate this point, figure 4 shows the histograms of maximum principal curvature and mean curvature of the cortical surface shown in figure 3 (a). Obviously, compared to the histogram distribution of mean curvature, which is more like a single Gaussian distribution (was also observed in [15]), it is much easier to determine the threshold for sulcal and gyral region segmentation from the histogram distribution of maximum principal curvature which acts as a distribution of two Gaussian mixtures. We don't adopt sulcal depth as feature because, firstly, the outer hull of cortical surface is not easy to define since the cortex can be concave; secondly, both the sulcal regions and buried ridges in sulcal regions are very deep, therefore, sulcal depth can not distinguish between them. To encode both statistical and spatial information into the Gaussian mixture model, we extended the hidden Markov random field and the expectation maximization (HMRF-EM) framework, which is an elegant method originally developed for tissue segmentation in human brain MR images [16], on triangular cortical surfaces as follows.

Let y_i be the maximum principal curvature and $x_i \in \{0, 1\}$ be the class label at vertex i, where 0 represents sulcal region and 1 represents gyral region. According to

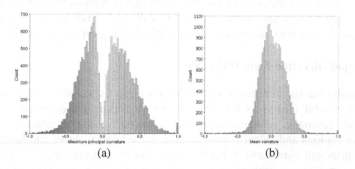

(a)   (b)

Fig. 4. The histogram distributions of curvatures on the cortical surface as in Fig. 3 (a). (a) The histogram of maximum principal curvatures; (b) The histogram of mean curvatures.

the Bayes theory and MAP criterion [16], the problem of sulcal and gyral region segmentation can be formulated as seeking the true class label $\hat{X} = (\hat{x}_1,...,\hat{x}_n)$, which satisfies:

$$\hat{X} = \arg\max_{X}\{P(Y\mid X)P(X)\}$$
(1)

where $X = (x_1,...,x_n)$ and $Y = (y_1,...,y_n)$ and n is the total vertex number on the cortical surface. Given a label $x_i = l$, the observed values of y_i follow a Gaussian distribution with the parameter $\theta = (\mu_l, \sigma_l)$. In the Gaussian hidden Markov random field (GHMRF) model, the distribution of y_i dependent on the parameter θ and x_{N_i} is calculated as:

$$p(y_i \mid x_{N_i}, \theta) = \sum_{l \in L} g(y_i; \theta_l) p(l \mid X_{N_i})$$
(2)

where x_{N_i} is the set of neighborhood of vertex i, L represents all of the possible labels and $g(y_i; \theta_l)$ is a Gaussian function:

$$g(y; \theta_l) = \frac{1}{\sqrt{2\pi\sigma_l^2}}\exp(-\frac{(y-\mu_l)^2}{2\sigma_l^2})$$
(3)

According to the Hammersley-Clifford theorem, a Markov random field (MRF) can equivalently be characterized by a Gibbs distribution [16], and its energy function is the sum of clique potential of all possible cliques. In the paper, a clique is defined as a vertex pair in which the vertices are neighbors and only cliques of a size up to two are considered. The clique potential function is defined as:

$$V_c(X) = -\left\|v_i - v_j\right\|^{-1}$$
(4)

where v_i and v_j are the spatial locations of a pair of vertex neighbors in a clique.

To estimate both of the class label and model parameters, we adopt the expectation maximization (EM) algorithm. The iterated conditional modes (ICM) is employed for solving MRF-MAP estimation. After sulcal region segmentation, we use connective component analysis on the extracted sulcal regions to label each connective sulcal region as a unique value, which will be further used for sulcal basin segmentation. Figure 8 (a) shows an example of sulcal region segmentation results.

2.3 Principal Direction Field Diffusion

After obtaining the sulcal regions, we further partition the cortical surface into sulcal basins. The central idea is as follows. As the maximum principal directions point towards the maximum principal curvature steep decreasing directions, meanwhile gyral crown regions and sulcal bottom regions have large positive and large negative maximum principal curvatures respectively, we follow the maximum principal directions from gyral crown regions until to sulcal bottom regions. The set of vertices flowing to the same sulcal bottom are naturally grouped together as a sulcal basin. However, the principal directions are noisy and unreliable at flat cortical areas. To deal with this issue, inspired by the gradient vector field diffusion method for intensity images [18, 21], we design a novel principal direction field diffusion method on the cortical surface to produce a smoothing principal direction flow field.

Given a triangular cortical surface, the principal direction flow field $\mathbf{v}(\mathbf{x}) = (u(\mathbf{x}), v(\mathbf{x}), w(\mathbf{x}))$ is defined as the solution that minimizes an energy function:

$$\varepsilon = \int_{\mathbf{x} \in S} \lambda |\nabla \mathbf{v}(\mathbf{x})|^2 + f(\mathbf{x}) |\mathbf{v}(x) - \mathbf{p}(x)|^2 \, d\mathbf{x} \tag{5}$$

with subject to: $\mathbf{v}(\mathbf{x}) \cdot \mathbf{n}(\mathbf{x}) = 0$, where λ is a weighting parameter and ∇ is the gradient operator. $\mathbf{p}(\mathbf{x})$ is the maximum principal direction at vertex $\mathbf{x}$ and $f(\mathbf{x})$ is set to be: $f(\mathbf{x}) = |c(\mathbf{x})|$, where $c(\mathbf{x})$ is the maximum principal curvature. $\mathbf{n}(\mathbf{x})$ is the normal vector, and S indicates the set of all of the vertices on the cortical surface. The formula $\mathbf{v}(\mathbf{x}) \cdot \mathbf{n}(\mathbf{x}) = 0$ constrains the flow field in the tangent planes of the surface. According to the energy function, at flat cortical regions, where the magnitudes of maximum principal curvatures are small, the energy is dominated by the first partial derivatives term to enforce that the flow field varies smoothly. While at regions with large magnitudes of maximum principal curvatures, corresponding to sulcal bottoms and gyral crowns with reliable and informative principal directions, the energy is dominated by the second term to enforce that the flow field is close to the original principal direction field. The parameter λ determines the tradeoff between the first smoothing term and the second fidelity term. We set λ as 0.1 in all of our experiments and the optimal parameter λ will be investigated in future.

To minimize the above energy function, we use calculus of variation to obtain the following partial differential equation (PDE):

$$\lambda \nabla^2 \mathbf{v}(\mathbf{x}) - (\mathbf{v}(\mathbf{x}) - \mathbf{p}(\mathbf{x})) f(\mathbf{x}) = 0 \tag{6}$$

Above PDE is solved by treating $\mathbf{v}$ as a function of time:

$$\mathbf{v}_t(\mathbf{x}, t) = \lambda \nabla^2 \mathbf{v}(\mathbf{x}, t) - (\mathbf{v}(\mathbf{x}, t) - \mathbf{p}(\mathbf{x})) f(\mathbf{x}) \tag{7}$$

where $\mathbf{v}_t(\mathbf{x}, t)$ denotes the partial derivative of $\mathbf{v}(\mathbf{x}, t)$ with respect to time t, and ∇^2 is the Laplacian term on the surface. The equation can be further decoupled as:

$$u_t(\mathbf{x}, t) = \lambda \nabla^2 u(\mathbf{x}, t) - (u(\mathbf{x}, t) - \mathbf{p}_u(\mathbf{x})) f(\mathbf{x})$$

$$v_t(\mathbf{x}, t) = \lambda \nabla^2 v(\mathbf{x}, t) - (v(\mathbf{x}, t) - \mathbf{p}_v(\mathbf{x})) f(\mathbf{x}) \tag{8}$$

$$w_t(\mathbf{x}, t) = \lambda \nabla^2 w(\mathbf{x}, t) - (w(\mathbf{x}, t) - \mathbf{p}_w(\mathbf{x})) f(\mathbf{x})$$

The algorithm of principal direction field diffusion is summarized as follows:

1. According to $\mathbf{v}(\mathbf{x}, t)$ $(t = 0, 1, 2...)$, solve the decoupled PDE equations to obtain the diffused principal direction field $\mathbf{v}(\mathbf{x}, t+1)$;
2. Project $\mathbf{v}(\mathbf{x}, t+1)$ into the tangent plane;
3. Normalize the projected $\mathbf{v}(\mathbf{x}, t+1)$;
4. Replace $\mathbf{v}(\mathbf{x}, t)$ with the normalized and projected $\mathbf{v}(\mathbf{x}, t+1)$ and repeat steps 1-3 until enough iterations have been carried out.

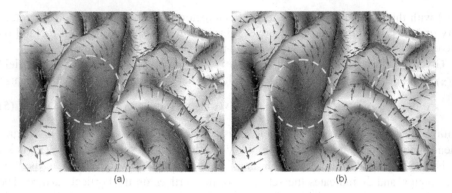

(a)   (b)

Fig. 5. An example of principal direction field diffusion on a cortical region cropped from the cortical surface shown in Figure 3 (a). (a) is the original principal direction field. (b) is the principal direction flow field. The yellow circles highlight two regions in which the vectors flow much more smoothly towards sulcal bottom regions in the principal direction flow field.

Figure 5 shows a comparison between the original principal direction field and the diffused principal direction field on a cortical surface. Apparently, in the diffused principal direction field, vectors flow much more smoothly from gyral crowns towards sulcal bottoms. This elegant property greatly contributes to the success of sulcal basin segmentation based on the flow field tracking method as described later.

2.4   Sulcal Basin Segmentation Based on Flow Field Tracking

In the principal direction flow field, the vectors flow smoothly toward the sinks of the flow field, corresponding to sulcal bottom regions on the cortical surface. To follow the vectors until stopping at the sulcal bottom regions, the flow field tracking procedure on the cortical surface is performed as follows. From a given vertex $\mathbf{X}$ with the diffused principal direction $\mathbf{v}(\mathbf{x})$, the next vertex $\mathbf{x}'$ that $\mathbf{X}$ flows through in the flow field is computed as:

$$\mathbf{x}' = \min_{\mathbf{x}_i}(\arccos\langle \mathbf{v}(\mathbf{x}) \cdot \mathbf{x}\mathbf{x}_i / \|\overrightarrow{\mathbf{x}\mathbf{x}_i}\| \rangle) \qquad (9)$$

where $\mathbf{x}_i$ is the one-ring adjacent vertices of $\mathbf{X}$. It means that the next vertex $\mathbf{x}'$ is the vertex in the one-ring neighborhood of $\mathbf{X}$ which minimizes the angle between vector $\mathbf{v}(\mathbf{x})$ and the direction of edge $\overrightarrow{\mathbf{x}\mathbf{x}_i}$. The angle between two consecutive vectors in the flow path is determined as: $\theta = \arccos\langle \mathbf{v}(\mathbf{x}) \cdot \mathbf{v}(\mathbf{x}') \rangle$. If the angle between two consecutive vectors is less than $\pi/2$ (the inner product between two consecutive vectors is positive), the flow tracking procedure continues. Otherwise, two consecutive vectors will point to each other and the inner product between them will be negative, which is a necessary condition for valley detection in the triangular surface mesh [19, 20], and the flow tracking procedure will be stopped. As a result, a sulcal bottom region is reached. In this way, the vectors at vertices along the flow tracking trajectory define a smooth path leading to a sulcal bottom region. The partition of cortical surface into different sulcal basins can be achieved by starting this flow tracking

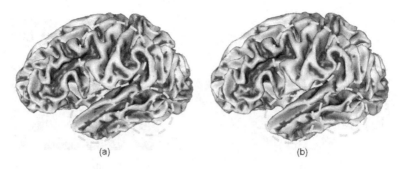

(a)   (b)

Fig. 6. A comparison of the termination vertices on flow tracking trajectories before and after principal direction field diffusion on a cortical inner surface. The red color vertices in (a) and (b) are the set of termination vertices in the original principal direction field and the diffused principal direction field respectively. The yellow circles highlight some regions where noisy flow tracking termination vertices at flat cortical regions are removed in the flow field.

procedure from each vertex on the cortical surface. All the vertices flowing to the same sulcal region are grouped as a sulcal basin. Figure 6 provides a comparison of the termination vertices on flow tracking trajectories before and after principal direction diffusion on a cortical surface. Clearly, after the diffusion procedure, some noisy termination vertices of flow tracking at flat cortical regions are removed effectively. Meanwhile, the termination vertices at sulcal bottom regions are well preserved. This further demonstrates that the principal direction diffusion procedure is quite important for producing robust and reliable sulcal basin segmentation. However, it is time-consuming to run the flow tracking procedure for every vertex to achieve sulcal basin segmentation. Actually, it is not necessary to apply the flow tracking procedure to the vertices that have already been on the flow trajectories of any previously passed vertices. Instead, these passed vertices can be directly associated with the sulcal region to which the path flows. This improvement not only speeds up the method, but also yields reproducible segmentation results. After flow field tracking, we may obtain some very small basins, therefore, we prune these small basins and combine them with adjacent sulcal basins. Figure 7 shows an example of vector view of the flow field tracking result on a cortical surface. Figure 8 shows an example of the final sulcal region and sulcal basin segmentation result on a cortical surface.

The flow tracking algorithm on the cortical surface is summarized as follows:

1. Start from a not passed vertex $\mathbf{X}$ as the initial vertex $\mathbf{x}^0$;
2. Obtain $\mathbf{x}^{n+1}$ ($n = 0, 1, 2...$) based on Eq. (9) and $\mathbf{x}^n$;
3. Calculate the angle θ_n between diffused vectors at $\mathbf{x}^{n+1}$ and $\mathbf{x}^n$. If θ_n is larger than $\pi/2$, stop. Otherwise, if the $\mathbf{x}^{n+1}$ is already on a flow path, associate vertices from $\mathbf{x}^0$ to $\mathbf{x}^n$ to the corresponding termination vertex of $\mathbf{x}^{n+1}$ and stop.
4. Replace $\mathbf{x}^n$ with $\mathbf{x}^{n+1}$. Return to step 2.

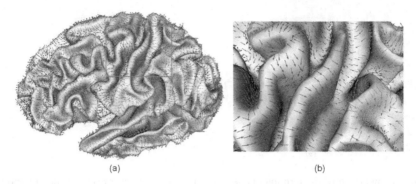

(a)   (b)

Fig. 7. An example of vector view of flow field tracking result on a cortical surface, in which the set of vectors flowing to the same sulcal region are labeled with the same color. (a) is the vector view of the result. (b) is the zoomed view of the bounded rectangular region in (a).

3 Results

We have applied the method to brain MR images of twelve normal subjects. All the topologically correct and geometrically accurate cortical surfaces used in this section were reconstructed by the BrainVISA software [22]. Figure 9 shows the sulcal region and basin segmentation results on the inner cortical surfaces of the left hemisphere of the 12 subjects. It is striking that all of the twelve cortical surfaces are consistently segmented into anatomically meaningful sulcal regions and basins by the proposed method. For example, the central and superior temporal sulcal basins in these twelve subjects, represented by purple and green colors respectively, are quite visually reasonable. Each sulcal region and basin in each subject is randomly assigned a color in Fig. 9, except that the colors for the central and superior temporal sulcal regions and sulcal basins are interactively identified by experts for visualization purpose.

To quantitatively evaluate the sulcal region and sulcal basin segmentation results, we use two metrics: the over-segmentation and under-segmentation. The over-segmentation denotes that a sulcal region has been wrongly separated into more than one sulcal region. The under-segmentation denotes that multiple adjacent sulcal regions have not been appropriately divided. In the paper, we use three major sulci, including central, post-central and superior temporal sulci for validation. In the left hemispheres of the 12 subjects, all of the central and superior temporal sulcal regions are segmented correctly. Therefore, there is no over-segmentation and under- segmentation error. There exists only one over-segmentation error and one under-segmentation error in the post-central sulcal regions of the 12 hemispheres. Since one sulcal basin corresponds to one sulcal region, we have the same performance for sulcal basin segmentation in these 12 subjects. In conclusion, those results indicate good performance of the proposed method.

To further quantitatively evaluate the sulcal basin segmentation results, the central sulcal basins on the inner cortical surfaces of left hemispheres of the twelve subjects are manually annotated by two experts and this manual segmentation is as a standard.

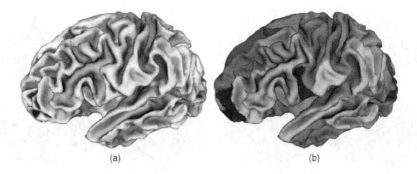

        (a)   (b)

Fig. 8. An example of sulcal region and sulcal basin segmentation results on a cortical surface. (a) is the sulcal region segmentation result, in which each sulcal region is labeled with a unique color. (b) is the corresponding sulcal basin segmentation result.

We applied the area overlap measurement to validate the method. The area overlap is defined as:

$$O(R_a, R_m) = \frac{S(R_a \cap R_m)}{(S(R_a) + S(R_m))/2} \tag{10}$$

where R_a is the automatically extracted sulcal basin and R_m is the manually labeled sulcal basin. The $\cap$ operator takes the intersection of the two regions. $S(.)$ is the area of the region. Figure 10 shows the details of the area overlap measurement for the left central sulcal basins of the 12 subjects. The average area overlap with annotations done by both experts for the 12 subjects is above 0.96, indicating the relatively accurate performance of our sulcal basin segmentation method. Figure 11 shows an example of comparison of the automatically extracted and manually labeled central sulcal basins on a cortical surface.

In order to evaluate the reproducibility of the proposed method, we employ simulated T1-weighted normal brain images with different noise levels obtained from the BrainWeb website [23]. We generated three simulated images with 1mm slice thickness, 20% intensity non-uniformity, and $181 \times 217 \times 181$ voxel resolution. The noise levels of the three images are set as 3%, 5% and 7%, respectively. The topologically correct and geometrically accurate cortical surfaces in this section were generated by in-house tools. As each simulated image has its own independently reconstructed cortical surface with different vertices and triangle faces, it is not convenient to evaluate the results using area overlap measurement. Instead, we calculated the area agreement of several major sulci, including central, post-central and superior temporal sulci on the inner cortical surface of left hemisphere between each pair of the images. The area agreement is computed as:

$$A(S_a, S_b) = \left| 1 - \frac{|S_a - S_b|}{S_a + S_b} \right| \tag{11}$$

where S_a and S_b refer to the areas of the sulcal basins or sulcal regions obtained by the proposed method on different images. The average area agreement of the three

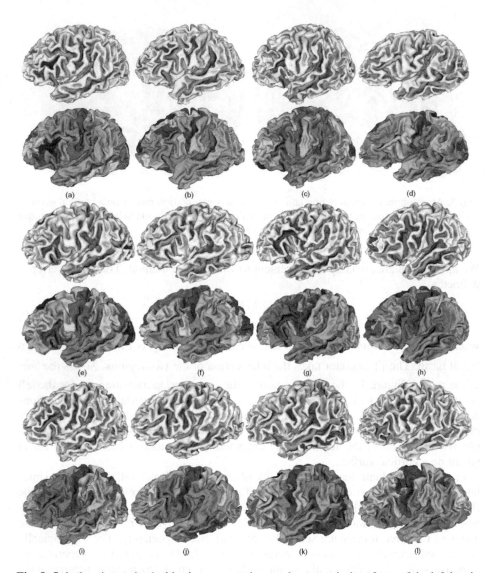

Fig. 9. Sulcal region and sulcal basin segmentation results on cortical surfaces of the left hemispheres of the twelve normal subjects. For each case, the top row image shows the sulcal region segmentation result, and the bottom row image shows the sulcal basin segmentation result. Each sulcal region and its corresponding sulcal basin are labeled with the same color in each cortical surface. It is noted that anatomically corresponding sulcal regions and sulcal basins in different cases may have different colors, except that the colors for the central and superior temporal sulcal regions and sulcal basins of these twelve subjects which are interactively identified by experts for visualization purpose.

sulci on the three simulated images is around 0.98, indicating the good reproducibility of our method.

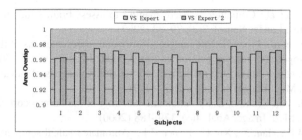

Fig. 10. The area overlap measurement of the left central sulcal basins of the twelve subjects

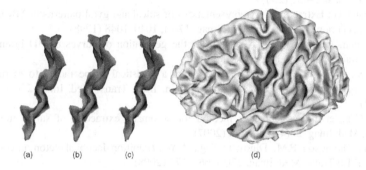

Fig. 11. A comparison of the automatically extracted and the manually labeled left central sulcal basins on a cortical surface. (a) and (b) The manually labeled sulcal basins by two experts. (c) The automatically extracted sulcal basin. (d) The (c) overlaid on the cortical surface.

4 Conclusion

In this paper, a novel method for automatic sulcal parcellation on cortical surfaces is proposed. The method has been applied to 12 normal human brain MR images. Our preliminary results demonstrate that the method is able to segment sulcal region and sulcal basin on cortical surfaces accurately and effectively. Our future work will include further validation of the method on more subjects and development of methods for automatic recognition of the segmented sulcal regions and sulcal basins.

References

1. Ono, M., Kubick, S., Abernathey, C.: Atlas of the Cerebral Sulci. Thieme, New York (1990)
2. Thompson, P.M., Toga, A.W.: A surface-based technique for warping three-dimensional images of the brain. IEEE Trans. Med. Imag. 15(4), 402–417 (1996)
3. Davatzikos, C.: Spatial transformation and registration of brain images using elastically deformable models. Comput. Vis. Image Underst. 66(2), 207–222 (1997)
4. Fillard, P., et al.: Measuring brain variability by extrapolating sparse tensor fields measured on sulcal lines. NeuroImage 34(2), 639–650 (2007)

5. Ashburner, J., et al.: Computer-assisted imaging to assess brain structure in healthy and diseased brains. Lancet Neurol. 2(2), 79–88 (2003)
6. Mangin, J.-F., et al.: From 3D MR images to structural representations of the cortex topography using topology preserving deformations. J. Math. Imaging Vis. 5, 297–318 (1995)
7. Le Goualher, et al.: Automated extraction and variability analysis of sulcal neuroanatomy. IEEE. Trans. Med. Imag. 18(3), 206–217 (1999)
8. Lohmann, G., von Cramon, D.Y.: Automatic labelling of the human cortical surface using sulcal basins. Med. Image. Anal. 4(3), 179–188 (2000)
9. Rettmann, M.E., Han, X., Xu, C., Prince, J.L.: Automated sulcal segmentation using watersheds on the cortical surface. NeuroImage 15(2), 329–344 (2002)
10. Yang, F., Kruggel, F.: Automatic segmentation of human brain sulci. Med. Image. Anal. 12(4), 442–451 (2008)
11. Lohmann, G.: Extracting line representations of sulcal and gyral patterns in MR images of the human brain. IEEE Trans. Med. Imag. 17(6), 1040–1048 (1998)
12. Bartesaghi, A., Sapiro, G.: A system for the generation of curves on 3D brain images. Hum. Brain. Mapp. 14(1), 1–15 (2001)
13. Tao, X., Prince, J.L., Davatzikos, C.: Using a statistical shape model to extract sulcal curves on the outer cortex of the human brain. IEEE Trans. Med. Imag. 21(5), 513–524 (2002)
14. Kao, C.Y., et al.: A geometric method for automatic extraction of sulcal fundi. IEEE Trans. Med. Imag. 26(4), 530–540 (2007)
15. Shi, Y., Thompson, P.M., Dinov, I., Toga, A.W.: Hamilton-Jacobi skeleton on cortical surfaces. IEEE Trans. Med. Imag. 27(5), 664–673 (2008)
16. Zhang, Y., Brady, M., Smith, S.: Segmentation of brain MR image through a Hidden Markov Random Field model and the Expectation-Maximization algorithm. IEEE Trans. Med. Imag. 20(1), 45–57 (2001)
17. Rusinkiewicz, S.: Estimating curvatures and their derivatives on triangle meshes. In: Proc. Symposium on 3D Data Processing, Visualization and Transmission, pp. 486–493 (2004)
18. Xu, C., Prince, J.L.: Snakes, shapes, and gradient vector flow. IEEE Trans. Image Proc. 7(3), 359–369 (1998)
19. Thirion, J.-P.: The extermal mesh and understanding of 3D surfaces. Int. J. Comput. Vis. 19(2), 115–128 (1996)
20. Li, G., et al.: A novel method for cortical sulcal fundi extraction. In: Metaxas, D., Axel, L., Fichtinger, G., Székely, G. (eds.) MICCAI 2008, Part I. LNCS, vol. 5241, pp. 270–278. Springer, Heidelberg (2008)
21. Li, G., et al.: 3D cell nuclei segmentation based on gradient flow tracking. BMC Cell Biol. 8, 40 (2007)
22. http://www.brainvisa.info/
23. http://www.bic.mni.mcgill.ca/brainweb/

A New Information-Theoretic Measure to Control the Robustness-Sensitivity Trade-Off for DMFFD Point-Set Registration

Nicholas J. Tustison, Suyash P. Awate, Gang Song, Tessa S. Cook, and James C. Gee

University of Pennsylvania, Penn Image Computing and Science Laboratory

Abstract. An essential component of many medical image analysis protocols is the establishment and manipulation of feature correspondences. These image features can assume such forms spanning the range of functions of individual or regional pixel intensities to geometric structures extracted as a preprocessing segmentation step. Many algorithms focusing on the latter set of salient features attempt to reduce these structures to such geometric primitives as surfaces, curves and/or points for correspondence-based study. Although the latter geometric primitive forms the basis of many of these algorithms, unrealistic constraints such as assumptions of identical cardinality between point-sets hinder general usage. Furthermore, the local structure for certain point-sets derived from segmentation processes is often ignored. In this paper, we introduce a family of novel information-theoretic measures for poointset registration derived as a generalization of the well-known Shannon entropy known as the Havrda-Charvat-Tsallis entropy. This divergence measure permits a fine-tuning between robustness and sensitivity emphasis. In addition, we employ a directly manipulated free-form deformation (DMFFD) transformation model, a recently developed variant of the well-known FFD transformation model.

1 Introduction

Feature correspondence analysis is an important element in many medical image analysis scenarios. This vast field of research encompasses such problems as intensity-based image registration as well as the establishment of geometrically-based correspondences. The principal contribution that we make in this paper is a novel set of point-set similarity measures based on the local structure intrinsic to the point-sets themselves without exact cardinality constraints. In addition, we present a unique transformation model for point-set registration based on B-splines which we call *directly manipulated free-form deformation* (DMFFD) which overcomes the problematic energy topographies associated with standard FFD approaches [1]. Of most practical consequence is that this work is freely available as open source built within the Insight Toolkit framework [2].

J.L. Prince, D.L. Pham, and K.J. Myers (Eds.): IPMI 2009, LNCS 5636, pp. 215–226, 2009.
© Springer-Verlag Berlin Heidelberg 2009

2   Previous Work: Information-Theoretic Strategies for Point-Set Correspondence

Recent work for point-set correspondence has drawn upon the rich information-theoretic research literature for inspiration of new metrics for assessing point-set correspondence. Tsin and Kanade use a kernel density estimation scheme for approximating a smoothed probability density function (PDF) from a point-set [3]. Correspondence with other similarly constructed PDFs are assessed utilizing correlation. Independently formulated yet employing a similar strategy, Singh et al., dub their correspondence measure *kernel density correlation* [4].

In order to increase robustness over previous approaches, Jian and Vemuri formulate an L_2 distance between two PDFs generated from distinct point-sets using nonparametric density estimation with Gaussian kernels [5]. As an interesting theoretical contribution, they elicit the connection between their L_2 distance and ML-based estimation not only for a pair of PDFs but for multiple PDFs as well. Such investigation draws interesting relationships to an actual distance metric. An L_2 distance is also used by Guo et al. who match point-sets in the space of diffeomorphisms [6].

Wang et al. generalize the Kullback-Leibler (KL) divergence measure to the Jensen-Shannon divergence measure for the construction of unbiased atlases [7] using a thin-plate spline transformation model. This generalization accommodates the unbiased registration of multiple point-sets. Basu et al. propose a class of estimators, known as the *density power divergence* (DPD), between pairs of PDFs which are mutually distinguished by a single, tunable parameter, $\phi \in [0, 1]$ [8]. The authors demonstrate that at the lower extreme, i.e. $\phi = 0$, the DPD reduces to the KL divergence whereas at the upper extreme, i.e. $\phi = 1$, the DPD is equivalent to the L_2 measure between the two PDFs thus allowing a control mechanism for oscillating between sensitivity and robustness.

The paper offers the next stage of development of assessing point-set correspondence. The proposed measure is a generalization of the Jenson-Shannon divergence known as the Jensen-Havrda-Charvat-Tsallis divergence. It is also tunable by a single parameter which modulates between degrees of robustness and sensitivity. Furthermore, in contrast to previous approaches, we encode the local neighborhood configuration of the point-sets within the proposed measure for closer representation to the underlying structure represented by certain types of point-sets.

3   Application of the Jensen-Havrda-Charvat-Tsallis Divergence for Point-Set Correspondence

3.1   Overview

The Havrda-Charvat-Tsallis (HCT) entropy was introduced in [9] and further developed in [10,11]. For a random variable $X : \Omega \mapsto \Re^D$, on sample space Ω, taking values $x \in \Re^D$ and with probability density function $\mathbf{P}(X)$, the HCT entropy [12] (parameterized by a variable, $\alpha > 0$) is defined to be

$$H_\alpha(\mathbf{P}(X)) = \frac{1}{1-\alpha}\left[\int_{\Re^D}[\mathbf{P}(x)]^\alpha dx - 1\right] \approx \frac{1}{1-\alpha}\left[\sum_{x\sim\mathbf{P}(X)}[\mathbf{P}(x)]^{\alpha-1} - 1\right] \quad (1)$$

where $x \sim \mathbf{P}(X)$ denotes that x is randomly drawn from the PDF $\mathbf{P}(X)$. It is well known that $H_\alpha(\cdot)$ reduces to the well-known Shannon entropy as $\alpha \to 1$ [11,12].

Similar to the Jensen-Shannon (JS) divergence, given the HCT entropy one can define a generalized mutual information measure for a set of random variables. This measure is known as the Jensen-Havrda-Charvat-Tsallis (JHCT) divergence [12] and is calculated from K PDFs as follows:

$$\mathrm{JHCT}_\alpha(\mathbf{P}_1,\ldots,\mathbf{P}_K,\alpha,\gamma_1,\ldots,\gamma_K) = H_\alpha\left(\sum_{k=1}^K \gamma_k\mathbf{P}_k(X_k)\right) - \sum_{k=1}^K \gamma_k H_\alpha\left(\mathbf{P}_k(X_k)\right)$$

$$(2)$$

where the set of γ_k can be construed as a prior weighting on the point-sets. The values of these weights are constrained such that $\gamma_k \geq 0$ and $\sum_{k=1}^K \gamma_k = 1$.

3.2   Properties of the JHCT$_\alpha$ Divergence

Several salient properties are associated with the HCT generalized entropy and its Jensen divergence. Burbea and Rao demonstrate that the JHCT$_\alpha$ divergence is convex if and only if $\alpha \in [1,2]$ [12]. Additionally, the mutual information defined via the JS or JHCT$_\alpha$ divergences is not a distance metric due to their failure to satisfy the triangular inequality [12]. Nevertheless, extending that which is demonstrated in [13] with respect to the JS divergence, Majtey et al. show that the square root of the JHCT$_\alpha$, $\alpha \in [1,2]$ is indeed a distance metric [14]. For a similarity measure, this is is a desirable property that allows one to treat the measure with the usual intuitive notions of distance in Euclidean space.

3.3   Assessing Local Point-Set Structure via Manifold Parzen Windowing

Each point-set is represented as a PDF via a Gaussian mixture model (GMM). Assuming K point-sets denoted by $\{X_k, k \in \{1,\ldots,K\}\}$, the kth point-set is comprised of N_k points and is denoted by $\{x_1^k,\ldots,x_{N_k}^k\}$. The kth PDF is calculated from the kth point-set as

$$\mathbf{P}_k(X_k) = \frac{1}{N_k}\sum_{i=1}^{N_k} G(x_i^k, C_i^k) \quad (3)$$

where $G(x_i^k, C_i^k)$ is a Gaussian with mean x_i^k and covariance C_i^k.

Whereas previous work used isotropic Gaussians, e.g. [7], we use the local point-set neighborhood to estimate an appropriate covariance matrix where the local structure of the point-set is reflected in the anisotropy of that covariance using a technique called *manifold Parzen windowing* [15]. For each point, x_i, the associated weighted covariance matrix, $C_{\mathcal{K}_i}$, is given by

$$C_{\mathcal{K}_i} = \frac{\sum_{x_j \in \mathcal{N}_i, x_j \neq x_i} \mathcal{K}(x_i; x_j)(x_i - x_j)^{\mathrm{T}}(x_i - x_j)}{\sum_{x_j \in \mathcal{N}_i, x_j \neq x_i} \mathcal{K}(x_i; x_j)} \tag{4}$$

where $\mathcal{N}_i$ is the local neighborhood of the point x_i and $\mathcal{K}$ is a user-selected neighborhood weighting kernel. We use an isotropic Gaussian for $\mathcal{K}$ with variance $\sigma^2_{\mathcal{K}_i}$ as well as a k-d tree structure for efficient determination of $\mathcal{N}_i$.

Calculation of the gradient requires the inverse of each covariance matrix. Determination of $C_{\mathcal{K}_i}$ from Eqn. (4) could potentially result in an ill-conditioned matrix problematizing the calculation of the gradient. For this reason, we use the modified covariance,

$$C_i = C_{\mathcal{K}_i} + \sigma^2_n I \tag{5}$$

where I is the identity matrix and σ_n is a parameter denoting added isotropic Gaussian noise. This particular aspect of our point-set matching formulation will be explained in a later section as it is incorporated into a deterministic annealing strategy during optimization.

3.4 Calculation of the JHCT$_\alpha$ Divergence Measure and Gradient from Point-Sets

Subsequent to calculation of the covariances, sample sets are generated for calculation of both the JHCT$_\alpha$ measure and its gradient. Both evaluations require the generation of a set of sample points from each of the K PDFs. For each PDF, we generate a random sample by first selecting, at random, a single Gaussian function comprising the GMM. Normal random variate generation from that single Gaussian provides a single random sample. We designate the number of sample points generated for each of the K probability density functions as $\{M_1, \ldots, M_K\}$ and the kth set of samples as $\{s^k_1, \ldots, s^k_{M_k}\}$. Eqn. (2) is then calculated using the sets of samples and the formula

$$\mathrm{JHCT}_\alpha(\mathbf{P}_1, \ldots, \mathbf{P}_K) = \frac{1}{1-\alpha} \left[\frac{1}{M} \left(\sum_{k=1}^{K} \sum_{j=1}^{M_k} \left[\mathbf{P}^*(s^k_j) \right]^{\alpha-1} - 1 \right) \right.$$
$$\left. + \frac{1}{N} \sum_{k=1}^{K} \frac{N_k}{M_k} \left(\sum_{j=1}^{M_k} \left[\mathbf{P}_k(s^k_j) \right]^{\alpha-1} - 1 \right) \right] \tag{6}$$

where

$$\mathbf{P}^*(X) = \frac{1}{N} \sum_{k=1}^{K} \sum_{i=1}^{N_k} G(x; x^k_i, C^k_i), \quad N = \sum_{k=1}^{K} N_k, \quad \text{and} \quad M = \sum_{k=1}^{K} M_k. \tag{7}$$

The prior weighting values are calculated from $\gamma_k = N_k/N$ such that the larger point-sets are weighted more heavily.

For many optimization routines the gradient with respect to the individual points is also required. This is calculated in a straightforward manner from Eqn. (6):

$$\frac{\partial \mathrm{JHCT}_\alpha}{\partial x_i^k} = -\frac{1}{M_k N} \sum_{j=1}^{M_k} \frac{G(s_j^k; x_i^k, C_i^k)(C_i^k)^{-1}(x_i^k - s_j^k)}{[\mathbf{P}_k(s_j^k)]^{2-\alpha}}$$

$$+ \frac{1}{MN} \sum_{k'=1}^{K} \sum_{j=1}^{M_{k'}} \frac{G(s_j^{k'}; x_i^k, C_i^k)(C_i^k)^{-1}(x_i^k - s_j^{k'})}{[\mathbf{P}^*(s_j^{k'})]^{2-\alpha}}. \tag{8}$$

4   Deformable Point-Set Registration

The JHCT_α divergence measure introduced in the previous sections can be used as a correspondence measure within a point-set registration framework. In this section we describe the remaining two components—the transformation model and the optimization strategy.

Associating each point-set with a continuous mapping function, $\mathcal{T}_k$, and minimizing the JHCT_α divergence with respect to the parameters of all K transformation models brings the point-sets into correspondence. Assuming the L parameters for the kth transformation model are denoted by the set $\{\phi_1^k, \ldots, \phi_L^k\}$, the derivative of the JHCT_α divergence with respect to the lth transformation parameter of the kth transformation model is given by

$$\frac{\partial \mathrm{JHCT}_\alpha}{\partial \phi_l^k} = \sum_{i=1}^{N_k} \frac{\partial \mathrm{JHCT}_\alpha}{\partial x_i^k} \frac{\partial \mathcal{T}_k}{\partial \phi_l^k} \tag{9}$$

where the term on the right is derived from the selected transformation model.

4.1   The Directly Manipulated Free-Form Deformation Transformation Model

The transformation model of our point-set registration algorithm is defined by directly manipulated free-form deformations (DMFFD) which were recently introduced in [1] for intensity-based image registration. It demonstrated superiority over the traditional FFD image registration approach [16] due to the problematic energy topographies inherent in the traditional FFD framework. We extended that result to encompass point-set registration using the JHCT_α divergence measure.

For n-D domains the traditional B-spline FFD transformational model is defined as

$$\mathcal{T} = \sum_{i_1=1}^{M_1} \cdots \sum_{i_n=1}^{M_n} \phi_{i_1,\ldots,i_n} \prod_{j=1}^{n} B_{i_j,d_j}(u_j) \tag{10}$$

where $\phi_{i_1,\dots,i_n}$ is an n-D grid of control points and $B_{i_j,d_j}(u_j)$ is the B-spline in the i_j^{th} direction of order d_j. Traditional gradient-based optimization approaches which are intrinsically susceptible to hemstitching during the gradient ascent/descent calculate $\frac{\partial \mathcal{T}_k}{\partial \phi_l^k}$ as

$$\frac{\partial \mathcal{T}_k}{\partial \phi_l^k} = \prod_{j=1}^n B_{l_j,d_j}(u_j) \tag{11}$$

where the control point values are the parameters over which the energy is minimized. In contrast, we calculate a preconditioned version of the gradient

$$\frac{\partial \mathcal{T}_k}{\partial \phi_l^k} = \frac{\prod_{j=1}^n B_{l_j,d_j}(u_j) \cdot \prod_{j=1}^n B_{l_j,d_j}^2(u_j)}{\sum_{k_1=1}^{d_1+1} \cdots \sum_{k_n=1}^{d_n+1} \prod_{j=1}^n B_{k_j,d_j}^2(u_j)} \cdot \left(\frac{1}{\sum_{\forall u_j} \prod_{j=1}^n B_{l_j,d_j}^2(u_j)} \right) \cdot \tag{12}$$

Additional details discussing the deficiency of traditional gradient approaches as well as the derivation of Eqn. (12) can be found in [1].

4.2 Deterministic Annealing

Minimization of the divergence measure occurs via conjugate gradient descent. We placed this minimization routine within a deterministic annealing framework [17], both in terms of the transformation model as well as the JHCT$_\alpha$ divergence, which decreases the susceptibility to local minima.

At the initial stage of the optimization, the B-spline transformation model is defined by a low-resolution mesh to determine more global correspondence. At each subsequent level, the mesh-resolution is doubled for increased local, refined registration. In coordination with this hierarchical registration, we specify an annealing schedule for the isotropic Gaussian noise discussed previously. At the pth iteration the covariance is calculated as

$$C_i = C_{\mathcal{K}_i} + \lambda^p \sigma_n^2 I \tag{13}$$

where λ is the annealing rate (typical values are in the range $[0.93, 1.0]$). This also has the effect of increasing the localization during the course of the optimization.

5   Experimental Evaluation

Several experiments are used to develop the theoretical ideas discussed in previous sections. Our first set of synthetic experiments are meant to elucidate the sensitivity/robustness trade-off associated with the JHCT$_\alpha$ divergence measure. Anatomically-based pulmonary registration results are then given which take advantage of our newly developed point-set registration framework.

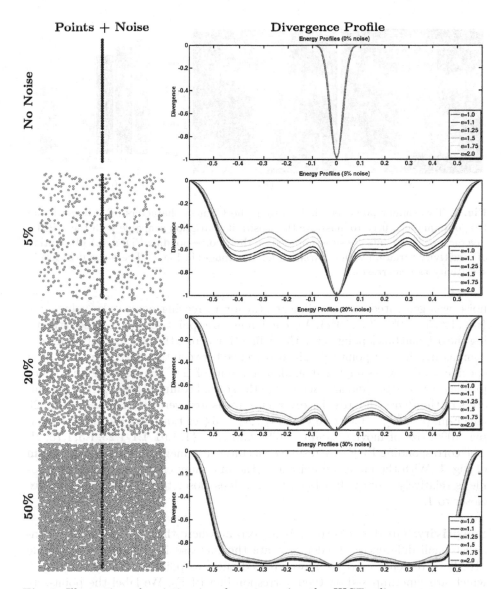

Fig. 1. Illustration of variation in robustness using the JHCT$_\alpha$ divergence measure. Top row: Noise free fixed point-set, the corresponding PDF, and the scaled divergence profiles for $\alpha = \{1, 1.01, 1.25, 1.5, 1.75, 2\}$. Note that the profiles are nearly identical for the noise-free case. Second row to last row: Noise levels of $\{5\%, 20\%, 50\%\}$ demonstrate an increase in robustness for $\alpha \to 2$.

5.1   Synthetic Experiments

Robustness. Fig. 1 illustrates the effects of varying the α values in the presence of increasing noise levels. A single vertical line was sampled to create the black point-set on the point-set domain $[-0.5, 0.5] \times [0, 1]$. Added random

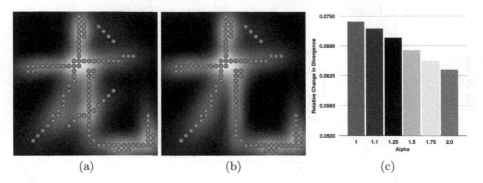

(a)   (b)   (c)

Fig. 2. Two similar point-sets derived from the Chinese characters (a) "dragon" and (b) "outstanding" used to illustrate the sensitivity variation available with the JHCT_α divergence. The points are superimposed on their corresponding PDFs. (c) Illustration of sensitivity variation with α variation for the images in Fig. 2. There is a decrease in sensitivity as α increases.

noise was generated on a rectilinear grid for increasing percentage values, i.e. $\{0\%, 1\%, 5\%, 10\%, 20\%, 50\%\}$. A second, noise-free point-set was created by shifting the original black point-set in the x direction across the width of the image encompassing the first point-set. The divergence between these two point-sets for a specific α value was sampled at small increments of Δx. The resulting divergence profiles were plotted and are included in the second column of Fig. 1. The parameters of the PDFs and JHCT_α divergence measures were as follows: $\sigma_n = 0.025$ (see Eqn. (5)), $\sigma_{\mathcal{K}_i} = 0.02$ (see Eqn. (4)), $\mathcal{N}_i = 3$ (see Eqn. (4)), size of fixed sample: 1000, size of moving sample: 1000, and $\alpha = \{1, 1.01, 1.1, 1.25, 1.5, 1.75, 2\}$. The corresponding PDFs are displayed as intensity images in the second column of Fig. 1. With the increased noise level the minimum energy in the energy profile is relatively more well-defined for α values closer to 2 than those α values closer to 1.

Sensitivity. Greater sensitivity is important where the problem domain concerns small differences. To demonstrate the increase in the sensitivity of the JHCT_α divergence as $\alpha \to 1$, we created the two point sets shown in Fig. 2 which are superimposed on their corresponding PDFs. We label the point-sets in Fig. 2(a) and 2(b) as X_d and X_o, respectively. The PDFs were generated using the following parameters: $\sigma_n = 1$ (see Eqn. (5)), $\sigma_{\mathcal{K}_i} = 3$ (see Eqn. (4)), $\mathcal{N}_i = 8$ (see Eqn. (4)), point-set domain: $[0, 30] \times [0, 30]$ and $\alpha = \{1, 1.1, 1.25, 1.5, 1.75, 2\}$.

The divergences $\text{JHCT}_\alpha(X_d, X_o)$, $\text{JHCT}_\alpha(X_d, X_d)$, and $\text{JHCT}_\alpha(X_d, \mathcal{T}_\infty(X_d))$ were calculated where $\mathcal{T}_\infty(X_d)$ denotes a large translation of the point-set X_d. This was to obtain a baseline measurement for comparison between the other two calculated divergence values such that the entropy measure is entirely dominated by the second term of the JHCT_α entropy (Eqn. (2)). The relative change in divergence is derived from the following sensitivity calculation

Table 1. Total cardinality of the left and right lung surface and blood vessel tree point-sets. Note that only a percentage of these points are used during the point-set registration.

	Left Lung	Right Lung	Left Vessel Tree	Right Vessel Tree
N02 (ins)	260,019	247,199	296,676	226,527
N02 (exp)	220,329	207,739	314,932	229,643

$$S = \frac{\mathrm{JHCT}_\alpha(X_d, X_d) - \mathrm{JHCT}_\alpha(X_d, X_o)}{\mathrm{JHCT}_\alpha(X_d, X_d) - \mathrm{JHCT}_\alpha(X_d, \mathcal{T}_\infty(X_d))}. \tag{14}$$

The generated values are displayed graphically for comparison in Fig. 2(c). Intuitively, these results can be understood by looking at the extreme cases involved. For an extremely insensitive measurement ($S = 0$) there would be no difference between $\mathrm{JHCT}_\alpha(X_d, X_d)$ and $\mathrm{JHCT}_\alpha(X_d, X_o)$ despite the subtle discrepancy between X_d and X_o. At the other end of the spectrum, an extremely sensitive measurement would produce the maximally possible difference (hence the baseline measurement $\mathrm{JHCT}_\alpha(X_d, \mathcal{T}_\infty(X_d))$ in the denominator) resulting in $S = 1$. The sensitivity values for the example in Fig. 2 with $\alpha = \{1, 1.1, 1.25, 1.5, 1.75, 2\}$ are given in Fig. 2(c). These values show an increased sensitivity with decreased α values.

5.2   Pulmonary Registration Experiments

The motivating research aim of the theoretical framework described in the previous sections is the move towards anatomically-based registration for CT lung kinematic and morphometry studies. This direction is meant to take advantage

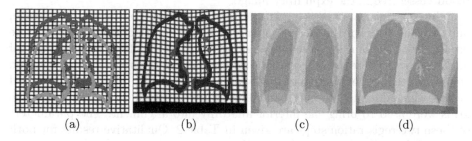

| (a) | (b) | (c) | (d) |

Fig. 3. Image (a) illustrates the lung boundaries for a mid-coronal 2-D image slice before the global point-set registration step. Image (b)illustrate the aligned boundaries of the lungs after the global registration step ($\alpha = 2$). The lung boundaries (red = inspiration, green/blue = expiration before/after registration) are superimposed over grid images to illustrate the initial deformation. Image (c) illustrate the same coronal slice before point-set registration. Image (d) illustrates the registered image after the refined registration step ($\alpha = 2$) using faux-colormapped inspiratory image superimposed on the grayscale expiratory image.

Table 2. Registration parameters for the global and local point-set registration steps

Global	Local
– B-spline order: cubic	– B-spline order: cubic
– number of levels: 1	– number of levels: 3
– control point grid: $5 \times 5 \times 4$	– level 1 (control point grid: $35 \times$
– iterations: 100	35×19, iterations: 30)
– $\sigma_{\mathcal{K}_i} = 20.0$ (see Eqn. (4))	– level 2 (control point grid: $67 \times$
– $\mathcal{N}_i = 5$ (see Eqn. (4))	67×35, iterations: 20)
– $\sigma_n = 30.0$ (see Eqn. (5))	– level 3 (control point grid:
– $\lambda^2 = 0.97$ (see Eqn. (13))	$131 \times 131 \times 67$, iterations: 10)
– lung surface points: 10%	– $\sigma_{\mathcal{K}_i} = 5.0$ (see Eqn. (4))
	– $\mathcal{N}_i = 5$ (see Eqn. (4))
	– $\sigma_n = 10.0$ (see Eqn. (5))
	– $\lambda^2 = 0.93$ (see Eqn. (13))
	– lung surface points: 25%
	– vessel points: 50%

of the wealth of segmentation techniques specifically for segmentation of CT lung imagery (e.g. whole lungs, fissures, blood vessels, small and large airways). A single 3-D inspiratory/expiratory CT lung image volume pair (denoted as N02) was acquired. The left and right lung surfaces were segmented along with the left and right blood vessel trees. The number of points comprising these four point sets for inspiration and expiration are given in Table 1. Thus for this registration scenario we have four distinct labels and our registration framework is implemented such that only identically-labeled point-sets are registered, e.g. the gradient of the divergence measure for the points comprising the left blood vessel tree in the inspiratory image employ only the points comprising the left blood vessel tree in the expiratory image.

Point-set registration was performed in two stages. During the first stage, only a small fraction the surface points of both the left and right lungs were used to bring the lung surfaces into alignment. The results from this more global alignment stage were then used as the initialization of a more refined registration step in which a larger fraction of the two labeled point sets taken from the blood vessels were added to the lung boundary points and higher resolution B-spline grids were used to bring the interior anatomy into alignment. The parameters of these two registration steps are given in Table 2. Qualitative results for both stages of the registration are given in Fig. 3.

More relevant to the theoretical content of this paper is an additional series of Monte Carlo additive noise experiments meant to illustrate the advantage of the fine-tuning capabilities of our approach. For each $\alpha \in \{1, 1.5, 2\}$, we repeat the global registration step outlined above for a maximum of ten gradient descent iterations for four different noise levels, $\{0.001\%, 0.01\%, 0.1\%, 1\%\}$, where we added random noise points to both point sets at different image voxel locations. This experiment was performed five times for each alpha value/noise

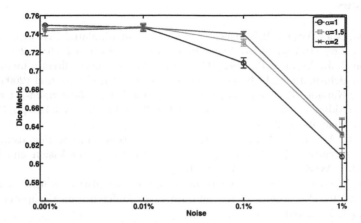

Fig. 4. N02 Additive Noise Experimental Results. Performance was evaluated using the Dice metric on the lung surface boundaries. Also shown are the error bars which reflect one standard deviation over the five experiments performed for that point. At low noise levels, the performance for $\alpha = 1$ exceeds those of the other two alpha values whereas greater noise levels demonstrate the superiority of higher α values for those conditions.

level combination for a total of sixty additional additive noise registration experiments. Accuracy was assessed by extracting the boundary surfaces from the lung segmentations using standard morphological operations (radius $= 5$) and the overlapping Dice metric was calculated for each registration solution. The results are plotted in Fig. 4 and demonstrate the robustness/sensitivity spectrum alluded to throughout this paper. As expected, at lower noise levels, the performance is very similar between the three α values with the ordering reflecting the priority of degree of sensitivity. However, as the noise level increases, the relatively greater degree of robustness for higher α values translates into a superior performance.

6   Discussion and Conclusions

We have described a technique for point-set correspondence based on a generalization of the Jensen-Shannon divergence. To accommodate the local structure of many extracted point-sets, we incorporated structural quantitation into the actual point-set divergence measure for a more accurate representation of the features of interest. We have also presented this point-set measure within a relatively novel transformation model based on B-splines. This DMFFD transformation model takes advantage of many of the salient properties of B-splines without the problematic energy topographies associated with the traditional FFD transformation model.

References

1. Tustison, N.J., Avants, B.B., Gee, J.C.: Directly manipulated free-form deformation image registration. IEEE Trans. Image Process. 18(3), 624–635 (2009)
2. Tustison, N.J., Awate, S.P., Gee, J.C.: Information-theoretic directly manipulated free-form deformation labeled point-set registration. Insight Journal (2009)
3. Tsin, Y., Kanade, T.: A correlation based approach for robust point-set registration. In: Pajdla, T., Matas, J(G.) (eds.) ECCV 2004. LNCS, vol. 3023, pp. 558–569. Springer, Heidelberg (2004)
4. Singh, M., Arora, H., Ahuja, N.: Robust registration and tracking using kernel density correlation. In: Proceedings of the IEEE Computer Vision and Pattern Recognition Workshop, pp. 174–182 (2004)
5. Jian, B., Vemuri, B.: A robust algorithm for point set registration using mixture of Gaussians. In: Proceedings of the International Conference on Computer Vision, pp. 1246–1251 (2005)
6. Guo, H., Rangarajan, A., Joshi, S.: Diffeomorphic Point Matching. In: Handbook of Mathematical Models in Computer Vision, pp. 205–220. Springer, Heidelberg (2005)
7. Wang, F., Vemuri, B., Rangarajan, A., Eisenschenk, S.: Simultaneous nonrigid registration of multiple point sets and atlas construction. IEEE Transactions on Pattern Analysis and Machine Intelligence 30(11), 2011–2022 (2008)
8. Basu, A., Harris, I., Hjort, N., Jones, M.: Robust and efficient estimation by minimizing a density power divergence. Biometrika 85, 549–559 (1998)
9. Havrda, M., Charvat, F.: Quantification method of classification processes: concept of structural alpha-entropy. Kybernetica 3, 30–35 (1967)
10. Tsallis, C.: Possible generalization of Boltzmann-Gibbs statistics. Journal of Statistical Physics 52, 479–487 (1988)
11. Gell-Mann, M., Tsallis, C.: Nonextensive Entropy. Oxford University Press, Oxford (2004)
12. Burbea, J., Rao, C.R.: On the convexity of some divergence measures on entropy functions. IEEE Transactions on Information Theory 28, 489–495 (1982)
13. Endres, D., Schindelin, J.: A new metric for probability distributions. IEEE Transactions on Information Theory 49, 1858–1860 (2003)
14. Majtey, A., Lamberti, P., Plastino, A.: A monoparametric family of metrics for statistical mechanics. Physica A 344, 547–553 (2004)
15. Vincent, P., Bengio, Y.: Manifold parzen windows. In: Thrun, S., Becker, S., Obermayer, K. (eds.) Advances in Neural Information Prcessing Systems, pp. 825–832. MIT Press, Cambridge (2003)
16. Rueckert, D., Sonoda, L., Hayes, C., Hill, D., Leach, M., Hawkes, D.: Nonrigid registration using free-form deformations: application to breast MR images. IEEE Trans. Med. Imaging 18(8), 712–721 (1999)
17. Rose, K.: Deterministic annealing for clustering, compression, classification, regression, and related optimization problems. Proceedings of the IEEE 86(11), 2210–2239 (2000)

Generalized L2-Divergence and Its Application to Shape Alignment⋆

Fei Wang[1], Baba Vemuri[2], and Tanveer Syeda-Mahmood[1]

[1] IBM Almaden Research Center, San Jose, CA, USA
[2] Department of CISE, University of Florida, Gainesville, FL, USA

Abstract. This paper proposes a novel and robust approach to the groupwise point-sets registration problem in the presence of large amounts of noise and outliers. Each of the point sets is represented by a mixture of Gaussians and the point-sets registration is treated as a problem of aligning the multiple mixtures. We develop a novel divergence measure which is defined between any arbitrary number of probability distributions based on L2 distance, and we call this new divergence measure "*Generalized L2-divergence*". We derive a closed-form expression for the Generalized-L2 divergence between multiple Gaussian mixtures, which in turn leads to a computationally efficient registration algorithm. This new algorithm has an intuitive interpretation, is simple to implement and exhibits inherent statistical robustness. Experimental results indicate that our algorithm achieves very good performance in terms of both robustness and accuracy.

1 Introduction

The need for groupwise shape matching occurs in diverse sub-domains of engineering and science e.g., computer vision, medical imaging, sports science, archaeology, and others. In model-based image segmentation for example, constructing an atlas typically requires us to bring the pre-segmented shapes into alignment. Shape features are frequently used in image retrieval as well, and need a shape alignment algorithm. And in cardiac applications, if the shapes of the heart chamber are extracted, the septal wall motion tracking problem requires us to solve for shape correspondences in the cardiac cycle.

However, matching multiple shapes can be a daunting task due to the lack of the *correspondence* information across the shapes. Typically correspondences can be estimated once the point-sets are properly aligned with appropriate spatial transformations. If the objects under consideration are deformable, the adequate transformation would obviously be a non-rigid spatial mapping. Solving for nonrigid deformations between point-sets with unknown correspondence is a challenging problem. A second problem we face in multiple shape matching context is the *robustness* issue. Some of the raw features present in one image may not be present in the other. Finally, it is desirable for a registration to be

---

⋆ This research was in part funded by the NIH grant RO1-NS046812.

J.L. Prince, D.L. Pham, and K.J. Myers (Eds.): IPMI 2009, LNCS 5636, pp. 227–238, 2009.

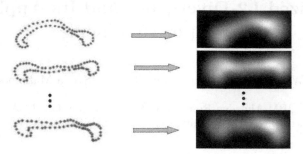

Fig. 1. Illustration of corpus callosum shapes (point-sets) represented as density functions.

unbiased, i.e., if one arbitrarily chooses any one of the given data sets as a reference, the estimated transformation would be biased toward this chosen reference and it would be desirable to avoid such a bias.

One possible solution for such situations to apply probabilistic shape matching techniques. A recent approach models each point-set by a probability density function, and then quantify the distance between these probability densities using an information-theoretic measure[1,2,3]. Figure 1 illustrates this idea, wherein the right column of the figure depicts the density functions corresponding to the point-sets (representing the boundary and shape) drawn from corpus callosum shapes shown in the left column. Using this approach, the correspondence issue is avoided since we now draw comparisons between density functions instead of point features. The robustness problem is also alleviated since we are matching holistic density functions making it robust to the point-sets of different sizes and the presence of missing features/data. Furthermore, if an unbiased information theoretic measure is chosen to quantify the multiple densities representing the shapes, the matching results can potentially be unbiased to any of the given point-sets [3].

In this paper, we develop a new non-rigid registration method for multiple point-sets. It is based on a novel information theoretic matching criterion called Generalized $L2$ (GL2) divergence, which is used measure the similarity between the probability densities representing the shapes. Both the Jensen-Shannon (JS) divergence [2] and our Generalized L2-divergence are shown to belong the so-called *Generalized Linear Divergence* family. In this paper, we use Generalized L2-divergence for achieving non-rigid registration between multiple shapes represented using the points features. We show that the Generalized L2 divergence can be expressed in a closed-form expression for registering mixtures of Gaussians. We also derive the analytic gradient of this match measure in order to achieve efficient and accurate non-rigid registration. The GL2 measure is then minimized over a class of smooth non-rigid transformations expressed in a thin-plate spline basis. The key strengths of our proposed nonrigid registration scheme are: (1) The cost function and its derivative can be expressed in closed form for the point-sets represented as Gaussian Mixtures, and they are computationally less expensive than the rival approaches; (2) The Generalized L2 divergence is inherently more robust than the rival Jensen-Shannon divergences; (3) it can accommodate point-sets to be registered of varying size.

2   Previous Work

Several articles have been reported on point-set alignment in the recent literature that utilizing the information-theoretic measures. For instance, in Wang et al. [4], the relative entropy measure (Kullback-Leibler distance) is used to find a similarity transformation between two point-sets. Their approach only solves the pairwise rigid matching problem, which is a lot easier than the non-rigid matching problem that we tackle in this paper. Jian et al. [1] introduced a novel and robust algorithm for rigidly and non-rigidly registering pairs of data sets using the L2 distance between mixtures of Gaussians representing the point-set data. They derived a closed form expression for the L2 distance between the mixtures of Gaussians, and their algorithm is very fast in comparison to existing methods on point-set registration and the results shown are quantitatively satisfactory. However, they do not actually fit a mixture density to each point-set, choosing instead to allow each point in each set be a cluster center. Consequently, their method is actually more similar to the image matching method of [5] discussed below, but with the advantage of not having to evaluate a cost function involving spatial integrals numerically, since a closed form expression is derived for the same. Roy et al. [6] used a similar approach as in [1], except that they fit a density function to the data via maximum likelihood before the registration step. Both of the methods however have not been extended to the problem of unbiased simultaneous matching of multiple point-sets being addressed in this paper. These methods are similar to our work since we also model each of the point-sets by a kernel density function and then quantify the (dis)similarity between them using an information-theoretic measure. This is followed by an optimization of a (dis)similarity function over a space of coordinate transformations yielding the desired transformation. The difference lies in the fact that GL2-divergence used in our work can be shown to be more general than the information-theoretic measures used in [1,4], and can easily cope with multiple point-sets. Recently, in [5], Glaunes et al. represent points as delta functions and match them using the dual norm in a reproducing kernel Hilbert space. The main problem with this technique is that it needs the numerical evaluation of a 3D spatial integral. In contrast, we compute the GL2-divergence using an empirical framework where the computations converge in the limit to the true values. We will show that our method when applied to matching point-sets, achieves very good performance in terms of both robustness and accuracy. Finally, a related work by Twining et al. [7] has used minimum description length (MDL) for groupwise image registration where contiguity constraints between pixels could be utilized.

Perhaps the methods that are closest in spirit to our approach are the recent work in [2,3]. They minimize the Jensen-Shannon divergence and the CDF-based Jensen-Shannon divergence respectively between the feature point-sets with respect to non-rigid deformation. The divergence measures are then estimated using the law of large numbers, which is computationally expensive and takes large amount of storage (memory). In contrast, the proposed method in this paper is much simpler, and thus less time-consuming than the previously reported methods. Furthermore, the JS-divergence and CDF-JS cannot be computed in closed form for a mixture model. In sharp contrast, our distance between the densities is expressed in closed form, making it computationally attractive. More importantly, Generalized L2 divergence is a special case to a family of divergence measures, which is called Generalized Linear Divergence, and JS-divergence is one of its special case (when we choose D to be KL-divergence in the expression of the Generalized Linear divergence).

3   Generalized L2 Divergence: A New Divergence Measure between Distributions

In this section, we define our new information theoretic measure and present some of its' property/theorems. To motivate the derivation of generalized L2 divergence, we observe that an earlier divergence measure called Jensen-Shannon (JS) divergence had addressed the groupwise point-sets registration problem [2], where each point-set X^i is modeled as probability density functions.

The JS-divergence between probability density functions p_i can be written as

$$JS_\pi(p_1, p_2, ..., p_n) = H(\sum \pi_i p_i) - \sum \pi_i H(p_i), \qquad (1)$$

where $\pi = \{\pi_1, \pi_2, ..., \pi_n | \pi_i > 0, \sum \pi_i = 1\}$ are the weights of the probability densities p_i and $H(p_i)$ is the Shannon entropy.

The JS-divergence and popular Kullback-Leibler (KL) divergence are related by the following equation

$$JS_\pi(p_1, p_2, ..., p_n) = \sum_{i=1}^{n} \pi_i D_{KL}(p_i, p), \qquad (2)$$

where p is the convex combination of the n probability densities, $p = \sum \pi_i p_i$.

If we extend the Jensen-Shannon divergence by replacing the KL-divergence with a general distance measure between two densities, we get a generalized divergence measure between multiple distributions, which we call Generalized Linear (GL) divergence,

$$GL(p_1, p_2, ..., p_n) = \sum_{i=1}^{n} \pi_i D(p_i, p) \qquad (3)$$

In particular, if we use the $L2$ distance to quantify the distance between two density function in Eqn. 3 because of its proven robustness property (Jian & Vemuri [1]), we get

$$GL2(p_1, p_2, ..., p_n) = \sum_{i=1}^{n} \pi_i L_2(p_i, \sum_i \pi_i p_i). \qquad (4)$$

For example, when $n = 2$, the Generalized L2-divergence become $L2$ distance between two density functions, $GL2(p_1, p_2) = \sum_{i=1}^{2} \pi_i L_2(p_i, \pi_1 p_1 + \pi_2 p_2) = \pi_1 \pi_2 L_2(p_1, p_2)$.

3.1   Properties of the Generalized Linear Divergence

Definition 1: *Recall the definition of the Density Power Divergence between two PDFs p and q,*

$$P_\alpha(p, q) = \int \left\{ \frac{1}{\alpha} p^{1+\alpha} - (1 + \frac{1}{\alpha} pq^\alpha) + q^{1+\alpha} \right\} dx$$

when $\alpha = 1$, then $P_1(p, q) = L_2(p, q)$, and when $\alpha = 0$, then $P_0(p, q) = D_{KL}(p, q)$.

Definition 2: *If we choose the pairwise distance measure D to be the Density Power Divergence in definition of the Generalized Linear divergence in Eqn. (3), and we get the Generalized Power Divergence between multiple PDFs,*

$$GP_\alpha(p_1, p_2, ..., p_n) = \sum_{i=1}^{n} \pi_i P_\alpha(p_i, p) \tag{5}$$

where p is the convex combination of the n probability densities, $p = \sum \pi_i p_i$, and $P_\alpha(\cdot)$ is the density power divergence.

Theorem 1. *When $\alpha \to 0$, generalized Power Divergence will converge to Jensen-Shannon divergence; When $\alpha \to 1$, generalized Density Divergence converges to GL2-divergence, i.e.*

$$\begin{cases} \lim_{\alpha \to 0} GP_\alpha(p_1, p_2, ..., p_n) = JS(p_1, p_2, ..., p_n) \\ \lim_{\alpha \to 1} GP_\alpha(p_1, p_2, ..., p_n) = GL2(p_1, p_2, ..., p_n) \end{cases} \tag{6}$$

Proof: The theorem can be derived easily from the property of Density Power Divergence. We will omit it for brevity.

For general $0 < \alpha < 1$, the class of generalized power divergences provides a smooth bridge between the JS divergence and the $GL2$ divergence. Furthermore, this single parameter α controls the trade-off between robustness and asymptotic efficiency of the parameter estimators which are the minimizers of this family of divergences. The fact that the $L2E$ is inherently superior to MLE in terms of robustness can be well explained by viewing the minimum density power divergence estimators as a particular case of M-estimators [8]. For in-depth discussion on this issue, we refer the reader to [9].

Proposition 1. *For a convex symmetric distance function D, the generalized divergence $\sum_{i=1}^{n} D(p_i, p)$ is a convex function of $p_1, p_2, \cdots, p_n$; conversely, if D is a concave function, the generalized divergence $\sum_{i=1}^{n} D(p_i, p)$ is a concave function of $p_1, p_2, \cdots, p_n$.*

4   Multiple Point-Sets Registration with Generalized-L2 Divergence

We now present the framework of simultaneous non-rigid shape matching of multiple point-sets using the Generalized L2-divergence. The main idea is to measure the similarity between multiple finite point-sets by considering their continuous approximations. In this context, one can relate a point-set to a probability density function. Considering the point set as a collection of Dirac Delta functions, it is natural to think of Gaussian Mixture Model as representation of a point-set, which is defined as a convex combination of Gaussian component densities $G(x - \mu_i, \Sigma_i)$, where μ_i is the mean vector and Σ_i is the covariance matrix. The probability density function is explicitly given as $p(x) = \sum_{i=1}^{k} w_i G(x - \mu_i, \Sigma_i)$ where

$$G(x - \mu_i, \Sigma_i) = \frac{exp[-\frac{1}{2}(x - \mu_i)^T \Sigma_i^{-1}(x - \mu_i)]}{\sqrt{(2\pi)^d |det(\Sigma_i)|}} \qquad (7)$$

and w_i is the weights associate with the components. In a simplified setting, the number of components is the number of the points in the set. And for each component, the mean vector is given by the location of each point. For a dense point cloud, a mixture model-based clustering or grouping may be performed as preprocessing procedure.

Let the N point-sets to be registered be denoted by $\{X^a, a \in \{1, ..., N\}\}$. Each point-set X^a consists of points $\{x_i^a \in \mathbb{R}^d, i \in \{1, ..., k_a\} \}$, where k_a is the total number of points contained in the ath point-set. Each point set is represented by a probability density function $\mathbf{P}_a$. Let the atlas or the mean shape be denoted by Z. Each point set is related to the atlas through a nonrigid transformation f^i parameterized by a set of transformation parameters μ^i. We now pose the simultaneous registration of multiple point sets as the problem of determining the transformation parameters μ^i such that the Generalized-$L2$ (GL2) divergence between the probability density functions of the transformed points is minimized. The groupwise registration problem can then be formulated as the problem of minimizing

$$\min_{\boldsymbol{\mu}^i} GL2(\mathbf{P}_1, \mathbf{P}_2, ..., \mathbf{P}_N) + \lambda \sum_{i=1}^{N} ||Lf^i||^2, \qquad (8)$$

where Lf^i is a regularization term to control the nature of deformation. Having introduced the cost function, now the task is to design an efficient way to estimate the empirical GL2-divergence from the Gaussian mixtures and derive the analytic gradient of the estimated divergence in order to achieve the optimal solution efficiently.

4.1   Estimating Empirical Generalized L2-Divergence with GMMs

Using the Gaussian Mixture model, the density function for the ath point-set can be expressed as $\mathbf{P}_a = \frac{1}{k_a} \sum_{j=1}^{k_a} G(x - x_j^a, \sigma_a^2 \mathbf{I})$. Assume $M := \sum_{i=1}^{N} k_i$ is the total number of points contained in the N point-sets, the pooled points in all point-sets can be expressed as $\{x_1, x_2, ..., x_M\} \equiv \{x_1^1, ..., x_j^i, ..., x_{k_N}^N\}$.

For the convex combination $\sum \pi_i \mathbf{P}_i$, if we choose $\pi_i = \frac{k_i}{M}$, we have the following,

$$
\sum_{i=1}^{N} \pi_i \mathbf{P}_i = \sum_{i=1}^{N} \pi_i \sum_{a=1}^{K_i} \frac{1}{k_i} G(x - x_a^i, \sigma_i^2 \mathbf{I}) = \frac{1}{M} \sum_{i=1}^{N} \sum_{a=1}^{K_i} G(x - x_a^i, \sigma_i^2 \mathbf{I})
$$
$$
= \frac{1}{M} \sum_{j=1}^{M} G(x - x_j, \sigma_{\tau(j)}^2 \mathbf{I}), \tag{9}
$$

where $\tau : \{1, ..., M\} \rightarrow \{1, ..., N\}$ is a mapping function that maps the index of a point to the index of the point-set. Therefore the linear combination of the GMMs can be expressed as a single Gaussian Mixture centered on the pooled point-sets. Consequently, we have the $L2$ distance between $\mathbf{P} = \sum \pi_i \mathbf{P}_i$ and $\mathbf{P}_i$

$$
L_2(\sum_{i=1}^{N} \pi_i \mathbf{P}_i, \mathbf{P}_i) = \int \Big(\sum_{i=1}^{N} \pi_i \mathbf{P}_i - \mathbf{P}_i \Big)^2 dx = \int \Big(\mathbf{P}^2 + \mathbf{P}_i^2 - 2\mathbf{P}\mathbf{P}_i \Big) dx. \tag{10}
$$

Use the fact that

$$
\int_{+\infty}^{+\infty} G(x - v_i, \Sigma_i) G(x - v_j, \Sigma_j) dx = G(v_i - v_j, \Sigma_i + \Sigma_j) \tag{11}
$$

the $L2$ distance can be expressed as

$$
L_2(\sum_{i=1}^{N} \pi_i \mathbf{P}_i, \mathbf{P}_i) = \int \Big(\mathbf{P}^2 + \mathbf{P}_i^2 - 2\mathbf{P}\mathbf{P}_i \Big) dx
$$
$$
= \frac{1}{M^2} \sum_{i=1}^{M} \sum_{j=1}^{M} G(x_i - x_j, (\sigma_{\tau(i)}^2 + \sigma_{\tau(j)}^2)\mathbf{I}) + \frac{1}{k_i^2} \sum_{j=1}^{k_i} \sum_{l=1}^{k_i} G(x_j^i - x_l^i, 2\sigma_i^2 \mathbf{I}) \tag{12}
$$
$$
- \frac{2}{k_i M} \sum_{j=1}^{M} \sum_{l=1}^{k_i} G(x_j - x_l^i, (\sigma_i^2 + \sigma_{\tau(j)}^2)\mathbf{I}).
$$

Let us introduce a Gaussian kernel matrix $\mathbf{G}$ with $G_{ij} = G(u_i - u_j, (\sigma_{\tau(i)}^2 + \sigma_{\tau(j)}^2)\mathbf{I})$, and define an indicator vectors I_a (of length M) for a^{th} point-set, i.e. $I_a(i) = 1$ if u_i is from the ath point-set (therefore $\tau(i) = a$). I_M is a vector of length M whose elements are all ones. Eqn. (12) can be rewritten as

$$
L_2(\sum_{i=1}^{N} \pi_i \mathbf{P}_i, \mathbf{P}_i) = \frac{I_M G I_M}{M^2} + \frac{I_i G I_i}{k_i^2} - \frac{2 I_M G I_i}{k_i M}. \tag{13}
$$

Therefore, the final closed-form Generalized L2-divergence becomes

$$
\sum_{i=1}^{N} \pi_i L_2(\sum_{i=1}^{N} \pi_i \mathbf{P}_i, \mathbf{P}_i) = \sum_{i=1}^{N} \frac{k_i}{M} \Big(\frac{I_M G I_M}{M^2} + \frac{I_i G I_i}{k_i^2} - \frac{2 I_M G I_i}{k_i M} \Big)
$$
$$
= \sum_{i=1}^{N} \frac{I_i G I_i}{k_i M} - \frac{I_M G I_M}{M^2}. \tag{14}
$$

Based on Eqn. (14), we can derive the gradient of the GL2-divergence with respect to the transformation parameters μ^a, which can be expressed as

$$\frac{\partial GL2}{\partial \mu^a} = \sum_{i=1}^{N} \frac{I_i^T \frac{\partial \mathbf{G}}{\partial \mu^a} I_i}{k_i M} - \frac{I_M^T \frac{\partial \mathbf{G}}{\partial \mu^a} I_M}{M^2}. \tag{15}$$

The details of the derivation are omitted here due to space limitations. Once we have the analytical gradient, the cost function optimization of Eqn. (8) is achieved very efficiently using a quasi-Newton method.

The Gaussian Kernel in matrix $\mathbf{G}$ can be replaced by other kernels (e.g. radial-basis-function, cauchy kernel etc.) leading to a "Generalized L2 divergence family". Using Gaussian mixtures keeps the complexity $O(L^2)$ and the estimation computationally simple. Since GL2 is a generalization of the popular L2 measure, our method is equivalent to the algorithms presented in Jian et al.[1] and Roy et al. [6] when applied to align pairwise pointsets.

5 Experiment Results

We now present experimental results on the application of our algorithm to both synthetic and real data sets. First, to demonstrate the robustness and accuracy of our algorithm, we show the alignment results by applying the GL2 divergence to the matching of pairs of point-sets. Then, we will present the groupwise registration results achieved for the shapes from cardiac echocardiographic videos as well as human brain MRI. For the non-rigid registration experiments, we choose the thin-plate spline (TPS) to represent the deformation, which is similar to [2].

5.1 Pair-Wise Point-Sets Alignment

Next, we validate our method based on comparing the recovered motion parameters against the synthetical transformation parameters. We begin with a 2D range data set X of a road (Figure 2) consisting of 277 points (which was also used in Jian & Vemuri's experiment [1]). 30 randomly generated rigid transformations were applied to transform the range pointsets to obtain a transformed pointset Y, and we then remove 20% of the points in Y to get a reduced set and this is done so that the two mixture densities have a large discrepancy in the number of centroids. Different level of noise is then added to perturb reduced set. We then match X to the reduced Y using both GL2 and Jensen-Shannon algorithms. From the error plots in Figure 2, we observe that our method exhibits stronger resistance to noise than the JS method. Furthermore, the average running time for all synthetic examples are $2.151s$ of our methods compared with $3.738s$ with the Jensen-Shannon algorithm, and both algorithms are tested on the same laptop with a 1.66 GHZ processor.

5.2 Multipoint Registration of Cardiac Echo Videos

Our next experiments were conducted over cardiac echo videos. The data sets depicted over 500 heart beat cycles chosen from over 50 patients with a number

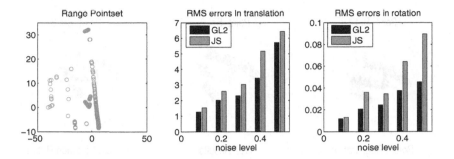

Fig. 2. Left: 2D range road pointset; Middle & Right: Errors in estimated rigid transform vs. noise strength

of cardiac diseases including cardiomyopathy, hypokinesia, mitral regurgitation, etc. For each disease class, we collected videos depicting similar views (long axis, short axis, four chamber views). An Active Shape Model (ASM) was used to characterize each such view, feature points corresponding to identifiable landmarks on heart wall boundaries were automatically extracted and tracked again as described in [10] to obtain a 3D point set.

For a set of Parasternal Long Axis (PLA) views, the points from all frames of a single cycle are then stacked together for five patients to form a 3D pointset, and the time axis is normalized. The point-sets are different in size, with the number of points $1026, 988, 988$ in each point-set respectively. As shown in Figure 3, the recovered deformation between each point-set ('o') and the mean shape ('+') are superimposed on the first row in Figure 3. The point-sets before and after registration results are shown in second and third image of the second row of Figure 3. The registration results generated using GL2 is shown in the lower-right for comparison, from which we can observe that the results generated using our algorithm exhibits more similarity than the JS approach. This example clearly demonstrates that our joint matching and atlas construction algorithm can simultaneously align multiple shapes (modeled by sample point-sets) and compute a meaningful mean shape.

The advantage of GL2 over JS in registering point sets also exists within each disease categories. In Table 1, we show the remaining point variance after registration of videos from a number of diseases: regional wall motion abnormality (RWMA), mitral regurgitation (MR), and myocardial infarction (MI). For all diseases, the GL2 variance is lower than the corresponding JS variance, showing that GL2 performs a superior registration of the point sets. As in Figure 3, the pointsets are drawn from ASM tracking of wall boundaries in PLA views of the heart.

5.3   Nonrigid Registration of Point-Sets from Human Brain MRI

In this we show examples of our algorithm for 2D corpus callosum atlas estimation and describe a 3D implementation on real hippocampal data sets. The

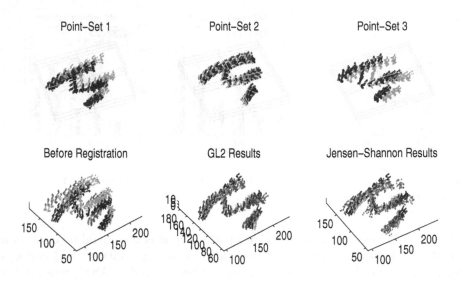

Fig. 3. Experimental results on three 3D echocardiogram point-sets (see text for details).

structure we are interested in this experiment is the corpus callosum as it appears in MR brain images. Constructing an atlas for the corpus callosum and subsequently analyzing the individual shape variation from "normal" anatomy has been regarded as potentially valuable for the study of brain diseases such as agenesis of the corpus callosum(ACC), and fetal alcohol syndrome(FAS).

We manually extracted points on the outer contour of the corpus callosum from nine normal subjects, (as shown Figure 4, indicated by 'o'). The recovered deformation between each point-set and the mean shape are superimposed on the first two rows in Figure 4. The resulting atlas (mean point-set) is shown in third row of Figure 4, and is superimposed over all the point-sets. As we described earlier, all these results are computed simultaneously and automatically.

Next, we present results on 3D hippocampal point-sets. Four 3D point-sets were extracted from epilepsy patients with right anterior temporal lobe foci identified with EEG. An interactive segmentation tool was used to segment the hippocampus from the 3D brain MRI scans of 4 subjects. The point-sets differ in

Table 1. Within different cardiac diseases, registration variance is lower with our GL2 approach compared with JS, showing we achieve a better overall registration

	Cardiac disease		
	RWMA	MR	MI
GL2 variance	0.1051	0.1194	0.1103
JS variance	0.1212	0.1384	0.1222

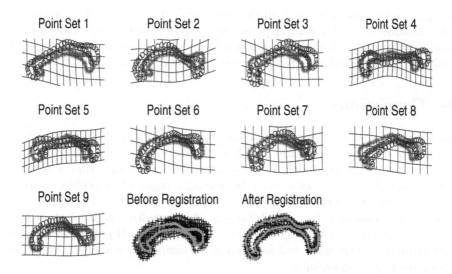

Fig. 4. Experiment results on nine 2D corpus callosum point-sets (see text for details)

shape, with the number of points $412, 763, 573, 644$ in each point-set respectively. In the first four images of Figure 5, the first row and the left image in second row shows the deformation of each point-set to the atlas (represented as cluster centers), superimposed with initial point set (show in 'o') and deformed point-set (shown in '+'). In second row of the Figure 5, we also show the scatter plot of

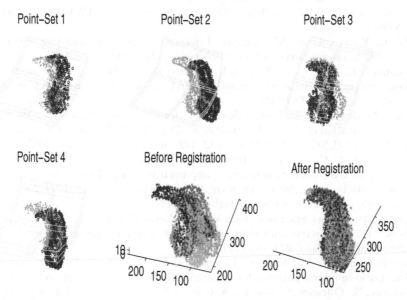

Fig. 5. Registration of four 3D hippocampal point sets (see text for details)

original point-sets along with all the point-sets after the non-rigid warping. An examination of the two scatter plots clearly shows the efficacy of our recovered non-rigid warping. Note that validation of an atlas shape for real data sets is a difficult problem and is a problem to be addressed in future.

6   Conclusions

In this paper, we presented a new and robust algorithm that utilizes a novel information theoretic measure, namely Generalized L2-divergence, to simultaneously register multiple unlabeled point-sets. We have shown that it is possible to obtain a closed form solution to the non-rigid registration problem leading to computational efficiency in registration. While we used Gaussian kernels to represent the probability density of point sets, the formalism holds for other kernels as well. Experiments were depicted with both 2D and 3D point sets from medical domain. Future work will focus on generalizing the non-rigid deformations to diffeomorphic mappings.

References

1. Jian, B., Vemuri, B.: A robust algorithm for point set registration using mixture of gaussians. In: ICCV 2005, pp. 1246–1251 (2005)
2. Wang, F., Vemuri, B.C., Rangarajan, A., Eisenschenk, S.J.: Simultaneous nonrigid registration of multiple point sets and atlas construction. IEEE Trans. Pattern Anal. Mach. Intell. 30(11), 2011–2022 (2008)
3. Wang, F., Vemuri, B.C., Rangarajan, A.: Groupwise point pattern registration using a novel CDF-based Jensen-Shannon divergence. In: CVPR, pp. 1283–1288 (2006)
4. Wang, Y., Woods, K., McClain, M.: Information-theoretic matching of two point sets. IEEE Transactions on Image Processing 11(8), 868–872 (2002)
5. Glaunes, J., Trouvé, A., Younes, L.: Diffeomorphic matching of distributions: A new approach for unlabelled point-sets and sub-manifolds matching. In: CVPR 2004 (2), pp. 712–718 (2004)
6. Roy, A., Gopinath, A., Rangarajan, A.: Deformable density matching for 3d non-rigid registration of shapes. In: Ayache, N., Ourselin, S., Maeder, A. (eds.) MICCAI 2007, Part I. LNCS, vol. 4791, pp. 942–949. Springer, Heidelberg (2007)
7. Twining, C.J., Cootes, T.F., Marsland, S., Petrovic, V.S., Schestowitz, R., Taylor, C.J.: A unified information-theoretic approach to groupwise non-rigid registration and model building. In: Christensen, G.E., Sonka, M. (eds.) IPMI 2005. LNCS, vol. 3565, pp. 1–14. Springer, Heidelberg (2005)
8. Huber, P.: Robust Statistics. John Wiley & Sons, Chichester (1981)
9. Scott, D.: Parametric statistical modeling by minimum integrated square Error. Technometrics 43(3), 274–285 (2001)
10. Syeda-Mahmood, T., Wang, F., Beymer, D., London, M., Reddy, R.: Characterizing spatio-temporal patterns for disease discrimination in cardiac echo videos. In: Ayache, N., Ourselin, S., Maeder, A. (eds.) MICCAI 2007, Part I. LNCS, vol. 4791, pp. 261–269. Springer, Heidelberg (2007)

Fully-Automated White Matter Hyperintensity Detection with Anatomical Prior Knowledge and without FLAIR

Christopher Schwarz[1], Evan Fletcher[2], Charles DeCarli[2], and Owen Carmichael[1,2]

[1] Computer Science Department, University of California, Davis, CA 95618
[2] Neurology Department, University of California, Davis, CA 95618

Abstract. This paper presents a method for detection of cerebral white matter hyperintensities (WMH) based on run-time PD-, T1-, and T2-weighted structural magnetic resonance (MR) images of the brain along with labeled training examples. Unlike most prior approaches, the method is able to reliably detect WMHs in elderly brains in the absence of fluid-attenuated (FLAIR) images. Its success is due to the learning of probabilistic models of WMH spatial distribution and neighborhood dependencies from ground-truth examples of FLAIR-based WMH detections. These models are combined with a probabilistic model of the PD, T1, and T2 intensities of WMHs in a Markov Random Field (MRF) framework that provides the machinery for inferring the positions of WMHs in novel test images. The method is shown to accurately detect WMHs in a set of 114 elderly subjects from an academic dementia clinic. Experiments show that standard off-the-shelf MRF training and inference methods provide robust results, and that increasing the complexity of neighborhood dependency models does not necessarily help performance. The method is also shown to perform well when training and test data are drawn from distinct scanners and subject pools.

1 Introduction

Relevance of WMHs. White matter foci that are hyperintense on FLAIR images of the human brain are indicative of focal dysfunction of underlying axonal tracts. Common in a variety of clinical conditions, including multiple sclerosis, cerebrovascular disease, and depression, WMHs are important clinical measures in the elderly because their prevalence is strongly associated with cognitive function, longevity, disease progression, and the effects of disease-modifying treatments [1][2][3]. Because semi-quantitative manual grading of WMH severity is time-consuming and variable due to human subjectivity [4], a variety of fully-automated methods have been developed to detect WMHs on FLAIR images in a robust, efficient, and objective manner [5][6].

Need for Detecting WMH without FLAIR. However, while FLAIR images provide optimal contrast between WMHs and all other tissues, the detection of

J.L. Prince, D.L. Pham, and K.J. Myers (Eds.): IPMI 2009, LNCS 5636, pp. 239–251, 2009.

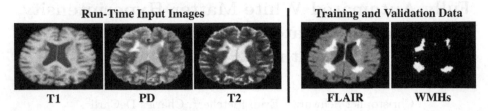

Fig. 1. A representative axial slice from the input images used for detecting WMHs at run time (left) and ground-truth data used for training the WMH detection method and validating the results (right)

WMHs when no FLAIR is available is an increasingly important problem. Large-scale imaging studies are under pressure to collect a wide range of MR imaging sequences, including T1, T2, proton density (PD), diffusion tensor, functional, and perfusion MR, to capture the broadest possible range of biological phenomena in the brains of participants. Simultaneously, the studies are under pressure to scan each subject for the shortest amount of time possible due to scanner resource costs and the increases in head motion and subject discomfort that occur over the course of the scan session. Therefore, a growing list of large-scale imaging studies that have a strong interest in white matter dysfunction have nonetheless chosen to forgo FLAIR acquisition [3][7][8].

WMH Detection without FLAIR Using Spatial and Contextual Priors. Because T1-weighted and double echo PD/T2-weighted acquisitions are nearly ubiquitous in large-scale imaging studies, we focus on WMH detection based solely on T1, T2, and PD input images. We use FLAIR exclusively for training data and the validation of automated methods (Fig. 1). WMHs are hyperintense on PD and T2, and hypointense on T1, but none of these modalities provide sufficient contrast between normal white matter (WM) and WMHs (Fig. 1). Therefore, we combine image intensity information with prior anatomical knowledge about where WMHs are known to occur in the brain and how they progress over time from one part of the brain to another. In particular, we employ a **spatial prior**– the prior probability of a WMH occurring at a given pixel, irrespective of imaging data– and a **contextual prior**– the conditional probability of a WMH occurring at a given pixel, given that WMHs have occurred at neighboring pixels. In elderly subjects, the spatial and contextual priors are highly structured and capture a characteristic spatial distribution of WMH occurrence and progression; specifically, WMHs in Alzheimer's Disease and healthy aging tend to begin in periventricular zones and spread upward and outward (see Fig. 2 and [9]). The prior models that capture this progression are learned from FLAIR-based ground-truth WMH detections in a training phase, and are combined with intensity information at run-time in an MRF framework to detect WMHs in novel sets of coregistered (PD, T1, T2) test image sets.

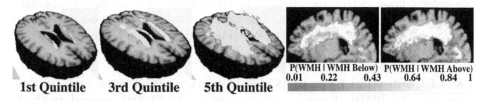

1st Quintile   3rd Quintile   5th Quintile

P(WMH | WMH Below) P(WMH | WMH Above)
0.01   0.22   0.43   0.64   0.84   1

Fig. 2. Left: ADC subjects were divided into quintiles based on total WMH volume; voxels that had WMHs in more than 5% of subjects in the quintile are shown in red. Note that WMHs appear to progress systematically upwards and outwards from periventricular zones. **Right:** The contextual prior captures the characteristic inferior-to-superior progression of WMHs in elderly subjects. Each pixel is colored according to the probability that it is WMH, given that the pixel below it, *vs.* above it, is WMH. $P(WMH|WMHBelow)$ is moderate at most pixels because if a downward neighbor is WMH, the upward propagation of WMHs may have arrived there and stopped; or it may have continued upward to include the pixel in question. Meanwhile $P(WMH|WMHAbove)$ is generally high because if the upward progression of WMHs has already reached a particular pixel, it is likely to have already passed through the pixels below it. The WMH detection method uses this known spatial progression of WMH to help determine which pixels are WMH, based on the absolute position of the pixel and the presence of neighboring WMHs.

1.1   Prior Work

WMH Detection without FLAIR. Few papers to date have dealt with the problem of automated WMH detection in the absence of FLAIR images, each using a comparatively simple model of WMH spatial distribution. One such method detected WMHs using a MRF system with a 2D and spatially invariant isotropic smoothing prior [10]. In another, the authors detected WMHs as outliers to models of other tissue classes instead of modelling them explicitly [11]. One method used boosted classifiers and Support Vector Machines to perform detection from PD and T1 images using spatially invariant isotropic smoothing and radial distance from center as a spatial prior. It also required separate training sets for mild, moderate, and severe WMH cases [12]. Finally, another used several run-time steps, including segmentations of grey matter, white matter, and CSF; segmentation of the thalamic nuclei; morphological post-processing to fix segmentation problems; and separation of WMHs into sub-classes based on image contrast [13]. The key difference between these methods and the current one is that the current method uses training data to directly capture the anatomical distribution and progression of WMHs in a model that allows spatial dependencies in WMH occurrence to vary arbitrarily across the image. Our method leverages this additional prior knowledge to directly model WMHs using a relatively straightforward run-time procedure that requires few steps or arbitrary parameter settings since it only fits parameters to a 3D intensity distribution and runs an existing, widely available MRF solver. Additionally, we focus on the elderly brain, whose morphological characteristics can be highly heterogeneous across a population due to diverse aging-related biological phenomena; the heterogeneity provides challenges to WMH detection that may differ from those associated with multiple sclerosis [10] and [11].

Use of Contextual Cues in WMH Detection. While little attention has been paid to WMH detection in the absence of FLAIR, several methods have used neighborhood information during FLAIR-based WMH detection (*e.g.*, [6][5]). Usually the use of contextual information amounts to fully-isotropic smoothing– that is, WMHs are considered more likely at a given pixel if they occur at neighboring pixels, regardless of their absolute positions or the directions in which neighboring WMHs do or do not occur. We extend these prior contextual methods by allowing the associations between neighboring WMH detections to vary with pixel position and direction of neighbors. As suggested above, the spatially- and directionally-variable nature of associations between neighboring WMHs in our contextual model allows us to more accurately capture the neurobiological course of spreading WMHs over the course of brain aging.

2   Methods

Data. We tested our method on a diverse pool of 114 elderly individuals who received a full clinical workup and structural MR scans including T1-weighted, double-echo PD/T2 weighted, and FLAIR scans at their times of enrollment into the University of California, Davis Alzheimer's Disease Center (ADC). Subjects were 70-90 years of age; the subject pool included individuals with normal cognition, mild cognitive impairment, and dementia.

Pre-processing. All scans were pre-processed through a standardized pipeline. T1, T2, PD, and FLAIR were rigidly coregistered using cross-correlation as a similarity measure and previously-presented optimization methods [14]. Non-brain tissues were manually separated from the brain on all scans. A strongly-validated, semi-automated method was used to detect WMHs based solely on the FLAIR scans and human input [15]. The skull-stripped T1-weighted image was then nonlinearly aligned to a minimum deformation template (MDT) based on moving control points in a multi-scale grid and using cubic spline interpolation to move image pixels between the control points [16][17]. The warp was constrained using hard limits on the magnitude of local deformation field expansion and contraction. This prevented voxels from collapse entirely. The T1, T2, PD, FLAIR, and map of ground-truth FLAIR-based WMH pixels were then warped to the space of the MDT image using the nonlinear alignment. Warping to MDT provided an implicit normalization of WMH volumes to total brain volume.

MRF Approach. We take a Bayesian MRF approach to WMH detection. Let y_i denote a vector of three image intensities– PD, T1, and T2– associated with image pixel i. Our goal is to determine a binary label x_i for each image pixel i: $x_i = 1$ denotes the presence of a WMH at pixel i and $x_i = 0$ denote the absence of WMH there, *i.e.* to find a set of labels $X = \{x_1, x_2, \cdots x_k\}$ corresponding to image intensity vectors $Y = \{y_1, y_2 \cdots y_k\}$ that maximizes the posterior probability of the labels given the image data, $P(X|Y)$. By Bayes' theorem, $P(X|Y) \propto \Pi(X) * L(Y|X)$, where $\Pi(X)$ is the prior probability of a particular set of labels X irrespective of imaging data and $L(Y|X)$ is the likelihood of observing image intensities Y given that the underlying labels are X. The prior probability of a specific label x_i depends on a spatial prior– the prior probability that WMHs occur at pixel i– as well as a contextual prior– the conditional probability of x_i given the labels at neighbors of pixel i. The likelihood depends on the statistical distribution of the (PD, T1, T2) image intensities Y relative to the underlying labels X.

MRF Prior: $\Pi(x)$. The MRF label prior involves spatial and contextual prior models whose parameters are learned from training data. We write the MRF prior as a Gibbs field:

$$\Pi(X) = Z^{-1} * exp(-H(X))$$

where Z, the partition function, is the sum of $exp(-H(X))$ over all possible labelings, and $H(X)$ is an energy function that takes on lower values when the label field X is more probable *a priori*. This Gibbs prior is equivalent to an MRF prior under straightforward technical restrictions [18]. The energy function is a sum of terms that represent energies from the spatial and contextual priors: $H(X) = H_s(X) + H_c(X)$. The spatial prior penalizes pixel i if it is labeled as WMH but WMHs are deemed unlikely there according to a prior probability, α_i (see sec. 2), of a WMH occurring at pixel i:

$$H_s(X) = \sum_{x_i \in X} \alpha_i r_i + (1 - \alpha_i)(1 - x_i)$$

The contextual prior $H_c(X)$ penalizes a label x_i when it differs from the labels of its neighbors. Recall that the MRF formulation utilizes a graph in which all pixels in the image are attached to some arbitrary set of their immediate spatial neighbors (see Sec. 3 for more information); there is one term in H_c for each clique in this graph. Let δ be one such clique of nodes, Δ be the set of all such cliques, and X^δ be the assignment of labels (*i.e.*, WMH or non-WMH) that X provides to the nodes of δ. Then, H_c is given by:

$$H_c(X) = \sum_{\delta \in \Delta} \beta_{X^\delta}$$

This is a Potts model in which neighboring labels within a group δ incur a fixed penalty of β_{X^δ} [19]. Generally, these β parameters encourage neighboring pixels to have the same label, but in some locations of the brain, they may actually be encouraged to be different. These β parameters are calculated from the training data (Sec. 2).

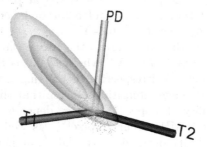

Fig. 3. The intensity distributions of WM and WMH intensities empirically follow "comet-like" patterns. Pictured: WMH intensities and the fit distribution for them in one ADC subject.

MRF Likelihood. The likelihood of a given set of image intensity vectors, given the underlying labels, comes from a tissue mixture model with one lognormal distribution for WM and one for WMH:

$$L(Y|X) = exp(-H_L(Y|X))$$

$$H_L(Y|X) = \sum_{x_i \in X} \frac{\pi_{x_i} f(y_i; \mu_{x_i}, \Sigma_{x_i})}{\sum_{x_i \in \{0,1\}} \pi_{x_i} f(y_i; \mu_{x_i}, \Sigma_{x_i})}$$

$$f(y; \mu, \Sigma) = \frac{1}{C} * exp(-.5 * (log(y) - \mu)^T \Sigma^{-1} (log(y) - \mu))$$

$$C = |\Sigma|^{.5}(2\pi)^{1.5}|log(y)|$$

where π_0 and π_1 are mixture coefficients for non-WMH and WMH respectively, with $\pi_0 + \pi_1 = 1$ and $log(y)$ is the component-wise log of vector y. We estimate π_1, by taking the proportion of pixels in Y_H that are inliers to the distribution found for the pixels in Y_L.

A lognormal mixture model was chosen because the distributions of 3D intensity vectors for WM and WMH empirically followed asymmetric, "comet-like" patterns (Fig. 3). Normal distributions failed to accurately capture this asymmetry. As we explain below, the μ and Σ parameters are estimated at run time by an unsupervised method that fits the two lognormal distributions to (PD, T1, T2) triples sampled from a large number of pixels.

Combining the equations for Π and L and taking the log, we have

$$log(P(X|Y)) \propto -H_s(X) - H_c(X) + H_L(Y|X)$$

In the following sections, we describe the Training phase that determines the values of α and β, followed by the Inference phase where the best set of labels X is determined for an input image Y.

Training. In the training phase the parameters α_i and β_{X^δ} governing H_s and H_c respectively are estimated from the ground-truth FLAIR-based WMH detection. The α_i values are the empirical probabilities of WMHs at each pixel in labeled training examples, i.e. sets of (X, Y) pairs gathered from ground-truth FLAIR-based WMH detection. That is, α_i is the proportion of training examples that have a WMH at pixel i.

The β_{X^δ} values are calculated using the same training data as the α_i values using Iterative Proportional Fitting (IPF) [20]. For each δ and for each possible label assignment to X^δ, IPF iteratively computes an estimate for β_{X^δ} using the following fixed point equation:

$$\beta_{X^\delta}^n = \beta_{X^\delta}^{n-1} \times R\left(\frac{M_{X^\delta}^e}{M_{X^\delta}^m}\right)$$

where $\beta_{X^\delta}^n$ is the value of β_{X^δ} at the nth iteration of IPF, $M_{X^\delta}^e$ is the empirical marginal probability of $\delta = X^\delta$ calculated as the proportion of the training data in which that label configuration occurred in δ, and $M_{X^\delta}^m$ denotes the model marginal probability of X^δ: the integral of $\Pi(X)$ over all X in which the assignment X^δ occurs. The model marginal is calculated through Sum-Product BP (Sec. 2). $R(x)$ is a sigmoid regularization function that prevents divergence of the fixed point iteration.

Run-Time Inference Fitting the MRF Likelihood Distributions. Run-time processing of a novel image set begins by using an MLESAC-based procedure to robustly estimate the means and covariances of the lognormal distributions associated with the WM and WMH classes [21]. Specifically, we generate k random samples of 10 pixels each from among those pixels that are most likely to contain WMHs *a priori*, *i.e.* from among the 5% of pixels i with the highest α_i. Similarly we generate k 10-pixel samples from among the 5% of pixels with the lowest α_i. From each high-α_i sample we estimate a candidate μ_1 and Σ_1 from the corresponding y_i, and similarly a candidate μ_0 and Σ_0 is estimated from each low-α_i sample . Let Y_L and Y_H be the y_i corresponding to the low-α_i pixels and high-α_i pixels respectively. Let X_L contain a WM label for each low-α_i pixel and X_H contain a WMH label for each high-α_i pixel. Each candidate $(\mu_0, \mu_1, \Sigma_0, \Sigma_1)$ is assigned a numerical score that summarizes how well it fits the high-α_i and low-α_i y_i, as well as how many of the $y_i \in \{Y_L, Y_H\}$ are outliers. The score is

$$\sum_{X \in \{X_L, X_H\}} \sum_{x_i \in X} \delta(i) f(y_i; \mu_{x_i}, \Sigma_{x_i}) + (1 - \delta(i))\nu$$

where ν is a fixed penalty for outliers and $\delta(i)$ indicates whether y_i is an outlier, *i.e.* it is 1 when $f(y_i; \mu_{x_i}, \Sigma_{x_i}) > T$ and 0 when $f(y_i; \mu_{x_i}, \Sigma_{x_i}) < T$. In our experiments, we set k, T, and ν to 100, 10^{-6}, and -0.1 respectively. The highest-scoring $(\mu_0, \mu_1, \Sigma_0, \Sigma_1)$ are our parameter estimates for the distributions. Given the parameters needed to calculate the likelihood and contextual prior, we then use Belief Propagation to infer labels X that maximize $log(P(X|Y))$ [22].

MRF Inference. In Belief Propagation (BP), inference is performed by propagating local evidence (beliefs) as messages. Here, we use the Factor Graph formulation of BP in order to simplify notation. Factor Graphs represent undirected graphs in a bipartite fashion with two types of nodes: factor nodes and variable nodes. In our method, variable nodes directly correspond with pixel labels x_i and factor nodes each correspond to a $\delta \in \Delta$. In each BP iteration, each variable node sends a message to each factor node that represents a clique it is a member of, and each factor node sends a message to the variable nodes of the clique member nodes. These messages are called variable messages $x_i \rightarrow \delta(x)$ and factor messages $\delta \rightarrow x_i(x)$ respectively. For Max-Product BP, the version used to compute a set of *maximum a posteriori* labels, the messages are:

$$x_i \rightarrow \delta(x) = O(i,x) \sum_{\alpha \in \Delta_i \setminus \{\delta\}} \alpha \rightarrow x_i(x)$$

$$\delta \rightarrow x_i(x) = \max_{X^\delta : x_i = x} C(X^\delta) \sum_{x_m \in \delta \setminus \{x_i\}} x_m \rightarrow \delta(x)$$

where x is a candidate label for x_i, Δ_i denotes the set of δ containing i, the observation term

$$O(i,x) = [x\alpha_i + (1-x)\alpha_i][L(x_i = x|y_i)],$$

and the compatibility term $C(X^\delta) = S(\beta_{X^\delta})$ where $S(u)$ is a regularization function that smoothes across values of K to avoid numerical implementation issues introduced by extreme-valued weightings. When computing the β terms using Sum-Product BP as referenced in Sec. 2, the sums in the above terms are replaced with products, the max is replaced with a sum, and $O(x) = 1$. The model marginals are then computed by:

$$M_{X^\delta}^m = C(X^\delta) \prod_{x_i \in \delta} x_i \rightarrow \delta(x_i)$$

for each possible configuration of labels X^δ for the given δ to form $M_{X^\delta}^m$ [23].

3   Experiments

In this section, we test the method's performance under varying training/ inference conditions, training set sizes, neighborhood connectivity, and training data sources.

Training and Inference Methods. In these tests, we use leave-one-out cross-validation to evaluate MRF-based WMH detection on the ADC data set; for each subject, we estimate the α and β parameters from the remainder of the subjects

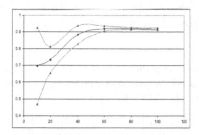

Fig. 4. Plotted mean μ and $\mu \pm \sigma$ of ICC values between ground-truth WMH volume and WMH volume estimated by our method using differently-sized random subsets of the training set in cross validation. Note that these values are absolute, not percents, and are out of a maximum of 114 (training with all data). *Each of the size-10 ICC measures is without 1-2 test subjects for whom IPF did not converge.

and use them to detect WMHs on the left-out subject. Agreement between the ground-truth WMH volumes and our computed volumes is evaluated using the intraclass correlation coefficient (ICC). We compute these ICC values for our method under each of these conditions: In the **No MRF** method, we do not use an MRF-based system and instead simply threshold the Posterior probabilities deduced from the H_s and H_L terms alone. In the **6-MRF Without Training** method, we use the empirical marginals $M_{X^\delta}^e$ for the β_{X^δ} terms instead of performing a proper training method. Finally, the **6-MRF With Training** method uses our complete system with its designed proper IPF-based training. The results of these experiments are available in Table 1 and an example is given in Fig. 5.

In our experiments, our MRF-based method outperforms the No-MRF and untrained MRF versions.

Contextual Prior Connectivity. One variable parameter of the method is the connectivity of its Contextual Prior information, ie. what size groupings of neighboring pixels influence each other in the MRF system. Higher values allow the system to model more complex spatial patterns. In 2D images, this choice is generally whether or not diagonal pixels are considered neighbors. In 3D, neighborhoods are described in values between 6, ie. a pixel's 4 nearest neighbors within the plane and 2 nearest in the Z direction; and 26, ie. all of a pixel's neighbors in a 3x3x3 pixel box around it. Results of testing our method

Table 1. Intraclass correlation coefficients (ICCs) between ground-truth WMH volume and WMH volume estimated by our method on the ADC data set with several variations

	No MRF	6-MRF Without Training	6-MRF with Training
ICC	0.909	0.872	0.916

under varying connectivities are presented in Table 2. For these tests, as in the previous, we used the ADC dataset and leave-one-out cross validation.

Table 2. Intraclass correlation coefficients (ICCs) between ground-truth WMH volume and WMH volume estimated by our method using various degrees of spatial prior directional connectivity for the ADC data set

	6-MRF	10-MRF	18-MRF	24-MRF
ICC	0.916	0.909	0.898	0.862

In these experiments, we found that our method performs best using 6-connected neighborhoods, the smallest logical size within 3D space.

Training Set Size. One important property of any training-based classification method is the amount of training data it requires to give good results on test data. To test this property, we trained upon three different randomly selected subsets of the ADC dataset for each size: 10, 20, 40, 60, 80, and 100 subjects. We then ran the method to classify the dataset using these subsets as training data (Fig. 4).

For this dataset our method performs better when using more training data up until about 60 images, after which there is little improvement.

Training and Test Sets from Different Populations and Scanners. To test our method's performance using a completely different dataset from that upon which it was trained, we employed ground-truth WMH map data of 51 subjects from the Chicago Health and Aging Project (CHAP), a longitudinal Epidemiological study of individuals with risk factors for Alzheimer's Disease [24]. These images were preprocessed in the same fashion as the ADC data (Sec. 2) and used for training. We then tested (using 6-connected neighborhoods

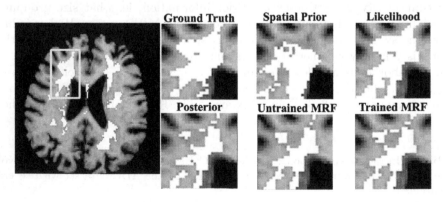

Fig. 5. Comparison of WMH detection results for a selected brain region (see green box, left, and ground-truth). Detected WMHs are shown in yellow.

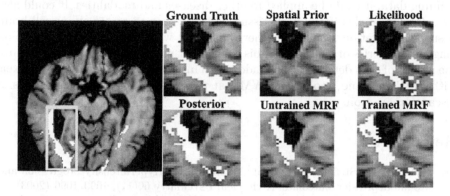

Fig. 6. Comparison of WMH detection results for a selected brain region (see green box, left, and ground-truth). Detected WMHs are shown in yellow.

and standard training/inference) our dataset of 114 ADC subjects using this training data and obtained results with an ICC of **0.841**, demonstrating our method's ability to perform reasonably when classifying images from a dataset from an entirely different MRI scanner, study type (epidemiological vs. clinic-based cohorts), and population.

4   Discussion and Future Work

Summary of Results. Our method performs robust WMH detection with no FLAIR when using at least 60 training images and standard MRF training/ inference, including when the sources of training and testing data differ significantly. While our method performs strongly in these experiments, there exist several routes through which it can be improved in the future. Specifically, we discuss why the method performed worse using higher connectivities and possible new applications such as longitudinal WMH detection and multi-class segmentation.

Higher Degrees of Neighborhood Connectivity. Increased complexity can model more complex spatial dependencies among WMHs, but did not perform well in our experiments (Sec. 3). This drop in performance can be explained by a combination of factors. Higher connectivities subdivide the training data into a larger set of parameters, requiring a larger amount of training data. Additionally, it is possible that higher connectivities result in overfitting to the training data. Finally, BP, used here in both training and inference, is technically not guaranteed to perform well in loopy graphs but empirically does for 4-connected 2D latices. As the connectivity of our model increases, so does the proportion of loops in the graph, which may decrease performance. Future work should determine which combination of factors causes the decrease.

Other Applications. In addition to improving the method itself, future work will test and extend it for use in other applications. Simply by using appropriate training data, it could be applied to other diseases and modalities. It could also be extended to classify multiple tissue types at once to create an overall brain tissue segmentation system. Another possibility would be to detect WMHs on longitudinal series of MRIs. With this change our method could not only improve the results of each detection by the additional information (eg. encouraging pixels with WMH at time 1 to remain WMH at time 2) but also generate models of disease progression.

References

1. Taylor, W.D., Steffens, D.C., et al.: White Matter Hyperintensity progression and late-life depression outcomes. Arch. Gen. Psychiatry 60(11), 1090–1096 (2003)
2. Au, R., Massaro, J.M., et al.: Association of White Matter Hyperintensity volume with decreased cognitive functioning: the Framingham Heart Study. Arch. Neurol. (in press)
3. Dufouil, C., de Kersaint-Gilly, A., et al.: Longitudinal study of blood pressure and White Matter Hyperintensities: The EVA MRI cohort. Neurology 56(7) (April 2001)
4. van Straaten, E., Fazekas, F., et al.: Impact of White Matter Hyperintensities scoring method on correlations with clinical data: The LADIS study. Stroke 37(3) (2006)
5. Admiraal-Behloul, F., van den Heuvel, D., et al.: Fully automatic segmentation of White Matter Hyperintensities in MR images of the elderly. Neuroimage 28(3), 607–617 (2005)
6. Wu, M., Rosano, C., et al.: A fully automated method for quantifying and localizing White Matter Hyperintensities on MR images. Psychiatry Research: Neuroimag 148(2-3), 133–142 (2006)
7. Longstreth, W., Manolio, T.A., et al.: Clinical correlates of White Matter findings on cranial magnetic resonance imaging of 3301 elderly people: The Cardiovascular Health Study. Stroke 27, 1274–1282 (1996)
8. Mueller, S., Weiner, M., et al.: Ways toward an early diagnosis in Alzheimer's disease: The Alzheimer's disease neuroimaging initiative (ADNI). Alzheimers Dement. 1(1), 55–66 (2005)
9. Yoshita, M., Fletcher, E., et al.: Extent and distribution of White Matter Hyperintensities in normal aging, mci, and ad. Neurology 67(12), 2192–2198 (2006)
10. Van Leemput, K., Maes, F., Bello, F., Vandermeulen, D., Colchester, A.C.F., Suetens, P.: Automated segmentation of MS lesions from multi-channel MR images. In: Taylor, C., Colchester, A. (eds.) MICCAI 1999. LNCS, vol. 1679, pp. 11–21. Springer, Heidelberg (1999)
11. Van Leemput, K., Maes, F., Vandermeulen, D., Colchester, A., Suetens, P.: Automated segmentation of Multiple Sclerosis lesions by model outlier detection. IEEE Transactions on Medical Imaging 20(8), 677–688 (2001)
12. Azhar Quddus, P.F., Basir, O.: Adaboost and support vector machines for White Matter Lesion segmentation in MR images. Engineering in Medicine and Biology Society (2005)
13. Maillard, P., Delcroix, N., et al.: An automated procedure for the assessment of White Matter Hyperintensities by multispectral (T1, T2, PD) MRI and an evaluation of its between-centre reproducibility based on two large community databases. Neuroradiology 50(1), 31–42 (2008)

14. Maes, F., Collignon, A., et al.: Multimodality image registration by maximization of mutual information. IEEE Trans. Med. Imaging 16, 187–198 (1997)
15. Yoshita, M., Fletcher, E., et al.: Current concepts of analysis of cerebral White Matter Hyperintensities on Magnetic Resonance Imaging. Top Magn. Reson. Imaging 16(6), 399–407 (2005)
16. Kochunov, P., Lancaster, J., et al.: Regional spatial normalization: toward an optimal target. J. Comp. Assist. Tomog. 25(5), 805–816 (2001)
17. Otte, M.: Elastic registration of fMRI data using bezier-spline transformations. IEEE Trans. Med. Imaging 20, 193–206 (2001)
18. Hammersley, J., Clifford, P.: Markov fields on finite graphs and lattices (1971)
19. Besag, J.: On the statistical analysis of dirty pictures. Journal of the Royal Statistical Society. Series B 48(3), 259–302 (1986)
20. Jirousek, R., Preucil, S.: On the effective implementation of the iterative proportional fitting procedure. Computational Statistics & Data Analysis 19(2), 177–189 (1995)
21. Torr, P., Zisserman, A.: MLESAC: A new robust estimator with application to estimating image geometry. CVIU 78(1), 138–156 (2000)
22. Freeman, W.T., Pasztor, E.C., Owen, T., Carmichael, Y.: Learning low-level vision. International Journal of Computer Vision 40 (2000)
23. Bishop, C.M.: Pattern Recognition and Machine Learning. Springer Science+Business Media, Heidelberg (2006)
24. Bienias, J.L., Beckett, L.A., Bennett, D.A., Wilson, R.S., Evans, D.A.: Design of the chicago health and aging project (CHAP). J. Alzheimers Dis. 5, 349–355 (2003)

Identification of Growth Seeds in the Neonate Brain through Surfacic Helmholtz Decomposition

Julien Lefèvre[1], François Leroy[2], Sheraz Khan[3], Jessica Dubois[2],
Petra S. Huppi[4], Sylvain Baillet[3,5], and Jean-François Mangin[1]

[1] LNAO, Neurospin, CEA, Saclay, France
{julien.lefevre,jean-francois.mangin}@cea.fr
[2] INSERM, U562, Neurospin
[3] Cognitive Neuroscience and Brain Imaging Laboratory,
CNRS UPR640–LENA, Université Pierre et Marie CURIE–Paris6, Paris, France
[4] Division of Child Development and Growth, Department of Pediatrics, Geneva
University Hospitals 1211, Geneva 4, Switzerland
[5] Department of Neurology, Medical College of Wisconsin, Milwaukee

Abstract. We report on a new framework to investigate the rapid brain development of newborns. It is based on the analysis of depth maps of the cortical surface through the study of a displacement field estimated by surfacic optical flow methods. This displacement field shows local evolution of sulci directly on the cortical surface. Detection of its critical points is performed with the Helmholtz decomposition which allows us to identify sources of the developmental process. They can be viewed as growth seeds or in other terms points around which the sulcal growth organizes itself. We show the reproducibility of such growth seeds across 4 neonates and make a link of this new concept to the "sulcal roots" one proposed to explain the variability of human brain anatomy.

1 Introduction

Recent studies in MRI have described precisely the ontogenesis of the cortical folding during early phases of development [5],[18]. Thank to these studies it becomes now possible to follow the evolution of brain structures during the period of gyrification, to detect potential cerebral lesions [5] or to follow step by step the complex processes of sulci and gyri formation whose physiological bases are yet not well deciphered [15] [16] [17]. Through image postprocessing tools [5] our group has extracted the surface between gray and white matter of preterm newborns at critical ages for cortical folding namely 26-36 weeks gestational age. Another group has presented [19] a registration algorithm in order to align cortical surfaces in longitudinal studies and to track the cortical development. This tracking has been evaluated on sulci which are 3D structures but very few methods have been previously performed directly on the surfaces. In our prior work [3] a primal sketch of the cortical mean curvature provides elementary cortical folds and fold merging during brain development.

Further in a study of functional brain activations [10] we have shown the possibility to follow evolving texture – MEG neural activities in the present case

J.L. Prince, D.L. Pham, and K.J. Myers (Eds.): IPMI 2009, LNCS 5636, pp. 252–263, 2009.

– directly on the cortical surfaces through optical flow algorithms. Moreover the knowledge of such a deformation field reveals local patterns of growth in particular focal point around which the growth spreads [6]. This last study rises future possibilities for validating models of cortical growth such as the "sulcal roots" model in which "atoms" of future sulci are supposed to preexist in the developing fetus [14].

The aim of our study is to propose a framework which allows us to track the changes in the sulcation of neonates along time and directly on the cortical surface. The advantage of working on surfaces is twofold since there is a gain in computation time with respect to 3D analysis and since we offer a practical visualization of displacement fields.

We will define a quantity of interest which is based on depth maps projected to cortical surfaces. Then using non linear registration technique based on iconic feature [4] we will align brain surfaces of neonates and their depth maps longitudinally. Next we apply a recent methodology to track evolutions of scalar measures on surfaces through generalized optical flow [9]. At last we perform a helmholtz decomposition of the resulting deformation field that will enable us to identify robust features such as sources of growth. Using this approach we will demonstrate that the evolution field of the developing brain has a radial structure and organizes itself into growth seeds.

We evaluate the reproducibility of these growth seeds using a rigid registration of the cortical surfaces and show that we find some clusters of seeds that can be compared to anatomical features ("sulcal roots") previously described in the literature.

2   Optical Flow on Surfaces

In this part we recall the formalism introduced in a prior study [9] based on differential geometry to extend the computation of optical flow equation on Riemannian manifolds. This theoretical development will allow us to deduce a vector field that represents the evolution of a scalar quantity defined on a surface (typically the depth maps in the next application) along time.

2.1   Notations

Here are some notations : $\mathcal{M}$ is a 2-Riemannian manifold representing the imaging support (i.e. the cortical surfaces) and $I(p,t)$ a scalar quantity defined on a 2-dimensional surface and in time . We note $\mathbf{e}_\alpha = \partial_{x_\alpha} p$, the canonical basis – with respect to a coordinate system x_α– of the tangent space $T_p\mathcal{M}$ at a point p of the manifold, and $T\mathcal{M} = \bigcup_p T_p\mathcal{M}$ the tangent bundle of $\mathcal{M}$.

$\mathcal{M}$ is equipped with a Riemannian metric, that is there exists a positive-definite form: $g_p : T_p\mathcal{M} \times T_p\mathcal{M} \to \mathbb{R}$. A natural choice for g_p is the restriction of the Euclidian metric to $T_p\mathcal{M}$, which we have adopted for subsequent computations. For concision purposes, we will now only refer to g_p as g.

The classical hypotheses for computing optical flow [8] leads to the equation:

$$\partial_t I + g(\mathbf{V}, \nabla_\mathcal{M} I) = 0. \tag{1}$$

Since only the component of the flow $\mathbf{V}$ in the direction of the gradient is accessible to estimation (aperture problem) [8], additional constraints on the flow are needed to yield a unique solution. This approach classically reduces to minimizing an energy functional such as in [8]:

$$\mathcal{E}(\mathbf{V}) = \int_{\mathcal{M}} \left(\frac{\partial I}{\partial t} + g(\mathbf{V}, \nabla_{\mathcal{M}} I) \right)^2 d\mu + \lambda \int_{\mathcal{M}} \mathcal{C}(\mathbf{V}) d\mu, \qquad (2)$$

The first term is a measure of fit of the optical flow model to the data, while the second one acts as a spatial regularizer of the flow. The smoothness term can be expressed as a Frobenius norm:

$$\mathcal{C}(\mathbf{V}) = \mathrm{Tr}(^t \nabla \mathbf{V}.\nabla \mathbf{V}) \text{ and } (\nabla \mathbf{V})_\alpha^\beta = \partial_\alpha V^\beta + \sum_\gamma \Gamma_{\alpha\gamma}^\beta V^\gamma \qquad (3)$$

$(\nabla \mathbf{V})$ is the covariant derivative of $\mathbf{V}$, a generalization of vectorial gradient. $\partial_\alpha V^\beta$ is the classical Euclidian expression of the gradient, and $\sum_\gamma \Gamma_{\alpha\gamma}^\beta V^\gamma$ reflects local deformations of the tangent space basis since the Christoffel symbols $\Gamma_{\alpha\gamma}^\beta$ are the coordinates of $\partial_\beta \mathbf{e}_\alpha$ along $\mathbf{e}_\gamma$. This expression ensures the tensoriality property of $\mathbf{V}$, i.e. the invariance with parametrization changes.

2.2   Variational Formulation

Deriving a variational formulation from the minimization of (2) ensures the well-posedness of the problem – existence and unicity of the solution in a specific and convenient function space – and allows us to solve numerically the problem on discrete irregular surfacic tessellations.

$\Gamma^1(\mathcal{M})$ is the working space of vector fields on which functional $\mathcal{E}(\mathbf{V})$ will be minimized. We chose a space of vector fields in which the coordinates of each element are located in $C^1(\mathcal{M})$ (the space of differentiable functions on the manifold):

$$\Gamma^1(\mathcal{M}) = \left\{ \mathbf{V} : \mathcal{M} \to T\mathcal{M} \ / \ \mathbf{V} = \sum_{\alpha=1}^2 V^\alpha \mathbf{e}_\alpha, \ V^\alpha \in C^1(\mathcal{M}) \right\},$$

with the scalar product :

$$< \mathbf{U}, \mathbf{V} >_{\Gamma^1(\mathcal{M})} = \int_{\mathcal{M}} g(\mathbf{U}, \mathbf{V}) \ d\mu + \int_{\mathcal{M}} \mathrm{Tr}(^t \nabla \mathbf{U} \nabla \mathbf{V}) \ d\mu.$$

$\mathcal{E}(\mathbf{V})$ can be simplified from (2) as a combination of a constant $K(t)$, a linear and a bilinear form :

$$f(\mathbf{U}) \quad = \quad - \int_{\mathcal{M}} g(\mathbf{U}, \nabla_{\mathcal{M}} I) \partial_t I \ d\mu,$$

$$a(\mathbf{U}, \mathbf{V}) \quad = \quad \int_{\mathcal{M}} g(\mathbf{U}, \nabla_{\mathcal{M}} I) g(\mathbf{V}, \nabla_{\mathcal{M}} I) d\mu + \lambda \int_{\mathcal{M}} \mathrm{Tr}(^t \nabla \mathbf{U} \nabla \mathbf{V}) \ d\mu.$$

Minimizing $\mathcal{E}(\mathbf{V})$ on $\Gamma^1(\mathcal{M})$ is then equivalent to the following problem :

$$\min_{\mathbf{V} \in \Gamma^1(\mathcal{M})} \left(a(\mathbf{V}, \mathbf{V}) - 2f(\mathbf{V}) + K(t) \right). \qquad (4)$$

It has been proved in [9] that there exists a unique solution. Moreover, this solution $\mathbf{V}$ to (4) satisfies:

$$a(\mathbf{V}, \mathbf{U}) = f(\mathbf{U}), \forall\, \mathbf{U} \in \Gamma^1(\mathcal{M}). \tag{5}$$

3   Helmholtz Decomposition of a Vector Field

Helmholtz decomposition is a classical way to decompose a vector field into the sum of a rotational part and a divergential part as illustrated on Fig.1. This technique enables to detect the singularities of a vector field, that is, source, sink or rotation center [13]. It has been recently used [7] in cardiac video analysis in order to track the critical points in the heart which can lead to a better understanding of the dynamics of the cardiac electrical activity and its anomalies. Identification of such points for a brain growth field seems to be of highest importance to characterize the underlying spatiotemporal evolution.

More formally we have the following theorem :

Theorem: Given $\mathbf{V}$ a vector field in $\Gamma^1(\mathcal{M})$, there exists unique functions U and A in $L^2(\mathcal{M})$ and a vector field $\mathbf{H}$ in $\Gamma^1(\mathcal{M})$ such as :

$$\mathbf{V} = \nabla_{\mathcal{M}} U + \mathbf{Curl}_{\mathcal{M}} A + \mathbf{H} \tag{6}$$
$$\mathrm{div}_{\mathcal{M}} \mathbf{H} = 0 \qquad \mathrm{curl}_{\mathcal{M}} \mathbf{H} = 0 \tag{7}$$

Notations: In our applications $\mathcal{M}$ is a surface (or submanifold) thus it is possible to get a normal vector in each point:

$$\mathbf{n}_p = \frac{\partial}{\partial x_1} \wedge \frac{\partial}{\partial x_2}.$$

The normal does not depend on the choice of the parametrization (x_1, x_2). Then we define the divergence operator through duality:

$$\int_{\mathcal{M}} U \mathrm{div}_{\mathcal{M}} \mathbf{H} = - \int_{\mathcal{M}} g(\mathbf{H}, \nabla_{\mathcal{M}} U)$$

Scalar and vectorial curl are at last :

$$\mathbf{Curl}_{\mathcal{M}} A = \nabla_{\mathcal{M}} A \wedge \mathbf{n} \qquad \mathrm{curl}_{\mathcal{M}} \mathbf{H} = \mathrm{div}_{\mathcal{M}} (\mathbf{H} \wedge \mathbf{n})$$

With these formulas we have intrinsic expressions which do not depend on the parametrization of the surface.

Proof: The proof of the existence of a solution follows a classical construction. It can be shown that if U and A minimize the two functionals:

$$\int_{\mathcal{M}} ||\mathbf{V} - \nabla_{\mathcal{M}} U||^2$$

$$\int_{\mathcal{M}} ||\mathbf{V} - \mathbf{Curl}_{\mathcal{M}} A||^2$$

$\mathbf{V} - \nabla_{\mathcal{M}} U - \mathbf{Curl}_{\mathcal{M}} A$ is solution of (7).

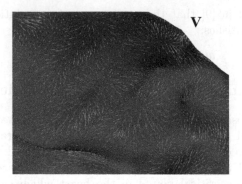

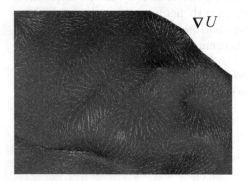

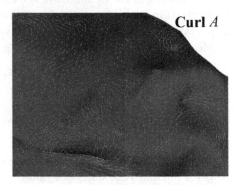

Fig. 1. First line: Vector field on a cortical mesh. Second line : divergential and rotational parts of the vector field. We can note that the vector field is mainly divergential and we can identify visually that it has only sources and no sinks.

These two previous functionals are convex therefore they have unique minimum on $L^2(\mathcal{M})$ which satisfies:

$$\forall \phi \in L^2(\mathcal{M}), \int_{\mathcal{M}} g(\mathbf{V}, \nabla_{\mathcal{M}}\phi) \;=\; \int_{\mathcal{M}} g(\nabla_{\mathcal{M}} U, \nabla_{\mathcal{M}}\phi) \qquad (8)$$

$$\forall \phi \in L^2(\mathcal{M}), \int_{\mathcal{M}} g(\mathbf{V}, \mathbf{Curl}_{\mathcal{M}}\phi) \;=\; \int_{\mathcal{M}} g(\mathbf{Curl}_{\mathcal{M}} A, \mathbf{Curl}_{\mathcal{M}}\phi) \qquad (9)$$

4   Numerical Aspects

Once proved the well-posedness of the regularized optical flow problem and the Helmholtz decomposition, we derive numerical methods from the variational formulations (5), (8) and (9).

Optical flow: First we consider the vector space of continuous piecewise affine vector fields which belong to the tangent space at each node of a mesh $\widehat{\mathcal{M}}$. A basis is:

$$\mathbf{W}_{\alpha,i} = w(i)\mathbf{e}_{\alpha}(i) \text{ for } 1 \leq i \leq \mathrm{Card}(\widehat{\mathcal{M}}), \ \alpha \in \{1,2\},$$

where $w(i)$ stands for the continuous piecewise affine function which is 1 at node i and 0 at all other triangle nodes, and $\mathbf{e}_{\alpha}(i)$ is a basis of tangent space at node i.

The variational formulation in (5) yields the linear system:

$$\left[a(\mathbf{W}_{\alpha,i}, \mathbf{W}_{\beta,j})\right]_{(\alpha,i),(\beta,j)} \left[\mathbf{V}\right] = \left[f(\mathbf{W}_{\alpha,i})\right]_{\alpha,i} \tag{10}$$

where $\left[\mathbf{V}\right]$ are the components of the velocity field $\mathbf{V}$ in the basis $\mathbf{W}_{\alpha,i}$. The matricial coefficient $a(\mathbf{W}_{\alpha,i}, \mathbf{W}_{\beta,j})$ and $f(\mathbf{W}_{\alpha,i})$ can be explicitly computed with first-order finite elements by estimating the integrals on each triangle T of the mesh and summing the different contributions.

$\nabla_{\widehat{\mathcal{M}}} I$ is obtained on each triangle $T = [i,j,k]$ from the linear interpolation:

$$\nabla_{\widehat{\mathcal{M}}} I = I(i)\nabla_T w(i) + I(j)\nabla_T w(j) + I(k)\nabla_T w(k).,$$

with

$$\nabla_T w(i) = \frac{\mathbf{h_i}}{\parallel \mathbf{h_i} \parallel^2},$$

where $\mathbf{h_i}$ is the height of triangle T from vertex i.

Helmholtz decomposition: Equations 8) and (9) hold when we replace ϕ by the basis function w_i so we have the two systems :

$$\left[\int_{\widehat{\mathcal{M}}} g(\nabla_{\mathcal{M}} w(i), \nabla_{\mathcal{M}} w(j))\right]_{i,j} \left[\mathbf{U}\right] = \left[\int_{\widehat{\mathcal{M}}} g(\mathbf{V}, \nabla_{\mathcal{M}} w(i))\right]_i \tag{11}$$

$$\left[\int_{\widehat{\mathcal{M}}} g(\mathbf{Curl}_{\mathcal{M}} w(i), \mathbf{Curl}_{\mathcal{M}} w(j))\right]_{i,j} \left[\mathbf{A}\right] = \left[\int_{\widehat{\mathcal{M}}} g(\mathbf{V}, \mathbf{Curl}_{\mathcal{M}} w(i))\right]_i \tag{12}$$

Similarly to (10) we can compute each coefficient of the matrix on each triangle. So the two previous equations have the following expressions:

$$\sum_{T\ni i,j} \frac{\mathbf{h_i}}{\parallel \mathbf{h_i} \parallel^2} \cdot \frac{\mathbf{h_j}}{\parallel \mathbf{h_j} \parallel^2} \mathcal{A}(T) = \sum_{T\ni i} \mathcal{A}(T)\mathbf{V} \cdot \frac{\mathbf{h_i}}{\parallel \mathbf{h_i} \parallel^2}$$

$$\sum_{T\ni i,j} \left(\frac{\mathbf{h_i}}{\parallel \mathbf{h_i} \parallel^2} \wedge \mathbf{n}\right) \cdot \left(\frac{\mathbf{h_j}}{\parallel \mathbf{h_j} \parallel^2} \wedge \mathbf{n}\right) \mathcal{A}(T) = \sum_{T\ni i} \mathcal{A}(T)\mathbf{V} \cdot \left(\frac{\mathbf{h_i}}{\parallel \mathbf{h_i} \parallel^2} \wedge \mathbf{n}\right)$$

5   Application to the Growth of the Neonatal Brain

5.1   Preprocessing

Acquisition. The dataset consists of 4 healthy term born infants. MR scans were acquired two times with T2 weighted sequence on a 3T MRI system. The first acquisition was respectively, 40.6, 40.7, 41.4 and 39.3 weeks of gestational age and the second one, 43.2, 44.6, 43.1 and 42 weeks. Slice resolution was 0.7 × 1.5 × 0.7 mm for subjects 1,3,4 and 0.78 × 1.2 × 0.78 mm for subject 2.

Brain segmentation. The segmentation of white and gray matter in neonate MRI is a challenging issue because of the inversion of contrast regarding adult MRI and the ongoing myelination process. We have used a dedicated algorithm to overcome this problem [11]. It is based on a characterization of tissue using features based on geometrical properties and the evolution of two surfaces located on each side of the GM-WM interface.

Depth maps. Once the cortical surfaces have been segmented we use a specific treatment of BrainVisa [1] to compute their depth maps. They are obtained from the geodesic distance of the surface to a binary mask of the brain that has been dilated and eroded (respectively 5 and 2 voxels). Fig. 2 illustrates the resulting depth maps for two cortical surfaces of the same neonate taken at two different ages (birth, birth + 4 weeks).

5.2   Registration of Cortical Surfaces

We have used two kinds of registration techniques.

First we have used iconic based non rigid registration [4] to match the brain surfaces of each subject longitudinally. This method estimates a transformation C between two 3D images I and J that must minimize iteratively the following energy:

$$S(I, J, C) + \sigma||C - T||^2 + \lambda R(T) \tag{13}$$

where S is a similarity measure, R is a quadratic regularization energy, T an intermediate transformation and σ, λ are parameters. The resulting volumic transformation is then applied to cortical surfaces.

After having registered the less mature cortical surface on the more mature one we interpolate the depth maps by a nearest neighbors method. So we have

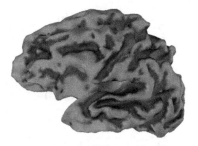 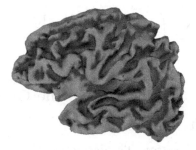

Fig. 2. Depth maps of two surfaces of the same subject at two different ages (birth, birth + 4 weeks)

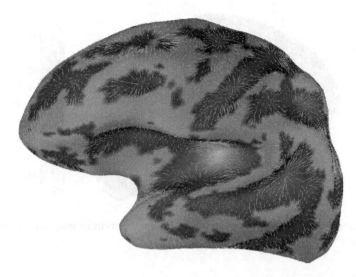

Fig. 3. Optical flow (green) on the smooth surface of the second time step and Depth maps of the first time step

two depth maps at different time steps projected on the same surface. It becomes now possible to track the evolution of this map from a time step to another.

Secondly we have used a coarser method to make correspond the growth seeds across the subjects. It is based on the iterative closest point (ICP) algorithm [2] in order to register rigidly one surface onto another one chosen as a template. The initialization of the algorithm is done by matching the principal directions of the two surfaces. We use also a nearest neighbors projection to resample the registered depth map.

5.3 Identification of Growth Seeds

Optical Flow Computation. For visualization purposes we compute the optical flow between the two depth maps on a smooth version of the more mature cortical surface. On Fig. 3 we display the result of the computation in green and the depth map of the less mature cortical surfaces for the subject 1.

We can see the radial structure of the vector field which has suggested the use of the Helmholtz decomposition in order to locate points of big divergence.

Helmholtz decomposition. We compute the two scalar potentials U and A involved in the Helmholtz decomposition. On Fig 4 we show only the divergential part of the field which is simply given by ∇U. We elicit also the local minima of the potential U which corresponds to sources of the optical flow.

Such sources correspond to locations in the brain around which the depth maps tend to grow.

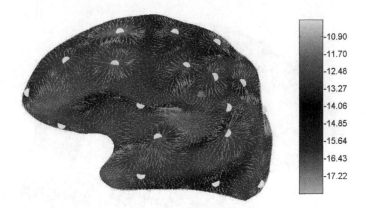

Fig. 4. Divergential part of the optical flow (green), potential map and local minima of U in yellow

Evaluation

- First we analyze the relative contribution of the divergential and rotational parts to the displacement field. We can see on Fig 5 the histograms of the norms of the divergential and rotational parts for one subject. It is interesting to compute the ratio of the norms to get the proportion of points where the divergential part is greater than the rotational part. We give the mean of this ratio for each subject on table 1. It confirms that the displacement field is mainly divergential and justify to use only the local extrema of the potential function U.
- On Fig 6 we display the superposition of seeds computed for four subjects and rigidly registered on one of the four surfaces. For a better visualization we only show clusters of seeds that belong to spheres of radius 1.5 cm. We also represent an average depth maps defined as the mean of the four depth maps after the nearest neighbors interpolation.

We can observe that despite the variability we can isolate a certain number of clusters (inside spheres). They can be compared to sulcal regions previously defined in the literature [14], [12] and called sulcal roots or sulcal pits, anatomical structures in the sulcus fundi that are supposed to be strong reproducible landmarks. We suggest the following classification based on [14] : 1 : Centralis superior, 2 : Centralis inferior, 3 : Frontalis superior posterior or Precentralis superior, 4 : fissura intraparietalis occipitalis superior, 5 : Frontalis inferior posterior or Precentralis inferior, 6 : Fronto-orbitalis, 7

Table 1. Ratio of divergential and rotational norms (Log) for 4 subjects

	S_1	S_2	S_3	S_4
Left hemisphere	0.75± 0.89	0.13 ± 0.88	0.58 ± 0.93	0.76 ± 0.95
Right hemisphere	0.61± 0.93	0.34 ± 0.91	0.35 ± 0.96	0.71 ± 0.9

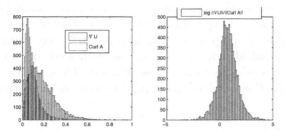

Fig. 5. Left: two histograms showing the norms of divergential part (blue) and rotational part (red). Right: Log ratio of the norms.

: Temporal superior posterior, 8 : Temporal inferior posterior or Temporal inferior ascendens, 9 : Frontalis inferior anterior.

Discussion. Two concepts have been introduced recently to try to overcome the variability of the folding patterns through a focus on the deepest part of the folds. The first dimples appearing on the cortical surface are called "sulcal roots" [14] while the deepest locations in the bottom of the folds at adult stage are called "sulcal pits" [12]. While these two concepts merge into only one corresponding to the dimples at the earliest stages of the folding process, there is a lack of data to assess if the sulcal pits remain at a fixed position on the cortical surface during growth. Our map of the growth seeds share striking similarities with the

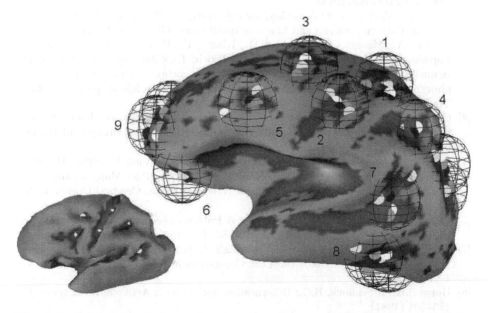

Fig. 6. Left : Left hemisphere of a premature infant at 30 weeks. The yellow dots indicate the deepest parts of the sulci. Right : Superposition of seeds for four subjects after affine registration and clustering. See text for legend.

sulcal roots mapped on the cortex of a highly premature baby [5] on Fig 6 left. This observation lead us to speculate that these seeds play a very specific role in the dynamic of the folding process. This idea needs further validation but could lead to merge the sulcal root / sulcal pits/ growth seed concepts into only one kind of entity that could be stable across subjects. These entities would become very important for the search of meaningful correspondence across brains.

6   Conclusion

We have introduced the concept of Helmholtz decomposition on manifolds. We have seen how, from a vector field, to extract potential functions that represent sources, sinks and rotation centers. We have applied this methodology to the displacement field computed from the evolution of depth maps of neonatal brains between birth and four weeks later. We have shown that the displacement field organizes itself into growth centers or growth seeds that offer a certain reproducibility across four subjects. In future developments we propose to use a bigger cohort to yield statistical tests and comparisons between different classes of subjects and to identify disorders in the brain development. Moreover we plan to apply our method for aging where we could expect to detect sinks rather than sources in the evolution of depth maps.

References

[1] http://brainvisa.info/
[2] Besl, P.J., McKay, N.D.: A method for registration of 3-d shapes. IEEE Transactions on Pattern Analysis and Machine Intelligence 14(2), 239–256 (1992)
[3] Cachia, A., Mangin, J.F., Riviere, D., Kherif, F., Boddaert, N., Andrade, A., Papadopoulos-Orfanos, D., Poline, J.B., Bloch, I., Zilbovicius, M., Sonigo, P., Brunelle, F., Regis, J.: A primal sketch of the cortex mean curvature: a morphogenesis based approach to study the variability of the folding patterns. IEEE Trans. Medical Imaging 22(6), 754–765 (2003)
[4] Cachier, P., Bardinet, E., Dormont, D., Pennec, X., Ayache, N.: Iconic feature based registration: the pasha algorithm. Computer Vision and Image Understanding 89(2-3), 272–298 (2003)
[5] Dubois, J., Benders, M., Cachia, A., Lazeyras, F., Ha-Vinh Leuchter, R., Sizonenko, S.V., Borradori-Tolsa, C., Mangin, J.F., Huppi, P.S.: Mapping the Early Cortical Folding Process in the Preterm Newborn Brain. Cerebral Cortex 18(6), 1444–1454 (2008)
[6] Grenander, U., Srivastava, A., Saini, S.: A Pattern-Theoretic Characterization of Biological Growth. IEEE Transactions on Medical Imaging 26(5), 648–659 (2007)
[7] Guo, Q., Mandal, M.K., Liu, G., Kavanagh, K.M.: Cardiac video analysis using Hodge–Helmholtz field decomposition. Computers in Biology and Medicine 36(1), 1–20 (2006)
[8] Horn, B.K.P., Schunck, B.G.: Determining optical flow. Artificial Intelligence 17, 185–204 (1981)
[9] Lefèvre, J., Baillet, S.: Optical Flow and Advection on 2-Riemannian Manifolds: A Common Framework. IEEE Transactions on pattern analysis and machine intelligence, 1081–1092 (2008)

[10] Lefèvre, J., Obozinski, G., Baillet, S.: Imaging brain activation streams from optical flow computation on 2-riemannian manifolds. In: Karssemeijer, N., Lelieveldt, B. (eds.) IPMI 2007. LNCS, vol. 4584, pp. 470–481. Springer, Heidelberg (2007)

[11] Leroy, F., Mangin, J.F., Rousseau, F., Glasel, H., Hertz-Pannier, L., Dubois, J., Dehaene-Lambertz, G.: Cortical Surface Segmentation in Infants by Coupled Surfaces Deformation across Feature Field. In: Imaging the Early Developing Brain: Challenges and Potential Impact, Workshop at MICCAI (2008)

[12] Lohmann, G., von Cramon, D.Y., Colchester, A.C.F.: Deep sulcal landmarks provide an organizing framework for human cortical folding. Cerebral Cortex 18(6), 1415–1420 (2008)

[13] Polthier, K., Preuss, E.: Identifying vector fields singularities using a discrete hodge decomposition. Visualization and Mathematics 3, 113–134 (2003)

[14] Régis, J., Mangin, J.F., Ochiai, T., Frouin, V., Riviére, D., Cachia, A., Tamura, M., Samson, Y.: "Sulcal Root" Generic Model: a Hypothesis to Overcome the Variability of the Human Cortex Folding Patterns. Neurologia medico-chirurgica 45(1), 1–17 (2005)

[15] Richman, D.P., Stewart, R.M., Hutchinson, J.W., Caviness Jr., V.S.: Mechanical Model of Brain Convolutional Development. Science 189(4196), 18–21 (1975)

[16] Toro, R., Burnod, Y.: A Morphogenetic Model for the Development of Cortical Convolutions. Cerebral Cortex 15(12), 1900–1913 (2005)

[17] Van Essen, D.C.: A tension-based theory of morphogenesis and compact wiring in the central nervous system. Nature 385(6614), 313–318 (1997)

[18] Xue, H., Srinivasan, L., Jiang, S., Rutherford, M., Edwards, A.D., Rueckert, D., Hajnal, J.V.: Automatic cortical segmentation in the developing brain. Inf. Process. Med. Imaging 20, 257–269 (2007)

[19] Xue, H., Srinivasan, L., Jiang, S., Rutherford, M.A., Edwards, A.D., Rueckert, D., Hajnal, J.V.: Longitudinal Cortical Registration for Developing Neonates. In: Ayache, N., Ourselin, S., Maeder, A. (eds.) MICCAI 2007, Part II. LNCS, vol. 4792, pp. 127–135. Springer, Heidelberg (2007)

Active Imaging with Dual Spin-Echo Diffusion MRI

Jonathan D. Clayden[1], Zoltan Nagy[2], Matt G. Hall[3,4], Chris A. Clark[1], and Daniel C. Alexander[3,4]

[1] Institute of Child Health
[2] Wellcome Trust Centre for Neuroimaging
[3] Department of Computer Science
[4] Centre for Medical Image Computing, University College London, UK
j.clayden@ucl.ac.uk

Abstract. Active imaging is a recently developed approach to model-based optimisation of imaging protocols. In the application we discuss here, a diffusion magnetic resonance imaging (dMRI) protocol is optimised for directly measuring aspects of biological tissue microstructure, subject to appropriate scanner hardware and acquisition time constraints. We present the theoretical basis for active imaging with the dual spin-echo (DSE) dMRI pulse sequence, which is more complex than the standard sequence, but widely used due to its robustness to image distortion. The new formulation provides the basis for future active imaging studies using DSE. To demonstrate the approach, we optimise DSE sequences for estimating parameters in a simple model of neural white matter, specifically axon density and diameter. Results show that sensitivity to these important parameters is at least as good as with more traditional pulse sequences that are not robust to image distortion.

1 Introduction

Diffusion magnetic resonance imaging (dMRI) is an umbrella term for a set of magnetic resonance acquisition and processing techniques in which MRI is sensitised to the random movement of particles in a sample or subject [1]. In living subjects, the diffusing species is almost invariably water. By characterising the diffusion process, information about the microstructure and connectivity of the underlying tissue can be obtained; and in the brain, in particular, dMRI has proven to be a practical and versatile tool for clinical and neuroscientific work. By applying diffusion sensitivity along one or more directions, diffusion weighted images are produced, and these have been particularly valuable in the study of stroke [2]. However, the later development of diffusion tensor imaging (DTI) [3] has broadened the usefulness of dMRI considerably. DTI uses diffusion weighted measurements along at least six noncollinear directions to estimate a rank-two diffusion tensor at each point in the image, which is proportional to the covariance matrix of a 3D Gaussian distribution over molecular displacements. A scalar value commonly derived from the tensor is fractional anisotropy, a

J.L. Prince, D.L. Pham, and K.J. Myers (Eds.): IPMI 2009, LNCS 5636, pp. 264–275, 2009.
© Springer-Verlag Berlin Heidelberg 2009

measure of dispersion in the tensor eigenvalues, which has been shown to be locally or globally reduced in a number of diseases [4], as well as some psychiatric disorders such as schizophrenia [5], reflecting changes in the underlying tissue. The principal eigenvector of the tensor, indicating the direction of greatest mean-squared displacement, was the original basis for dMRI-based white matter fibre tracking, which has provided insights in basic neuroscience with regard to the connectivity of the brain (e.g. [6]).

As useful as simple, DTI-derived measures of diffusion magnitude, direction and anisotropy have proven to be, they do not provide specific information about tissue microstructure. In reality, several distinct populations of water molecules, both inside and outside of neural cells, contribute to the dMRI signal, and so the displacement distribution is more complex than the Gaussian model used in DTI. However, analytical expressions for the displacement distribution and dMRI signal in a number of regular, bounded geometries are now well established [7], allowing more sophisticated approaches to construct geometric tissue models and combine these expressions to obtain better signal models [8,9]. These models potentially include a wide variety of parameters relating directly to microstructure, such as the radius and density of neuronal axons and other cellular structures, diffusivities in various parts of the tissue, permeabilities of different cell types, myelin thickness or the relative proportions of white matter and other tissue types in the imaged region—since all of these parameters affect water mobility and thus the dMRI signal. This exciting new area of development for dMRI offers the possibility of measuring these parameters in live tissue, thereby providing new insight into the workings of the brain and the mechanisms of disease, as well as important new biomarkers.

Previous work has demonstrated the viability of estimating microstructure parameters both in simulation and in real tissue [10,11,12]. For example, Stanisz et al. [11] used a white matter model incorporating two cell types, axons (modelled with prolate ellipsoids) and glia (spheres), with permeable membranes; and they fitted their model to image data acquired from excised optic nerve tissue. More recently, Assaf et al. [10] used a model incorporating cylindrical axons with radii following a gamma distribution, whose parameters were fitted to data from ex vivo optic and sciatic nerves. The imaging protocols in these studies are, however, impractical for use on live humans, due to the large gradient strengths and scan times required: the former up to $1400\,\mathrm{mT\,m^{-1}}$ (compared to the $32\,\mathrm{mT\,m^{-1}}$ available on a typical clinical scanner), and the latter often on the order of many hours to days. Moreover, they exploit a priori knowledge of white matter tract orientation, which is not generally available in vivo.

Active imaging optimises imaging protocols for sensitivity to specific parameters of a tissue model, subject to scan hardware and time constraints [13,14]. The term "active imaging" comes from active learning, which is a branch of machine learning that aims to identify the minimum set of enquiries required to determine the state of a system [15]. Optimising an imaging paradigm for estimating tissue microstructure parameters reduces to the same problem. In [16], an active imaging algorithm is constructed for optimising dMRI protocols when the fibre orientation is unknown. Simulations using a signal model similar to that in [10] demonstrate the feasibility of measuring axon size and density in live human subjects on current systems. The technique generalises to more complex models incorporating a variety of useful microstructural parameters and provides the opportunity, for the first time, to map these parameters over the live human brain.

A limitation of the approach in [16] is that it assumes the dMRI measurements come from the standard pulsed-gradient spin-echo (PGSE) pulse sequence. Here, we extend the method to the more complex dual spin-echo (DSE) sequence, which is more useful in practice as it is more robust to distortion effects. In §2 we give some background on how MRI is sensitised to diffusion, and on microstructural models of the dMRI signal. In §3 we develop a full parameterisation of the DSE pulse sequence, and establish bounds on each parameter; we extend a previous model of the dMRI signal arising from cylindrical axons to the DSE case; and we integrate the new encoding into the optimisation framework in [16]. In §4, we demonstrate the approach, comparing optimised DSE and PGSE protocols for estimating axon density and diameter in simulation. We conclude in §5. This study provides the foundational techniques for the future development of DSE pulse sequences optimised for any suitable tissue model, with recovered parameters as specific as the data admit.

2   Background

In this section we provide relevant background material on dMRI pulse sequences and the nature of diffusion in white matter.

2.1   Pulse Sequences

There are a number of ways of using magnetic gradient pulses to achieve diffusion sensitivity in an MRI experiment. The original PGSE sequence was described by Stejskal & Tanner [17], and is shown schematically in Fig. 1a. It consists of a pair of gradient pulses of equal magnitude and length δ, either side of a radio frequency (RF) inversion, or 180°, pulse. The first gradient applies a spatially varying phase shift to diffusing spins, which is reversed by the second pulse if the molecules do not move. However, molecular movement results in a residual phase offset, which manifests as an attenuation in the signal. The greater the aggregate distance moved due to diffusion along the direction of the gradient, the more greatly attenuated is the signal measured.

Unfortunately this sequence has a practical problem: electric eddy currents are induced by the onset and offset of the gradient pulses, causing distortion effects in the acquired image data. Some of these effects decay with time constants comparable to the length of the sequence, and so in practice they tend to accumulate. The recently developed DSE sequence [18]—shown in Fig. 1b— works similarly, but has much improved robustness to eddy current effects. In fact, the sequence can be configured to eliminate entirely eddy current effects

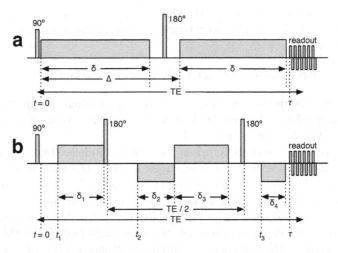

Fig. 1. Schematic representations of the standard pulsed-gradient spin-echo (a) and dual spin-echo (b) dMRI pulse sequences. The axis represents time.

with a particular time constant. For this reason, it is becoming the standard diffusion sequence on commercial MRI scanners. In DSE, the initial phase shift is provided by a combination of the first two gradient pulses, with lengths δ_1 and δ_2. (These pulses appear with opposite sign in the figure, but the phase effect of all gradients is inverted between the two 180° RF pulses.) Rephasing is effected by the remaining two pulses, and there is therefore a "balance" requirement that

$$\delta_1 + \delta_2 = \delta_3 + \delta_4 . \tag{1}$$

Since large gradient magnitudes are usually required for measuring tissue microstructure features, and eddy current effects scale with gradient strength, the DSE sequence is particularly appealing for this application. However, the sequence has not previously been used for estimating tissue model parameters, due to the relative difficulty of designing by hand a suitable protocol based on this more complex sequence, combined with an absence of analytical signal models. This paper provides an encoding of the DSE sequence, enabling optimisation of the protocol with active imaging. We also derive models of the DSE signal from water in simple restricted geometries, which allows us to extend the microstructural dMRI models in [10,11,16] for DSE. In combination, these novel contributions enable microstructure imaging protocols free of image distortion, which is an essential step towards their realisation in practice.

2.2   Hindered and Restricted Diffusion

Under the simple model used in [8], neural white matter tissue consists of two compartments: a homogeneous substrate, and a set of impermeable cells with regular geometry embedded within the substrate. Diffusion within the cells is therefore restricted by their geometry, while extracellular diffusion is merely hindered. In common with the CHARMED model [9], it is assumed that the total normalised signal, E, arising from the two compartments is a linear combination of contributions from each, viz.

$$E(\mathbf{G}, \Theta, \Phi) = fE_r(\mathbf{G}, \Theta, \Phi) + (1 - f)E_h(\mathbf{G}, \Theta, \Phi) , \tag{2}$$

where $f \in [0, 1]$ is the volume fraction of the intracellular compartment, $\mathbf{G}$ is the diffusion gradient direction, Θ is a set of sequence parameters, and Φ is a set of parameters for the tissue model.

The signal due to hindered diffusion, E_h, can be modelled by assuming a standard Gaussian displacement distribution, as in DTI. Diffusion in the restricted compartment is far from Gaussian, however, and depends on the geometry of the cells. By solving the diffusion equation subject to suitable boundary conditions, Neuman [7] derives expressions for the displacement distributions in spheres and cylinders. He then calculates approximations for the signal, E_r, within these restricted domains in the presence of a single continuous gradient, based on the assumption of a Gaussian distribution over *phases* among the diffusing molecules. The equivalent expression for cylindrical domains with the PGSE sequence was given by van Gelderen [19], and we give the new DSE solution below.

3 Methods

This section begins with our parameterisation of the DSE pulse sequence. We then derive a model for the restricted signal arising from a dMRI experiment under this parameterisation.

3.1 Parameterisation and Constraints

Figure 1b shows the DSE pulse sequence. It involves four individual diffusion-sensitising pulses of lengths δ_1, δ_2, δ_3 and δ_4, split into three blocks separated by two 180° RF pulses. The first gradient pulse occurs at a time t_1 after the initial excitation (90°) RF pulse. The second occurs at time t_2, the third immediately after the second, and the fourth at time t_3. Additionally, we choose to arrange that the first 180° pulse occurs immediately after the first gradient pulse.

The diffusion sensitisation pulses cannot take up the whole echo time (TE) of a DSE sequence, because time is required for the 180° pulses; and for excitation and "readout", or signal measurement, at the beginning and end of the sequence respectively. We denote the total amount of time actually available for the diffusion pulses with $\tau = \text{TE} - T_{\text{prep}} - T_{\text{read}}$, and the time required for each 180° pulse with P_{180}. The time between the two 180° pulses, within which the second and third diffusion gradients must fit, is exactly $T_{\text{inner}} = \text{TE}/2 - P_{180}$. The time available for the outer two pulses is therefore $T_{\text{outer}} = \tau - \text{TE}/2 - P_{180}$. It should be noted that as TE increases, the basic signal-to-noise ratio (SNR) of the sequence will decrease because of spontaneous dephasing due to spin relaxation.

We encode the sequence with the parameter set $\Theta = \{\text{TE}, T, t_s, \delta_1, t_1, t_2, t_3, G\}$, where $T = \delta_1 + \delta_2 + \delta_3 + \delta_4$ and $t_s = \delta_2 + \delta_3 - \delta_1 - \delta_4$. We include T and t_s rather than δ_2 and δ_3 for convenience when nulling eddy currents in §3.2. The fourth pulse length need not be included because of the balancing constraint in (1). A number of constraints on these parameters must be satisfied in order to ensure that the diffusion weighting properties of the sequence remain intact, and that all pulse lengths are nonnegative. These are outlined below.

The time available for the outer two pulses, δ_1 and δ_4, must be nonnegative; and so it follows directly from the definitions of T_{outer} and τ above that

$$\mathrm{TE} \geq 2(P_{180} + T_{\mathrm{prep}} + T_{\mathrm{read}}) \,. \tag{3}$$

Due to the balancing constraint, we can write $T = 2(\delta_1 + \delta_2)$, which has bounds

$$0 \leq T \leq \mathrm{TE} - 2(P_{180} + T_{\mathrm{prep}} + T_{\mathrm{read}}) = 2\tau - \mathrm{TE} - 2P_{180} \,. \tag{4}$$

It follows from the balancing constraint and the definitions of T and t_s that $T + t_s = 2(\delta_2 + \delta_3)$, which is bounded by the time available for the inner two pulses. Similarly, $T - t_s = 2(\delta_1 + \delta_4)$, so we have

$$T + t_s \leq 2T_{\mathrm{inner}} \quad \text{and} \quad T - t_s \leq 2T_{\mathrm{outer}} \,. \tag{5}$$

Moreover, since no single diffusion pulse can be longer than $T/2$, or negative in length, the absolute difference between δ_3 and δ_1 also cannot exceed $T/2$. As a result, $|t_s|$ cannot exceed T. The full bounds on t_s are therefore

$$\max\{-T, \mathrm{TE} - 2\tau + 2P_{180} + T\} \leq t_s \leq \min\{T, \mathrm{TE} - 2P_{180} - T\} \,. \tag{6}$$

Given valid choices of T and t_s, subject to these bounds, we will be able to recover the lengths of the second and third pulses as

$$\delta_2 = T/2 - \delta_1 \quad \text{and} \quad \delta_3 = t_s/2 + \delta_1 \,, \tag{7}$$

subject to first choosing δ_1. The latter must be constrained such that none of the other three pulse lengths will be negative:

$$\max\{0, -t_s/2\} \leq \delta_1 \leq \min\{T/2, (T - t_s)/2\} \,. \tag{8}$$

The times of onset are also constrained. They must all be nonnegative, and must leave room for each pulse. The upper bound on t_3 is set by the requirement that the last pulse must finish before $t = \tau$, but it must occur after the second refocussing pulse. We therefore have

$$0 \leq t_1 \leq T_{\mathrm{outer}} - 2\delta_1 - \delta_2 + \delta_3 \,; \tag{9}$$

$$t_1 + \delta_1 + P_{180} \leq t_2 \leq t_1 + \delta_1 + \mathrm{TE}/2 - \delta_2 - \delta_3 \,; \tag{10}$$

$$t_1 + \delta_1 + P_{180} + \mathrm{TE}/2 \leq t_3 \leq \tau - (\delta_1 + \delta_2 - \delta_3) \,. \tag{11}$$

The final relevant parameter is G, the magnitude of the gradient pulses, but this is independent of the other quantities and bounded simply by $0 \leq G \leq G_{\mathrm{max}}$, for some G_{max} appropriate to the scanner being used. All four gradient pulses in each arrangement use the same G.

3.2   Nulling Eddy Current Effects

The ability to null eddy current induced distortion effects is the major benefit of DSE over PGSE. Heid [20] established that eddy current effects proportional to $e^{-\lambda_0 t}$ will vanish exactly if

$$\delta_1 = \frac{1}{\lambda_0} \ln \left(\frac{1 + \cosh \frac{\lambda_0 T}{2}}{\exp \frac{\lambda_0 t_s}{2} + \exp \frac{-\lambda_0 T}{2}} \right) . \tag{12}$$

Off-design eddy current effects, with time constants different from λ_0, will also be reduced, although not totally nulled. We can substitute this fixed form for the bounds given by (8), thus improving the eddy current distortion properties of the sequence further, at the cost of losing one degree of freedom in the parameterisation. In this case, the bounds on T, t_1, t_2 and t_3 remain exactly as before, although the limits on t_s take a different form. The right hand side of (12) must be nonnegative, so we constrain

$$t_s \leq \frac{2}{\lambda_0} \ln \left(1 + \sinh \frac{\lambda_0 T}{2} \right) . \tag{13}$$

In addition, we observe from (7) that δ_2 is negative unless $\delta_1 \leq T/2$. This condition imposes the additional constraint

$$t_s \geq \frac{2}{\lambda_0} \ln \left(\frac{1 + e^{-\lambda_0 T}}{2} \right) . \tag{14}$$

The limits described by (5) also continue to apply.

3.3   Signal Model

The model of neural white matter that we use here to demonstrate active imaging with DSE consists of nonabutting cylinders of radius R, representing neural axons, in a homogeneous substrate [8]. The signal model takes the form of (2), assuming cylindrically symmetric Gaussian diffusion in the hindered, extracellular compartment. Here we derive an expression for the DSE signal in the intracellular compartment.

We decompose the intracellular signal into components parallel and perpendicular to the axons. In the parallel case, diffusion is assumed to be univariate Gaussian with diffusivity $d_\parallel$; and the effective gradient strength is $G \cos \beta$, where β is the angle between the gradient direction, $\mathbf{G}$, and the fibre direction, $\mathbf{n}$. The perpendicular component, however, exhibits restricted diffusion due to the inner walls of the axons. Following Neuman [7], assuming a Gaussian distribution of phases in the tissue, we integrate over molecular displacements during the course of the sequence to arrive at the form

$$E_{r\perp}(\mathbf{G}, \Theta, \Phi) = -2\gamma^2 (G \sin \beta)^2 \sum_{m=1}^{\infty} \frac{\zeta_m}{\alpha_m^6 d_\perp^2 (\alpha_m^2 R^2 - 1)} , \tag{15}$$

where

$$
\begin{aligned}
\zeta_m = {} & 2\alpha_m^2 d_\perp (\delta_1 + \delta_2) - \big[5 + Y_m(t_2 - t_1) - Y_m(t_3 - t_1) - Y_m(t_3 - t_2) - Y_m(\delta_1) \\
& - Y_m(t_2 - t_1 - \delta_1) + Y_m(t_3 - t_1 - \delta_1) - 2Y_m(\delta_2) - 2Y_m(t_2 - t_1 + \delta_2) \\
& + 2Y_m(t_2 - t_1 + \delta_2 - \delta_1) + 2Y_m(t_3 - t_2 - \delta_2) - 2Y_m(\delta_3) + Y_m(\delta_2 + \delta_3) \\
& + Y_m(t_2 - t_1 + \delta_2 + \delta_3) - Y_m(t_2 - t_1 + \delta_2 + \delta_3 - \delta_1) \\
& - 2Y_m(t_3 - t_2 + \delta_1 - \delta_3) - Y_m(t_3 - t_1 + \delta_2 - \delta_3) - Y_m(\delta_1 + \delta_2 - \delta_3) \\
& + Y_m(t_3 - t_1 + \delta_1 + \delta_2 - \delta_3) + Y_m(t_3 - t_2 + \delta_1 + \delta_2 - \delta_3) \\
& - Y_m(t_3 - t_2 - \delta_2 - \delta_3) + Y_m(t_3 - t_2 + \delta_1 - 2\delta_3)\big] \quad (16)
\end{aligned}
$$

and

$$
Y_m(x) = \exp(-\alpha_m^2 d_\perp x) . \tag{17}
$$

The term α_m represents the mth smallest α solving the equation $J_1'(\alpha R) = 0$, where J_1' is the derivative of the Bessel function of the first kind, order one. The total signal from the restricted compartment is finally

$$
E_r(\mathbf{G}, \Theta, \Phi) = E_{r\parallel}(\mathbf{G}, \Theta, \Phi) E_{r\perp}(\mathbf{G}, \Theta, \Phi) . \tag{18}
$$

The full set of model parameters is therefore $\Phi = \{f, R, \mathbf{n}, d_\parallel, d_\perp\}$.

4   Experiments and Results

In all our experiments, we use parameter settings similar to the natural values in human white matter, and sequence constraints which are easily achievable on most clinical MRI scanners. Specifically, we choose $f = 0.7$, $d_\parallel = 1.7 \times 10^{-9}$ m^2 s^{-1} and $d_\perp = 1.2 \times 10^{-9}$ m^2 s^{-1}. We take $G_{\max} = 32$ mT m^{-1} and assume a base SNR of 10 at TE = 90 ms—both of which are well within reach of most scanners.

We constrain the protocol to contain M different sets of sequence parameters, each of which are applied along N noncollinear gradient directions. We use the optimisation framework and cost function described in [16], based on the Cramér–Rao Lower Bound (CRLB) and a Rician noise model, which is appropriate for MRI images [21]. The noise level used to calculate the cost function is adjusted in line with the optimised TE, as in [16], which we choose to fix over all pulse arrangements, leaving $7M+1$ parameters to optimise over. Again following [16], we use $M = 4$ and $N = 90$ throughout, for a total of 360 measurements, which is achievable in under an hour with a modern human system.

The first experiment compares the sensitivity of the PGSE and DSE sequences to the parameters of the tissue model, as indicated by the cost function itself. We optimise both sequences for each $R \in \{1, 3, 5, 10, 20\}$ μm separately. The DSE sequence is optimised both without and with the eddy current nulling constraint in (12). For the latter, we set $\lambda_0 = 0.7/\tilde{T}$ as in [20], where $\tilde{T}$ is the maximal T across all pulse arrangements. The means and coefficients of variation (CVs) of the cost function over 500 fibre orientations equally distributed on the sphere

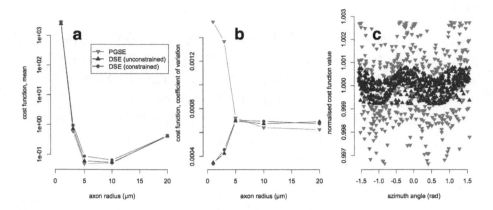

Fig. 2. Trends in the cost function with axon radius (a,b) and azimuth angle (c). $R = 3$ μm in c; base SNR $= 10$ in all cases.

[22], are shown in Fig. 2. It can be seen from Fig. 2a that the mean values vary by several orders of magnitude over the five axon radii, but there is little difference between the three pulse sequences. On the other hand, the CVs are slightly smaller for the PGSE case at large R, but substantially larger at small R, suggesting that the DSE sequence has better orientation invariance when R is small. (This effect persists when the base SNR is higher.) Figure 2c shows the dependence of the cost function value on the azimuthal orientation of the fibre: the spread is much larger for the PGSE sequence at $R = 3$ μm, whereas it is almost identical at $R = 5$ μm (not shown). The absolute magnitude of the variance is, however, small in all cases. Data for the constrained DSE sequence is omitted from this subfigure for clarity, but the pattern is very similar to the unconstrained sequence.

Additionally, we investigated the ability of the method to recover tissue parameters from a synthetic data set. We obtain very accurate synthetic signal data using a simulation of 10,000 molecules undergoing Brownian motion, by tracking the phase of each molecule through the optimised sequences to calculate the final signal [23]. The geometric environment in the simulation was the same as in the tissue model, although with uniform diffusivity. Cylinder radius was fixed to 5 μm and cylinder separation adjusted to produce an intracellular volume fraction of 0.7. Rician noise was added. We used Markov chain Monte Carlo (MCMC) to sample from posterior distributions over the tissue parameters of interest, using Metropolis–Hastings samplers with zero-mean Gaussian proposal distributions. Variances of these proposal distributions were tuned by hand to give reasonable acceptance rates. Priors were uninformative within appropriate bounds. A burn-in period of 10,000 iterations was used, after which 100 samples were taken with a sampling interval of 1000 iterations. Parameters were initialised with their true values to speed up convergence. This process was repeated for ten generative fibre orientations, **n**, equally spaced on the sphere.

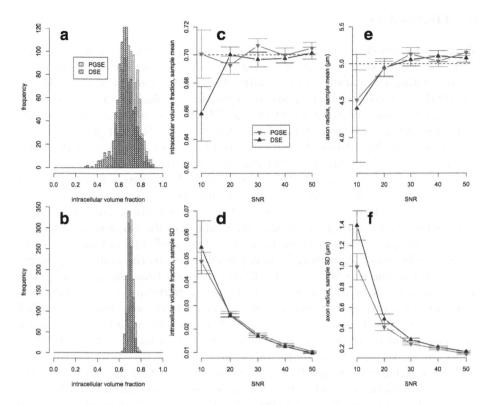

Fig. 3. Results from MCMC sampling of tissue model parameters: histograms of samples from the posterior distribution over f at base SNR 10 (a) and 30 (b), and relationships between SNR and the means and standard deviations of these histograms for f (c,d) and R (e,f). Error bars indicate mean $\pm$ standard error over ten fibre directions. Generating values are $f = 0.7$ and $R = 5$ μm throughout (dashed lines in c,e).

PGSE and unconstrained DSE sequences were tested, and sampling was repeated with protocols optimised using base SNRs of 20, 30, 40 and 50.

Figure 3 shows the results of the MCMC experiments. The sampled posterior distributions over intracellular volume fraction, f, a proxy for axon density, are broad at a base SNR of 10 (Fig. 3a); and although both modes are close to the generating value of 0.7, they differ slightly from one another. By contrast, at a base SNR of 30 (Fig. 3b), both distributions are far tighter. Figure 3c shows that DSE tends to underestimate f at SNR = 10, although it is generally both more accurate and more stable where SNR $\geq$ 20. DSE also has a slight precision advantage at these lower noise levels (Fig. 3d). Both sequences produce underestimates of axon radius, R, at low SNR, and their accuracies are largely similar; although PGSE exhibits somewhat greater precision for this parameter over the whole SNR range (Fig. 3e,f). Overall, the differences between the two sequences are small, and neither is consistently superior.

5   Discussion

We have developed the analytical infrastructure needed for active imaging with DSE, facilitating the optimisation of this widely deployed dMRI pulse sequence for estimating the parameters of arbitrarily complex models of living tissue. The DSE sequence has been shown to perform very similarly to PGSE, both in terms of a cost function based on the CRLB, and in terms of its ability to recover generative parameters from simulated data. However, it has a major practical benefit in its reduced sensitivity to eddy currents, which are particularly significant at the large gradient strengths used for experiments of this type. We have shown that eddy current effects can be nulled completely for a particular time constant with little impact on the cost function.

The exact performance of the two dMRI sequences discussed in this paper has been shown to depend on the SNR achievable and the parameter of interest. For the example tissue model we have described, DSE appears to have some advantage for small axon radii. This is probably due to the ability to position pulses next to one another, making effective diffusion times short (cf. Fig. 1b). The noise level is clearly an important factor in performance, and there is a substantial improvement in accuracy and precision in the step from a base SNR of 10 to 20 with both sequences. The latter is quite achievable for *in vivo* work. We have found no evidence of a consistent noise penalty with DSE, which is sometimes thought to be a problem with the sequence.

A very significant avenue for future work will be the application of DSE-based active imaging to other tissue models and related problems. DSE may prove to be more flexible than PGSE due to the extra degrees of freedom in the parameterisation ($7M + 1$ parameters rather than $3M$). We also intend to investigate the effect of eddy currents in acquired images on estimates of tissue model parameters. Implementation of our protocol will be complex due to the substantial number of parameters, but it will be essential to quantify the full benefits of the DSE sequence in active imaging applications.

Acknowledgments. Support for this work was provided through EPSRC grants EP/C536851/1 and EP/E007748. ZN is supported by the Wellcome Trust.

References

1. Le Bihan, D.: Looking into the functional architecture of the brain with diffusion MRI. Nature Reviews Neuroscience 4, 469–480 (2003)
2. Baird, A., Warach, S.: Magnetic resonance imaging of acute stroke. Journal of Cerebral Blood Flow & Metabolism 18, 583–609 (1998)
3. Basser, P., Mattiello, J., Le Bihan, D.: Estimation of the effective self-diffusion tensor from the NMR spin echo. Journal of Magnetic Resonance, Series B 103, 247–254 (1994)
4. Horsfield, M., Jones, D.: Applications of diffusion-weighted and diffusion tensor MRI to white matter diseases - a review. NMR in Biomedicine 15, 570–577 (2002)
5. Lim, K., Helpern, J.: Neuropsychiatric applications of DTI - a review. NMR in Biomedicine 15, 587–593 (2002)

6. Behrens, T., Johansen-Berg, H., Woolrich, M., Smith, S., Wheeler-Kingshott, C., Boulby, P., Barker, G., Sillery, E., Sheehan, K., Ciccarelli, O., Thompson, A., Brady, J., Matthews, P.: Non-invasive mapping of connections between human thalamus and cortex using diffusion imaging. Nature Neuroscience 6, 750–757 (2003)
7. Neuman, C.: Spin echo of spins diffusing in a bounded medium. Journal of Chemical Physics 60, 4508–4511 (1974)
8. Alexander, D.: Axon radius measurements in vivo from diffusion MRI: a feasibility study. In: Proceedings of the IEEE 11th International Conference on Computer Vision. IEEE, Los Alamitos (2007)
9. Assaf, Y., Basser, P.: Composite hindered and restricted model of diffusion (CHARMED) MR imaging of the human brain. NeuroImage 27, 48–58 (2005)
10. Assaf, Y., Blumenfeld-Katzir, T., Yovel, Y., Basser, P.: Axcaliber: A method for measuring axon diameter distribution from diffusion MRI. Magnetic Resonance in Medicine 59, 1347–1354 (2008)
11. Stanisz, G., Szafer, A., Wright, G., Henkelman, R.: An analytical model of restricted diffusion in bovine optic nerve. Magnetic Resonance in Medicine 37, 103–111 (1997)
12. Weng, J.C., Chen, J.H., Kuo, L.W., Wedeen, V., Tseng, W.Y.: Maturation-dependent microstructure length scale in the corpus callosum of fixed rat brains by magnetic resonance diffusion-diffraction. Magnetic Resonance Imaging 25, 78–86 (2007)
13. Andersson, J.: Maximum a posteriori estimation of diffusion tensor parameters using a Rician noise model: Why, how and but. NeuroImage 42, 1340–1356 (2008)
14. Cercignani, M., Alexander, D.: Optimal acquisition schemes for in vivo quantitative magnetization transfer MRI. Magnetic Resonance in Medicine 56, 803–810 (2006)
15. MacKay, D.: Information-based objective functions for active data selection. Neural Computation 4, 590–604 (1992)
16. Alexander, D.: A general framework for experiment design in diffusion MRI and its application to measuring direct tissue-microstructure features. Magnetic Resonance in Medicine 60, 439–448 (2008)
17. Stejskal, E., Tanner, J.: Spin diffusion measurements: spin echoes in the presence of a time-dependent field gradient. Journal of Chemical Physics 42, 288–292 (1965)
18. Reese, T., Heid, O., Weisskoff, R., Wedeen, V.: Reduction of eddy-current-induced distortion in diffusion MRI using a twice-refocused spin echo. Magnetic Resonance in Medicine 49, 177–182 (2003)
19. van Gelderen, P., DesPres, D., van Zijl, P., Moonen, C.: Evaluation of restricted diffusion in cylinders. Phosphocreatine in rabbit leg muscle. Journal of Magnetic Resonance, Series B 103, 255–260 (1994)
20. Heid, O.: Eddy current-nulled diffusion weighting. In: Proceedings of the ISMRM 8th Scientific Meeting & Exhibition, International Society for Magnetic Resonance in Medicine, p. 799 (2000)
21. Henkelman, R.: Measurement of signal intensities in the presence of noise in MR images. Medical Physics 12, 232–233 (1985)
22. Rakhmanov, E., Saff, E., Zhou, Y.: Minimal discrete energy on the sphere. Mathematical Research Letters 1, 647–662 (1994)
23. Hall, M., Alexander, D.: A tissue model of white matter undergoing tissue swelling. In: Proceedings of the MICCAI Workshop on Computational Diffusion MRI (2008)

Voxel-by-Voxel Functional Diffusion Mapping for Early Evaluation of Breast Cancer Treatment*

Bing Ma[1], Charles R. Meyer[1], Martin D. Pickles[2], Thomas L. Chenevert[1],
Peyton H. Bland[1], Craig J. Galbán[1], Alnawaz Rehemtulla[3],
Lindsay W. Turnbull[2], and Brian D. Ross[1]

[1] Department of Radiology, University of Michigan Medical School,
Ann Arbor, MI, 48109, USA
[2] Centre for Magnetic Resonance Investigations, Division of Cancer,
Postgraduate Medical School, University of Hull, HU3 2JZ Hull, UK
[3] Department of Radiation Oncology, University of Michigan Medical School,
Ann Arbor, MI, 48109, USA
bingm@umich.edu

Abstract. Quantitative isotropic diffusion MRI and voxel-based analysis of the apparent diffusion coefficient (ADC) changes have been demonstrated to be able to accurately predict early response of brain tumors to therapy. The ADC value changes measured during pre- and post-therapy interval are closely correlated to treatment response. This work was demonstrated using a voxel-based analysis of ADC change during therapy in the brains of both rats and humans, following rigidly registering pre- and post-therapeutic ADC MRI exams. The primary goal of this paper is to extend this voxel-by-voxel analysis to assess therapeutic response in breast cancer. Nonlinear registration (with higher degrees of freedom) between the pre- and post-treatment exams is needed to ensure that the corresponding voxels actually contain similar cellular partial contributions due to soft tissue deformations in the breast and compartmental tumor changes during treatment as well. With limited data sets, we have observed the correlation between changes of ADC values and treatment response also exists in breast cancers. With diffusion scans acquired at three different timepoints (pre-treatment, early post-treatment and late post-treatment), we have also shown that ADC changes across responders within 5 weeks are a function of time interval after the initiation of treatment. Comparison of the experimental results with pathology shows that ADC changes can be used to evaluate early response of breast cancer treatment.

1 Introduction

Breast cancer patients may elect to receive neoadjuvant chemotherapy before surgery. If the patient elects to have surgery as soon as possible to remove the

---

* This work is supported in part by NIH grants 1P01CA85878, 1P01CA87634, and P50CA93990.

tumor following diagnosis, neoadjuvant chemotherapy may be performed while the patient waits for the surgery. For the patient who chooses to undergo a longer course of neoadjuvant chemotherapy before surgery, usually several complete treatment cycles will be conducted and the surgery will remove whatever tumor mass remains. A demonstrated benefit of such neoadjuvant chemotherapy for responders is the achievement of tumor shrinkage, allowing breast conservation surgery for a proportion of the patients. Unfortunately 20 − 25% of all breast cancer patients do not respond to chemotherapy. It would be beneficial to identify those patients who are not responding to their neoadjuvant chemotherapy so that a change in treatment management may be introduced earlier, sparing patients from potentially ineffective and toxic treatment. Some existing methods of detecting response, e.g., clinical palpation or radiological RECIST measurements, typically support accurate detection of response only after 8 − 10 weeks of chemotherapy. Identifying surrogates that can predict therapeutic outcome earlier or more accurately than current methods would be valuable to tailor treatment to individual patients.

Large clinical trials assume that the degree of response of the primary tumor to neoadjuvant chemotherapy correlates with patient survival [1,2,3,4]. This suggests tumor response may be a surrogate for evaluating the effect of chemotherapy and could therefore be an important prognostic indicator of treatment outcome.

Imaging modalities can be used to track tumor changes resulting from response to a particular chemotherapy regimen. Several imaging modalities have been used in assessing the extent of response to primary breast cancer treatment. These modalities include mammography, ultrasound, and anatomical magnetic resonance imaging (MRI). Unfortunately, the sensitivity of these imaging technologies is inadequate in predicting pathological complete response (pCR) when compared to clinical examination [5].

Given that diffusion MRI is sensitive to structure at the cellular level, it has the potential to detect and quantify cellular changes that occur in response to successful therapeutic intervention [6]. It has been increasingly used to predict the magnitude of response of cancer to chemotherapy [6,7,8,9]. Diffusion MRI, combined with voxel-based analysis of the apparent diffusion coefficient (ADC) changes during treatment has been used to predict early response to cancer treatment. Researchers have demonstrated a fundamental correlation between ADC changes within the tumor measured over the pre- to early post-treatment interval and the response of various brain tumors to therapies [6,7,8,9,10,11,12,13,14,15]. This correlation has been shown both in primary and metastatic tumors of multiple organ systems in both rats and humans. In this paper we extend the voxel-by-voxel analysis to assess early response of breast cancer treatment and establish that the same correlation exists in breast cancer and can be used as an early biomarker of cell death and a potential surrogate for clinical outcome.

In previous work on tracking changes in ADC values over the pre- to early post-treatment interval for brain tumors, affine registration was performed on the interval exams. A functional diffusion map (fDM), i.e., a voxel-by-voxel

scatter plot of the registered pre- vs. post-therapy ADC values, was then constructed assuming that the voxels in the registered pre- and post-treatment
volumes contain approximately the same cells. FDM analysis has been shown
to provide a strikingly accurate early biomarker for determining therapy response in the brain tumor patients. Affine registration works remarkably well
in these brain tumors because the tumor's geometry changes during treatment
are constrained and thus well modeled by rigid body deformation (rotation and
translation) or at most include some shearing due to the high gradients used in
diffusion echo planar imaging.

However, the scenario is completely different for breast tumors. The breast
consists of soft, deformable tissue and thus nonlinear warping is definitely needed
to accomplish accurate alignment of pre- and post-treatment volumes so that corresponding voxels in the registered pre- and post-treatment volumes contain similar cellular partial contributions. Automatic nonlinear registration algorithms
are within reach with only modest effort if the breast in question is cropped
down to the approximate boundaries of the lesion by the user, which is common
practice in image processing.

2   Methods

2.1   Diffusion MRI for Assessing Cancer Treatment Response

Diffusion weighted MRI allows quantitative investigation of the changes in the
Brownian motion of water [16]. Intracellular water is tightly bound and high density cellular packing in cancers has low diffusivity. During an effective treatment
cancerous cells are killed and lyse increasing the ADC in the affected regions.

Each diffusion-weighted image series is comprised of 2 images per anatomic
slice: b_0 ($b = 0$) which has relatively high signal-to-noise ratio (SNR) and no
diffusion-weighting, and b_{high} (e.g., $b = 700$ or 800 s/mm^2) which has heavy
diffusion weighting and lower SNR. The diffusion weighted imaging (DWI) is
rotationally invariant, i.e., isotropic. That is, the diffusion weighted images are
insensitive to the directionality of water mobility by combination of DWI along
three orthogonal directions. ADC maps were calculated by simply taking the
logarithm of the ratio of images acquired at two diffusion weightings and then
scaling by the inverse of the difference in b-values (assuming low SNR pixels are
properly eliminated):

$$ADC = \frac{1}{b_{high} - b_0} \log \frac{S_{b_0}}{S_{b_{high}}}, \tag{1}$$

where S_{b_0} and $S_{b_{high}}$ are the signal intensities recorded at $b = 0$ and $b = b_{high}$ s/mm^2, respectively.

A functional diffusion map (fDM) is constructed from the registered pre- and
post-treatment image volumes. It consists of a color overlay image of therapeutic-
induced ADC change (post-treatment minus pre-treatment) within the tumor
(Fig. 1, right column) and the scatter plot of corresponding pre- and post-
treatment ADC values (Fig. 1, left column). The fDM provides the ability to

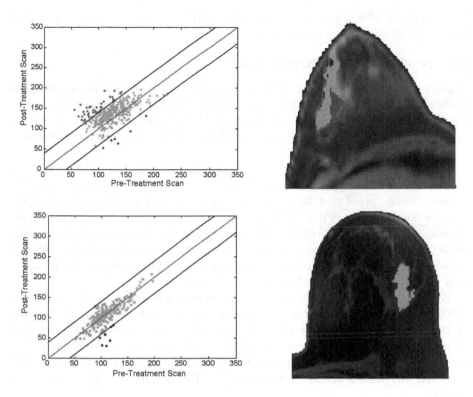

Fig. 1. Functional diffusion maps for responsive and non-responsive breast treatment. Top and bottom rows respectively show from left to right the treatment effect, and fDM treatment overlay on one anatomical slice. Patient on the top was found to be ER+ while the bottom patient was ER-.

objectively segment the tumor into three colored regions based on the magnitude and direction of ADC change. Red region includes voxels whose ADC values have increased significantly during treatment, represented by "V_i"; blue region includes voxels whose ADC values have decreased significantly, represented by "V_d"; and green region includes voxels whose ADC values have not changed significantly compared with the null hypothesis, represented by "V_0". The scatter plots (Fig. 1, left column) were found to correlate with subsequent tumor response.

The voxel-by-voxel fDM approach has a significant advantage over volumetric summary metrics (i.e., mean change in ADC values). Mean ADC change within the entire tumor during therapy can be an early response estimator, but it has its limitations. Therapeutic response is usually quite complex including often opposite and competing effects: some cells die causing increased extracellular water and associated increased ADC values while some other cells proliferate at a high rate leading to decreased extracellular water and ADC values. Averaging the ADC changes over the entire tumor cancels out some (if not most) of these opposite effects and thus makes mean ADC change insensitive to spatial heterogeneity of treatment response.

2.2 Nonlinear Image Registration

A prerequisite for proper fDM analysis using pre- and post-therapy breast examinations is that the corresponding pre- and post-treatment image voxels contain similar cellular partial volume contributions. Mutual information (MI) based image registration algorithms are employed to align the pre- and post-treatment scans.

Tumor volumes of interest (VOI) were drawn on the high resolution anatomical image volumes and were warped from the anatomical volumes onto the pre-treatment (pre-Tx) diffusion volumes denoted as the reference; a warping registration is necessary due to the susceptibility artifacts in the diffusion, echo-planar acquisitions not present in the anatomical, spin echo acquisitions. Subsequent registrations between the pre- and post-treatment (post-Tx) diffusion scans are also warped to account for repositioning deformations to the breast as well as any compartmental changes to the tumor.

Warping is accomplished using thin plate splines where the degrees of freedom (DOF) of the warp is related to the local mutual information density and volume of the tumor. The user only picks the loci of 3 control points in the floating tumor volume that approximate their loci in the reference tumor volume. The multiscale registration first implements rigid body registration, then low DOF warping, and finally full DOF warping [17]. The details of registration are as follows:

1. Automatically generate a distance sorted set of hexagonal close-pack control points in the cropped reference volume based on the highest density of control points supported by the mutual information of the dataset pairs to be registered. Let N be the total number of control points in this pre-generated set and these control points are sorted according to decreasing pairwise distances.
2. Choose the first 3 control points from the pre-generated point set in the reference volume.
3. Provide 3 approximate homologous control points in the floating volume that correspond to the positions of the first 3 control points in the reference set, again based on the resultant cropping of the user.
4. Apply rigid body registration to roughly align the floating exam to the reference.
5. More points from the pre-generated control point set in the reference volume are chosen for warping registration where the number of points is set in the registration schedule. The corresponding control points in the floating exam are generated using the resultant geometric transformation from the previous registration schedule. Since the reference control points are distance sorted in order from most distant to nearest, iteratively increasing the number of points not only implements an increasing DOF warping, but also a decreasing scale space registration.

6. Repeat step 5 until all N control points have been used in the last schedule line which yields the final solution, subject to no folding. Folding is prevented by checking the sign of the Jacobian deformation after each optimization. If negative, the reference and corresponding homologous control point pair closest to the loci of the most negative Jacobian value are removed, and the optimization is repeated until no negative Jacobian values occur in the solution. This strategy allows the algorithm to locally decrease the DOF and control point density to follow local MI density variations.

2.3   Determination of Thresholds

After registration is accomplished, the voxel-by-voxel fDM analysis will be applied to estimate treatment response based on the changes in ADC values during treatment. A primary task in fDM analysis is to set appropriate thresholds which determine how much ADC change can be treated as significantly increased/decreased. Due to the complicated nature of noise distribution, analytical derivation of the thresholds is impossible. Instead, we utilize a small set of patient data as the training data to experimentally determine the appropriate thresholds to segment the tumor areas. These thresholds are then applied to the data acquired by the University of Hull MRI Centre for early evaluation of treatment response.

The training set comes from an ongoing double-blinded feasibility study at the University of Michigan investigating the role of diffusion MRI and functional diffusion maps as an early biomarker to predict therapeutic response for breast cancer. In the imaging protocol patients with breast cancer that have elected neoadjuvant chemotherapy prior to surgery receive 2 baseline exams (affectionately named "coffee-break" exams), typically within a 15 minute interval where the patient is removed from the scanner and then repositioned for the second scan; these short interval exams are used to observe the null change distribution since no macroscopic changes have occurred to the tumor in this interval. The initiation of the first cycle of chemotherapy (adriamyacin/cyclophosphamide) typically follows within one day of the short interval exams. In this acquisition the high b value is 800 s/mm^2. ADC maps are computed from the interleaved b_0 and b_{800} diffusion weighted MRI acquisitions by substituting b_{high} with b_{800} in Equation (1).

For each pair of registered ADC images a 128×128 joint density histogram (JDH) is constructed by incrementing the count of the 2D histogram defined by the two ADC values of the registered tumor (a demonstration is shown in Fig. 2(a)). Ideally the resulting JDH will be symmetric about the diagonal assuming no tumor growth/recession in such a short period. However, in practice for each experimental sample of the null distribution JDH is slightly biased. To remove this inevitable bias, the sum of the JDH and its transpose is used to derive the variance of the null change, now unbiased distribution. A 95% confidence interval is applied to the null hypothesis test: If a test value is outside the interval, the test rejects the null. With currently available 5 patients' pre-treatment coffee-break exams, the average 95% confidence interval for ADC changes is

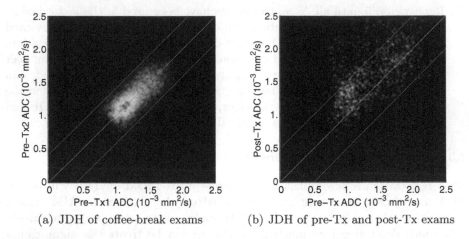

(a) JDH of coffee-break exams   (b) JDH of pre-Tx and post-Tx exams

Fig. 2. Joint distribution histograms. (a) JDH of a pair of pre-treatment coffee-break exams. The green line represents the linear regression of the JDH, which is the diagonal line in this case. The magenta lines represent the 97.5^{th} and 2.5^{th} percentile, respectively; i.e., the area between the magenta lines is 95% confidence interval for the null distribution. (b) JDH of a pair of pre- and post-treatment exams. The green line represents the diagonal line and the magenta lines represent the 97.5^{th} and 2.5^{th} percentile lines of the null distribution, respectively. Note that the magenta lines in (a) and (b) are of different intercepts. The magenta lines in (a) are the 97.5^{th} and 2.5^{th} percentile for this specific coffee-break exam pair. The magenta lines in (b) are the average 97.5^{th} and 2.5^{th} percentile for the 5 pairs of coffee-break exams in the training data sets.

$[-0.5, 0.5] \times 10^{-3} \text{mm}^2/\text{s}$ rounded to one decimal place. Since the increased ADC values associated with cell death and increased diffusion in extracellular water are our primary interest in predicting therapy response, the 97.5^{th} percentile threshold corresponding to an ADC change of $0.5 \times 10^{-3} \text{ mm}^2/\text{s}$ is the threshold we choose for evaluating the treatment response in the University of Hull data. In other words, if the ADC change of a voxel is larger than $0.5 \times 10^{-3} \text{ mm}^2/\text{s}$, this voxel belongs to the region of significantly increased ADC values, i.e., V_i.

2.4   FDM Analysis on the University of Hull Data [18]

We evaluate the diffusion weighted MRI combined with functional diffusion mapping analysis as an imaging response biomarker using the clinical data provided by the University of Hull clinical trial [18]. Together 27 patients with biopsy-proven breast cancer were scanned prior to and after the first, second and fourth (final scheduled) cycle of neoadjuvant chemotherapy to allow monitoring tumor changes by using diffusion weighted MRI. Treatment cycles consisted of epirubicin (90 mg/m^2) and cyclophosphamide (600 mg/m^2) administered at 3 week intervals. Patients were scanned either on a 3.0 or 1.5T scanner (GE Healthcare,

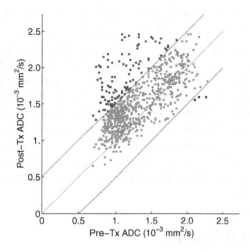

Fig. 3. fDM analysis in assessing treatment response based on registered diffusion scans obtained shortly after and before the initiation of neoadjuvant therapy for a patient

Milwaukee, WI, USA) in combination with dedicated bilateral breast coils. Different field strengths do not affect the study results as ADC values, in principle, are not dependant on B0 field strength.

Diffusion weighted MRI was acquired axially with a water-only excitation, singleshot, dual spin-echo EPI sequence with the following parameters: TR, 4000 ms, fractional TE, 74 ms (3.0 T) or 98 ms (1.5 T); FOV, 340×340 mm; matrix, 128×128; slice, 5 mm; gap, 1 mm; 10 averages; b values, 0 and 700 s/mm^2, applied in all three orthogonal directions. DWI scans were acquired in 2 min 40 s at both field strengths. A dual spinecho EPI sequence was utilized since this sequence reduces eddy currents and, therefore, image distortions with the addition of an extra refocusing pulse after the conventional refocusing pulse.

Not all 27 data sets were used to study the correlation between ADC changes and treatment response. Some diffusion scans only include partial tumor scans and are treated as inadequate for assessing the treatment efficacy and therefore excluded from this study. Eventually we have 14 complete data sets.

To test the capability of ADC changes in assessing early treatment response, the joint distribution histogram of registered pre-treatment and post-treatment ADC values was investigated. An example of JDH is shown in Fig. 2(b). This distribution represents the treatment effect distribution and clearly reveals that ADC values have increased in several ways: first the mean has moved upwards, and secondly there is a larger portion of voxels above the 97.5[th] percentile line derived from the null distribution based on the training data sets. The corresponding scatter plot is shown in Fig. 3. Here red indicates the presence of voxels whose ADC changes (post-treatment minus pre-treatment) are greater than the 97.5[th] percentile of the null distribution (i.e. regions of cell kill and limited noise, "V_i"); green indicates voxels whose changes are within the

$2.5^{th} - 97.5^{th}$ percentiles (regions of no significant change, "V_0"); and blue indicates changes that are below the 2.5^{th} percentile of the null (regions of continued tumor growth and limited noise, "V_d"). The voxels in the "red" region (V_i) count for 12.25% of the entire tumor volume in Fig 2(b). Note that while 2.5% of these voxels are expected noise and distributed as spatially uncorrelated, single voxels, the treatment effect increment above 2.5% is typically seen as spatially correlated, i.e., connected voxels. We repeated this functional diffusion mapping analysis on each of the data set in this study and percentage_V_i (the percentage of the V_i volume over the entire tumor volume) was calculated. We subtracted 2.5% from percentage_V_i to remove the effect of the noise inherent in the null distribution so that percentage_V_i reflects the actual percentage of voxels with increased ADC values.

3   Experimental Results

The pathological outcome was used to remove 4 non-responding patients from the regression fit to the response of neoadjuvant therapy. The chemotherapeutic agent for the first two cycles of neoadjuvant therapy was exactly the same and consistent response was expected during this time period. The first post-therapy data acquisition took place within 2-12 days after the initiation of the first cycle of treatment. The second post-therapy data acquisition took place within 11-19 days after the initiation of the second cycle of treatment and within 32-39 days after the initiation of the first treatment cycle. Note that the post-treatment scans were acquired within different numbers of days after the initiation of therapy. To study the role of ADC changes between pre- and post-therapy examinations as an early indicator of treatment effectiveness, we focus on the relationship between ADC changes and time intervals after the initiation of treatment. In our study post-treatment scans include the diffusion scans obtained after both the first and the second cycle of treatment.

Percentage_V_i as a function of the number of days after treatment for responders is shown in Fig. 4. Responders are indicated by "×" while non-responders by "o". For most responder cases, their percentage_V_i is above zero, which means that there are voxels in the tumor whose ADC values have increased significantly during treatment.

To investigate the correlation of ADC changes and interval lengths after the initiation of treatment, linear regression was performed and the regression line (red line) with p-value 0.03 was shown in Fig. 4. We clearly observe that these five-week-post-treatment exams exhibit a larger effect size in ADC change compared to their one-week-post-treatment counterparts. After some duration we would expect the treatment effect on diffusion level to off or even drop back to the null effect after most cancer cells have been killed.

A blue line was drawn to connect the two time points for each patient. Please note that the post-first-treatment scans for cases 07 and 10 were obtained only 5 days after the initiation of treatment and it is highly likely that it is too soon to see any cellular change in the tumor. However, it was 33 days after the initiation

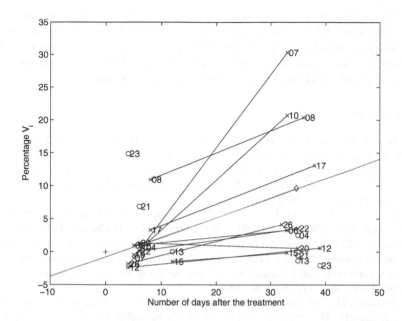

Fig. 4. Percentage_V_i versus number of days after the initiation of treatment. The red line represents linear regression of all (percentage_V_i, number of days after treatment) pairs. A blue line connects the two different time points for each patient. The (0, 0) point is plotted with a "+"; Ideally after a zero length time interval there should be no measured response to therapy.

of therapy that post-second-treatment exams were taken and the interval was long enough for the treatment to take effect. Therefore, these two cases exhibit large increases in the ADC values in the post-second-treatment exams compared to their pre-treatment scans.

Logistic regression analysis was performed to further examine the correlation of ADC changes during treatment with clinical outcomes. A logistic regression fit with $p = 0.009$ at five weeks post-treatment demonstrated that the probability of a responsive treatment is strongly associated with increased ADC values. We observed 1 false positive and 1 false negative for a sensitivity of 90% and a specificity of 75%. On the other hand, logistic regression at one week post-treatment showed no capability of separating responders from non-responders.

4   Conclusion

We have extended voxel-by-voxel functional diffusion mapping analysis to assess early response to breast cancer treatment. The thresholds of significant ADC changes were derived from short interval exams and were used to evaluate treatment efficacy based on ADC changes during treatment. With limited data sets, experimental results have shown that ADC changes have the potential to be used to assess treatment effectiveness and are likely an increasing function of the temporal interval after the initiation of treatment within an as yet unknown time limit. Clearly the ratio of therapeutic effect size to noise at one week post-therapy is small; at 5 weeks post-therapy the opposite appears to be true. Logistic regression analysis has further revealed that ADC changes at five weeks post-therapy are highly correlated with treatment response.

References

1. Fisher, B., Bryant, J., Wolmark, N., Mamounas, E., Brown, A., Fisher, E.R., Wickerham, D.L., Begovic, M., DeCillis, A., Robidoux, A., Margolese, R.G., Cruz Jr., A.B., Hoehn, J.L., Lees, A.W., Dimitrov, N.V., Bear, H.D.: Effect of preoperative chemotherapy on the outcome of women with operable breast cancer. Journal of Clinical Oncology 6, 2672–2685 (1998)
2. Kuerer, H.M., Newman, L.A., Smith, T.L., Ames, F.C., Hunt, K.K., Dhinga, K., Theriault, R.L., Singh, G., Binkley, S.M., Sneige, N., Buchholz, T.A., Ross, M.I., McNeese, M.D., Buzdar, A.U., Hortobagyi, G.N., Singletary, S.E.: Clinical course of breast cancer patients with complete pathologic primary tumor and axillary lymph node response to doxorubicin-based neoadjuvant chemotherapy. Journal of Clinical Oncology 17, 460–469 (1999)
3. Bonadonna, G., Valagussa, P., Brambilla, C., Ferrari, L., Moliterni, A., Terenziani, M., Zambetti, M.: Primary chemotherapy in operable breast cancer: eight-year experience at the Milan cancer institute. Journal of Clinical Oncology 16, 93–100 (1998)
4. Buchholz, T.A., Hill, B.S., Tucker, S.L., Frye, D.K., Kuerer, H.M., Buzdar, A.U., McNeese, M.D., Singletary, S.E., Ueno, N.T., Pusztai, L., Valero, V., Hortobagyi, G.N.: Factors predictive of outcome in patients with breast cancer refractory to neoadjuvant chemotherapy. Cancer J. 7, 413–420 (2001)
5. Schott, A.F., Roubidoux, M.A., Helvie, M.A., Hayes, D.F., Kleer, C.G., Newman, L., Pierce, L.J., Griffith, K.A., Murray, S., Hunt, K.A., Paramagul, C., Baker, L.H.: Clinical and radiologic assessments to predict breast cancer pathologic complete response to neoadjuvant chemotherapy. Breast Cancer Res. Treat 92, 231–238 (2005)
6. Chenevert, T.L., Stegman, L.D., Taylor, J.M.G., Robertson, P.L., Greenberg, H.S., Rehemtulla, A., Ross, B.D.: Diffusion magnetic resonance imaging: an early surrogate marker of therapeutic efficacy in brain tumors. J. Natl. Cancer Inst. 92(24), 2029–2036 (2000)
7. Moffat, B.A., Chenevert, T.L., Lawrence, T.S., Meyer, C.R., Johnson, T.D., Dong, Q., Tsien, C., Mukherji, S., Quint, D., Gebarski, S.S., Robertson, P.L., Junck, L.R., Rehemtulla, A., Ross, B.D.: Functional diffusion map: a noninvasive MRI biomarker for early stratification of clinical brain tumor response. Proc. Natl. Acad. Sci. USA 102(15), 5524–5529 (2005)
8. Ross, B.D., Moffat, B.A., Lawrence, T., Mukherji, S., Gebarski, S., Quint, D., Johnson, T.D., Junck, L., Robertson, P., Muraszko, K., Dong, Q., Meyer, C.R., Bland, P., McConville, P., Geng, H., Rehemtulla, A., Chenevert, T.L.: Evaluation of cancer therapy using diffusion magnetic resonance imaging. Mol. Cancer Therapy 2, 581–587 (2003)
9. Hamstra, D.J., Chenevert, T.L., Moffat, B.A., Johnson, T.D., Meyer, C.R., Mukherji, S., Quint, D.J., Gebarski, S.S., Xiaoying, F., Tsiena, C., Lawrence, T.S., Junck, L.R., Rehemtulla, A., Ross, B.D.: Evaluation of the functional diffusion map as an early biomarker of time-to-progression and overall survival in high grade glioma. Proc. Natl. Acad. Sci. USA 102(46), 16759–16764 (2005)

10. Chenevert, T.L., Meyer, C.R., Moffat, B.A., Rehemtulla, A., Mukherji, S.K., Gebarski, S.S., Quint, D.J., Robertson, P.L., Lawrence, T.S., Junck, L., Taylor, J.M., Johnson, T.D., Dong, Q., Muraszko, K.M., Brunberg, J.A., Ross, B.D.: Diffusion MRI: a new strategy for assessment of cancer therapeutic efficacy. Mol. Imaging 1(4), 336–343 (2002)

11. Lee, K.C., Hall, D.E., Hoff, B.A., Moffat, B.A., Sharma, S., Chenevert, T.L., Meyer, C.R., Leopold, W.R., Johnson, T.D., Mazurchuk, R.V., Rehemtulla, A., Ross, B.D.: Dynamic imaging of emerging resistance during cancer therapy. Cancer Res. 66(9), 4687–4692 (2006)

12. Lee, K.C., Moffat, B.A., Schott, A.F., Layman, R., Ellingworth, S., Juliar, R., Khan, A.P., Helvie, M.A., Meyer, C.R., Chenevert, T.L., Rehemtulla, A., Ross, B.D.: Prospective early response imaging biomarker for neoadjuvant breast cancer chemotherapy. Clin. Cancer Res. 13(2), 443–450 (2007)

13. Lee, K.C., Sud, S., Meyer, C.R., Moffat, B.A., Chenevert, T.L., Rehemtulla, A., Pienta, K.J., Ross, B.D.: An imaging biomarker of early treatment response in prostate cancer that has metastasized to the bone. Cancer Res. 67(8), 3524–3528 (2007)

14. Lee, K.C., Bradley, D., Hussain, M., Meyer, C., Chenevert, T., Jacobson, J., Johnson, T., Galbán, C., Rehemtulla, A., Pienta, K., Ross, B.: A feasibility study evaluating the functional diffusion map as a predictive imaging biomarker for detection of treatment response in a patient with metastatic prostate cancer to the bone. Neoplasia 9(12), 1003–1011 (2007)

15. Hamstra, D.A., Galbán, C.J., Meyer, C.R., Johnson, T.D., Sundgren, P.C., Tsien, C., Lawrence, T.S., Junck, L., Ross, D.J., Rehemtulla, A., Ross, B.D., Chenevert, T.L.: Functional Diffusion Map as an early imaging biomarker for high-grade glioma: Correlation with conventional radiologic response and overall survival. J. Clin. Oncol. 26(20), 3387–3394 (2008)

16. Ross, B.D., Chenevert, T.L., Kim, B., Ben-Joseph, O.: Magnetic resonance imaging and spectroscopy: Application to experimental neuro-oncology. Q. Magn. Reson. Biol. Med. 1, 89–106 (1994)

17. Meyer, C.R., Boes, J.L., Kim, B., Bland, P.H., Zasadny, K.R., Kison, P.V., Koral, K., Frey, K.A., Wahl, R.L.: Demonstration of accuracy and clinical versatility of mutual information for automatic multimodality image fusion using affine and thin-plate spline warped geometric deformations. Medical Image Analysis 1, 195–206 (1997)

18. Pickles, M.D., Gibbs, P., Lowry, M., Turnbull, L.W.: Diffusion changes precede size reduction in neoadjuvant treatment of breast cancer. Magnetic Resonance Imaging 24(7), 843–847 (2006)

MRI Tissue Classification and Bias Field Estimation Based on Coherent Local Intensity Clustering: A Unified Energy Minimization Framework

Chunming Li[1,*], Chenyang Xu[2], Adam W. Anderson[1], and John C. Gore[1]

[1] Vanderbilt University Institute of Imaging Science, Nashville, TN 37232, USA
[2] Siemens Corporate Research, Princeton, NJ 08540, USA
lchunming@gmail.com

Abstract. This paper presents a new energy minimization method for simultaneous tissue classification and bias field estimation of magnetic resonance (MR) images. We first derive an important characteristic of local image intensities — the intensities of different tissues within a neighborhood form separable clusters, and the center of each cluster can be well approximated by the product of the bias within the neighborhood and a tissue-dependent constant. We then introduce a coherent local intensity clustering (CLIC) criterion function as a metric to evaluate tissue classification and bias field estimation. An integration of this metric defines an energy on a bias field, membership functions of the tissues, and the parameters that approximate the true signal from the corresponding tissues. Thus, tissue classification and bias field estimation are simultaneously achieved by minimizing this energy. The smoothness of the derived optimal bias field is ensured by the spatially coherent nature of the CLIC criterion function. As a result, no extra effort is needed to smooth the bias field in our method. Moreover, the proposed algorithm is robust to the choice of initial conditions, thereby allowing fully automatic applications. Our algorithm has been applied to high field and ultra high field MR images with promising results.

1 Introduction

Magnetic resonance imaging (MRI) is a ubiquitous and powerful medical imaging technique, which provides detailed images with high contrast between different soft tissues; MRI thus has significant advantages over other medical imaging modalities for many applications, making it especially useful for neurological, musculoskeletal, cardiovascular, and oncological imaging. However, there are commonly substantial artifacts in real MR images, such as image nonuniformities caused by inhomogeneities in the B1 or B0 fields, especially in high field (e.g. 3T) MR images. The intensity inhomogeneity may severely challenge quantitative image analysis algorithms, such as those used for image segmentation and registration. Intensity inhomogeneities are particularly severe in MRI at ultra high field strengths (e.g. 7T) and sometimes make it difficult even for expert human observers to view the images.

---

* Corresponding author.

J.L. Prince, D.L. Pham, and K.J. Myers (Eds.): IPMI 2009, LNCS 5636, pp. 288–299, 2009.
© Springer-Verlag Berlin Heidelberg 2009

It is commonly assumed that intensity inhomogeneities can be ascribed to a spatially varying field that is a multiplicative component of the measured image. This multiplicative component, known as a *bias field*, varies spatially because of inhomogeneities in the B0 and B1 fields. *Bias field correction* refers to a procedure to estimate the bias field from the measured image so that its effect can be eliminated. There are two main types of methods for bias correction: prospective and retrospective methods. Prospective methods aim to avoid intensity inhomogeneities in the image acquisition process. These methods, while capable of correcting intensity inhomogeneity induced by the imaging device, are not able to remove object-induced effects. In contrast, retrospective methods rely only on the information in the acquired images, and thus they can remove intensity inhomogeneities regardless of their sources. Retrospective methods include those based on filtering [1, 2, 3, 4], surface fitting [5, 6, 7, 8], histogram [9, 10], and segmentation [11, 12, 13, 14, 15, 16, 17].

Most retrospective methods assume that the bias field is smooth (i.e. slowly varying). The smoothness of the bias field is not only consistent with its physical origins in the MR imaging process, but also necessary to make the bias field correction problem tractable. However, the bias fields computed by direct implementation of most of the well-known methods are in general not smooth. This then requires an extra effort to maintain the smoothness of the computed bias field, which is often performed in an ad-hoc manner. For example, in the method of Wells *et al.* [11], an extra step of moving-average low pass filtering is introduced to smooth the computed bias field. In the method proposed by Sled *et al.* [9], the estimated bias field has to be replaced by a linear combination of smooth B-spline basis functions to generate a smooth field.

In [14], Pham and Prince proposed an energy minimization method for adaptive segmentation and estimation of the bias field. The smoothness of the bias field is ensured by adding a smoothing constraint term into the energy in their method. However, this introduces a highly computationally expensive procedure to solve a space-varying difference equation for a smooth bias field. In parametric methods (e.g. [10, 12]), which model the bias field as a linear combination of polynomial basis functions, the computed bias field is always smooth. However, such parametric methods are not able to capture bias fields that cannot be well approximated by polynomials, such as the bias field in the 7T MR images shown in Section 3.2.

Among retrospective methods, segmentation-based approaches are particularly attractive, as they unify the tasks of segmentation and bias correction into a single framework. Segmentation-based methods have been one of the most popular type of bias correction methods according to a recent review by Vovk *et al.* [18]. In these methods, segmentation and bias field estimation are interleaved to benefit each other, thereby allowing both to be refined iteratively until convergence to an optimal solution. In this process, the segmentation is usually achieved by using maximum likelihood [12, 19] or maximum a posteriori based methods [11, 13]. Fuzzy-C-Means based methods have also been used in [14, 20].

In this paper, we propose a new energy minimization method for simultaneous tissue classification and bias field estimation of MR images. We first describe an important characteristic of local image intensities — the intensities of different tissues within a neighborhood form separable clusters, and the center of each cluster can be well approximated by the product of the bias within the neighborhood and a tissue-dependent constant. This characteristic provides an effective metric to evaluate the classification of the tissues and the estimation of the bias field in terms of a *coherent local intensity clustering (CLIC)* criterion function. This CLIC criterion is an energy on a bias field, membership functions of the tissues, and the parameters that approximate the true signal from the corresponding tissues. Tissue classification and bias field estimation are simultaneously achieved by minimizing this energy. The CLIC energy has two desirable properties: it is convex in each of its variables, which renders the proposed method robust to initialization, thereby allowing fully automatic applications; the smoothness of the derived estimate of the bias field is intrinsically ensured by the spatial coherent nature of the CLIC criterion function. As a result, no extra effort is needed for the bias field smoothing. Finally, our method is able to estimate bias fields of more general profiles, including those in high and ultra high field MR images.

2   Method

2.1   Problem Formulation

We consider the following model of MR image formation with multiplicative bias and additive noise:

$$I = bJ + n, \tag{1}$$

where I is the measured image intensity, J is the true signal to be restored, b is an unknown bias field, and n is additive noise. The goal of bias correction is to estimate the bias field b from the measured intensity I. This is obviously an underdetermined problem, as neither b nor J is known. To make the problem tractable, it is necessary to make assumptions on the unknowns b and J. The generally accepted assumption on the bias field is that it is slowly varying. Ideally, the intensity J in each tissue should take a specific value c_i of the physical property being measured (e.g. the proton density for MR images). This property, in conjunction with the spatially coherent nature of each tissue's distribution, implies that the true signal J is approximately a piecewise constant map. In addition, the additive noise n can be assumed to be zero-mean Gaussian noise.

To be specific, we assume that there are N types of tissues in the image domain Ω, and these tissues are located in N disjoint regions $\Omega_1, \cdots, \Omega_N$ in Ω. Then, the above assumptions on the true signal J and the bias field b can be formally stated as follows:

(A1) The true signal J from the i-th tissue is approximately a constant c_i, i.e. $J(\mathbf{x}) \approx c_i$ for $\mathbf{x} \in \Omega_i$. The constants $c_1, \cdots, c_N$ are assumed to be distinct from each other, as they characterize a physical property of N different tissues.

(A2) The bias field b is slowly varying in the entire image domain Ω.

Tissue classification can be achieved by partitioning the image domain Ω into N disjoint regions $\Omega_1, \cdots, \Omega_N$. Alternatively, in view of the possibility of partial volume effects, it is more advisable to perform tissue classification by seeking membership functions $u_1, \cdots, u_N$ of the tissues, which take values between 0 and 1 and satisfy

$$\sum_{i=1}^{N} u_i(\mathbf{x}) = 1, \quad \text{for all } \mathbf{x}. \tag{2}$$

The values of $u_i(\mathbf{x})$ can be interpreted as the percentage of the i-th tissue in voxel $\mathbf{x}$.

Based on the above assumptions, tissue classification and bias field estimation can be achieved by: 1) seeking the membership functions $u_1, \cdots, u_N$; 2) estimating the parameters c_i that approximate the true signal from the i-th tissue for $i = 1, \cdots, N$; 3) estimating the bias field b. In these three tasks, the membership functions $u_1, \cdots, u_N$, the parameters $c_1, \cdots, c_N$, and the bias field b can be obtained to satisfy a specified optimality criterion. For convenience, the membership functions $u_1, \cdots, u_N$ and the constants $c_1, \cdots, c_N$ are denoted by a vector valued membership function $U = (u_1, \cdots, u_N)$, and a vector $\mathbf{c} = (c_1, \cdots, c_N)$, respectively. In our proposed energy minimization framework, optimal U, $\mathbf{c}$, and b are obtained by minimizing an energy $\mathcal{F}(U, \mathbf{c}, b)$ in terms of the variables U, $\mathbf{c}$, and b.

2.2   Statistical Property of Local Intensities

The proposed algorithm is based on the properties that the bias field is slowly varying and the true signal J is piecewise approximately constant. From these basic properties, we are able to see the problem of tissue classification and bias field correction from a local viewpoint of the image intensities. These properties imply a key statistical characteristic of local intensities, which leads to an effective scheme to solve the problem of tissue classification and bias field correction.

We consider a circular neighborhood of each point $\mathbf{x} \in \Omega$, defined by $\mathcal{O}_\mathbf{x} \triangleq \{\mathbf{y} : |\mathbf{y} - \mathbf{x}| \leq \rho\}$, where ρ is the radius of the circular neighborhood. For a slowly varying bias field b, the values $b(\mathbf{y})$ for all $\mathbf{y}$ in the circular neighborhood $\mathcal{O}_\mathbf{x}$ can be well approximated by $b(\mathbf{x})$. On the other hand, the neighborhood $\mathcal{O}_\mathbf{x}$ consists of N subregions $\mathcal{O}_\mathbf{x} \cap \Omega_i$, $i = 1, \cdots, N$, where Ω_i is the region corresponding to the i-th tissue. According to the assumption (A1), the true signal J from the i-th tissue is approximately a constant c_i. Thus, the intensities $b(\mathbf{y})J(\mathbf{y})$ in each subregion $\mathcal{O}_\mathbf{x} \cap \Omega_i$ can be approximated by $b(\mathbf{x})c_i$. Thus, we have the following approximation

$$b(\mathbf{y})J(\mathbf{y}) \approx b(\mathbf{x})c_i \quad \text{for } \mathbf{y} \in \mathcal{O}_\mathbf{x} \cap \Omega_i \tag{3}$$

From the image model (1), we have

$$I(\mathbf{y}) \approx b(\mathbf{x})c_i + n(\mathbf{y}) \quad \text{for } \mathbf{y} \in \mathcal{O}_\mathbf{x} \cap \Omega_i$$

where $n(\mathbf{y})$ is additive zero-mean Gaussian noise.

The above arguments show that the measured intensities within the neighborhood $\mathcal{O}_\mathbf{x}$ can be considered as samples from N Gaussian distributions with means $b(\mathbf{x})c_i$, $i = 1, \cdots, N$. In the other words, the intensities in the neighborhood $\mathcal{O}_\mathbf{x}$ form N clusters $\{I(\mathbf{y}) : \mathbf{y} \in \mathcal{O}_\mathbf{x} \cap \Omega_i\}$, $i = 1, \cdots, N$, and the cluster center m_i of the i-th cluster can be well approximated by $m_i \approx b(\mathbf{x})c_i$. Furthermore, these clusters can be assumed to be well separated, as the cluster centers $m_i \approx b(\mathbf{x})c_i$ are distinct from each other according to the assumption (A1). This property of local intensities allows us to apply standard clustering techniques, such as K-means and fuzzy C-means algorithms, to classify the local intensities in a neighborhood into N classes.

Standard K-means or fuzzy C-means clustering are processes of minimizing a clustering criterion function. In particular, for the intensities in the neighborhood $\mathcal{O}_\mathbf{x}$, the fuzzy C-means clustering criterion function can be expressed as:

$$\mathcal{J}_{\mathbf{x}}^{\text{loc}} = \int_{\mathcal{O}_{\mathbf{x}}} \sum_{i=1}^{N} u_i^q(\mathbf{y})|I(\mathbf{y}) - m_i|^2 d\mathbf{y}, \tag{4}$$

where $q > 1$ is the fuzzifier, $u_1, \cdots, u_N$ are the membership functions satisfying $\sum_{i=1}^{N} u_i = 1$, and $m_1, \cdots, m_N$ are the cluster centers of the N clusters.

The above clustering criterion function characterizes how well the membership functions $u_1, \cdots, u_N$ give a classification of the intensities $I(\mathbf{y})$ within the neighborhood $\mathcal{O}_{\mathbf{x}}$ into N clusters or classes with cluster centers $b(\mathbf{x})c_i$. The smaller the clustering criterion function, the better the classification. Minimizing the above clustering criterion function results in an optimal set of cluster centers and membership functions as the desired classification results. However, classifying the intensities in a single neighborhood $\mathcal{O}_{\mathbf{x}}$ does not achieve our ultimate goal of bias field estimation and segmentation of the entire image. To achieve our ultimate goal, we need further development as described below.

2.3 Coherent Local Intensity Clustering

Recall that the analysis in Section 2.2 has shown that the intensities in the neighborhood $\mathcal{O}_{\mathbf{x}}$ form N separate clusters with distinct cluster centers $m_i \approx b(\mathbf{x})c_i$, $i = 1, \cdots, N$, with $c_1, \cdots, c_N$ being constants that approximate the true signal from N tissues. For the intensities $I(\mathbf{y})$ in the neighborhood $\mathcal{O}_{\mathbf{x}}$, we define a similar clustering criterion function as in Eq. (4), with the clustering centers m_i replaced by $b(\mathbf{x})c_i$. In addition, we introduce a weight for each intensity $I(\mathbf{y})$ to control its influence on the clustering criterion function. The intensity $I(\mathbf{y})$ at location $\mathbf{y}$ far away from the neighborhood center $\mathbf{x}$ should have less influence in the clustering criterion function than the locations close to $\mathbf{x}$. More specifically, we define the following clustering criterion function

$$\mathcal{J}_{\mathbf{x}}^{\text{loc}}(U, \mathbf{c}, b(\mathbf{x})) \triangleq \sum_{i=1}^{N} \int_{\mathcal{O}_{\mathbf{x}}} u_i^q(\mathbf{y})K(\mathbf{x} - \mathbf{y})|I(\mathbf{y}) - b(\mathbf{x})c_i|^2 d\mathbf{y} \tag{5}$$

where $u_1, \cdots, u_N$ are the membership functions for N regions (tissues), and $K(\mathbf{x} - \mathbf{y})$ is the weight assigned to the intensity $I(\mathbf{y})$.

The weighting function $K(\mathbf{x} - \mathbf{y})$ is preferably designed so that its value decreases as the distance from $\mathbf{y}$ to the neighborhood center $\mathbf{x}$ increases. In this paper, the weighting function K is chosen as a truncated Gaussian kernel

$$K(\mathbf{u}) = \begin{cases} \frac{1}{a} e^{-|\mathbf{u}|^2/2\sigma^2} & \text{for } |\mathbf{u}| \le \rho; \\ 0 & \text{else,} \end{cases} \tag{6}$$

With such a truncated Gaussian kernel $K(\mathbf{x} - \mathbf{y})$, the above clustering criterion function $\mathcal{J}_{\mathbf{x}}^{\text{loc}}$ can be written as

$$\mathcal{J}_{\mathbf{x}}^{\text{loc}}(U, \mathbf{c}, b(\mathbf{x})) = \sum_{i=1}^{N} \int u_i^q(\mathbf{y})K(\mathbf{x} - \mathbf{y})|I(\mathbf{y}) - b(\mathbf{x})c_i|^2 d\mathbf{y} \tag{7}$$

as $K(\mathbf{x} - \mathbf{y}) = 0$ for $\mathbf{y} \notin \mathcal{O}_{\mathbf{x}}$.

The above clustering criterion characterizes the local performance of the tissue classification associated with the membership functions $u_1, \cdots, u_N$, which are defined on the entire image domain. The desired tissue classification on the entire image domain should have good local performance in terms of the above clustering criterion for every neighborhood $\mathcal{O}_{\mathbf{x}}$. Therefore, we seek the membership function U, constant $\mathbf{c}$, and bias field b such that $\mathcal{J}_{\mathbf{x}}^{\text{loc}}(U, \mathbf{c}, b(\mathbf{x}))$ is minimized for all $\mathbf{x} \in \Omega$.

We have defined the above local clustering criterion function $\mathcal{J}_{\mathbf{x}}^{\text{loc}}$ based on the smoothness of the bias field b. The definition of such local clustering criterion function $\mathcal{J}_{\mathbf{x}}^{\text{loc}}$ intrinsically implies the smoothness of the optimal field estimator b that minimizes $\mathcal{J}_{\mathbf{x}}^{\text{loc}}$ for all $\mathbf{x} \in \Omega$. The optimal field b is denoted by $\hat{b}$. The smoothness of $\hat{b}$ can be intuitively explained as follows. The clustering criterion function $\mathcal{J}_{\mathbf{x}}^{\text{loc}}$ involves all the intensities $I(\mathbf{y})$ in the neighborhood $\mathcal{O}_{\mathbf{x}}$. Therefore, the value of $b(\mathbf{x})$ that minimizes $\mathcal{J}_{\mathbf{x}}^{\text{loc}}$ depends on all the intensities $I(\mathbf{y})$ in the neighborhood $\mathcal{O}_{\mathbf{x}}$. As the neighborhood center moves from $\mathbf{x}$ to a point $\mathbf{x}' = \mathbf{x} + \Delta\mathbf{x}$ for a small displacement $\Delta\mathbf{x}$, the majority of points in the neighborhood $\mathcal{O}_{\mathbf{x}}$ remain in the neighborhood $\mathcal{O}_{\mathbf{x}'}$. Therefore, the value of $\hat{b}(\mathbf{x}')$ is close to $\hat{b}(\mathbf{x})$, which indicates the smoothness of $\hat{b}$. The smoothness of the optimal bias field estimator $\hat{b}$ will be clearly seen from its closed form solution in Section 2.4.

The above argument shows the spatial coherence of the minimization of the local clustering criterion $\mathcal{J}_{\mathbf{x}}^{\text{loc}}$ for all $\mathbf{x} \in \Omega$ — the local clustering criterion functions $\mathcal{J}_{\mathbf{x}}^{\text{loc}}$ for different $\mathbf{x}$ are not minimized independently. There is a strong relationship between the local clustering criterion functions $\mathcal{J}_{\mathbf{x}}^{\text{loc}}$ for neighboring points $\mathbf{x}$ and the corresponding results of minimization, due to the overlap of the neighborhoods. Therefore, we call the minimization of the local clustering criterion functions $\mathcal{J}_{\mathbf{x}}^{\text{loc}}$ for all $\mathbf{x} \in \Omega$ a process of *coherent local intensity clustering (CLIC)*.

Minimization of $\mathcal{J}_{\mathbf{x}}^{\text{loc}}$ for all $\mathbf{x} \in \Omega$ can be achieved by minimizing the integral of $\mathcal{J}_{\mathbf{x}}^{\text{loc}}$ over Ω. Therefore, we define an energy $\mathcal{J}(U, \mathbf{c}, b) \triangleq \int \mathcal{J}_{\mathbf{x}}^{\text{loc}}(U, \mathbf{c}, b(\mathbf{x}))d\mathbf{x}$, i.e.

$$\mathcal{J}(U, \mathbf{c}, b) \triangleq \int \sum_{i=1}^{N} \int u_i^q(\mathbf{y}) K(\mathbf{x} - \mathbf{y}) |I(\mathbf{y}) - b(\mathbf{x})c_i|^2 d\mathbf{y} d\mathbf{x} \tag{8}$$

By changing the order of integration, the above energy $\mathcal{J}(U, \mathbf{c}, b)$ can be written in the form:

$$\mathcal{J}(U, \mathbf{c}, b) = \int \sum_{i=1}^{N} u_i^q(\mathbf{y}) d_i(I(\mathbf{y})) d\mathbf{y} \tag{9}$$

where

$$d_i(I(\mathbf{y})) \triangleq \int K(\mathbf{x} - \mathbf{y}) |I(\mathbf{y}) - b(\mathbf{x})c_i|^2 d\mathbf{x} \tag{10}$$

The minimization of the energy $\mathcal{J}(U, \mathbf{c}, b)$ is subject to the constraint

$$\sum_{i=1}^{N} u_i = 1.$$

The minimization of the above energy $\mathcal{J}(U, \mathbf{c}, b)$ is described in Section 2.4. The algorithm for minimizing this energy is simply referred to as the *coherent local intensity clustering (CLIC)* algorithm. The estimated bias field and true signal are given by $\hat{b}$, and $I/\hat{b}$, respectively. We note that the proposed method can provide a solution only up to a scaling factor. In fact, for any bias field $\hat{b}$ and vector $\hat{c}$ that minimize the energy $\mathcal{J}(U, \mathbf{c}, b)$, the bias field $s\hat{b}$ and vector $\hat{c}/s$ for any constant s also minimize the energy.

2.4   Energy Minimization

The energy $\mathcal{J}(U, \mathbf{c}, b)$ is convex in each of its variables. Therefore, there is a unique minimizer of the energy $\mathcal{J}(U, \mathbf{c}, b)$ in each variable, given the other two variables remain fixed. Thus, minimization of the energy $\mathcal{J}(U, \mathbf{c}, b)$ can be performed by an interleaving process of minimization with respect to the variables U, $\mathbf{c}$, and b. Moreover, the energy minimization algorithm is robust to the initialization of the variables U, $\mathbf{c}$, and b.

For the case $q > 1$, the above constrained energy minimization results in a fuzzy membership function $\hat{u}_1, \cdots, \hat{u}_N$, which take values between 0 and 1, yielding a result of *soft segmentation*. For the case $q = 1$, the constrained energy minimization results in binary maps $\hat{u}_1, \cdots, \hat{u}_N$, with values being either 0 or 1, yielding a result of *hard segmentation*. The segmentation results can be visualized by showing the image $\sum_{i=1}^{N} \hat{c}_i \hat{u}_i$.

2.5   Minimization with Respect to Variables c and b

For any $q \geq 1$, the solutions to the minimization of the energy $\mathcal{J}(U, \mathbf{c}, b)$ with respect to the variables $\mathbf{c}$ and b are given as below:

– For fixed U and b, there is a unique minimizer of the energy $\mathcal{J}(U, \mathbf{c}, b)$ with respect to $\mathbf{c}$, denoted by $\hat{\mathbf{c}} = (\hat{c}_1, \cdots, \hat{c}_N)$. It can be shown that

$$\hat{c}_i = \frac{\int (b * K) I u_i^q d\mathbf{x}}{\int (b^2 * K) u_i^q d\mathbf{x}}, \quad i = 1, \cdots, N. \tag{11}$$

where $*$ is the convolution operation.
– Given U and $\mathbf{c}$, there is a unique minimizer of the energy $\mathcal{J}(U, \mathbf{c}, b)$ with respect to b, denoted by $\hat{b}$. It can be shown that

$$\hat{b} = \frac{(I J^{(1)}) * K}{J^{(2)} * K} \tag{12}$$

where $J^{(1)} = \sum_{i=1}^{N} c_i u_i^q$ and $J^{(2)} = \sum_{i=1}^{N} c_i^2 u_i^q$.

Note that the convolutions with a kernel K in the expression of $\hat{b}$ in Eq. (12) confirms the smoothness of the derived optimal bias field $\hat{b}$, which has been explained from the definition of the clustering criterion function $\mathcal{J}_\mathbf{x}^{\text{loc}}$ in the previous section.

2.6   Minimization with Respect to the Membership Function U

The minimization of $\mathcal{J}(U, \mathbf{c}, b)$ with respect to the membership function U should be considered for the cases of $q > 1$ and $q = 1$ separately, which correspond to soft segmentation and hard segmentation, respectively. We first consider the case $q > 1$. For fixed c and b, there is a unique minimizer of the energy $\mathcal{J}(U, c, b)$ with respect to U. We denote this minimizer by $\hat{U} = (\hat{u}_1, \cdots, \hat{u}_N)$. It can be shown that

$$\hat{u}_i(\mathbf{y}) = \frac{1}{\sum_{k=1}^{N} \left(\frac{d_i(I(\mathbf{y}))}{d_k(I(\mathbf{y}))} \right)^{\frac{1}{q-1}}} \tag{13}$$

For the case of $q = 1$, given the variables c and b fixed, the energy $\mathcal{J}(U, c, b)$ is minimized when $U = \hat{U} = (\hat{u}_1, \cdots, \hat{u}_N)$ as below:

$$\hat{u}_i(\mathbf{x}) = \begin{cases} 1, & i = i_{\min}(\mathbf{x}); \\ 0, & i \neq i_{\min}(\mathbf{x}). \end{cases} \tag{14}$$

where

$$i_{\min}(\mathbf{x}) = \arg\min_i \{d_i(I(\mathbf{x}))\}.$$

3 Experimental Results

In this section, we apply the proposed CLIC algorithm to 3T and 7T MR images to demonstrate its effectiveness. As mentioned above, the CLIC algorithm is robust to initialization of the variables U, c, and b. To demonstrate the robustness, the initializations of these variables for the experiments in this paper are all generated as random numbers (for c) and random fields (for b and U). The parameter σ in the truncated Gaussian kernel K can be chosen from the range of $4 \leq \sigma \leq 7$ for 3T MR images, while we set $\sigma = 4$ for 7T MR images. The fuzzifier q is set to 2 for all the images in this paper.

3.1 Application to 3T MR Images

We first show the results for MR images obtained at 3T in Fig. 1. Inhomogeneity of the image intensity can be clearly seen in the original images in Fig. 1(a). The extracted bias field and the corresponding bias corrected image are shown in Figs 1(b) and 1(c), respectively. Note that we usually display the extracted bias field only on a mask of the brain. In the bias corrected image, the intensities within each tissue become quite homogeneous.

The improvement of the image quality in terms of intensity homogeneity can also be demonstrated by comparing the histograms of the original images and the bias corrected images, as shown in Fig. 1(f). There are three well-defined and well-separated peaks in the histograms of the bias corrected image, corresponding to the background, gray matter (GM), and white matter (WM). The peak for the cerebrospinal fluid (CSF) is not so well-defined (the one between the peaks for the background and the GM), as the volume of the CSF is relatively small. The histograms of the original images do not have such well-separated or well-defined peaks due to the mixture of the intensity distributions for different tissues caused by the bias.

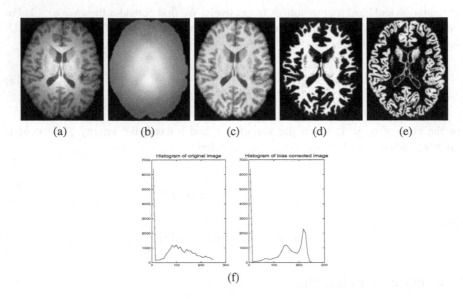

(a)   (b)   (c)   (d)   (e)

(f)

Fig. 1. Applications of our method to a 3T MR image. (a) Original image; (b) Extracted bias field (displayed on the brain mask); (c) Bias corrected image; (d) Membership function for WM; (e) Membership function for GM; (f) Comparison of histograms of the original image (left) and bias corrected image (right).

It is worth noting that the proposed algorithm does not rely on skull stripping. For example, we apply the CLIC algorithm to a 3T MR image of a brain shown in Fig. 2(a) without stripping the skull. Desirable results of bias corrected image and tissue segmentation are obtained as shown in Figs. 2(b) and 2(c), respectively. Comparison of the histograms of the original images in Fig. 2(d) further demonstrates the improved image quality.

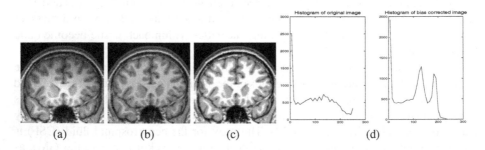

(a)   (b)   (c)   (d)

Fig. 2. Applications of our method to a 3T MR image. (a) Original image; (b) Bias corrected image; (c) Segmentation result; (d) Comparison of histograms of the original image (left) and bias corrected image (right).

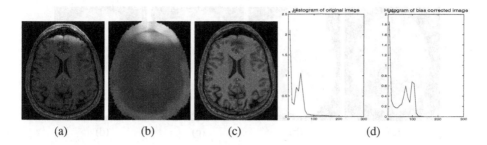

Fig. 3. Applications of our method to a 7T MR image. (a) Original image; (b) Extracted bias field (displayed on the brain mask); (c) Bias corrected image; (d) Comparison of histograms of the original image (left) and bias corrected image (right).

3.2 Application to 7T MR Images

The CLIC algorithm has also been tested on 7T MR images, where attenuation of the RF fields and standing wave effects are more pronounced than at lower fields. In addition, susceptibility-induced gradients, which scale with the main field, cause signal dephasing and more local signal bias. Such effects are most pronounced at air/tissue interfaces, as can be seen from the 7T MR image in Fig. 3(a), which appear as highly localized and strong biases. The extracted bias field of this image and the bias corrected image are shown in Figs. 3(b) and 3(c), respectively. Comparison of the histograms of the original image (left in Fig. 3(d)) and the bias corrected image (left in Fig. 3(d)) further demonstrates the improved image quality after bias field correction.

3.3 Validation and Method Comparisons

To quantitatively evaluate and compare the proposed CLIC algorithm with other algorithms. we use the synthetic MR images with ground truth from BrainWeb: http://www.bic.mni.mcgill.ca/brainweb/. We use Jaccard similarity (JS) as the metric to quantitatively evaluate the segmentation accuracy. The JS is defined as

$$J(S_1, S_2) = \frac{|S_1 \cap S_2|}{|S_1 \cup S_2|} \tag{15}$$

Table 1. Evaluation of tissue segmentation in terms of Jaccard Similarity Coefficients

		Wells	Leemput	CLIC
	WM	90.60%	85.17%	**95.76%**
Synthetic image 1	GM	80.90%	71.12%	**88.37%**
	CSF	84.53%	81.38%	**89.87%**
	WM	91.05%	82.30%	**92.55%**
Synthetic image 2	GM	80.02%	65.37%	**82.19 %**
	CSF	82.49%	79.07%	**86.33 %**

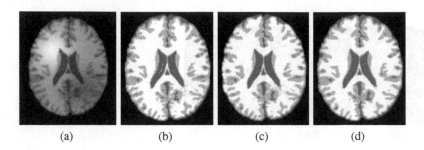

| (a) | (b) | (c) | (d) |

Fig. 4. Segmentation results for a synthetic image. (a) Original image; (b) Result of Wells *et al.*'s method. (c) Result of Leemput *et al.*'s method. (d) Result of our method.

where $| \cdot |$ represents the area of a region, S_1 is the region segmented by the algorithm, and S_2 is the corresponding region in the ground truth. The closer the JS values to 1, the better the segmentation and bias correction. We applied the algorithms of Wells *et al.* [11] and Leemput *et al.* [12] on two synthetic images. The tissue segmentation for the noisy images is shown in Fig. 4 as an example. The resulting JS values for the three methods are listed in Table 1. It can be seen that the JS valics of our method are higher than the other two methods.

4   Conclusion

We have introduced a coherent local intensity clustering (CLIC) criterion function as a metric to evaluate tissue classification and bias field estimation based on an important characteristic of local intensities in MR images. An integration of this metric defines an energy on a bias field, membership functions of the tissues, and the parameters that approximate the true signal from the corresponding tissues. Tissue classification and bias field estimation are simultaneously achieved by minimizing this energy. The smoothness of the derived optimal bias field is intrinsically ensured by the spatially coherent nature of the CLIC criterion function. As a result, no extra effort is needed to smooth the bias field in our method. Moreover, the proposed CLIC algorithm is robust to the choice of initial conditions, thereby allowing fully automatic applications. The CLIC algorithm has been applied to high field and ultra high field MR images with promising results.

References

1. Lewis, E., Fox, N.: Correction of differential intensity inhomogeneity in longitudinal MR images. Neuroimage 23(1), 75–83 (2004)
2. Johnston, B., Atkins, M.S., Mackiewich, B., Anderson, M.: Segmentation of multiple sclerosis lesions in intensity corrected multispectral MRI. IEEE Trans. Med. Imag. 15(2), 154–169 (1996)

3. Brinkmann, B., Manduca, A., Robb, R.: Optimized homomorphic unsharp masking for MR grayscale inhomogeneity correction. IEEE Trans. Med. Imag. 17(2), 161–174 (1998)
4. Cohen, M., DuBois, R., Zeineh, M.: Rapid and effective correction of RF inhomogeneity for high field magnetic resonance imaging. Hum. Brain Mapp. 10, 204–211 (2000)
5. Vokurka, E., Thacker, N., Jackson, A.: A fast model independent method for automatic correction of intensity nonuniformity in MRI data. J. Magn. Reson. Imag. 10, 550–562 (1999)
6. Meyer, C., Bland, P., Pipe, J.: Retrospective correction of intensity inhomogeneities in MRI. IEEE Trans. Med. Imag. 14(1), 36–41 (1995)
7. Milles, J., Zhu, Y.M., Chen, N., Panych, L.P., Gimenez, G., Guttmann, C.R.: MRI intensity nonuniformity correction using simultaneously spatial and gray-level histogram information. In: Proc. SPIE Med. Imag. 2004: Physiol., Function, Structure Med. Images, vol. 5370, pp. 734–742 (2004)
8. Vemuri, P., Kholmovski, E., Parker, D., Chapman, B.: Coil sensitivity estimation for optimal SNR reconstruction and intensity inhomogeneity correction in phased array MR imaging. In: Christensen, G.E., Sonka, M. (eds.) IPMI 2005. LNCS, vol. 3565, pp. 603–614. Springer, Heidelberg (2005)
9. Sled, J., Zijdenbos, A., Evans, A.: A nonparametric method for automatic correction of intensity nonuniformity in MRI data. IEEE Trans. Med. Imaging 17(1), 87–97 (1998)
10. Styner, M., Brechbuhler, C., Szekely, G., Gerig, G.: Parametric estimate of intensity inhomogeneities applied to MRI. IEEE Trans. Med. Imag. 19(3), 153–165 (2000)
11. Wells, W., Grimson, E., Kikinis, R., Jolesz, F.: Adaptive segmentation of MRI data. IEEE Trans. Med. Imag. 15(4), 429–442 (1996)
12. Leemput, V., Maes, K., Vandermeulen, D., Suetens, P.: Automated model-based bias field correction of MR images of the brain. IEEE Trans. Med. Imag. 18(10), 885–896 (1999)
13. Guillemaud, R., Brady, J.: Estimating the bias field of MR images. IEEE Trans. Med. Imag. 16(3), 238–251 (1997)
14. Pham, D., Prince, J.: Adaptive fuzzy segmentation of magnetic resonance images. IEEE Trans. Med. Imag. 18(9), 737–752 (1999)
15. Zhang, Y., Brady, M., Smith, S.: Segmentation of brain MR images through a hidden Markov random field model and the expectation-maximization algorithm. IEEE Trans. Med. Imag. 20(1), 45–57 (2001)
16. Liew, A., Yan, H.: An adaptive spatial fuzzy clustering algorithm for 3-D MR image segmentation. IEEE Trans. Med. Imag. 22(9), 1063–1075 (2003)
17. Li, C., Gatenby, C., Wang, L., Gore, J.: A robust parametric method for bias field estimation and segmentation of MR images. In: Proceedings of IEEE Conference on Computer Vision and Pattern Recognition (CVPR) (2009)
18. Vovk, U., Pernus, F., Likar, B.: A review of methods for correction of intensity inhomogeneity in MRI. IEEE Trans. Med. Imag. 26(3), 405–421 (2007)
19. Gispert, J., Reig, S., Pascau, J., Vaquero, J., Garcia-Barreno, P., Desco, M.: Method for bias field correction of brain t1-weighted magnetic resonance images minimizing segmentation error. Human Brain Mapping 22(2), 133–144 (2004)
20. Ahmed, M., Yamany, S., Mohamed, N., Farag, A., Moriarty, T.: A modified fuzzy c-means algorithm for bias field estimation and segmentation of MRI data. IEEE Trans. Med. Imaging 21(3), 193–199 (2002)

A Unified Framework for MR Based Disease Classification

Kilian M. Pohl[1,2] and Mert R. Sabuncu[2]

[1] Healthcare Informatics, IBM Almaden Research Center, San Jose, CA, USA
pohl@us.ibm.com
[2] Computer Science and Artificial Intelligence Lab,
Massachusetts Institute of Technology, Cambridge, MA, USA
msabuncu@csail.mit.edu

Abstract. In this paper, we employ an anatomical parameterization of spatial warps to reveal structural differences between medical images of healthy control subjects and disease patients. The warps are represented as structure-specific 9-parameter affine transformations, which constitute a global, non-rigid mapping between the atlas and image coordinates. Our method estimates the structure-specific transformation parameters directly from medical scans by minimizing a Kullback-Leibler divergence measure. The resulting parameters are then input to a linear Support Vector Machine classifier, which assigns individual scans to a specific clinical group. The classifier also enables us to interpret the anatomical differences between groups, as we can visualize the discriminative warp that best differentiates the two groups. We test the accuracy of our approach on a data set consisting of Magnetic Resonance scans from 16 first episode schizophrenics and 17 age-matched healthy control subjects. The data set also contains manual labels for four regions of interest in both hemispheres: superior temporal gyrus, amygdala, hippocampus, and para-hippocampal gyrus. On this small size data set, our approach, which performs classification based on the MR images directly, yields a leave-one-out cross-validation accuracy of up to 90%. This compares favorably with the accuracy achieved by state-of-the-art techniques in schizophrenia MRI research.

1 Introduction

Thanks to in-vivo imaging technologies like magnetic resonance images (MRI), the last few decades have witnessed a rapid growth in the amount of research that explores structural and functional abnormalities due to certain diseases (see e.g. [1]). Studies that investigate such inter-group differences rely heavily on the notion of cross-subject correspondence. They ensure cross-subject correspondence, for example, by extracting structure-specific features from labor-intensive manual segmentations [2,3]. An alternative strategy is to investigate thousands of local features, such as in [4,5,6], but determining an unbiased dense spatial correspondence across a heterogeneous population is challenging. In this paper,

J.L. Prince, D.L. Pham, and K.J. Myers (Eds.): IPMI 2009, LNCS 5636, pp. 300–313, 2009.

we propose an alternative methodology that employs local features, yet takes advantage of well-established structure-based correspondence across individuals.

In schizophrenia research, structural imaging studies have traditionally focused on showing differences between the sizes of certain brain regions [7]. Other studies have shown that various boundary and/or skeleton shape representations can also be employed for discriminating corresponding structures in two different groups [2,3]. These structure-based morphology methods typically require a *priori* knowledge about abnormal regions, which generally is extracted from manual segmentations [8]. Generating manual segmentations is labor intensive and therefore limits the size of datasets used by structure-based morphological methods. This shortcoming can be addressed by automatic segmentations but any bias or error in the segmentations will negatively impact the analysis.

As an alternative strategy, recent research has proposed automatic comparative analysis techniques that typically investigate thousands of features from each image. There are two flavors to this approach: voxel-based and deformation-based morphology. The first approach attempts to discover statistical differences in, for example, tissue density at various voxel locations between the groups [9]. This assumes a global spatial normalization of the images. Once voxel-wise correspondence is established, various local measurements are compared across subjects. The second approach is to employ a highly nonlinear registration algorithm to align the subjects with a template. A discriminative analysis then can be conducted based on the deformation fields [10] or both the deformation fields and residual images [11]. Rather than performing voxel-by-voxel univariate comparisons, other studies [4,5,6] have employed a large number of features to improve the statistical separation between two groups. These approaches provide the potential to design accurate classification algorithms that, in the future, can be used for diagnostic purposes. In these techniques, inter-subject spatial correspondence is often achieved using a non-linear intensity-based image registration algorithm, where the quality of alignment is quantified by the similarity between intensity values or local attribute vectors [12], and the warps that capture inter-subject anatomical variability are represented via arbitrary mechanical or probabilistic models. The high-dimensional nature of the problem and modeling assumptions made in the formulations can potentially bias inferences based on these registration results.

The community has suggested various dimensionality reduction methods (e.g. Principal Component Analysis [13]) and feature selection techniques (e.g. Recursive Feature Elimination [8]) to tackle the problem of learning in very high dimensions with a small training set. The outcome of these methods tend to be a complex mixture and/or a subset of the original feature space. Alternatively, researchers have proposed image features encoding local statistics or texture[6]. However, the complex nature of these features can obscure classification and make clinical interpretation difficult.

In this paper, we propose a population analysis methodology that takes advantage of the well-established structure-based correspondence across individuals. This approach is different from a majority of today's morphology methods that employ local descriptors and assume correspondence between these. In the proposed framework, we encode the inter-subject spatial mapping via structure-specific affine registration parameters. These parameters are global to each structure so that we do not introduce any further ambiguity to the correspondence problem.

Similar to [14,15], we compute the transformation parameters directly from the images by employing a Bayesian framework that models the relationship between the segmentation labels, transformation parameters and image intensities. Each structure-specific transformation is encoded by a global, 9-parameter affine model. Our method then uses a linear Support Vector Machine (SVM) [16] classifier to jointly examine subtle differences in the affine registration parameters across all structures while characterizing natural variability within the population. This analysis reveals the anatomical separation between two groups. The separation can be analyzed by generating warps based on the weights of the linear classifier [2]. We use these warps to visualize the most significant anatomical differences between the groups under study.

We test the accuracy of the proposed method on a data set consisting of 16 first episode schizophrenics and 17 age-matched healthy subjects [17]. The original morphometry study that used this data [17] studied volumetric measurements of eight temporal lobe structures, obtained from manual segmentations of the MR images. The goal of that study was to show statistical differences in independent volumetric measurements between first-order schizophrenics and controls. In the present paper, we show that a linear SVM trained on all eight volumetric measurements achieves a leave-one-out cross-validation accuracy of 69%. In comparison, the linear SVM based on our structure specific 9-parameter affine parameters achieves a cross-validation accuracy of up to 90%. This accuracy also compares favorably with state-of-the-art methods for schizophrenia classification based on MRI data [4].

The contributions of this paper are multi-fold: we present a new population analysis approach that takes advantage of unambiguous, well-established correspondences between anatomical structures to reduce the dimensionality of the problem. In the proposed framework, the discriminative features can be interpreted in anatomical terms. Furthermore, the integrated automatic segmentation procedure will allow us to deploy our analysis on large collections of image data, for which we may not have manual segmentations.

2   Classifying Images Based on Registration Parameters

Our population analysis methodology has two stages: the extraction of structure-specific image features and the discriminative statistical analysis of these feature samples. In the remainder of this section, we first derive a formulation for extracting structure-specific registration parameters from images. We then use a linear classifier to conduct a statistical analysis on these feature samples.

2.1   An Iterative Approach for Computing Warps

Let $\mathcal{T} \triangleq (\mathcal{T}_1, \ldots, \mathcal{T}_N)$ be the parameter set of structure-specific transformations, where N is the number of structures of interest (including a background label). In the following, we will assume the existence of an atlas and corresponding coordinate system, which we define in more detail in Section 2.2. For each structure $i \in \{1, \ldots, N\}$, $\mathcal{T}_i$ defines a mapping from the image coordinate frame to the atlas coordinate frame. We are interested in estimating $\mathcal{T}$ directly from the image $\mathcal{I}$ using a Maximum *A Posteriori* (MAP) formulation:

$$\hat{\mathcal{T}} = \arg\max_{\mathcal{T}} \log P(\mathcal{T}|\mathcal{I}) = \arg\max_{\mathcal{T}} \log P(\mathcal{I}, \mathcal{T}). \tag{1}$$

At this point, we introduce another random variable $\mathcal{L}$, which encodes the anatomical label at each voxel. As commonly done in the literature, we will factorize the joint probability on $P(\mathcal{I}, \mathcal{T}, \mathcal{L})$ using three distributions:

- a prior distribution on the transformation parameters: $P(\mathcal{T})$,
- a conditional label prior distribution: $P(\mathcal{L}|\mathcal{T})$, and
- the image likelihood, which we assume to be independent of $\mathcal{T}$:
  $P(\mathcal{I}|\mathcal{L}, \mathcal{T}) = P(\mathcal{I}|\mathcal{L})$.

Next, we can rewrite Equation (1) by marginalizing $P(\mathcal{I}, \mathcal{T}, \mathcal{L})$ over all possible label maps $\mathcal{L}$:

$$\hat{\mathcal{T}} = \arg\max_{\mathcal{T}} \log \sum_{\mathcal{L}} P(\mathcal{I}, \mathcal{L}, \mathcal{T}) = \arg\max_{\mathcal{T}} \log \sum_{\mathcal{L}} P(\mathcal{I}, \mathcal{L}|\mathcal{T}) + \log P(\mathcal{T})$$

$$= \arg\max_{\mathcal{T}} \log \sum_{\mathcal{L}} P(\mathcal{I}|\mathcal{L}) \cdot P(\mathcal{L}|\mathcal{T}) + \log P(\mathcal{T}) \tag{2}$$

where $\sum_A$ represents the sum over all possible values of A.

Equation (2) can be optimized using an Expectation Maximization (EM) strategy. Given a current estimate $\mathcal{T}'$ of $\hat{\mathcal{T}}$, we can expand Equation (2) with the posterior label probability $P(\mathcal{L}|\mathcal{T}', \mathcal{I})$

$$\hat{\mathcal{T}} = \arg\max_{\mathcal{T}} \log \sum_{\mathcal{L}} \frac{P(\mathcal{L}|\mathcal{T}', \mathcal{I}) \cdot P(\mathcal{I}|\mathcal{L}) \cdot P(\mathcal{L}|\mathcal{T})}{P(\mathcal{L}|\mathcal{T}', \mathcal{I})} + \log P(\mathcal{T})$$

and then apply Jensen's inequality to obtain an easier to optimize, tight lower bound:

$$\log \sum_{\mathcal{L}} P(\mathcal{L}|\mathcal{T}', \mathcal{I}) \cdot \frac{P(\mathcal{I}|\mathcal{L}) \cdot P(\mathcal{L}|\mathcal{T})}{P(\mathcal{L}|\mathcal{T}', \mathcal{I})} \geq \sum_{\mathcal{L}} P(\mathcal{L}|\mathcal{T}', \mathcal{I}) \cdot \log \left(\frac{P(\mathcal{I}|\mathcal{L}) \cdot P(\mathcal{L}|\mathcal{T})}{P(\mathcal{L}|\mathcal{T}', \mathcal{I})} \right),$$

which achieves equality for $\mathcal{T} = \mathcal{T}'$. We can then update $\mathcal{T}'$ by maximizing the lower bound:

$$\mathcal{T}' \leftarrow \arg\max_{\mathcal{T}} \sum_{\mathcal{L}} P(\mathcal{L}|\mathcal{T}', \mathcal{I}) \cdot \log \left(\frac{P(\mathcal{L}|\mathcal{T})}{P(\mathcal{L}|\mathcal{T}', \mathcal{I})} \right) + \log P(\mathcal{T})$$

$$= \arg\min_{\mathcal{T}} D_{KL}(P(\mathcal{L}|\mathcal{T}', \mathcal{I}) \| P(\mathcal{L}|\mathcal{T})) - \log P(\mathcal{T}), \tag{3}$$

where we have dropped terms that are independent of $\mathcal{T}$ and

$$D_{KL}(P||Q) = \sum_{\mathcal{L}} P(\mathcal{L}) \log \frac{P(\mathcal{L})}{Q(\mathcal{L})}$$

is the Kullback-Leibler divergence [18], a non-commutative measure of the difference between two probability distributions P and Q.

We note that this iterative scheme is an instance of the EM algorithm with the image $\mathcal{I}$ being the observed data, the label map $\mathcal{L}$ the unobserved data, and $\mathcal{T}$ the parameter. Similar to [14,15], the Expectation Step (E-Step) then computes the weights

$$\mathcal{W}(\mathcal{L}) \triangleq P(\mathcal{L}|\mathcal{T}', \mathcal{I}) \qquad (4)$$

and the Maximization Step (M-Step) updates the registration parameters by solving Equation (3).

2.2 An Example Implementation

Let us now instantiate the probabilistic model of the previous section. We will denote the stacked up image voxels as $\mathcal{I} \triangleq (\mathcal{I}_1, \ldots, \mathcal{I}_K)$, where K is the number of voxels. Similarly, the (possibly unknown) label map $\mathcal{L} \triangleq (\mathcal{L}_1, \ldots, \mathcal{L}_K)$ is a vector with K entries, where $\mathcal{L}_j \in \{1, \ldots, N\}$ denotes the label at voxel j (including a label for background). For simplicity, we will assume a suitable interpolator and treat the atlas $\mathcal{A} \triangleq (\mathcal{A}_1, \ldots, \mathcal{A}_N)$ as a collection of N continuous label probability images defined in the atlas coordinate frame, where at each location $k \in \{1, \ldots, K\}$, $\mathcal{A}_i(k)$ encodes the prior probability of structure $i \in 1, \ldots, N$. The structure-specific registration parameters $\{\mathcal{T}_i\}$ are length-9 vectors (which include 3 translational, 3 rotational and 3 scaling parameters) that define an affine mapping from the image coordinates to the atlas $\mathcal{A}_i$. Abusing notation, we will use $\mathcal{T}_i(k)$ to denote the mapped point of the image voxel k.

We now make several assumptions that allow us to simplify Equation (3):

– The registration parameters $\{\mathcal{T}_i\}$ have independent uniform priors:

$$P(\mathcal{T}) = \prod_i P(\mathcal{T}_i), \; P(\mathcal{T}_i) = \text{const.}$$

– The image likelihood is spatially independent $P(\mathcal{I}|\mathcal{L}) = \prod_k P(\mathcal{I}_k|\mathcal{L}_k)$ and $P(\mathcal{I}_k|\mathcal{L}_k)$ depends on the imaging modality.
– The conditional label distribution is spatially independent, $P(\mathcal{L}|\mathcal{T}) = \prod_k P(\mathcal{L}_k|\mathcal{T})$, and defined as $P(\mathcal{L}_k = i|\mathcal{T}) = \frac{A_i(\mathcal{T}_i(k))}{\sum_l A_l(\mathcal{T}_l(k))}$.

Based on these assumptions, we can rewrite the E-step of Equation (4) as

$$\mathcal{W}(\mathcal{L}) = \prod_k \mathcal{W}_k(\mathcal{L}_k) \text{ with } \mathcal{W}_k(\mathcal{L}_k) \propto P(\mathcal{I}_k|\mathcal{L}_k) \cdot A_{\mathcal{L}_k}(\mathcal{T}'_{\mathcal{L}_k}(k)). \qquad (5)$$

Using the uniform prior on $\mathcal{T}$ and inserting Equation (5) into Equation (3) yields:

$$\mathcal{T}' \leftarrow \arg\min_{\mathcal{T}} \sum_k D_{KL}(\mathcal{W}_k(\mathcal{L}_k)\|P(\mathcal{L}_k|\mathcal{T})) = \arg\min_{\mathcal{T}} \sum_k D_{KL}\left(\mathcal{W}_k(\mathcal{L}_k)\|\frac{A_{\mathcal{L}_k}(\mathcal{T}_{\mathcal{L}_k}(k))}{\sum_l A_l(\mathcal{T}_l(k))}\right)$$

$$= \arg\min_{\mathcal{T}} \sum_k \left(D_{KL}\left(P(I_k|\mathcal{L}_k)A_{\mathcal{L}_k}(\mathcal{T}'_{\mathcal{L}_k}(k))\|A_{\mathcal{L}_k}(\mathcal{T}_{\mathcal{L}_k}(k))\right) - \log\left(\sum_l A_l(\mathcal{T}_l(k))\right)\right), \quad (6)$$

where we abuse notation and only require that the second argument of the KL divergence normalizes to some constant, not necessarily 1. Note that in our implementation, we assume the image is globally aligned with the atlas coordinate frame, and thus fix the transformation associated with the background label to this global transformation.

In summary, the algorithm estimates the transformation parameters $\mathcal{T}$ by repeatedly solving Equation (2.2) until convergence. We note that the update equations do not specify the label likelihood $P(I_k|\mathcal{L}_k)$, as its definition depends on the type of medical scan, which in our case is MR data. Many methods in the literature that deal with MRI, such as [14,15,19,20], model $P(I_k|\mathcal{L}_k)$ using an independent Gaussian distribution with a mean modulated by a spatially varying multiplicative factor that captures MR inhomogeneity. For convenience, we use the same model and sequentially estimate its parameters within the EM algorithm (see also [21]).

2.3 Classification of Structure-Specific Transformation Parameters

In the second stage of our analysis, the estimated transformation parameters $\hat{\mathcal{T}}$ are fed into a linear Support Vector Machine (SVM) classifier [16]. In the following, we use $\mathcal{T}$ to denote a vector obtained by concatenating the structure-specific transformation parameters $\mathcal{T}_i$ (excluding the background label). Given a collection of transformation parameter values from two groups, the linear classifier searches for a weight vector λ that maximizes the "spread" between the projected scalar values $t \triangleq \lambda^T \cdot \mathcal{T}$ of the two groups. One advantage of using a linear classifier is that its weights can be interpreted as change along the normal of the separating hyperplane [2]: changing the value of a sample in the direction of λ will bring it closer to the positive class, while a change in the opposite direction will have the reverse effect. In our context, this allows us to illustrate the discriminating warp between the two groups of interest.

3   Classifying MR Images into Schizophrenic vs. Healthy

3.1   Data

We test the accuracy of our classifier on a data set that contains MR images of 33 subjects. Sixteen of the patients were diagnosed as first episode schizophrenia and the remaining seventeen are age-matched healthy control subjects. Because first episode patients are relatively free of confounds such as the long-term effects of medication, any difference between these two groups may be considered as a more direct indication of disease-specific abnormalities compared to, say, chronic cases. Each scan was acquired on 1.5 Tesla General Electric Scanner using a SPoiled Gradient-Recalled (SPGR) sequence with a voxel dimension of $0.9375 \times 0.9375 \times 1.5$ mm^3. Each scan was manually segmented into the (right and left) Superior Temporal Gyrus (STG) and three medial temporal lobe structures: Hippocampus (HIP), Amygdala (AMY) and Parahippocampal Gyrus (PHG). Further details about the data set can be found in [17].

3.2 Atlas Construction

Our framework requires the construction of an atlas from a collection of manually labeled training data. We first perform a global co-registration of all the 33 MRI volumes: each image is aligned with a dynamically evolving mean template [22,23]. The similarity measure is the mutual information between pixel intensities of the image and current estimate of the template, and the transformations are parameterized using a global 9 parameter affine model. We choose this approach based on our comparison of different atlas generation methods on the same data set [24].

Once all the images are spatially normalized, we compute the atlas $\mathcal{A}$. For each test subject, we construct a separate *leave-one-out* atlas: at each atlas voxel, we compute the frequency of each anatomical label, excluding the test subject. Figure 1 visualizes such an atlas, where we have rendered the 50% iso-probability surfaces for each one of the labels of interest and overlaid these on slices of the average MRI volume.

3.3 Transformation Parameters

The structure-specific transformations are parameterized using a 9 parameter affine model. The parameters include 3 transformations (t_x, t_y, t_z) along the

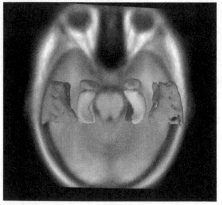
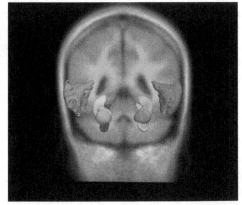

(a) Axial view	(b) Coronal view

Fig. 1. Three dimensional renderings of the 50% iso-probability surfaces for each structure overlaid on the average MRI scan: STG is shown in brown and blue; HIP in cyan and yellow; AMY in red and green; and PHG in pink and purple

	Axial	Coronal

Control (color) vs. Schiz. (gray)

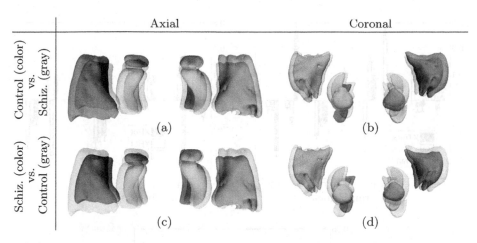

(a)   (b)

Schiz. (color) vs. Control (gray)

(c)   (d)

Fig. 2. Discriminating transformation between the two groups: Axial and coronal views of (a-b) the atlas warped towards the control group (in color) overlaid on the atlas warped towards the schizophrenic group (Schiz.) in semi-transparent gray; (c-d) the atlas warped towards the schizophrenic group (in color) overlaid on the atlas warped towards the control group (semi-transparent gray).

three axes:, 3 rotation angles $(\theta_x, \theta_y, \theta_z)$ around the x, y, z axes, and 3 scale coefficients (s_x, s_y, s_z) along the three axes. In our convention, the x coordinate represents the medial-lateral axis with increasing values indicating the left, increasing y denotes more superior and increasing z denotes more anterior. Formally, the transformation that maps the image coordinate $k \triangleq (x, y, z)$ to the atlas coordinate $\tilde{k} \triangleq (\tilde{x}, \tilde{y}, \tilde{z})$ is:

$$\tilde{k}^T = S \cdot R \cdot (x, y, z)^T + (t_x, t_y, t_z)^T, \tag{7}$$

where S is a diagonal matrix with diagonal elements defined by (s_x, s_y, s_z) and $R \triangleq R_x(\theta_x) \cdot R_y(\theta_y) \cdot R_z(\theta_z)$ is the rotation matrix with $R_u(\theta_u)$ being the rotation matrix around axis 'u'. We note that we use for the SVM the logarithm of the scale coefficients instead of the scale coefficient directly.

3.4   Automatic Segmentation of New Subject

Given a new subject with no manual labels, we run the EM-algorithm described in the previous section that jointly estimates the structure-specific registration parameters and segmentation labels. For each test subject we use its corresponding leave-one-out atlas. In practice, we have also found that treating the background label differently from the other labels improves segmentation accuracy: we fix the background label's transformation to a global transformation obtained through a pairwise image registration procedure, where the new subject is aligned with the atlas template using a B-spline transformation model [25,26]. We initialize our EM algorithm using segmentations obtained from an atlas-based method [21] that solves registration (with a B-spline model) and segmentation sequen-

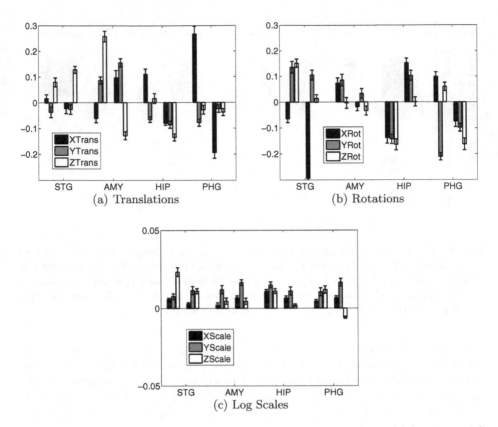

Fig. 3. The SVM weights for the affine parameters of the right and left anatomical structures of interest

tially. As we report in [24], this method, that we use for initialization, achieves accurate segmentation for all ROIs except PHG.

3.5   Statistical Analysis

The structure-specific transformation parameters of each new subject are then considered as samples for our statistical analysis. Figure 5 plots five features that demonstrate the highest individual separation (measured using an unpaired t-test) between schizophrenics and controls. Note that, even the feature with the lowest p-value (medial-lateral translation of the left PHG) does not demonstrate complete separation between the groups. We first train a linear SVM on all 33 subjects to analyze the separation between the groups. We achieve 100% training accuracy, which can be observed in Figure 5(f) that plots the transformation parameters linearly projected on to the normal of the SVM's separating hyperplane. Since the training data was linearly separable, the linear SVM classifier was parameter-free.

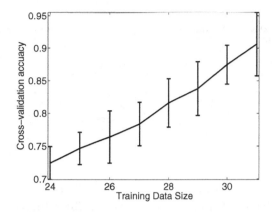

Fig. 4. Cross-validation accuracy versus training size.

As we previously discussed, the weights of the trained linear classifier can be used to analyze the discrimination between the groups. Let λ denote the weights of the classifier, such that $\lambda^T T$ is positive for age-matched healthy control subjects. If we apply a warp with $T = \alpha\lambda$, for some $\alpha > 0$, to the *total* atlas $\mathcal{A}$ computed on all subjects, this warped atlas will represent the "healthier" population. Similarly a warp in the opposite direction $-\alpha\lambda$ will represent a more "schizophrenic" population. We can therefore view λ as the discriminating transformation between schizophrenics and controls. Figure 2 overlays these warped atlases on top of each other to illustrate the discriminating transformation. Note that, in this figure we have chosen $\alpha = 5$, exaggerating the discrimination between the two groups for illustrative purposes.

Figure 3 shows the weights of the linear SVM classifier. Here, we performed 33 leave-one-out training procedures to obtain 33 different sets of weights. The plot shows the average over these cases and the error bars indicate the standard error, to illustrate the variability of the weights. In this analysis, the translational and scaling components are easier to interpret: e.g. a translation along the x-axis tells us whether a structure is more lateral or medial in one group and a scale along the y-axis indicates a length difference in inferior-superior direction. On the other hand, the rotational parameters are trickier to understand: a z-rotation represents a tilt of the sagittal plane. Some preliminary interpretations suggested by the analysis of Figure 3 are that in normal controls: the left STG is longer in the posterior-anterior direction, the left AMY is more posterior, and the left PHG is more lateral. Figure 2 visualizes these differences all together. We leave a detailed analysis of these results to future work.

To understand how generalization accuracy changes as a function of training data size we conducted the following jackknife experiment. We held out each subject and performed a repeated random sampling cross-validation on the remaining 32 subjects, while varying the training set size between 24 and 31. Thus, we obtained a cross-validation accuracy estimate for each hold-out subject and training set size. Figure 4 plots the average and standard deviation of these 33

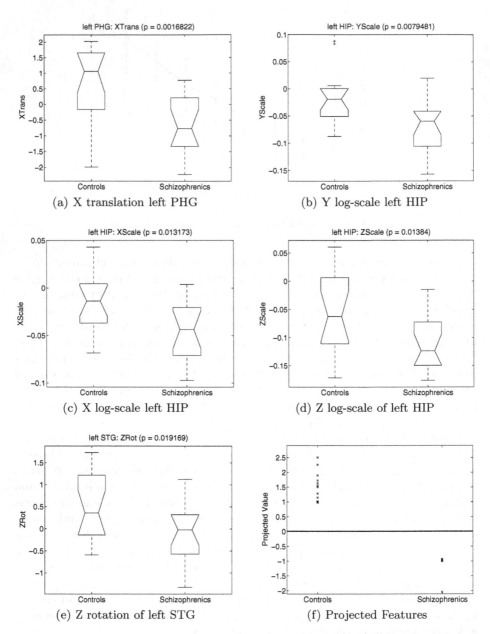

Fig. 5. (a-e): Boxplots of the top five structure-specific transformation parameters that demonstrate the highest separation between the two groups. p-values for unpaired t-tests are included in the title of each plot. (f) The transformation parameters when linearly projected on to the normal of the separating hyperplane of the SVM.

values as a function of training data size. We note that the standard deviation, indicated by the error bars, reflects our uncertainty in the generalization performance but is an underestimate of the underlying variance [27]. We observe that generalization accuracy continues to increase with the training data size, suggesting that more data would be helpful in building a better classifier for discriminating between schizophrenics versus controls. The final generalization accuracy reaches 90%.

As a further analysis, we trained separate linear SVMs on the 9 affine parameters of each structure. Only the parameters associated with left AMY, left and right HIPP, and left PHG yielded a significant discrimination of the two populations, with 61%, 70%, 54% and 60% as the respective leave-one-out (LOO) cross-validation accuracy values. We also trained linear SVMs on the parameters corresponding to each hemisphere independently. According to our LOO cross-validation, the two hemispheres manifested the same discriminative power, with 67% accuracy. To measure the discriminative power of volumetric measurements only and provide a benchmark against our results, we trained a linear SVM on the volumes of the manual segmentations. Thus each sample was a length-8 vector of the absolute sizes of the manually delineated regions of interest. LOO cross-validation accuracy for this feature set was 69%. This result suggests that the 9 parameter characterization of each structure obtained from our framework yields an improved discriminative power than size measurements of manual segmentations.

4   Conclusion

In this paper, we developed a deformation-based classifier that directly assigns a medical scan to a healthy or disease patient group. The assignment is based on an anatomical parameterization of the warp that leverages a structure-based correspondence across individuals. In our implementation, the parameters are a set of structure-specific affine registration parameters. These parameters are computed by minimizing the Kullback-Leibler divergence between the posterior label probability of the subject and structure prior probability of the atlas. The affine registration parameters are then fed into a linear support vector machine for classifying the image scan. The weights of this linear classifier can then be interpreted as a warp that discriminates the two groups. On an MR data set with 16 first episode schizophrenics and 17 age-matched healthy subjects, our approach achieves a promising cross-validation accuracy of up to 90%.

Acknowledgments. The authors would like to thank William Wells, Koen Van Leemput and Wanmei Ou for their feedback on this work, and Martha Shenton for providing the data. The research was partially supported by the following grants: NIH NIBIB NAMIC U54-EB005149, NIH NCRR NAC P41-RR13218, NIH NINDS R01-NS051826.

References

1. Shenton, M., Dickey, C., Frumin, M., McCarley, R.: A review of MRI findings in schizophrenia. Schizophrenia Research 49(1-2), 1–52 (2001)
2. Golland, P., Grimson, W., Kikinis, R.: Statistical shape analysis using fixed topology skeletons: Corpus callosum study. In: Kuba, A., Sámal, M., Todd-Pokropek, A. (eds.) IPMI 1999. LNCS, vol. 1613, pp. 382–387. Springer, Heidelberg (1999)
3. Styner, M., Lieberman, J.A., Pantazis, D., Gerig, G.: Boundary and medial shape analysis of the hippocampus in schizophrenia. Medical Image Analysis 8(3), 197–203 (2004)
4. Davatzikos, C., Shen, D., Gur, R.C., Wu, X., Liu, D., Fan, Y., Hughett, P., Turetsky, B.I., Gur, R.E.: Whole-brain morphometric study of schizophrenia reveals a spatially complex set of focal abnormalities. Archives of General Psychiatry 62, 1218–1227 (2005)
5. Lao, Z., Shena, D., Xuea, Z., Karacalia, B., Resnickb, S.M., Davatzikos, C.: Morphological classification of brains via high-dimensional shape transformations and machine learning methods. NeuroImage 21, 46–57 (2004)
6. Liu, Y., Teverovskiy, L., Carmichael, O., Kikinis, R., Shenton, M., Carter, C., Stenger, V.A., Davis, S., Aizenstein, H., Becker, J., Lopez, O., Meltzer, C.: Discriminative MR image feature analysis for automatic schizophrenia and alzheimer's disease classification. In: Barillot, C., Haynor, D.R., Hellier, P. (eds.) MICCAI 2004. LNCS, vol. 3216, pp. 393–401. Springer, Heidelberg (2004)
7. Pruessner, J., Li, L., Serles, W., Pruessner, M., Collins, D., Kabani, N., Lupien, S., Evans, A.: Volumetry of hippocampus and amygdala with high-resolution MRI and three-dimensional analysis software: Minimizing the discrepencies between laboratories. Cerebral Cortex 10, 433–442 (2000)
8. Fan, Y., Shen, D., Davatzikos, C.: Classification of structural images via high-dimensional image warping, robust feature extraction, and SVM. In: Duncan, J.S., Gerig, G. (eds.) MICCAI 2005. LNCS, vol. 3749, pp. 1–8. Springer, Heidelberg (2005)
9. Ashburner, J., Friston, K.: Voxel-based morphometry - the methods. NeuroImage 11, 805–821 (2000)
10. Volz, H., Gaser, C., Sauer, H.: Supporting evidence for the model of cognitive dysmetria in schizophreniaa structural magnetic resonance imaging study using deformation-based morphometry. Schizophrenia Research 46, 45–56 (2000)
11. Davatzikos, C., Genc, A., Xu, D., Resnick, S.: Voxel-based morphometry using the ravens maps: methods and validation using simulated longitudinal atrophy. NeuroImage 14, 1361–1369 (2001)
12. Shen, D., Davatzikos, C.: Hammer: Hierarchical attribute matching mechanism for elastic registration. IEEE Transactions on Medical Imaging 21, 1421–1439 (2002)
13. Narr, K.L., Bilder, R.M., Toga, A.W., Woods, R.P., Rex, D.E., Szeszko, P.R., Robinson, D., Sevy, S., Gunduz-Bruce, H., Wang, Y.P., DeLuca, H., Thompson, P.M.: Mapping cortical thickness and gray matter concentration in first episode schizophrenia. Cerebral Cortex 15(6), 708–719 (2005)
14. Ashburner, J., Friston, K.: Unified segmentation. NeuroImage 26(3), 839–851 (2005)
15. Pohl, K.M., Fisher, J., Grimson, W., Kikinis, R., Wells, W.: A Bayesian model for joint segmentation and registration. NeuroImage 31(1), 228–239 (2006)
16. Vapnik, V.: The Nature of Statistical Learning Theory. Springer, Heidelberg (1999)

17. Hirayasu, Y., Shenton, M.E., Salisbury, D., Dickey, C., Fischer, I.A., Mazzoni, P., Kisler, T., Arakaki, H., Kwon, J.S., Anderson, J.E., Yurgelun-Todd, D., Tohen, M., McCarley, R.W.: Lower left temporal lobe MRI volumes in patients with first-episode schizophrenia compared with psychotic patients with first-episode affective disorder and normal subjects. The American Journal of Psychiatry 155(10), 1384–1391 (1998)
18. Kullback, S., Leibler, R.: On information and sufficiency. The Annals of Mathematical Statistics 22, 79–86 (1951)
19. Van Leemput, K., Maes, F., Vandermeulen, D., Suetens, P.: Automated model-based bias field correction of MR images of the brain. IEEE Transactions on Medical Imaging 18(10), 885–895 (1999)
20. Zhang, Y., Brady, M., Smith, S.: Segmentation of brain MR images through a hidden Markov random field model and the expectation-maximization algorithm. IEEE Transactions on Medical Imaging 20(1), 45–57 (2001)
21. Pohl, K., Bouix, S., Nakamura, M., Rohlfing, T., McCarley, R., Kikinis, R., Grimson, W., Shenton, M., Wells, W.: A hierarchical algorithm for MR brain image parcellation. IEEE Transactions on Medical Imaging 26(9), 1201–1212 (2007)
22. Guimond, A., Meunier, J., Thirion, J.P.: Average brain models: A convergence study. Computer Vision and Image Understanding 77(2), 192–210 (1999)
23. Lorenzen, P., Prastawa, M., Davis, B., Gerig, G., Bullitt, E., Joshi, S.: Multi-modal image set registration and atlas formation. Medical Image Analysis 10(3), 440–451 (2006)
24. Zöllei, L., Shenton, M., Wells, W., Pohl, K.: The impact of atlas formation methods on atlas-guided brain segmentation, statistical registration. In: Pair-wise and Group-wise Alignment and Atlas Formation Workshop at MICCAI 2007: Medical Image Computing and Computer-Assisted Intervention, pp. 39–46 (2007)
25. Rueckert, D., Sonoda, L., Hayes, C., Hill, D., Leach, M., Hawkes, D.: Non-rigid registration using free-form deformations: Application to breast MR images. IEEE Transactions on Medical Imaging 18(8), 712–721 (1999)
26. Rohlfing, T., Maurer Jr., C.R.: Nonrigid image registration in shared-memory multiprocessor environments with application to brains, breasts, and bees. IEEE Transactions on Information Technology in Biomedicine 7(1), 16–25 (2003)
27. Bengio, Y., Grandvalet, Y.: No unbiased estimator of the variance of k-fold cross-validation. Journal of Machine Learning Research (5), 1089–1105 (2004)

MARM: Multiscale Adaptive Regression Models for Neuroimaging Data

Hongtu Zhu[1,3], Yimei Li[1], Joseph G. Ibrahim[1], Weili Lin[2,3], and Dinggang Shen[2,3]

[1] Departments of Biostatistics, [2] Radiology, [3] Biomedical Research Imaging Center, University of North Carolina at Chapel Hill

Abstract. We develop a novel statistical model, called *multiscale adaptive regression model (MARM)*, for spatial and adaptive analysis of neuroimaging data. The primary motivation and application of the proposed methodology is statistical analysis of imaging data on the two-dimensional (2D) surface or in the 3D volume for various neuroimaging studies. The existing voxel-wise approach has several major limitations for the analyses of imaging data, underscoring the great need for methodological development. The voxel-wise approach essentially treats all voxels as independent units, whereas neuroimaging data are spatially correlated in nature and spatially contiguous regions of activation with rather sharp edges are usually expected. The initial smoothing step before the voxel-wise approach often blurs the image data near the edges of activated regions and thus it can dramatically increase the numbers of false positives and false negatives. The MARM, which is developed for addressing these limitations, has three key features in the analysis of imaging data: being spatial, being hierarchical, and being adaptive. The MARM builds a small sphere at each location (called voxel) and use these consecutively connected spheres across all voxels to capture spatial dependence among imaging observations. Then, the MARM builds hierarchically nested spheres by increasing the radius of a spherical neighborhood around each voxel and combine all the data in a given radius of each voxel with appropriate weights to adaptively calculate parameter estimates and test statistics. Theoretically, we first establish that the MARM outperforms classical voxel-wise approach. Simulation studies are used to demonstrate the methodology and examine the finite sample performance of the MARM. We apply our methods to the detection of spatial patterns of brain atrophy in a neuroimaging study of Alzheimers disease. Our simulation studies with known ground truth confirm that the MARM significantly outperforms the voxel-wise methods.

1   Introduction

Anatomical and functional magnetic resonance imaging (MRI) are powerful tools for understanding the neural development of neuropsychiatric disorders, substance use disorders, and normal brains. Specifically, anatomical MRI has

J.L. Prince, D.L. Pham, and K.J. Myers (Eds.): IPMI 2009, LNCS 5636, pp. 314–325, 2009.

been widely used to segment the cortical and subcortical structures (e.g., hippocampus) of the human brain *in vivo* and to generate various morphological measures of their morphology for understanding neuroanatomical differences in brain structure across different populations [1]. Functional MRI (fMRI) has been widely used to understand functional integration of different brain regions in response to specific stimuli and behavioral tasks and detecting the association between brain function and covariates of interest, such as diagnosis, behavioral tasks, severity of disease, age, or IQ [2,3,4].

Much effort has been devoted to developing voxel-wise methods for analyzing various imaging measures including cortical thickness using numerical simulations and theoretical reasoning. The voxel-wise methods for analyzing imaging data are often sequentially executed in two steps. The first step involves fitting a general linear model (LM) (or a linear mixed model (LMM)) to imaging data from all subjects at each voxel and generating a statistical parametric map of test statistics (or p-values) [5,6]. The second step is to calculate adjusted p-values that account for testing the hypotheses across multiple brain regions or across many voxels of the imaging volume using various statistical methods (e.g., random field theory (RFT), false discovery rate, or permutation methods) [7,8]. Most of these methods have been implemented in existing neuroimaging software platforms, such as SPM (http://www.fil.ion.ucl.ac.uk), among many others.

The voxel-wise approach based on the LM (or LMM) and RFT has several obvious limitations for the analyses of imaging data, underscoring the great need for methodological development. (i) The voxel-wise approach essentially treats all voxels as independent units [9], whereas neuroimaging data are spatially correlated in nature and spatially contiguous regions of activation with rather sharp edges are usually expected. (ii) The initial smoothing step before the voxel-wise approach often blurs the image data near the edges of activated regions and thus it can dramatically increase the numbers of false positives and false negatives [11,12,13,9]. (iii) The voxel-wise approach is also based on a strong assumption that after an image warping procedure, the location of a voxel in the images of one person is assumed to be in precisely the same location as the voxel identified in another person——an assumption that is demonstrably false.

Spatially modeling imaging data in all voxels of the 3D volume (or 2D surface) represents both computational and theoretical challenges. Spatial dependencies were commonly characterized using conditional autoregressive (CAR) or Markov random field (MRF) priors, but estimating spatial correlation for the 3D volume, in which the number of voxels ranges from ten thousands to more than 500,000 voxels, is computationally prohibited. Moreover, given the complexity of imaging data, it can be restrictive to assume parametric spatial correlation such as CAR and MRF for the whole 3D volume (or 2D surface). Another method, called ROI analysis, is to model the imaging data from all voxels within multiple regions of interest (ROIs) [14]. The ROI method based on anatomically defined ROIs only models the spatial correlation among these ROIs [14], so it essentially ignores the spatial correlation structure in the neighboring voxels within each ROI.

Moreover, the ROI method is also based on a strong assumption that all voxels in the same ROI are homogeneous, and this assumption is largely false.

This paper aims to develop and apply a multiscale adaptive regression model (MARM) for the joint analysis of neuroimaging data with behavioral and clinical variables, and then to demonstrate its superiority over the voxel-wise approach using simulated and real imaging data. The MARM is a spatial, hierarchical and adaptive procedure. The MARM builds a small sphere at each voxel and use these consecutively connected spheres across all voxels to capture local and global spatial dependence among imaging observations. The MARM also builds hierarchically nested spheres by increasing the radius of a spherical neighborhood around each voxel and combine all the data in a given radius of each voxel with appropriate weights to adaptively calculate parameter estimates and test statistics. Thus, the MARM explicitly utilizes the spatial information to carry out statistical inference, while avoiding explicitly estimating spatial correlation. The hierarchical nature of the MARM can dramatically reduce the computational complexity in computing parameter estimates. The adaptive feature of the MARM can efficiently utilize all available information in the neighboring voxels to increase the precision of parameter estimates and the power of test statistics.

The MARM represents a novel generalization of the propagation separation (PS) approach, which was originally developed for nonparametric estimation of regression curves or surfaces [11,12], in several aspects. The MARM provides a general framework for carrying out statistical inference on imaging data, whereas the PS is applied to smooth the images of parameter estimates obtained from the voxel-wise approach based on classical linear models [9]. As shown in Section 2, it is inadequate to directly use the PS approach to smooth the images of parameter estimates, which are obtained from the voxel-wise method, for most regression models, such as nonlinear regression. Compared to the parametric assumptions in the PS method for the LM, the MARM is solely based on the pseudo-likelihood function, and thus it avoids specifying any parametric distribution for imaging data. This feature is desirable for the analysis of real neuroimaging data, including brain morphological measures, because the distribution of the univariate (or multivariate) neuroimaging measurements often deviates from the Gaussian distribution [15]. We also establish the theoretical properties of the MARM, which differs substantially from those of the original PS approach, which were developed for nonparametric estimation of regression curves or surfaces based on observations from the exponential family model [12]. Particularly, we show that the MARM outperforms the voxel-wise method theoretically.

Section 2 of this paper presents the MARM just described and establishes the associated theoretical properties. We establish the consistency and asymptotic normality of the adaptive estimators and the asymptotic distribution of the adaptive test statistics for the MARMs. In Section 3, we conduct simulation studies to examine the finite sample performance of the MARMs. Section 4 illustrates an application of the proposed methods in a neuroimaging dataset. We present concluding remarks in Section 5.

2   Multiscale Adaptive Regression Model

2.1   Data Structure and Model Formulation

Suppose we have 2D surfaces or 3D volumes of MRI measures and clinical variables from n subjects for $i = 1, \cdots, n$. MRI measures might be the shape representation of the surfaces of cortical or various subcortical regions, the determinant of the Jacobian matrices based on the deformation fields estimated by the registration algorithm, functional MRI signals, or diffusion tensors and their associated invariant measures, such as fractional anisotropy [1]. Clinical variables might include pedigree information, time, demographic characteristics (e.g., age, gender, height), and diagnoses, among others. Thus, for the i−th subject, we observe an $N_D \times 1$ vector of MRI measures, denoted by $\mathbf{Y}_{i,\mathcal{D}} = \{Y_i(d) : d \in \mathcal{D}\}$, and a $k \times 1$ vector of clinical variables $\mathbf{x}_i$, where $\mathcal{D}$ and d, respectively, represent a 3D volume (or 2D surface) and a voxel in $\mathcal{D}$ and N_D equals the number of points on $\mathcal{D}$.

Our primary scientific interest in the analysis of neuroimaging data is to identify important brain regions to characterize the neural development of neuropsychiatric disorders, substance use disorders, and normal brains. Statistically, we often use $\{\mathbf{Y}_{i,\mathcal{D}} : i = 1, \cdots, n\}$ as responses and establish their association with a set of covariates $\mathbf{x}_i$, such as age and gender. This requires the specification of the conditional distribution of

$$\mathbf{Y}_{\mathcal{D}} = \{\mathbf{Y}_{i,\mathcal{D}} = (\mathbf{Y}_{i,\mathcal{D}} : i = 1, \cdots, n\}$$

given $\mathbf{X} = \{\mathbf{x}_i : i = 1, \cdots, n\}$, that is, $p(\mathbf{Y}_{\mathcal{D}}|\mathbf{X})$. For MRI measures from the cross-sectional studies, it is natural to assume the independence across all subjects, that is given by

$$p(\mathbf{Y}_{\mathcal{D}}|\mathbf{X}) = \prod_{i=1}^{n} p(\mathbf{Y}_{i,\mathcal{D}}|\mathbf{X}_i).$$

Thus, we only need to specify $p(\mathbf{Y}_{i,\mathcal{D}}|\mathbf{X}_i)$ for each subject. However, even for a single observation within each cluster, the number of voxels in each brain region varies from thousands to more than 500,000 voxels, and at each voxel, the dimension of $Y_i(d)$ can be univariate or multivariate, thus totaling a billion or more data points in an entire study. In addition, imaging data $\mathbf{Y}_{i,\mathcal{D}}$ are spatially correlated in nature, and thus given the large number of voxels on each brain structure, it is statistically challenging to directly model the spatial correlations among all pairs of points [14].

The voxel-wise approach essentially assumes that

$$p(\mathbf{Y}_{i,\mathcal{D}}|\mathbf{X}_i) \approx \prod_{d \in \mathcal{D}} p(Y_i(d)|\mathbf{x}_i, \boldsymbol{\theta}(d)), \tag{1}$$

where $p(Y_i(d)|\mathbf{x}_i, \boldsymbol{\theta}(d))$ is the marginal density of $p(\mathbf{Y}_{i,\mathcal{D}}|\mathbf{X}_i)$ or a 'pseudo' density function for $Y_i(d)$ parameterized by an unknown parameter vector $\boldsymbol{\theta}(d) =$

$(\boldsymbol{\theta}_1(d), \cdots, \boldsymbol{\theta}_p(d))^T$ in an open subset Θ of R^p. Note that we use the pseudo density to emphasize the possible misspecification of $p(Y_i(d)|\mathbf{x}_i, \boldsymbol{\theta}(d))$. Model (1) comprises many statistical models such as the LM. For instance, for univariate measure, the LM assumes that

$$Y_i(d) = \mathbf{x}_i^T \boldsymbol{\beta}(d) + \epsilon_i(d) \quad \text{for all} \ \ i = 1, \cdots, n,$$

where $\boldsymbol{\beta}(d)$ is a $(p-1) \times 1$ regression coefficients, $\epsilon_{i1}(d) \sim N(0, \sigma(d)^2)$, and $\boldsymbol{\theta}(d) = (\boldsymbol{\beta}(d), \sigma(d))$. However, the linear link function $E[Y_i(d)|\mathbf{x}_i] = \mathbf{x}_i^T \boldsymbol{\beta}(d)$ and the Gaussian assumption are questionable in many applications [15]. Moreover, since the voxel-wise approach does not account for the fact that imaging data are spatially correlated and contain spatially contiguous regions of activation with rather sharp edges, it may lead to the loss of power in detecting statistical significance in the analysis of imaging data.

We formally introduce the multiscale adaptive regression model as follows. It is first assumed that for a relatively large radius r_0,

$$p(\mathbf{Y}_{i,\mathcal{D}}|\mathbf{X}_i) \approx \prod_{d \in \mathcal{D}} p(\{Y_i(d') : \ d' \in N(d, r_0)\}|\mathbf{x}_i), \tag{2}$$

where $N(d, r_0)$ denotes the set of all voxels in a spherical neighborhood of a voxel d with radius r_0. That is, we can approximate the joint distribution of $\mathbf{Y}_{i,\mathcal{D}}$ by the product of the joint distributions of $\{Y_i(d') : \ d' \in N(d, r_0)\}$. Using data in $N(d, r_0)$ for relatively large r_0 preserves the neighboring correlation structure in the imaging data (see the panel (a) in Figure 1 for an illustration). Moreover, since the spherical neighborhoods for all voxels are consecutively connected, equation (2) can capture a substantial amount of spatial information in the imaging data. Note that the right hand-side of equation (2) is essentially a composite likelihood [16,17].

Second, we consider the specification of $p(\{Y_i(d') : \ d' \in N(d, r_0)\}|\mathbf{x}_i)$. Since our primary interest is to make statistical inference about $\boldsymbol{\theta}(d)$, we avoid specifying spatial correlations among all the $\{Y_i(d') : d' \in N(d, r_0)\}$. Instead, we assume that $p(\{Y_i(d') : \ d' \in N(d, r_0)\}|\mathbf{x}_i)$ can be approximated by

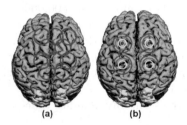

(a)   (b)

Fig. 1. Illustrating the key features of the multiscale adaptive regression model. For a relatively large radius r_0, panel (a) shows the spherical neighborhoods $N(d, r_0)$ of multiple points d on the cortical surface. Panel (b) shows the spherical neighborhoods with four different bandwidths h of the four selected points d on the cortical surface.

$$p(\{Y_i(d') : \quad d' \in N(d, r_0)\}|\mathbf{x}_i) \approx \left\{ \prod_{d' \in N(d, r_0)} p(Y_i(d')|\mathbf{x}_i, \boldsymbol{\theta}(d'))^{\omega(d, d'; r_0)} \right\}, \quad (3)$$

where $\omega(d, d'; h)$ is a weight function of two voxels and a radius h that character-izes the similarity between the data in voxels d and d'. We require that $\omega(d, d'; h)$ be independent of i just for simplicity. In imaging data, voxels, which are not on the boundary of regions of activation, often have a neighborhood in which $\boldsymbol{\theta}(d)$ is nearly constant. This assumption reflects the fact that imaging data are spatially correlated and contain spatially contiguous regions of activation with rather sharp edges. Incorporating this assumption leads to

$$p(\{Y_i(d') : \quad d' \in N(d, r_0)\}|\mathbf{x}_i) \approx \left\{ \prod_{d' \in N(d, r_0)} p(Y_i(d')|\mathbf{x}_i, \boldsymbol{\theta}(d))^{\omega(d, d'; r_0)} \right\}. \quad (4)$$

Equation (4) allows us to combine all data in $N(d, r_0)$ to make inference about $\boldsymbol{\theta}(d)$, which can substantially increase the efficiency in estimating $\boldsymbol{\theta}(d)$. More-over, the weights $\omega(d, d'; r_0)$ can prevent incorporating voxels whose data do not contain information on $\boldsymbol{\theta}(d)$, and thus preserve the edges of the regions of activation.

An important question that we need to address is how to determine $\omega(d, d'; r_0)$. We use a multiscale strategy to adaptively determine $\{\omega(d, d'; r_0) : d, d' \in \mathcal{D}\}$ and estimate $\boldsymbol{\theta}(d)$. Specifically, we select a sequence of bandwidths $h_0 = 0 < h_1 < \cdots < h_S = r_0$ ranging from the smallest scale $h_0 = 0$ to the largest scale $h_S = r_0$. By setting $\omega(d, d'; h_0 = 0) = 1$, we can estimate $\boldsymbol{\theta}(d)$ at scale h_0, denoted by $\tilde{\boldsymbol{\theta}}(d; h_0 = 0)$, and then we use some methods as detailed below to calculate $\omega(d, d'; h_1)$ at scale h_1 based on $\{\tilde{\boldsymbol{\theta}}(d; h_0 = 0) : d \in \mathcal{D}\}$. In this way, we can sequentially determine $\omega(d, d'; h_s)$ and adaptively update $\tilde{\boldsymbol{\theta}}(d; h_s)$ from $h_0 = 0$ to $h_S = r_0$ (see the panel (b) of Figure 1 for an illustration). A path diagram is given below:

$$
\begin{array}{ccccccc}
\omega(d, d'; h_0) & & \omega(d, d'; h_1) & & \cdots & & \omega(d, d'; h_S = r_0) \\
\Downarrow & \nearrow & \Downarrow & \nearrow \cdots \nearrow & & & \Downarrow \\
\tilde{\boldsymbol{\theta}}(d; h_0) & & \tilde{\boldsymbol{\theta}}(d; h_1) & & \cdots & & \tilde{\boldsymbol{\theta}}(d; h_S)
\end{array} \quad (5)
$$

At each iteration, the computation involved for the MARM is of the same order as that for the voxel-wise approach. Thus, this multiscale method provides an efficient method for adaptively exploring the neighboring areas of each voxel. Since this multiscale method sequentially includes more data at each voxel, it will adaptively increase the statistical efficiency in estimating $\boldsymbol{\theta}(d)$ in a homogenous region and decreases the variation of the weights $\omega(d, d'; h)$. This multiscale method distinguishes MARM from the composite likelihood methods proposed in the literature [16,17].

2.2   Estimation and Hypothesis Testing at a Fixed Scale

At a fixed scale h, we consider the weighted maximum likelihood estimates of $\boldsymbol{\theta}(d)$ across all voxels $d \in \mathcal{D}$ for given weights $\omega(d, d'; h)$. The weighted quasi-likelihood function $\ell_n(\boldsymbol{\theta}(d); h, \omega)$ is given by

$$\ell_n(\boldsymbol{\theta}(d); h, \omega) = \sum_{i=1}^{n} \sum_{d' \in N(d,h)} \omega(d, d'; h) \log p(Y_i(d') | \mathbf{x}_i, \boldsymbol{\theta}(d)). \tag{6}$$

The maximum weighted quasi-likelihood (MWQL) estimate of $\boldsymbol{\theta}$ is

$$\hat{\boldsymbol{\theta}}(d, h) = \operatorname{argmax}_{\boldsymbol{\theta}(d)} n^{-1} \ell_n(\boldsymbol{\theta}(d); h, \omega). \tag{7}$$

We use the Newton-Raphson algorithm to calculate $\hat{\boldsymbol{\theta}}(d, h)$ by iterating

$$\hat{\boldsymbol{\theta}}(d, h)^{(t+1)} = \hat{\boldsymbol{\theta}}(d, h)^{(t)} + \{-\partial^2_{\boldsymbol{\theta}(d)} \ell_n(\hat{\boldsymbol{\theta}}(d, h)^{(t)}; h, \omega)\}^{-1} \partial_{\boldsymbol{\theta}(d)} \ell_n(\hat{\boldsymbol{\theta}}(d, h)^{(t)}; h, \omega),$$

where $\partial_{\boldsymbol{\theta}(d)}$ and $\partial^2_{\boldsymbol{\theta}(d)}$ denote, respectively, the first- and second-order partial derivatives with respect to $\boldsymbol{\theta}(d)$ evaluated at $\hat{\boldsymbol{\theta}}(d, h)^{(t)}$. In practice, to stabilize the Newton-Raphson algorithm, we may approximate $-\partial^2_{\boldsymbol{\theta}(d)} \ell_n(\hat{\boldsymbol{\theta}}(d, h)^{(t)}; h, \omega)$ by $E[-\partial^2_{\boldsymbol{\theta}(d)} \ell_n(\hat{\boldsymbol{\theta}}(d, h)^{(t)}; h, \omega)]$. The Newton-Raphson algorithm stops when the absolute difference between consecutive $\hat{\boldsymbol{\theta}}(d, h)^{(t)}$s is smaller than a predefined small number, say 10^{-4}. After convergence, $\operatorname{Cov}[\hat{\boldsymbol{\theta}}(d, h)] = \Sigma_n(\hat{\boldsymbol{\theta}}(d, h))$ can be approximated by $[\Sigma_{n,1}(\hat{\boldsymbol{\theta}}(d, h))]^{-1} \Sigma_{n,2}(\hat{\boldsymbol{\theta}}(d, h)) [\Sigma_{n,1}(\hat{\boldsymbol{\theta}}(d, h))]^{-1}$, where $\Sigma_{n,1}(\boldsymbol{\theta}) = -\partial^2_{\boldsymbol{\theta}(d)} \ell_n(\boldsymbol{\theta}; h, \omega)$ and $\Sigma_{n,2}(\boldsymbol{\theta}) = \sum_{i=1}^{n} [\sum_{d' \in N(d,h)} \omega(d, d'; h) \partial_{\boldsymbol{\theta}(d)} \log p(Y_i(d') | \mathbf{x}_i, \boldsymbol{\theta})]^{\otimes 2}$, in which $\mathbf{a}^{\otimes 2} = \mathbf{a}\mathbf{a}^T$ for any vector $\mathbf{a}$.

Our choice of which hypotheses to test was motivated by either a comparison of brain structure across diagnostic groups or the detection of a change in brain structure across time [1]. These questions usually can be formulated as the testing of linear hypotheses about $\boldsymbol{\theta}(d)$

$$H_{0,\mu} : R\boldsymbol{\theta}(d) = \mathbf{b}_0 \quad \text{vs.} \quad H_{1,\mu} : R\boldsymbol{\theta}(d) \neq \mathbf{b}_0, \tag{8}$$

where $\mu = R\boldsymbol{\theta}(d)$, R is a $r \times k$ matrix of full row rank and $\mathbf{b}_0$ is an $r \times 1$ specified vector. We test the null hypothesis $H_{0,\mu} : R\boldsymbol{\theta}(d) = \mathbf{b}_0$ using the score test statistic

$$W_\mu(d, h) = [R\hat{\boldsymbol{\theta}}(d, h) - \mathbf{b}_0]^T [R\hat{\Sigma}_n(\hat{\boldsymbol{\theta}}(d; h))R^T]^{-1} [R\hat{\boldsymbol{\theta}}(d, h) - \mathbf{b}_0]. \tag{9}$$

To test whether $H_{0,\mu}$ holds in all voxels of the region under study, we consider the false discovery rate (FDR) method [10].

2.3   Adaptive Estimation and Testing Procedure

We develop an adaptive estimation and testing (AET) procedure for MARM. The AET procedure starts with a single voxel d and then successively increases the radius (or bandwidth) h of a spherical neighborhood around d. Each voxel d' in the neighborhood of d will be given a weight $\omega(d, d'; h_s)$ that depends on the distance between d and d' and the similarity between $\hat{\boldsymbol{\theta}}(d, h_{s-1})$ and $\hat{\boldsymbol{\theta}}(d', h_{s-1})$. Then, we use all the data in a given neighborhood of d with bandwidth h_s and the weight in each of these voxels to obtain updated estimates $\hat{\boldsymbol{\theta}}(d, h_s)$ and

$W_\mu(d, h_s)$ at d, respectively. Finally, we use a sequence of $\hat{\theta}(d, h_s)$ and $W_\mu(d, h_s)$ as a function of h to construct the final estimate for $\theta(d)$ and calculate the final test statistic $W_\mu(d)$ for testing hypotheses on $\theta(d)$ at d.

The AET procedure consists of five key steps as follows.

In the initialization step (i), we generate a geometric series $\{h_k = c_h^s : s = 1, \cdots, S\}$ of bandwidths with $h_0 = 0$, where c_h is a number in $(1, 2)$, say $c_h = 1.25$. At each voxel d, we calculate $\hat{\theta}(d, h_0)$ and $W_\mu(d, h_0)$, which are the same as those from the voxel-wise approach. We then set $s = 1$, and $h_1 = c_h$.

In the weights adaptation step (ii), we compute adaptive weights

$$\omega(d, d'; h_s) = K_{loc}(||d - d'||_2/h_s)K_{st}(D_\theta(d, d'; h_{s-1})), \tag{10}$$

where $K_{loc}(\cdot)$ and $K_{st}(\cdot)$ are two kernel functions with compact support, $|| \cdot ||_2$ denotes the Euclidean norm, and $D_\theta(d, d'; h_{s-1})$ denotes a weighted function based on the estimates of $\{\theta(d) : d \in \mathcal{D}\}$ at the $(s-1)$th iteration. The adaptive weights can downweight voxels d' in $\ell_n(\theta(d); h, d)$ if $D_\theta(d, d'; h_{s-1})$ is large.

In the estimation step (iii), we calculate $\hat{\theta}(d, h_s)$ and $W_\mu(d, h_s)$, which are defined in equations (7) and (10), respectively, at voxel d for the sth scale.

In the memory step (iv), we set $\tilde{\theta}(d, h_0) = \hat{\theta}(d, h_0)$ and then update $\tilde{\theta}(d, h_s)$ for $s > 0$ as

$$\tilde{\theta}(d, h_s) = \hat{\theta}(d, h_s)\eta_s/s + (1 - \eta_s/s)\tilde{\theta}(d, h_{s-1}), \tag{11}$$

where $\eta_s = K_{loc}(D_\theta(d, h_s)/C_0) \in (0, 1)$ and

$$D_\theta(d, h_s) = [\hat{\theta}(d, h_s) - \hat{\theta}(d, h_0)]^T \text{Cov}(\hat{\theta}(d, h_0))^{-1}[\hat{\theta}(d, h_s) - \hat{\theta}(d, h_0)]. \tag{12}$$

The $D_\theta(d, h_s)$ measures the difference between $\hat{\theta}(d, h_s)$ and $\hat{\theta}(d, h_0)$ at the same voxel d. Finally, we calculate an estimator of the covariance matrix of $\tilde{\theta}(d, h_s)$, denoted by $\text{Cov}(\tilde{\theta}(d, h_s))$ and compute the Wald test statistic as

$$\tilde{W}_\mu(d, h) = [R\tilde{\theta}(d, h_s) - \mathbf{b}_0]^T \text{Cov}(\tilde{\theta}(d, h_s))^{-1}[R\tilde{\theta}(d, h_s) - \mathbf{b}_0]. \tag{13}$$

In the stopping step (v), when $s = S$, we compute the p-values for $\tilde{W}_\mu(d, h)$, apply FDR to detect significant voxels and then stop, otherwise set $h_{s+1} = c_h h_s$, increase s by 1 and continue with the weight adaptation step (ii). The maximal step S can be taken to be relatively small, say 6, such that the largest spherical neighborhood of each voxel only contains a relatively small number of voxels compared with the whole volume.

Remark 1. The memory step in equation (11) differs substantially from that in the PS approach [12]. Equation (11) is exactly a stochastic approximation algorithm [18]. The sequence $\{1/s : s = 1, \cdots\}$ is introduced to cancel out the noise introduced in each iteration. Putting more weight $1/s$ at the beginning is very appealing in imaging analysis, because use of a local approximation often decreases the estimation error in the first few steps of the procedure and starts to slowly increase the estimation error as h_s gets large. In addition, compared with the memory step in the PS approach, we use the distance between $\hat{\theta}(d, h_s)$

and $\hat{\boldsymbol{\theta}}(d, h_0)$ to control the estimation error of $\tilde{\boldsymbol{\theta}}(d, h_0)$. Since $\hat{\boldsymbol{\theta}}(d, h_0)$ is a $\sqrt{n}$ consistent estimate of $\boldsymbol{\theta}(d)$, $\eta_s = K_{loc}(D_{\boldsymbol{\theta}}(d, h_s)/C_0)$ ensures that $\hat{\boldsymbol{\theta}}(d, h_s)$ is also a $\sqrt{n}$ consistent estimate of $\boldsymbol{\theta}(d)$ for all $s > 0$.

Remark 2. There is an efficient way for selecting the initial value $\boldsymbol{\theta}(d, h_s)^{(0)}$ for the Newton-Raphson algorithm by setting $\boldsymbol{\theta}(d, h_s)^{(0)} = \hat{\boldsymbol{\theta}}(d, h_{s-1})$ for each $s > 0$. Since the AET procedure always downweights voxels d' in $\ell_n(\boldsymbol{\theta}(d); h, d)$ if $D_{\boldsymbol{\theta}}(d, d'; h_{s-1})$ is large, $\hat{\boldsymbol{\theta}}(d, h_{s-1})$ and $\hat{\boldsymbol{\theta}}(d, h_s)$ should be close to each other. By starting from $\boldsymbol{\theta}(d, h_s)^{(0)} = \hat{\boldsymbol{\theta}}(d, h_{s-1})$, the Newton-Raphson algorithm converges very fast, and thus the additional computation involved for the MARM is very light compared to the voxel-wise approach.

3   Simulation Study

We only presented one set of Monte Carlo simulations to examine the finite sample performance of $\tilde{W}_\mu(d, h)$ with respect to different scales h at the levels of a single voxel and an entire brain region with known ground truth.

We applied a simulation model to automatically simulate realistic intra-individual deformations associated with tissue atrophy or growth on brain images from two groups [19]. We chose a specified location and a fixed radius in the white matter and then simulated spherical atrophy for all 20 subjects in each group (see Figure 2). The growth rates for each subject in the first and second groups were generated from $N(0.95, 0.01)$ and $N(1, 0.01)$, respectively.

We used simulated deformations and images with the known ground truth to demonstrate the superiority of the MARM over the voxel-wise approach. The true deformation area was highlighted in red (see the panel (a) of Figure 2). We applied the MARM with $c_h = 1.25$, $S = 6$ and computed the p-values of $\tilde{W}_\mu(d, h)$ across the 3D volume at each iteration. Note that the results obtained from $h_0 = 0$ correspond to those from the voxel-wise approach. Our results show a clear advantage of the MARM in detecting an accurate group difference as we increase the bandwidth h of the spherical neighborhood (compare the panels (b) and (c) of Figure 2). We calculated the ratio of voxels within the true deformation regions, whose p-values are smaller than 0.0001. The ratios for h_0 and h_6 are 49% and 68%, respectively. That is, the MARM based on h_6 leads to 19% improvement compared with the traditional voxel-wise approach with $h_0 = 0$.

4   Real Data Analysis

Alzheimer's disease (AD) is the most common form of dementia in people over 65 years of age. MRI has been used to develop imaging-based biomarkers for AD, measure spatial patterns of atrophy, and their evolution with disease progressions. We used a subset of a large MRI dataset obtained from the Alzheimer's Disease Neuroimaging Initiative (ADNI) database (www.loni.ucla.edu/ADNI). Our dataset includes 90 subjects, including 45 cognitively normal individuals

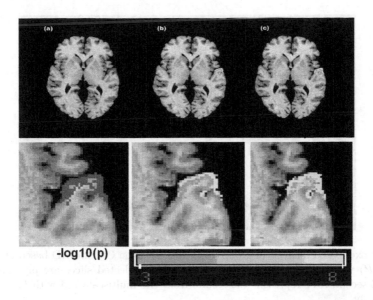

Fig. 2. Voxel-wise analysis of group difference. From left to right in the first row, it shows the true deformation region in red in panel (a), the raw $-\log_{10}(p)$ values of the Wald test statistics $\tilde{W}_\mu(d, h_0)$ in panel (b), and the raw $-\log_{10}(p)$ values of the Wald test statistics $\tilde{W}_\mu(d, h_6)$ based on a χ^2 distribution in panel (c). The second row shows the enlarged deformation regions of the corresponding figures in the first row.

(CN) (mean age S.D., 77.07 3.89), and 45 AD patients (77.32 6.01). The mini mental state examination (MMSE) scores (mean S.D.) of each group at baseline were 29.16 0.92, and 23.13 1.75, respectively. The two groups were relatively well-balanced in terms of gender (23,25 women in each of the 2 groups, respectively). The imaging data include standard T1-weighted MR images acquired sagittally using volumetric 3D MPRAGE with 1.25×1.25 mm^2 in-plane spatial resolution and 1.2 mm thick sagittal slices (8 flip angle).

The T1-weighted MRIs were preprocessed in six consecutive steps. These steps included (i) alignment to the AC-PC plane; (ii) removal of extra-cranial material (skull-stripping); (iii) tissue segmentation into grey matter (GM), white matter (WM), and cerebrospinal fluid (CSF) using a brain tissue segmentation method proposed; (iv) high-dimensional image warping to a standardized coordinate system, a brain atlas (template) that was aligned with the MNI coordinate space; (vi) formation of regional volumetric maps, named RAVENS maps, for GM, WM, and CSF using tissue preserving image warping.

We identify the spatial patterns of brain atrophy in Alzheimer's disease (AD) via the analysis of the RAVENS maps of GM and WM obtained from the ANDI dataset. To control for the effects of covariates (diagnosis, age, weight, and gender), we considered model $y_i(d) = \mathbf{x}_i^T \boldsymbol{\beta} + \epsilon_i(d)$ for respective RAVENS maps at each voxel. The $\mathbf{x}_i = (1, x_{1i}, x_{2i}, x_{3i}, x_{4i})^T$ is a 4×1 vector, in which x_{1i} is Age/10, x_{2i} is gender, x_{4i} denotes the weight, and x_{4i} denotes the diagnosis (1

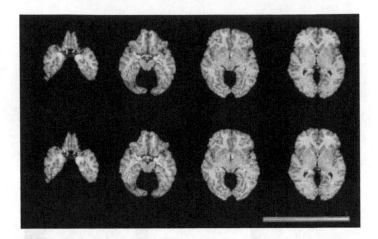

Fig. 3. Voxel-based analysis of group difference between CN and AD based on the raw $-\log_{10}(P)$ values of the Wald test statistics. Four selected slices are presented. The first and second rows represent the results from the multiscale LM with $h_0 =$ and h_6, respectively.

AD and 0 CN). We applied the AET procedure with $c_h = 1.25$ and $S = 6$ to carry out the statistical analysis. Figure 2 shows a clear advantage of the MARM in detecting more significant and smoothly area for the group differences between CN and AD as the bandwidth h increases. We observed the significant difference between CN and AD in the hippocampus and the entorhinal cortex.

5   Discussion

We have developed the MARM for spatial and adaptive analysis of imaging data. We have used simulation studies and real data to show that the MARM significantly outperforms the classical voxel-wise approach. Many issues still merit further research.

Acknowledgments. We thank the reviewers for their thoughtful comments. This work was supported in part by NSF grants SES-06-43663 and BCS-08-26844 and NIH grants UL1-RR025747-01 and R21AG033387 to Dr. Zhu, NIH grants GM 70335 and CA 74015 to Dr. Ibrahim, NIH grant R01NS055754 to Dr. Lin, and NIH grant R01EB006733 and R03EB008760 to Dr. Shen.

References

1. Thompson, P.M., Cannon, T.D., Toga, A.W.: Mapping Genetic Influences on Human Brain Structure. The Annals of Medicine 24, 523–536 (2002)
2. Friston, K.J.: Statistical Parametric Mapping: the Analysis of Functional Brain Images. Academic Press, London (2007)

3. Rogers, B.P., Morgan, V.L., Newton, A.T., Gore, J.C.: Assessing Functional Connectivity in the Human Brain by FMRI. Magnetic Resonance Imaging 25(10), 1347–1357 (2007)
4. Huettel, S.A., Song, A.W., McCarthy, G.: Functional Magnetic Resonance Imaging. Sinauer Associates, Inc. (2004)
5. Friston, K., Holmes, A.P., Worsley, K.J., Poline, J.B., Frith, C.D., Frackowiak, R.S.J.: Statistical Parametric Maps in Functional Imaging: a General Linear Approach. Human Brain Mapping 2, 189–210 (1995)
6. Beckmann, C.F., Jenkinson, M., Smith, S.M.: General Multilevel Linear Modeling for Group Analysis in fMRI. NeuroImage 20, 1052–1063 (2003)
7. Nichols, T., Hayasaka, S.: Controlling the Family-wise Error Rate in Functional Neuroimaging: a Comparative Review. Statistical Methods in Medical Research 12, 419–446 (2003)
8. Worsley, K.J., Taylor, J.E., Tomaiuolo, F., Lerch, J.: Unified Univariate and Multivariate Random Field Theory. NeuroImage 23, 189–195 (2004)
9. Tabelow, K., Polzehl, J., Voss, H.U., Spokoiny, V.: Analyzing fMRI Experiments with Structural Adaptive Smoothing Procedures. NeuroImage 33, 55–62 (2006)
10. Benjamini, Y., Hochberg, Y.: Controlling the False Discovery Rate: A Practical and Powerful Approach to Multiple Testing. Journal of the Royal Statistical Society, Ser. B 57, 289–300 (1995)
11. Polzehl, J., Spokoiny, V.G.: Image Denoising: Pointwise Adaptive Approach. Annals of Statistics 31, 30–57 (2003)
12. Polzehl, J., Spokoiny, V.G.: Propagation-Separation Approach for Local Likelihood Estimation. Probab. Theory Relat. Fields 135, 335–362 (2006)
13. Qiu, P.: Image Processing and Jump Regression Analysis. John Wiley & Sons, New York (2005)
14. Bowman, F.D.: Spatio-temporal Models for Region of Interest Analyses of Functional Mappping Experiments. Journal of American Statistical Association 102, 442–453 (2007)
15. Luo, W., Nichols, T.: Diagnosis and Exploration of Massively Univariate fMRI Models. NeuroImage 19, 1014–1032 (2003)
16. Lindsay, B.G.: Composite Likelihood Methods. Contemp. Math. 80, 221–240 (1988)
17. Varin, C.: On Composite Marginal Likelihoods. Advances in Statistical Analysis 92, 1–28 (2008)
18. Robbins, H., Monro, S.: A Stochastic Approximation Method. Annals of Mathematical Statistics 22, 400–407 (1951)
19. Xue, Z., Shen, D., Karacali, B., Stern, J., Rottenberg, D., Davatzikos, C.: Simulating Deformations of MR Brain Images for Validation of Atlas-based Segmentation and Registration Algorithms. NeuroImage 33, 855–866 (2006)

Automatic Segmentation of Brain Structures Using Geometric Moment Invariants and Artificial Neural Networks

Mostafa Jabarouti Moghaddam[1] and Hamid Soltanian-Zadeh[1,2]

[1] Control and Intelligent Processing Center of Excellence, Department of Electrical and Computer Engineering, University of Tehran, Tehran, Iran
[2] Image Analysis Laboratory, Department of Radiology, Henry Ford Hospital, Detroit, Michigan, USA
`m.jabarouti@ece.ut.ac.ir, hszadeh@ut.ac.ir, hamids@rad.hfh.edu`

Abstract. We propose an automatic method for the segmentation of the brain structures in three dimensional (3D) Magnetic Resonance Images (MRI). The proposed method consists of two stages. In the first stage, we represent the shape of the structure using Geometric Moment Invariants (GMIs) in 8 scales. For each scale, an Artificial Neural Network (ANN) is designed to approximate the signed distance function of a desired structure. The GMIs along with the voxel intensities and coordinates are used as the input features of the ANN and the signed distance function as its output. In the second stage, we combine the outputs of the ANNs of the first stage and design another ANN to classify the image voxels into two classes, inside or outside of the structure. We introduce a fast method for moment calculations. The proposed method is applied to the segmentation of caudate, putamen, and thalamus in MRI where it has outperformed other methods in the literature.

Keywords: Magnetic Resonance Images, Geometric Moments Invariants, Artificial Neural Network, automatic segmentation.

1 Introduction

Segmentation of the brain structures in Magnetic Resonance Images (MRI) is the first step in many medical image analysis applications and is useful for the diagnosis and evaluation of the neurological diseases such as autism, depression, fetal alcohol syndrome, Alzheimer's, and Parkinson's. Therefore, accurate, reliable, and automatic segmentation of the brain structures can improve diagnostic and treatment of the related neurological diseases. Manual segmentation by an expert is usually accurate but is impractical for large datasets because it is a tedious and time consuming process.

Until now, several methods have been developed for tissue segmentation and classification using MRI. These methods suffer from problems such as low contrast, discontinuous boundaries of the structures, ill-defined boundaries due to partial volume effect, intensity inhomogeneities [1], and low signal-to-noise ratio (SNR) [2]. On the

J.L. Prince, D.L. Pham, and K.J. Myers (Eds.): IPMI 2009, LNCS 5636, pp. 326–337, 2009.
© Springer-Verlag Berlin Heidelberg 2009

other hand, different subjects with different ages and genders have structures with a variety of different shapes and specifications. To solve these problems, the proposed methods should benefit from prior knowledge of the structures. In this direction, several approaches have been developed using shapes of the structures [3,4] into the deformable model equations [5], regional information such as histogram [6], relationships among the neighboring structures [7,8], probabilistic atlas priors [9,10], boundary information [11,12], multiscale Bayesian framework [25], pattern recognition techniques such as Artificial Neural Network (ANN) as classifiers [13,14], Support Vector Machine (SVM) [15], and fuzzy sets with deformable models [16,17].

We focus on the methods that use the ANN as a classifier to segment the brain structures. An earlier method developed by Magnotta et al [13] used voxel intensity values of the neighboring voxels as the input feature. Their task was to classify the voxels into two classes – being inside or outside of the structure. They designed one ANN for each structure. The input features did not contain any shape representations. This causes the need for large training data sets. On the other hand, voxel intensity values can solve the segmentation problem for the high-resolution MRI they utilized. Recently, Powell et al [14] developed their previous algorithm [13] and added 9 voxel intensity values along the largest gradient, one probabilistic map value, and voxel intensity values along each of the three orthogonal values as the input features. They used high-resolution images the same as [13] for the segmentation of the brain structures. They used 15 images as the training data sets that were collected using two protocols: T1-weighted and T2-weighted.

In [18], we proposed the use of a new input feature – Geometric Moment Invariants (GMIs) [19] to improve the differentiation between the brain regions compared to the image intensity values. The GMIs characterize the underlying anatomical structures calculated for each voxel [19]. They are eleven moment invariants that are calculated from the first-order, second-order, and third-order 3D-regular moments. They are invariant to translation and rotation. For the first time, Shen et al [20] used the GMIs for elastic registration of MRI. They utilized them to reflect the underlying anatomy at different scales. They defined similarity measures instead of using a classifier to identify the brain structures. They optimized an objective function to maximize the image similarity.

In [18], we utilized an ANN for the segmentation of the putamen. The input features were the GMIs along the neighboring voxel intensity values. We calculated the GMIs for one scale. The output of the ANN was a single node that took two values (-1, 1) for indicating inside of the structure or its outside. However, one scale was not sufficient to distinguish all parts of the putamen.

In this research, we propose a two-stage method for the segmentation of the brain structures. In the first stage, we consider the shape of the structures using the GMIs in different scales along with the neighboring voxels intensity values as the input features and the signed distance function of the structure as the outputs of the ANNs. In each scale, an ANN is designed to approximate the signed distance function of the structure. In the second stage, we combine the outputs of the ANNs by another ANN to classify the voxels. By calculating the GMIs in different scales and using them as input features, we are able to produce excellent results using significantly smaller training data sets.

Our method has multiple advantages compared to the previous methods. First, it does not need to solve the optimization problem that can be very time consuming. The use of the ANNs decreases the processing time of the algorithm. Calculation of the GMIs in different scales is time consuming but we decreased this time by using a proposed fast moment calculation method and multi-threaded programming. Therefore, our proposed method is sufficiently fast its excellent performance.

This paper is organized as follows. The next section (Method Section) describes the first stage of the method for representing the shapes of the structures. Then, it describes the second stage of the method for classifying the voxels into two classes. Next, the Results Section presents the results of our algorithm for the segmentation of caudate, putamen, and thalamus. It also compares the proposed method with a number of previously published methods and illustrates its superiority. Finally, the Conclusion Section concludes the work and presents future directions.

2 Method

The proposed method has two stages. The shape of the structure is represented in the first stage and the desired structure is segmented in the second stage.

2.1 First Stage – Shape Representation

In the first stage, the GMIs are used with the voxel intensity values as the input features and the signed distance function of the desired structure as the output of an ANN. In this stage, there is one ANN for each scale of the GMIs. The GMIs are defined later in this section.

Pre-processing. The proposed method requires the datasets to be registered to a template. We register the datasets to the Montreal Neurological Institute (MNI) atlas using the FSL software [21].

The atlas-based method allows generation of a mask that has a high probability to include pixels of the desired structure in it. To create this mask for each structure, we sum all of the training datasets and smooth the results using a mean filter with a kernel size of 4 in 3D. The voxels which have positive values define the mask. We utilize 12 subjects of the IBSR datasets [22] for the training datasets.

ANN Architecture. The Multi Layer Perceptron (MLP) neural network is used to establish the relation between the input and output features. Several configurations for the MLP network are investigated. A set of multiple MLP networks are used finally as a setting with a good generalization. There are 33 neurons (the dimension of the input features) in the input layer, 17 neurons in the first hidden layer, 7 neurons in the second hidden layer, and a single neuron in the output (Fig. 1). The activation function used in the MLP network is the sigmoid function in all layers. The ANNs in this stage are used for function approximation.

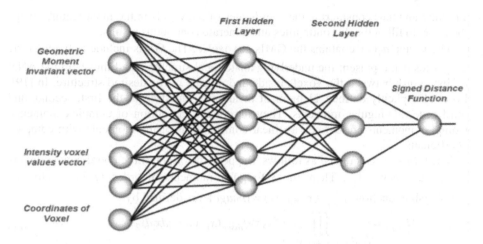

Fig. 1. ANN architecture of the first stage. Input features contain three components – GMIs, voxel intensity values, and coordinates of voxels. There are two hidden layers. There are 33 neurons in the input layer, 17 neurons in the first hidden layer, 7 neurons in the second hidden layer and a single neuron in the output. The output of the ANN is designed to approximate the singed distance function of the desired structure.

Input Features. Each input feature vector includes the neighbouring voxel intensity values, the GMIs, and the coordinates of the voxels. More formally, at voxel x, the input feature vector $a(x)$ is the concatenation of three row vectors, i.e., $a(x) = [a_1(x)\, a_2(x)\, a_3(x)]$ where $a_1(x)$ includes the voxel intensity values, $a_2(x)$ includes the coordinates of the voxel, and $a_3(x)$ includes the GMIs.

The vector $a_1(x)$ contains the neighbouring voxel intensity values of voxel x. We define $a_1(x)$ by considering the neighbouring voxels along the three orthogonal axes (± 3 voxels in each direction) in 3D. Therefore, the dimension of $a_1(x)$ **is** 19 including the intensity value of the voxel in the center (Fig 2.).

Fig. 2. Neighboring voxel intensity values that are considered for each voxel of the training datasets as a part of the input features

The vector $a_2(x)$ consists of the coordinates of the voxels in the Cartesian coordinate system. They help the ANN to find the relation between the voxels of the structure. The brain structures may have discontinuity in the image intensities inside the structure and thus considering the coordinates of the voxels in the input features helps the ANN to fill in the discontinuities and generate continuous results.

The vector $a_3(x)$ contains the GMIs at voxel x. The GMIs include rich geometric properties that represent the underlying anatomical structures and thus help the ANN to distinguish between the voxels inside and outside of the desired structure. In [19], Lo et al explicitly defined 11 moment invariants consisting of the first, second, and third order 3D-regular moments. They introduced the notion of complex moments. Complex moments are defined as linear combinations of the moments with complex coefficients.

The GMIs are calculated as follows. Suppose the origin of the coordinate system is shifted to the voxel x. Then, the 3D-regular moments of order $(p+q+r)$ for the membership function $f_{tissue}(x_1, x_2, x_3) = \{image\}$ are defined by

$$M_{p,q,r} = \iiint\limits_{(x_1)^2+(x_2)^2+(x_3)^2 < R^2} x_1^p x_2^q x_3^r f_{tissue}(x_1, x_2, x_3) dx_1 dx_2 dx_3 \tag{1}$$

where R is the radius of the spherical neighbourhood around the origin. Due to the complexity of the formulas, we only present the second order moments below. Other formulas can be found in [19].

$$I_1 = M_{2,0,0} + M_{0,2,0} + M_{0,0,2} \tag{2}$$

$$I_2 = M_{2,0,0}M_{0,2,0} + M_{2,0,0}M_{0,0,2} + M_{0,2,0}M_{0,0,2} - M_{1,0,1}^2 - M_{1,1,0}^2 - M_{0,1,1}^2 \tag{3}$$

$$I_3 = M_{2,0,0}M_{0,2,0}M_{0,0,2} - M_{0,0,2}M_{1,1,0}^2 + 2M_{1,1,0}M_{1,0,1}M_{0,1,1} - M_{0,2,0}M_{1,0,1}^2$$
$$- M_{2,0,0}M_{0,1,1}^2 \tag{4}$$

In this research, 8 scales have been considered for R={2,3,4,5,6,8,10,12}. Although more scales can be considered, this will substantially increase the computation time. Each scale can detect some parts of the structure of interest. In this case, in each scale, we collect more information from the structure which is desirable.

Considering the above, the input feature vector is made of 33 features including 19 features for the voxel intensity values, 11 features for the GMIs, and 3 features for the coordinates of the voxel in the center of the neighbourhood.

Fast Moment Calculation. Calculation of the moment invariants is time-consuming. There are algorithms in the literature for reducing the computational complexity of the moment invariants [23,24]. However, they are appropriate for binary and 2D data-sets. In our research, we use two tricks for fast moment calculation. First, we use the relation between successive voxels in the 3D datasets. Second, we use multithreading programming to reduce the processing time.

Usually, spheres with radius R are considered to calculate the regular moments using equation (1). This can be very time-consuming. The calculation complexity in this case is $O(R^3 \times M^3)$ where R is the radius used for the moment calculation and M is dimension of the volume over which to calculate the moments for each voxel inside it. We use the information of the previous voxel to calculate the moments. For voxel at position (x,y,z+1), we use the moment at position (x,y,z) with some consideration.

Instead of spheres, we use cubes for moment calculation. A cube can be divided into $2 \times R + 1$ planes along the z-axis. We define a buffer of size $2 \times R + 1$ and then we assign each entry as a weighted sum of each plane along the x and y coordinates. For moment calculation of voxels at position x, calculation of a weighted sum along the z-axis yields the 3D-regular moment for voxel at position (x,y,z). For the voxel at (x,y,z+1), we just update the buffer for the new plane when z increases by one. The entry of the buffer for the first plane of the previous voxel is removed. Therefore, for the moment calculation, we just need to update the weighted values along the z axis (Fig. 3). At the end of the line along the z axis, we increase the value of y and then update our buffer for the new position at (x,y+1,z). Hereby, all of the moments for the remaining voxels are calculated. In this case, the calculation complexity is $O(R^3 + R \times M^3)$. This shows that our algorithm is much faster than the regular calculation of the moments.

Another trick that we utilize for fast computation of the moments is multithreading. For the calculation of the GMIs, we need 12 orders of the 3D-regular moments. For fast calculation of GMIs, we divide these 12 orders into four groups and calculate each group with one core of the CPU. We use a computer with a quad core CPU and then use a thread for each group. Therefore, the speed for moment calculation is four times faster. For a volume with a dimension of $182 \times 218 \times 182$, calculation of a moment with a radius of 4 takes about two minutes.

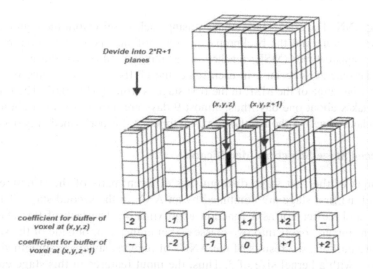

Fig. 3. Fast moment calculation method. In this figure, we demonstrate our method for the calculation of the moments with radius 2. For each voxel, we consider a cube with two voxels in each direction, therefore, the dimension of the cube is $5 \times 5 \times 5$. We show our method for two voxels at positions (x, y, z) and (x, y, z+1). At first, we construct the buffer for 5 planes of the first voxel. We assign each entry of the buffer as a weighted sum of each plane along the x- and y-coordinates. For moment calculation of the voxel at position (x, y, z), we multiply the coefficient vector (-2, -1, 0, 1, 2) by each entry of the buffer. For the next voxel at position (x, y, z+1), we calculate a weighted sum for a new plane and remove the first entry of the buffer and shift all entries by one to the right and then we calculate the new moment.

Fig. 4. An example of the signed distance function for the putamen in an image of the training datasets. Fig. *(a)* shows a segmented putamen. Fig. *(b)* shows the signed distance function of Fig. *(a)*. Positive voxel values are normalized to [0 1] and negative voxel values are normalized to [-1 0].

Output Feature. Another trick used in our research for shape representation is to consider the output feature as a signed distance function of the structure of interest. The signed distance function is a subset of implicit functions in shape representations. It is defined to be positive in the interior, negative in the exterior, and zero on the boundary. Near the boundaries, the absolute values decrease and far from the boundaries they increase. In Fig. 4, an example is shown for the putamen.

The signed distance function improves the training of the ANNs. In this case, both of the input and output have the ability to represent the shape of the structure of interest.

Training ANN. The ANNs were trained using each voxel within the region of interest of the structure and the backpropagation algorithm. The training continued until the Mean Square Error (MSE) reached an asymptotic value. We did not expect the MSE to become zero because in each scale, the GMIs can detect some parts of the structure. The range of the MSE in the first stage is from 0.02 to 0.03. The training of an ANN takes about one day, thus, almost 9 days are needed for the training of the ANNs in both stages. Although this is a long time but it is performed only once.

2.2 Second Stage-Structure Identification

Each output of the first stage distinguishes different parts of the structure. The 8 outputs of the first stage are combined by an ANN in the second stage. This ANN works as a classifier not as a function approximator. The task of this stage is to classify the image voxels into two classes – being inside or outside of the structure. To remove outliers, the results of the ANNs of the first stage are smoothed using a mean filter with a kernel size of 3. Thus, the input features in this stage consist of the smooth versions of the 8 outputs of the first stage, 19 image intensity values of the neighbouring voxels along the three orthogonal axes, and the voxel coordinates in the Cartesian coordinate system. Consequently, the dimension of input feature vector is 30 here. The ANN setting used in this stage is the same as the ANN setting in the first stage. The lower the error in this stage, the better the results. The resulting network activation function is thresholded at 0 to define the structure of interest. The voxels that have an output value larger than 0 are considered as the structure of interest and voxels that have an output smaller than 0 are considered as its outside.

Post-processing. There are small holes and outlier voxels that can be eliminated using morphological image processing methods. We utilize two morphological image processing methods: the image filling algorithm and the connected-component analysis. For filing the holes in the output of the ANN, we use the image filling algorithm and for eliminating the outlier voxels, we apply the connected-component analysis to find the largest connected component in 3D. This eliminates the outlier voxels.

Software. The training of the ANNs is implemented using the Matlab software ver. 2008a. The FSL software [21] is used for the registration algorithms. The calculation of the GMIs is performed by a program written in C programming language. The multi-threading is used to maximize the processing speed.

Datasets. We utilize 12 subjects of the IBSR datasets as the training datasets for all 6 structures. For the test datasets, we use three datasets. The first dataset includes the 6 remaining subjects of the IBSR and are used for the evaluation of the segmentation process on all of the 6 structures. The second datasets contains 8 subjects and is used for the evaluation of the segmentation process for the right and left putamen. The third dataset includes 6 subjects and is used for the evaluation of the segmentation process for the right and left caudate. All datasets include T1-weighted images. The second and third datasets are segmented by a local expert.

3 Results

Fig. 5 shows the outputs of the first stage for the putamen in the right hemisphere.

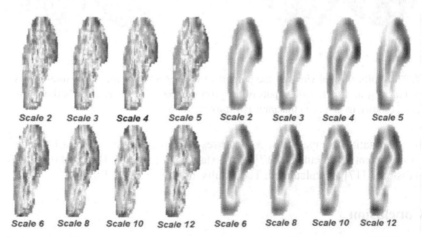

| Scale 2 | Scale 3 | Scale 4 | Scale 5 | Scale 2 | Scale 3 | Scale 4 | Scale 5 |

| Scale 6 | Scale 8 | Scale 10 | Scale 12 | Scale 6 | Scale 8 | Scale 10 | Scale 12 |

Fig. 5. Outputs of 8 ANNs of the first stage. Images on the left are outputs of ANNs in the first stage. Images on the right are the smoothed version of the images on the left.

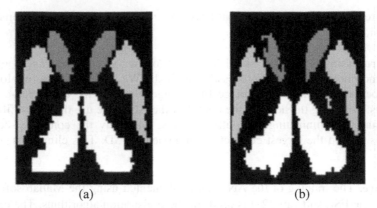

(a)   (b)

Fig. 6. The outputs of ANNs for three structures. *(a)* Manual segmentation by an expert. *(b)* Outputs of the second stage, i.e., the final segmentation by the proposed method.

Three-dimensional views of the putamen, caudate, and thalamus are shown in Figure 7.

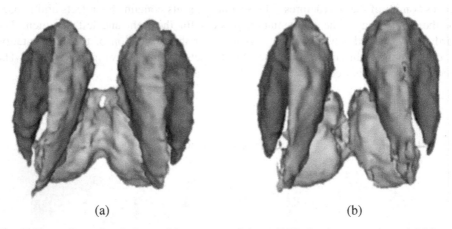

(a)   (b)

Fig. 7. Three dimensional views of the outputs of three ANNs for three structures. *(a)* Manual segmentation by an expert. *(b)* Outputs of the proposed method. The caudate is shown in green, putamen is shown in blue, and thalamus is shown in yellow.

For quantitative comparisons, 3 measures are utilized. As a similarity index, the Dice Coefficient is calculated [17]. As distance indices, the H95 distance [25] and mean distance [17] are calculated. The results are presented in Table 1.

4   Conclusion

We presented a new method for the segmentation of the brain structures using the Geometric Moments Invariants and artificial neural networks. The GMIs along with

Table 1. Dice Coefficient, H95 Distance, and Mean Distance. Data in the form of Mean (standard deviation) is reported.

	Putamen	Caudate	Thalamus
Our Method			
Dice Coefficient	0.88 (0.01)	0.86 (0.02)	0.89 (0.01)
H95	1.92 (0.48)	2.40 (1.2)	2.21 (0.38)
Mean Distance	0.70 (0.13)	0.75 (0.2)	0.90 (0.15)
Previous Method [18]			
Dice Coefficient	0.85 (0.02)	---	---
Multi-scale Bayesian Method (Akselrod-Ballin et al [25])			
Dice Coefficient	0.79	0.80	0.84
H95	3.36	3.07	2.90
Mean Distance	1.60	1.44	1.44
Akhondi-Asl et al [7]			
Dice Coefficient	0.82	0.76	---
ISCA Method [15] (results reported in [25])			
Dice Coefficient	0.78	0.74	0.80
H95	3.89	4.46	3.41
Mean Distance	1.72	1.84	1.59
Powell et al [14]*			
Dice Coefficient	0.92 (0.02)	0.91 (0.02)	0.93 (0.01)

* They have used their own datasets. Our method and other methods use the IBSR datasets.

the voxel intensities and coordinates and the signed distance function were the inputs and outputs of the ANNs, respectively, for shape representation in the first stage. The smoothed outputs of the first stage were used along with the voxel intensities and coordinates as the inputs of another ANN in the second stage. The output of this ANN defined the voxels inside the structure of interest.

The quantitative comparisons shown in Table 1 illustrate the superiority of the proposed method to other methods in the literature. Our previous method had a Dice Coefficient of about 0.85. This result was obtained when only 6 IBSR datasets were used for the testing of the ANNs, the region of interest was about one half of the region of interest in the new method, and the threshold of the output of the ANN was experimental. Also, for each structure only one ANN was used and the GMIs were calculated only for one scale.

In comparing our results with the method proposed by Powell et al [14], note that their Dice Coefficients are higher than ours. However, they used two high resolution MR images acquired in their institution by T1-weighted and T2-wieghted protocols (not the IBSR datasets). The IBSR datasets contain T1-weighted images only and for a variety of subjects with different ages and genders. The ages of the subjects range from 7 to 71 years. Having access to a single modality (instead of dual modality) and large range for the subjects' ages make the segmentation task hard. In addition, they utilized larger datasets. Their method did not contain any shape representation methods. On the other hand, they used two other methods, template-based method and probability method for constructing their input features. They utilized the voxel intensity values along the largest gradient. Obviously, in low-resolution images with intensity inhomogeneity inside the structure, this feature may not work well.

For further evaluation of our method, we compared the results with those of other methods in the literature that used the IBSR datasets. In all of the cases, our method is at least 5% superior to the others in terms of the Dice coefficient. Moreover, our H95 distances and mean distances are smaller than those of the other algorithms. Due to the nature of the neural network-based methods, we have more outlier voxels than the other methods. In spite of this limitation, our method is superior to the others. Sample results are shown in Figures 6-7 for visual inspection.

Akhondi-Asl et al [7] utilized 10 subjects for the training and 8 remaining subjects of the IBSR for the testing. Akselrod-ballin et al [25] incorporated the prior knowledge information into a multi-scale framework. In that work, the probability information constructed with the IBSR datasets was based on an atlas prior and on a likelihood function. 5 subjects of the IBSR datasets were used for constructing the atlas prior and 17 subjects were used for constructing the likelihood function. Their algorithm was tested on the 18 subjects of the IBSR. We tested our algorithm on 14 subjects for the putamen, 12 subjects for the caudate and 6 subjects for the thalamus.

Overall, we established a new framework for the segmentation of the brain structures in MRI. The proposed method can be extended to improve its performance. Alternative input features, a different number of scales for the first stage, and other design methods for the second stage can be investigated. For example, the level set method can be used in the second stage. Using the signed distance function available as the output of the first stage, the level set equations become simple. A framework can be established for combining all of the ANNs to develop a single network for the segmentation process. For the input feature, the use of the probability information such as prior atlas [14,25] and the use of the logarithm of the odds ratio, which encodes shapes of multiple anatomical structures with capturing some information concerning uncertainty [26], can be useful. Last but not least, the proposed method can be applied to the segmentation of other brain structures in MRI and other organs in other medical images.

References

1. Macovski, A.: Noise in MRI. Magnetic Resonance in Medicine 36(3), 494–497 (1996)
2. Simmons, A., Tofts, P.S., Baker, G.J., Arridge, S.R.: Sources of Intensity Nonuniformity in Spin Echo Images at 1.5T. Magnetic Resonance in Medicine 32(1), 121–128 (1994)
3. Leventon, M.E., Grimson, W.E.L., Faugeras, O.: Statistical Shape Influence in Geodesic Active Contours. In: IEEE International Conference on Computer Vision and Pattern Recognition, vol. 1, pp. 1316–1323 (2000)
4. Jehan-Besson, S., Herbulot, A., Barlaud, M., Aubert, G.: Shape Gradient for image and Video Segmentation. Mathematical Models in Computer Vision, The Handbook (2005)
5. Kass, M., Witkin, A., Terzopoulos, D.: Snakes: Active Contour Models. In: First International Conference on Computer Vision, pp. 259–268 (1987)
6. Woolrich, M.W., Behrens, T.E.: Variational Bayes Inference of Spatial Mixture Models for Segmentation. IEEE Transaction on Medical Imaging 25(10), 1380–1391 (2006)
7. Akhondi-Asl, A.R., Soltanian-Zadeh, H.: Constrained Optimization of Nonparametric entropy-based Segmentation of brain Structures. In: IEEE ISBI 2008, pp. 4–44 (2008)
8. Tsai, A., Wells, W., Tempany, C., Grimson, E., Willsky, A.: Mutual Information in Coupled Multi-Shape Model for medical Image Segmentation. Medical Image Analysis 8(4), 429–445 (2004)

9. Gouttard, S., Styner, S., Joshi, S., Smith, R.G., Cody, H., Gerig, G.: Subcortical Structure Segmentation using Probabilistic Atlas priors. In: Proc. SPIE, vol. 6512 (2007)
10. Liu, J., Chelberg, D., Smith, C., Chebrolu, H.: Automatic Subcortical Structure Segmentation Using probabilistic Atlas. In: Bebis, G., Boyle, R., Parvin, B., Koracin, D., Paragios, N., Tanveer, S.-M., Ju, T., Liu, Z., Coquillart, S., Cruz-Neira, C., Müller, T., Malzbender, T. (eds.) ISVC 2007, Part I. LNCS, vol. 4841, pp. 170–178. Springer, Heidelberg (2007)
11. Angelini, E.D., Jin, Y., Laine, A.F.: State-of-the-Art of levelset Methods in Segmentation and Registration of Medical Imaging Modalities. In: The handbook of Medical Image Analysis. Registration Models, vol. 3. Kluwer Academic/Plenum publishers, New York (2005)
12. Jacob, M., Blu, T., Unser, M.: Efficient energies and algorithms for parametric snakes. IEEE Transactions on Image Processing 13(9), 1231–1244 (2004)
13. Magnotta, V.A., Heckel, D., Andreasen, N.C., Cizadlo, T., Corson, P.W., Ehrhardt, J.C., Yuh, W.T.: Measurement of brain Structures with Artificial neural Network: two and three-dimensional applications. Radiology 211(3), 781–790 (1999)
14. Powell, S., Magnotta, V.A., Johnson, H., Jammalamadaka, V.K., Prerson, R., Anderasen, N.C.: Registration and Machine Learning-based Automated Segmentation of Subcortical and Cerebellar brain Structures. NeuroImage 39, 238–247 (2008)
15. Akselrod-Ballin, A., Galun, M., Gomori, M.J., Basri, R., Brandt, A.: Atlas Guided Identification of Brain Structures by Combining 3D Segmentation and SVM Classification. In: Larsen, R., Nielsen, M., Sporring, J. (eds.) MICCAI 2006. LNCS, vol. 4191, pp. 209–216. Springer, Heidelberg (2006)
16. Amini, L., Soltanian-Zadeh, H., Lucas, C., Gity, M.: Automatic Segmentation of Thalamus from brain MRI Integrating fuzzy clustering and dynamic contours. IEEE Transactions on Biomedical Engineering 51, 800–811 (2004)
17. Ciofolo, C., Barillot, C.: Brain Segmentation with Competitive level sets and fuzzy control. In: Christensen, G.E., Sonka, M. (eds.) IPMI 2005. LNCS, vol. 3565, pp. 333–344. Springer, Heidelberg (2005)
18. Jabarouti Moghaddam, M., Rahmani, R., Soltanian-Zadeh, H.: Automatic Segmentation of Putamen using Geometric Moment Invariants. In: The 15th Iranian Conference on Biomedical Engineering, Mashad, Iran (2009)
19. Lo, C.H., Don, H.S.: 3-D Moment Forms: Their Construction and Application to Object Identification and Positioning. IEEE Trans. on Pattern Analysis and Machine Intelligence 11(10), 1053–1064 (1989)
20. Shen, D., Davatzikos, D.: HAMMER: Hierarchical Attribute Matching Mechanism for elastic Registration. IEEE Trans. Med. 21(11), 1421–1439 (2002)
21. Jenkinson, M., Bannister, P., Brady, M., Smith, S.: Improved Methods for the Registration and Motion Correction of Brain Images. NeuroImage 17(2), 825–841 (2002)
22. The Internet Brain Segmentation Repository,
    http://www.cma.mgh.harvard.edu/ibsr
23. Shen, B.C., Shen, J.: Fast Computation of Moment Invariants. Pattern Recognition 24, 801–806 (1991)
24. Zakaria, M.F., Vroomen, L.J., Zsomhar-Murray, P.J.A., Kessel, M.H.M.V.: Fast Algorithm for Computation of Moment Invariants. Pattern Recognition 20, 634–643 (1987)
25. Akselrod-Ballin, A., Galun, M., Gomori, M.J., Basri, R., Brandt, A.: Prior Knowledge Driven Multiscale Segmentation of Brain MRI. In: Ayache, N., Ourselin, S., Maeder, A. (eds.) MICCAI 2007, Part II. LNCS, vol. 4792, pp. 118–126. Springer, Heidelberg (2007)
26. Pohl, K.M., Fisher, J., Bouix, S., Shenton, M., McCarley, R.W., Grimson, W.E.L., Kikinis, R., Wells, W.M.: Using the Logarithm of Odds to Define a Vector Space. Medical Image Analysis 11, 465–477 (2007)

Adaptive Kernels for Multi-fiber Reconstruction*

Angelos Barmpoutis[1], Bing Jian[2], and Baba C. Vemuri[1]

[1] CISE Department, University of Florida, Gainesville FL 32611, USA
[2] Siemens Healthcare, IKM CKS, Malvern, PA 19355, USA
abarmpou@cise.ufl.edu, bing.jian@siemens.com, vemuri@cise.ufl.edu

Abstract. In this paper we present a novel method for multi-fiber reconstruction given a diffusion-weighted MRI dataset. There are several
existing methods that employ various spherical deconvolution kernels
for achieving this task. However the kernels in all of the existing methods rely on certain assumptions regarding the properties of the underlying fibers, which introduce inaccuracies and unnatural limitations in
them. Our model is a non trivial generalization of the spherical deconvolution model, which unlike the existing methods does not make use
of a fix-shaped kernel. Instead, the shape of the kernel is estimated simultaneously with the rest of the unknown parameters by employing a
general adaptive model that can theoretically approximate any spherical deconvolution kernel. The performance of our model is demonstrated
using simulated and real diffusion-weighed MR datasets and compared
quantitatively with several existing techniques in literature. The results
obtained indicate that our model has superior performance that is close
to the theoretic limit of the best possible achievable result.

1 Introduction

Many diffusion MR reconstruction methods are based on the Stejskal-Tanner
equation $S = S_0 \exp(-bd)$ which describes the signal S observed in a diffusion
MR image at a voxel scale, where b is the diffusion weighting factor depending
on the strength as well as the effective time of diffusion, S_0 is the signal in the
absence of any diffusion weighting, and d is called *apparent diffusion coefficient*
(ADC) [1]. In the diffusion tensor imaging (DTI)[2], d is assumed to take a
quadratic form $d = \mathbf{g}^T \mathbf{D} \mathbf{g}$, where $\mathbf{D}$ is a 3×3 positive definite matrix, and $\mathbf{g}$ is the
diffusion gradient direction. However, the inability of DTI to deal with regions
containing intra-voxel orientational heterogeneity has been widely reported in
literature [3, 4, 5, 6] making it a well-known and challenging problem.

To overcome the single fiber orientation limitation inherent with the unimodal
quadratic functions, higher order models [3, 4, 7] have been proposed to model

* This research was supported by the NIH grant EB007082 to Baba Vemuri and fund-
ing for data acquisition was provided by the NIH grant P41-RR16105 to Stephen
Blackband. Authors thank Drs. Timothy M. Shepherd and Evren Özarslan for data
acquisition. Implementation is available at http://www.cise.ufl.edu/research/cvgmi.

J.L. Prince, D.L. Pham, and K.J. Myers (Eds.): IPMI 2009, LNCS 5636, pp. 338–349, 2009.
© Springer-Verlag Berlin Heidelberg 2009

the diffusivity function. However, the flexibility brought by these methods does not solve the problem that the peaks of the ADC profile do not necessarily yield the fiber orientations in the case of fiber crossings [8, 9].

The ensemble-average diffusion propagator P(r,t) can be computed using the q-space methods by exploiting the Fourier relation between the signal attenuation and the diffusion propagator. Diffusion spectrum imaging (DSI) [10] performs a discrete Fourier transform to obtain P(r,t), which requires a time-intensive Cartesian sampling in q-space and hence is impractical for routine clinical use. Instead of the Cartesian sampling, the Q-ball imaging (QBI) method takes measurements on a q-space ball and approximates the radial integral of the displacement probability distribution function by the spherical Funk-Radon transform [11]. In more recent studies, the analytic solution of QBI's Funk-Radon transform has been derived by using a spherical harmonic basis [12, 13, 14]. One problem with QBI is that the estimated diffusion ODF is modulated by a zeroth-order Bessel function that induces spectral broadening of the diffusion peaks. Another technique called the diffusion orientation transform (DOT) [8] computes the displacement probability profile at a fixed radius by expressing the Fourier transform in spherical coordinates and evaluating the radial part of the integral analytically. DOT assumes signals decay can be described by either a mono- or a multi-exponential model, the latter of which requires data acquisition over multiple concentric spheres, a time consuming proposition.

Another research direction in the multi-fiber reconstruction literature is to describe the signal attenuation by multi-compartment models beyond the mono-exponential Stejskal-Tanner equation. The approach in [6] assumes the signal in each voxel can be split into a weighted sum of contributions from different diffusion tensors individually. Various partial volume models have been studied in [15, 16] and were extended in [17, 18]. The model selection problem in these methods usually requires complicated solution techniques and computationally intensive simulations to infer the optimal model parameters properly.

To avoid the model-selection problem several spherical deconvolution techniques have been proposed in which the DW-MRI signal can be expressed as the convolution over the sphere of a fiber bundle response (also known as kernel function k) with a probability density function [19, 21, 20, 22]. In this spherical deconvolution approach there is no limitation on the number of the estimated distinct fiber populations within a voxel. However, all of these methods employ a predefined fix-shaped function such as Gaussian [19, 21, 23], von Mises [22], Rigaut-type [20], each of which is treated as a spherical basis, whose shape parameters are chosen based on certain assumptions relating to the properties of the underlying fibers. Such assumptions introduce inaccuracies and unnatural limitations in the methods since in a real DW-MRI dataset the properties of the underlying fibers may vary spatially.

In this paper we present a novel mathematical model for multi-fiber reconstruction using an adaptive deconvolution kernel, whose shape is not fixed and is estimated simultaneously with the rest of the unknowns of the model. The adaptive kernel is defined as a spline over the space of magnetic gradient directions and the diffusion weighting factor b, which can theoretically approximate any continuous function. We present extensive comparisons between the proposed method and other existing techniques demonstrating superior performance of our method. Furthermore we show that the results produced by the proposed model are close to the limit of the theoretically best possible result.

The main contribution of this paper is a novel mathematical model for multi-fiber reconstruction. To the best of our knowledge, it is the first method that employs an adaptively shaped spherical deconvolution kernel instead of a fixed one used by the existing techniques. Our model overcomes the limitations of the other methods and furthermore generalizes the spherical deconvolution framework, in which all the other existing methods can be expressed as special cases.

2   Mathematical Model

The DW-MRI signal response can be modeled as the convolution of a kernel function k, which corresponds to a single fiber response, with a mixing density function f as expressed in the following equation

$$S(b, \mathbf{g})/S_0 = \int f(\mathbf{p})k(b, \mathbf{g}|\mathbf{p})d\mathbf{p} \tag{1}$$

where the kernel k is a parametric function with parameter vector $\mathbf{p}$, which is also the random variable of the density function f, and the integration is over the domain of $\mathbf{p}$. S_0 is the zero gradient image, and $\mathbf{g}$ and b are the magnetic gradient field direction and the b-value respectively. In [24], it has been shown that several existing multi-fiber reconstruction models can be expressed in the above generalized fiber convolution model.

Two possible choices for the kernel function are the multivariate Gaussian function $k(b, \mathbf{g}|\mathbf{D}) = e^{-b\mathbf{g}^T \mathbf{D} \mathbf{g}}$ [19, 12, 20, 21], and the von Mises-Fisher function over the sphere given by $k(b, \mathbf{g}|\mu) = \frac{\kappa}{4\pi \sinh \kappa} e^{\kappa \mu^T \mathbf{g}}$ [22]. The integration space in the above examples is the space of 3×3 symmetric positive-definite matrices $\mathbf{D}$ and the space of 3-dimensional unit vectors μ respectively. The kernel functions as well as the mixing densities that correspond to several existing multi-fiber reconstruction models are reported and compared in [24].

Due to the spherical nature of the diffusion-weighted acquisition process, the mixing density function f can be parametrized using a discrete hemispherical lattice as follows

$$f(\mathbf{p}) = \sum_{j=1}^{N} w_j \phi(\mathbf{p}|\mathbf{v}_j) \tag{2}$$

where $\mathbf{v}_1 \ldots \mathbf{v}_N$ is a set of unit vectors uniformly distributed on the hemisphere, and $\phi(\mathbf{p}|\mathbf{v}_j)$ is a mixing density function that is treated here as a basis function weighted by the unknown mixing weights w_j. By substituting Eq. 2 into Eq. 1 and convolving these basis functions with the kernel over the space of the kernel's parameters as follows

$$\int \sum_{j=1}^{N} w_j \phi(\mathbf{p}|\mathbf{v}_j) k(b, \mathbf{g}|\mathbf{p}) d\mathbf{p} = \sum_{j=1}^{N} w_j K(b, \mathbf{g}|\mathbf{v}_j) \tag{3}$$

we obtain a continuous function $K(b, \mathbf{g}|\mathbf{v}_j) = \int \phi(\mathbf{p}|\mathbf{v}_j) k(b, \mathbf{g}|\mathbf{p}) d\mathbf{p}$. In several cases, this function can be computed analytically [20, 22] and corresponds to a multi-fiber reconstruction kernel K, employed in the following mixture model

$$S(b, \mathbf{g})/S_0 = \sum_{j=1}^{N} w_j K(b, \mathbf{g}|\mathbf{v}_j) \tag{4}$$

Different choices of $k(b, \mathbf{g}|\mathbf{p})$ in Eq.(1) and of $\phi(\mathbf{p}|\mathbf{v}_j)$ in Eq.(2) result in differently shaped kernel $K(b, \mathbf{g}|\mathbf{v}_j)$ in Eq.(4). Thus it is entirely possible for some kernels to be better suited to a particular data set than others in terms of reconstruction accuracy.

In all of the existing methods, the shape of the kernel K is assumed to be fixed, which is an unnecessary constraint and adds an unnatural restriction to the computed fiber reconstructions. For example the shape of the Rigaut-type kernel $K(b, \mathbf{g}|, \mathbf{T}_j) = (1 + (b\mathbf{g}^T \mathbf{T}_j \mathbf{g})/p)^{-p}$ derived in [20] is fixed by using certain predefined value of p as well as eigenvalues in the tensor $\mathbf{T}_j$, the diffusion basis kernel $K(b, \mathbf{g}|\mathbf{T}_j) = exp(-b\mathbf{g}^T \mathbf{T}_j \mathbf{g})$ in [19, 21] is also fixed by predefining the eigenvalues of the tensor, and the shape of the model employed in [22] is fixed by choosing a value for the parameter κ.

In this paper, we do not make any such assumptions instead, we develop a general adaptively shaped kernel, whose shape is simultaneously estimated with the mixing weights w_j in Eq.(4). The proposed kernel is expressed as a spline, which can theoretically approximate any continuous function. Furthermore, by considering the cylindrical geometry of the underlying fibers in the tissue [25] the spline model can be reduced to a 2-dimensional spline over the 2D domain $b \times |\mathbf{g} \cdot \mathbf{v}_j|$ as follows:

$$K(b, \mathbf{g}|\mathbf{v}_j) = \sum_{k} \sum_{l} c_{k,l} \psi_l(b) \psi_k(|\mathbf{g} \cdot \mathbf{v}_j|) \tag{5}$$

where $c_{k,l}$ are the so-called unknown control points, and $\psi_i(x)$ is a spline basis. In the special case of HARDI acquisition using a constant b-value, the formula for the corresponding adaptively shaped kernel is simplified to an 1-dimensional spline given by

$$K(\mathbf{g}|b, \mathbf{v}_j) = \sum_{k} c_k \psi_k(|\mathbf{g} \cdot \mathbf{v}_j|). \tag{6}$$

Figure 1 illustrates the 2D and 1D splines that correspond to Eq.(5) and Eq.(6) respectively computed from simulated DW-MRI data. As expected, the diffusion-weighted MR signal attenuation S/S_0 decreases while b-value increases and also decreases when the magnetic gradient direction $\mathbf{g}$ becomes parallel to the fiber orientation $\mathbf{v}$.

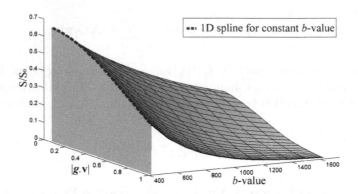

Fig. 1. Plot of the 2D spline that corresponds to $K(b, \mathbf{g}|\mathbf{v})$ computed from simulated DW-MRI data of a single fiber with orientation $\mathbf{v}$. The dashed line is a plot of the 1D spline that corresponds to $K(\mathbf{g}|b, \mathbf{v})$ for a constant b-value using the same simulated dataset.

By substituting Eq.6 into Eq.4 we derive our model which is given by Eq.(7).

$$S(\mathbf{g})/S_0 = \sum_{j=1}^{N} w_j \sum_k c_k \psi_k(|\mathbf{g} \cdot \mathbf{v}_j|) \tag{7}$$

The unknowns in this model are the weights w_j and the control points c_k. The number of the unknown weights w_j corresponds to the resolution of the hemisphere tessellation by the vectors $\mathbf{v}_j$, and the number of the control points c_k corresponds to the resolution of the discretization of the spline. Here we should emphasize that the adaptively shaped kernel employed in Eq. 7 can theoretically approximate any kernel function and therefore it does not add any kind of limitation related to the underlying fiber characteristics, which is one of the major advantages of our model when compared with the existing techniques. In the next section we estimate these unknowns from a given DW-MRI dataset.

3   Algorithm and Implementation Details

In this section we assume that a set of M diffusion-weighted MRI images S_i are given, along with the corresponding magnetic gradient directions $\mathbf{g}_i$. The underlying fiber populations in this dataset can be reconstructed by using our adaptively-shaped kernel model (Eq.7) in a least-square minimization framework, by minimizing the following objective function

$$E(\mathbf{w}, \mathbf{c}) = \sum_{i=1}^{M} \left(S_i/S_0 - \sum_{j=1}^{N} w_j \sum_{k=1}^{P} c_k \psi_k(|\mathbf{g}_i \cdot \mathbf{v}_j|) \right)^2 \tag{8}$$

where $\mathbf{w}$ and $\mathbf{c}$ are the two unknown vectors that consist of the unknown variables w_j and c_k.

Any spline basis function can be used for $\psi_k(x)$ in Eq.8. In our experiments we employed the B-spline basis of various orders due to their simple analytic form, and the corresponding control points were positioned on a uniform grid of knots. The number of control points P controls the flexibility of the estimated adaptive kernel, i.e. large P can accommodate more bumps in the approximated kernel function. However, in our particular application the kernel function should represent the diffusion-weighted MRI signal attenuation of a single fiber, which is a very smooth function (see Fig.1) and therefore can be well approximated by using a small number of control points ($P \sim 5$).

Additionally, the diffusion-weighted MRI signal attenuation of a single fiber is a monotonically decreasing function of $|\mathbf{g}_i \cdot \mathbf{v}_j|$, (or monotonically increasing function of $1 - |\mathbf{g}_i \cdot \mathbf{v}_j|$) due to the physics of DW-MRI acquisition. Hence the corresponding adaptively-shaped kernel should also be a monotonically increasing function of $1 - |\mathbf{g}_i \cdot \mathbf{v}_j|$, which can be incorporated into our parametrization by enforcing the corresponding unknown control points c_k to form a monotonically increasing sequence. This can be achieved by further parameterizing the sequence of control points as: $c_1 = a_1$, $c_2 = a_1 + a_2,..., c_k = \sum_{l=1}^{l=k} a_l$ where $a_1, \ldots, a_k$ is a sequence of non-negative numbers. By plugging the parameters a_k into Eq.8 we arrive at the following expression for the objective function

$$E(\mathbf{w}, \mathbf{a}) = \sum_{i=1}^{M} \left(S_i/S_0 - \sum_{j=1}^{N} w_j \sum_{k=1}^{P} a_k \sum_{l=k}^{P} \psi_l(1 - |\mathbf{g}_i \cdot \mathbf{v}_j|) \right)^2 \qquad (9)$$

where $\mathbf{a}$ is the unknown vector that consists of the parameters a_k. This minimization problem can be solved iteratively by first estimating $\mathbf{w}$ given $\mathbf{a}$ and then estimating $\mathbf{a}$ given $\mathbf{w}$. Note that all the unknown parameters should be non-negative real numbers and therefore they can be computed using the non-negative least squares method [26].

Both vectors $\mathbf{w}$ and $\mathbf{a}$ can be estimated by solving two linear systems. First we form the linear system $\mathbf{Aw} = \mathbf{b}$, where the matrix $\mathbf{A}$ is of size $M \times N$, and its elements are $A_{i,j} = \sum_{k=1}^{P} a_k \sum_{l=k}^{P} \psi_l(1 - |\mathbf{g}_i \cdot \mathbf{v}_j|)$ and the elements of $\mathbf{b}$ are $b_i = S_i/S_0$. After having solved this linear system using non-negative least squares, we form another linear system $\mathbf{A'a} = \mathbf{b}$, where the matrix $\mathbf{A'}$ is of size $M \times P$, and its elements are $A'_{i,k} = \sum_{j=1}^{N} w_j \sum_{l=k}^{P} \psi_l(1 - |\mathbf{g}_i \cdot \mathbf{v}_j|)$. This system should also be solved using a non-negative least squares approach. These two alternating steps are repeated until convergence of the algorithm. The convergence of the algorithm is guaranteed, due to the fact that both steps converge and reduce the same positive-valued objective function (Eq. 9).

The process for reconstructing fibers using adaptively-shaped kernels is summarized in Algorithm 1. As was previously discussed, *argmin* is implemented by solving a linear system using the non-negative least squares method. In order to increase the robustness of the adaptively-shaped kernel method to the presence of noise in the data, we can slightly modify our algorithm by penalizing the smallest weights from vector $\mathbf{w}$ when updating the vector $\mathbf{a}$. The dominant weights correspond to strong fiber responses, while the smallest weights capture high frequency details such as noise. In our experiments, in the step for updating vector **a**, we employed a penalizing function that scales down by a factor 0.5 those weights w_j that have less than half of the strength of the largest weight in **w**. Other penalizing functions can be employed as well. Note that the full vector **w** is used without penalization after the final reconstruction (line 1.5).

Algorithm 1. Adaptively-shaped kernels for multi-fiber reconstruction

---

    input : $S_1 \ldots S_M$, $\mathbf{g}_1 \ldots \mathbf{g}_M$, S_0, b-value, and a small tolerance value e
    output: the vector of weights **w** and the vector of control points **c**
1.1 **while** $\parallel a_t - a_{t-1} \parallel > e$ **do**
1.2 $\mathbf{w} \leftarrow argmin_{\mathbf{w}} E(\mathbf{w}, \mathbf{a})$ given **a** ;
1.3 $\mathbf{a} \leftarrow argmin_{\mathbf{a}} E(\mathbf{w}, \mathbf{a})$ given **w** ;
1.4 **end**
1.5 $\mathbf{w} \leftarrow argmin_{\mathbf{w}} E(\mathbf{w}, \mathbf{a})$ given **a** ;
1.6 **for** $k = 1 \ldots P$ **do**
1.7 $c_k \leftarrow \sum_{l=1}^{l=k} a_l$;
1.8 **end**

Finally, after having approximated the DW-MRI signal by using the proposed adaptively-shaped kernel model, we can estimate the fiber orientations by finding the maxima of the water molecule displacement probability given by the Fourier integral

$$P(\mathbf{r}) = \int \frac{S(\mathbf{q})}{S_0} e^{-2\pi i \mathbf{q}^T \mathbf{r}} d\mathbf{q} \tag{10}$$

where **q** is the reciprocal space vector, $S(\mathbf{q})/S_0$ is the approximated DW-MRI signal value associated with vector **q**, and **r** is the displacement vector. Note that vector **q** is a function of the b-value and the magnetic gradient direction **g**. However, if the adaptively-shaped kernel model is fitted to data that were acquired using a constant b-value, then the estimated kernel is given by Eq.6, which is not a function of b-value. In this case the fiber orientations can be computed by finding the maxima of the following approximated expression

$$P(\mathbf{r}) \simeq \sum_{j=1}^{N} w_j \sum_{k=1}^{P} c_k \int \psi_k(|\mathbf{g} \cdot \mathbf{v}_j|) e^{-2\pi i \|\mathbf{q}\| \mathbf{g}^T \mathbf{r}} d\mathbf{g} \tag{11}$$

where the integrals $\int \psi_k(|\mathbf{g} \cdot \mathbf{v}_j|) e^{-2\pi i \|\mathbf{q}\| \mathbf{g}^T \mathbf{r}} d\mathbf{g}$ form a new basis that can be precomputed numerically over a set of predefined displacement vectors **r**.

In the next section we demonstrate the results of application of our algorithm to synthetic and real DW-MRI datasets.

4   Experimental Results

This section is divided into two subsections: a) Synthetic data experiments and b) experiments using real DW-MRI data from excised rat hippocampus and optic chiasm.

4.1   Synthetic Data Experiments

The data employed in the experiments of this section were synthesized using the realistic simulation model proposed in [25]. This method simulates the DW-MRI signal attenuation from water molecules, whose diffusion is restricted inside a cylindrical fiber of radius ρ and length L. We employed this model to simulate a 2-fiber crossing (depicted in Fig. 2 left) using the parameters $\rho = 5\mu m$, $L = 5mm$, b-value $= 1500 s/mm^2$ which are typical values in rat brain datasets [8]. The dataset were simulated using 81 gradient directions computed as the 3rd-order tessellation of the icosahedron on the unit hemisphere.

First, in order to demonstrate the ability of our algorithm in estimating an accurate deconvolution kernel (i.e. single fiber response) from a 2-fiber crossing, we applied it to the simulated dataset using various orders of the b-spline basis $\psi_k(x)$ used in the kernel parametrization. By observing the recovered kernels (Fig. 2), we can see that for each order of the B-spline used, the recovered kernel was the closest possible approximation of the simulated signal from a single fiber (dotted line). In the 2nd-order case there was perfect match with the ground truth (floating precision degree error). Here we should emphasize that neither the number of fibers nor the shape of the deconvolution kernel (single fiber response) were known in our algorithm. This is in contrast to the existing methods, which employ a given fixed deconvolution kernel. The estimated control points c_k for order-2 are shown in Fig. 3.

In the next experiment, we added various levels of Riccian noise to the simulated 2-fiber crossing dataset and then tested the accuracy of several competing multi-fiber reconstruction techniques in estimating fiber orientations. The fiber orientations were estimated by finding the maxima of either the displacement probability or the ODF computed by the corresponding methods. We used four distinct noise levels and for each noise level the experiments were repeated 100 times. The obtained results are shown in Fig. 4 and for the particular noise level with std. dev.$= 0.08$ the errors are reported in the table. The results demonstrate the superiority of the proposed model. Furthermore, there was no significant difference between the results obtained by the 0th and the 2nd-order B-spline basis, both of which yielded more accurate results compared to the other methods.

The last entry in the table in Fig. 4 corresponds to results obtained using the simulated single fiber response as the deconvolution kernel K in the spherical deconvolution framework (Eq. 4). Since this kernel is identical to the simulated

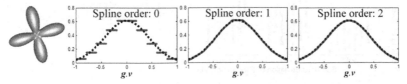

Fig. 2. Plots of the kernels computed by applying our algorithm to a synthetic dataset from a 2-fiber crossing (left) using various orders of the spline basis. The dotted line is the ground truth (simulated signal from a single fiber).

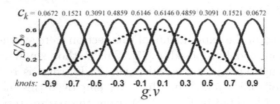

Fig. 3. The control points c_k computed by applying our algorithm to the simulated dataset. The plots of the b-spline basis are shown along with the evaluated kernel (dotted line). The centers of the basis (knots) are also marked.

single fiber response used in data generation, we will consider the multi-fiber reconstruction results produced by using it as the limiting case, which corresponds to the theoretic best possible result. Note that our method is the only method that produces average errors smaller than 1 degree compared to the limiting case. Finally we can further improve the results produced by all the methods by using post-processing tools such as ODF sharpening similar to that presented in [14], however in our experiments we compared the strength of each individual model without using any additional post-processing supplements.

4.2 Real Data Experiments

In this section we present experimental results obtained using real data set from excised rat hippocampus (shown in Fig. 5) and optic chiasm (shown in Fig. 6). The original DW-MRI data sets contained 22 images acquired using a pulsed gradient spin echo pulse sequence, with 21 different diffusion gradients and approximate b value of 1250 s/mm^2.

We applied the proposed method to the hippocampal dataset using 2nd-order b-spline and 5 control points c_k. In order to demonstrate the variability of the shape of the estimated deconvolution kernel across the dataset, we depict the

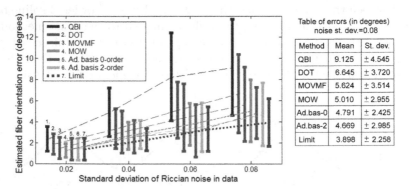

Fig. 4. Comparison of the estimated fiber orientation errors produced by several multi-fiber reconstruction models (QBI [11], DOT [8], MOVMF [22], MOW [20], and our adaptive kernel technique) using simulated 2-fiber crossing data

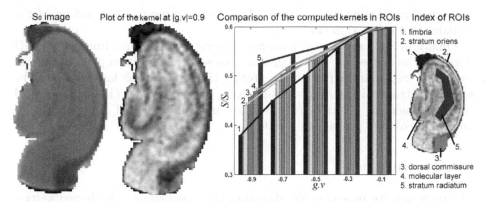

Fig. 5. The adaptively-shaped kernels estimated from a hippocampal DW-MRI dataset. The S_0 image is shown on the left and then the estimated kernel (Eq. 6) evaluated at $|\mathbf{g} \cdot \mathbf{v}| = 0.9$. The plot of the average adaptive kernel in various ROIs is shown as a bar chart on the right.

estimated kernel (eq. 6) evaluated at $|\mathbf{g} \cdot \mathbf{v}| = 0.9$ as an image in Fig. 5b. As we expected, the regions of high anisotropy appear darker, since the signal is more attenuated in such regions when the gradient direction $\mathbf{g}$ forms a small angle with the fiber orientation $\mathbf{v}$. This demonstrates that our method estimates clinically meaningful deconvolution kernels, which vary across the field, contrary to the existing methods, which employ a pre-defined fix-shaped kernel.

Furthermore, the plot in Fig 5 shows the average adaptively-shaped kernel estimated in various regions of interest (ROI) in hippocampus. By observing the plot we can see that fimbria contains more anisotropic fibers, which corresponds to steeper kernel shape, while stratum radiatum contains less anisotropic fibers, which corresponds to flattened kernel shape. These results are validated by the existing knowledge on hippocampal anatomy [27]. This motivates the use of our method, which is based on the cylindrical geometry of fibers as well as the physics of the DW-MRI acquisition, unlike othe existing techniques that require

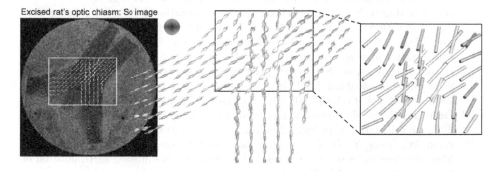

Fig. 6. The field of displacement probabilities estimated by the proposed technique using data from an excised rat's optic chiasm

the cylindrical geometry assumption but with prespecified dimensions of the cylinder (not required in our case).

Finally, in Fig. 6 we present multi-fiber reconstruction results from a DW-MRI dataset of an excised rat's optic chiasm. The spherical function plots depict the estimated displacement probability profiles (Eq. 11) at each lattice point. The region of interest is marked with a box in the S_0 image. The depicted field contains spherical plots that correspond to single fibers as well as fiber crossings and other complex probability profiles.

5   Conclusions

In this paper, we presented an algorithm that uses adaptively-shaped kernels for multi-fiber reconstruction. In this algorithm, we simultaneously estimate the shape of the kernel with the rest of the unknown parameters in the model. Our technique is motivated by the fact that the characteristics of the underlying fibers vary across a dataset, which corresponds to variations in the shape of the deconvolution kernel. The method was tested on synthetic and real DW-MRI datasets. The experimental results demonstrate the superiority of our model over existing techniques. We validated our algorithm by presenting quantitative as well as visual results. Our future efforts will be focused on employing the proposed method in multi-fiber tracking framework in order to study the changes on the shape of the estimated kernels along known fiber bundles in the brain.

References

[1] LeBihan, D., et al.: MR imaging of intravoxel incoherent motions: Application to diffusion and perfusion in neurologic disorders. Radiology 161, 401–407 (1986)

[2] Basser, P.J., et al.: Estimation of the effective self-diffusion tensor from the NMR spin echo. J. Magn. Reson. B 103, 247–254 (1994)

[3] Frank, L.: Characterization of Anisotropy in High Angular Resolution Diffusion Weighted MRI. Magn. Reson. Med. 47(6), 1083–1099 (2002)

[4] Alexander, D.C., et al.: Detection and modeling of non-Gaussian apparent diffusion coefficient profiles in human brain. MRM 48(2), 331–340 (2002)

[5] von dem Hagen, E.A.H., Henkelman, R.M.: Orientational diffusion reflects fiber structure within a voxel. Magn. Reson. Med. 48(3), 454–459 (2002)

[6] Tuch, D.S., et al.: High angular resolution diffusion imaging reveals intravoxel white matter fiber heterogeneity. MRM 48(4), 577–582 (2002)

[7] Barmpoutis, A., et al.: Symmetric positive 4th order tensors and their estimation from diffusion weighted MRI. In: Karssemeijer, N., Lelieveldt, B. (eds.) IPMI 2007. LNCS, vol. 4584, pp. 308–319. Springer, Heidelberg (2007)

[8] Özarslan, E., et al.: Resolution of complex tissue microarchitecture using the diffusion orientation transform. NeuroImage 36(3), 1086–1103 (2006)

[9] Zhan, W., Yang, Y.: How accurately can the diffusion profiles indicate multiple fiber orientations? a study on general fiber crossings in diffusion MRI. Journal of Magnetic Resonance 183(2), 193–202 (2006)

[10] Wedeen, V.J., et al.: Mapping complex tissue architecture with diffusion spectrum magnetic resonance imaging. MRM 54(6), 1377–1386 (2005)

[11] Tuch, D.S.: Q-ball imaging. Magn. Reson. Med. 52(6), 1358–1372 (2004)
[12] Anderson, A.W.: Measurement of fiber orientation distributions using high angular resolution diffusion imaging. MRM 54(5), 1194–1206 (2005)
[13] Hess, C.P., et al.: Q-ball reconstruction of multimodal fiber orientations using the spherical harmonic basis. MRM 56(1), 104–117 (2006)
[14] Descoteaux, M., Angelino, E., Fitzgibbons, S., Deriche, R.: Regularized, fast and robust analytical q-ball imaging. MRM 58, 497–510 (2007)
[15] Behrens, T., et al.: Characterization and propagation of uncertainty in diffusion-weighted MR imaging. Magn. Reson. Med. 50(2), 1077–1088 (2003)
[16] Assaf, Y., et al.: New modeling and experimental framework to characterize hindered and restricted water diffusion in brain white matter. MRM 52(5), 965–978 (2004)
[17] Hosey, T.P., et al.: Inference of multiple fiber orientations in high angular resolution diffusion imaging. MRM 54(6), 1480–1489 (2005)
[18] Behrens, T., et al.: Probabilistic tractography with multiple fibre orientations: What can we gain? NeuroImage 34, 144–155 (2007)
[19] Tournier, J.D., Calamante, F., Gadian, D.G., Connelly, A.: Direct estimation of the fiber orientation density function from diffusion-weighted MRI data using spherical deconvolution. NeuroImage 23(3), 1176–1185 (2004)
[20] Jian, B., et al.: A novel tensor distribution model for the diffusion weighted MR signal. NeuroImage 37(1), 164–176 (2007)
[21] Ramirez-Manzanares, A., et al.: Diffusion basis functions decomposition for estimating white matter intravoxel fiber geometry. IEEE Trans. Med. Imaging 26(8), 1091–1102 (2007)
[22] Kumar, R., et al.: Multi-fiber reconstruction from DW-MRI using a continuous mixture of von mises-fisher distributions. In: MMBIA (2008)
[23] Rathi, Y., Michailovich, O., Bouix, S., Shenton, M.: Directional functions for orientation distribution estimation. In: ISBI, pp. 927–930 (2008)
[24] Jian, B., Vemuri, B.C.: A unified computational framework for deconvolution to reconstruct multiple fibers from diffusion weighted MRI. IEEE Trans. Med. Imaging 26(11), 1464–1471 (2007)
[25] Soderman, O., Jönsson, B.: Restricted diffusion in cylindirical geometry. J. Magn. Reson. B 117(1), 94–97 (1995)
[26] Lawson, C.L., Hanson, R.J.: Solving Least Squares Problems. Prentice-Hall, Englewood Cliffs (1974)
[27] Shepherd, T.M., et al.: Structural insights from high-resolution diffusion tensor imaging and tractography of the isolated rat hippocampus. NeuroImage 32(4), 1499–1509 (2006)

Smooth 3-D Reconstruction for 2-D Histological Images

Amalia Cifor[1], Tony Pridmore[1], and Alain Pitiot[2]

[1] School of Computer Science, University of Nottingham, Nottingham, UK
[2] Brain and Body Centre, University of Nottingham, Nottingham, UK
{rzc, tpp}@cs.nott.ac.uk, alain.pitiot@nottingham.ac.uk

Abstract. We present an image driven approach to the reconstruction of 3-D volumes from stacks of 2-D post-mortem sections (histology, cryoimaging, autoradiography or immunohistochemistry) in the absence of any external information. We note that a desirable quality of the reconstructed volume is the smoothness of its notable structures (e.g. the gray/white matter surfaces in brain images). Here we propose to use smoothness as a means to drive the reconstruction process itself.

From an initial rigid pair-wise reconstruction of the input 2-D sections, we extract the boundaries of structures of interest. Those are then evolved under a mean curvature flow modified to constrain the flow within 2-D planes. Sparse displacement fields are then computed, independently for each slice, from the resulting flow. A variety of transformations, from globally rigid to arbitrarily flexible ones, can then be estimated from those fields and applied to the individual input 2-D sections to form a smooth volume.

We detail our method and discuss preliminary results on both real histological data and synthetic examples.

1 Introduction

In spite of rapid advances in 3-D imaging technologies (high-field magnetic resonance scanners, micro-CT, etc.), the spatial resolution, contrast and specificity of the acquired volumes still fall short of the level of anatomical or functional details afforded by post-mortem 2-D imaging technologies such as histology, cryoimaging, autoradiography or immunohistochemistry (hereafter referred to as "histology").

By fusing 2-D post-mortem sections with 3-D in vivo or post-mortem volumes, we can establish a one-to-one correspondence between the various modalities, with the 3-D volumes acting as an adequate anatomical framework. This enables researchers to view the complex anatomy of the organs or structures of interest in three dimensions (regardless of the modality), at multiple scale (anatomical, cellular, molecular) and multiple explanatory levels (structural or functional).

Due to the nature and high incidence of the distortions and artefacts that occur during the 2-D imaging process (shape changes during perfusion, fixation and tissue extraction; holes and tears during cutting; nonlinear shrinking

J.L. Prince, D.L. Pham, and K.J. Myers (Eds.): IPMI 2009, LNCS 5636, pp. 350–361, 2009.
© Springer-Verlag Berlin Heidelberg 2009

of tissues during preparation or dying; etc.) an accurate and robust fusion is difficult to achieve. The typical approach to fusion consists of (1) reconstructing a geometrically coherent 3-D volume by registering together the consecutive 2-D histological slices and (2) co-registering the reconstructed volume to the available 3-D modality (MR or CT for instance).

Often this first reconstruction involves registering successive pairs of 2-D slices with respect to a reference slice, generally taken as the middle one in the stack [1,2]. The available 2-D registration methods range from time-consuming manual techniques [3] or fiducial markers based ones [4], to more advanced geometrical approaches where features such as points [5], edges [6] or contours [7] are automatically extracted from the input slices. Iconic (i.e. intensity based) methods also proved very popular. For instance, Ourselin et al. [1] used a robust block-matching approach to linearly register histological sections of the rat brain with the correlation coefficient as similarity measure.

However, as argued at length in [2], restricting the reconstruction problem to a 2-D/2-D registration process is not likely to yield anatomically satisfactory results. Indeed, the 3-D conformation of a curved object is lost during the cutting process and cannot be accurately recovered in the absence of external information (the humorously nicknamed "banana problem"). Furthermore, considering slices only two at a time naturally gives rise to an aperture problem whose consequences are a general lack of robustness and a tendency to create wave patterns in the direction across slices.

Those issues can be alleviated in several ways. For instance, an external reference volume (e.g. MRI [8,2,9]) or the block-face images acquired during the histological process [10,11,12,13] can be used to guide the reconstruction. Recent approaches conjointly manipulate all the slices in the stack. In [14] for instance, the set of independent elastic transformations is globally optimized within a variational scheme, with the global sum of squared differences across all slices serving as fitness function. In [?], the linear transformations computed between each pairs of slices are filtered along the cutting axis. Yushkevitch et al. [15] use a graph-based approach to pick in the neighbourhood of each slice the registration path that will minimize the overall reconstruction error. In Guest et al.[16], springs are attached between corresponding points across consecutive slices, which are themselves modeled as thin elastic plates, and a finite element method evolves the system until equilibrium. In Tan et al. [17], three high-curvature points, extracted from tissue contours after an initial global reconstruction, are matched across slices and serve as surrogate fiducial markers. New affine transformations are estimated for each slice from the three displacement vectors computed between these feature points and the closest point in the same slice on an interpolating inter-slice cubic NURBS.

In this article, we focus on the reconstruction of a 3-D volume from 2-D slices, in the absence of an external reference. Indeed, the latter is not always available, or its resolution or contrast may not be sufficient to provide much help with the reconstruction. We note that a desirable quality for a reconstructed histological volume is the smoothness of its notable structures (e.g. the gray/white matter surface in a brain). In fact, it is common practice to qualitatively evaluate a reconstruction method by considering the smoothness, in the reconstructed volume, of some structures of interest in views orthogonal to the original 2-D histological sections. For instance, in [14] the quality of reconstructed histological volumes of rat brains was assessed by an expert who visually evaluated both the smoothness of the borders delimiting anatomical structures and the amount of recognizable small structures, such as the subcortical nuclei and the ventricles. In [16,18], the distance between corresponding points identified across slices was used to quantify the smoothness of the reconstruction: since histological slices are thin, the closer the corresponding points, the smoother the volume. In a recent work [19], Laissue et al. use the smoothness of crest-lines defined by high curvature points of the lateral ventricle in a reconstructed histological brain to assess the co-registration errors between MRI and the reconstructed volume.

Here we propose to use smoothness as a means to drive the reconstruction itself. The boundaries of structures of interest are automatically extracted from an initial rigid reconstruction of the input 2-D sections and smoothed by a constrained mean curvature flow. Arbitrarily flexible transformations can then be estimated, independently for each slice, from the computed flow and applied to the original sections to form a smooth volume. We build our method around the hypothesis that the histological sections are sufficiently thin to enable a smooth visual aspect of the reconstructed structures in the direction across slices.

Note that our approach bears some resemblance to the work of Tan et al. [17], in the sense that we also use smoothness to correct slice transformations. However, instead of focusing on an arbitrarily small number of feature points which have to be extracted and matched across slices (an error-prone process highly sensitive to segmentation errors), we use actual surfaces. This enables us to estimate a displacement field instead of just three displacement vectors, so arbitrarily flexible slice transformations can be accommodated. In turn, this gives us control over the desired smoothness of the reconstructed volume.

We first detail our method in the following section, before presenting some preliminary results on synthetic and real datasets in section 3. Finally, we conclude with some elements of validation regarding the robustness of the proposed approach.

2   Method

Our method consists of five steps. (1) We first reconstruct an estimate of the 3-D histological volume by rigidly registering consecutive 2-D sections, using a classic pair-wise approach. (2) Structures of interest (e.g. the gray/white matter boundary) are automatically extracted from the reconstructed volume. (3) The extracted surfaces are smoothed by evolving them under a modified version of the mean curvature flow restricted to 2-D planes. (4) A 3-D displacement field is estimated from the 3-D flow. A variety of transformations, from globally rigid to arbitrarily flexible ones, can then be estimated from the field. (5) Finally, a smooth reconstructed volume is obtained by applying the transformations to the original 2-D slices.

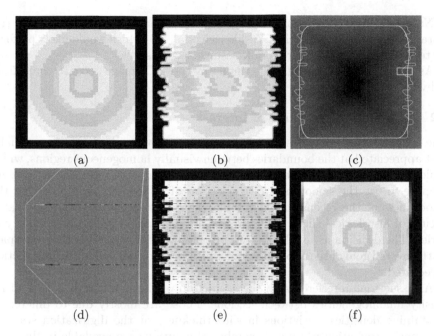

Fig. 1. Smooth reconstruction applied to a 2-D toy example: (a) source 2-D image: the structure of interest is a textured square; (b) source image after application of random translations to individual lines (gray) and extracted structure of interest (blue line); (c) signed distance map (gray), front before (blue line) and after (yellow line) application of flow, computed sparse displacement field (red); (d) magnified view of the trajectory of two points taken within the white square in (c) during the flow; (e) dense displacement field interpolated from the global rigid transformation (translations) estimated on sparse field of (c); (f) globally smoothed image

We illustrate on Fig. 1 the steps that will be described throughout this section. To facilitate visualization, we use a 2-D toy example rather than a 3-D one. The structure of interest is a textured square. In this example, the analogous of a 2-D histological slice is a horizontal line. We simulate the misalignments induced by the histological process by translating those lines horizontally by a random amount drawn from a zero-mean normal distribution (Fig. 1(b)). The goal of our approach is then to recover a smooth square, similar in shape to that of Fig. 1(a).

2.1 Approximating a 3-D Volume

We first need to estimate a globally coherent 3-D volume from the input stack of 2-D slices. We use the standard pair-wise reconstruction approach of Ourselin et al. [20], owing to its robustness to artifacts and noise. In this framework, consecutive pairs of 2-D slices are globally rigidly registered with a block-matching algorithm. We chose the middle slice as reference.

Note that any other global reconstruction approach could be used here (for instance, the robust approach of Yushkevich et al. [15] which would likely perform better if severe artifacts were to affect some sections).

As mentioned above, Fig. 1(b) simulates the 2-D image reconstructed from individual 1-D lines.

2.2   Extracting Structures of Interest

The roughness (as opposed to smoothness) of a reconstructed volume is usually best appreciated at the boundaries between visually homogeneous regions, which typically coincide with anatomical structures or sub-structures. Therefore, we propose to use the smoothness of a selection of boundaries as a proxy for the smoothness of the reconstructed volume. Note that because of the tessellated nature of histological slices, structures of interest can be found at a variety of scales. The decision as to which structure should be extracted is then informed by the overall goal of the application for which histological volume reconstruction is required.

An issue that interferes with the extraction of the boundaries is that of intensity inhomogeneities between sections. Those are mostly due to differences in staining densities, variations in slice thickness or the digitization stage of the image acquisition process. A number of solutions are available in the literature [21,22]. We picked the affine histogram matching approach of Malandain et al. [21] as it copes adequately with the anatomical differences and intensity variations across the stack of histological slices .

Once the intensities have been homogenized, we can extract the boundaries of the structures of interest. For the data presented in this paper, a simple intensity thresholding approach proved sufficient. Should the histological sections be more heavily textured, or if the noise level were higher, more sophisticated methods may become necessary. Note that the segmentation was done in 2-D, independently for each slice, which makes it independent from the quality of the initial 3-D reconstruction (although we may equally envision a 3-D segmentation approach). A completely accurate segmentation step is not mandatory here, since the extracted surfaces act as surrogates. Our method only requires approximately delineated boundaries of interest as long as their smoothness is representative for the smoothness of the initial volume reconstruction.

The blue line in Fig. 1(b) follows the boundary of the structure of interest in our toy example.

2.3   3-D Mean Curvature Flow Constrained to 2-D Planes

Because the initial rigid reconstruction is unlikely to generate a smooth volume, the extracted surfaces will be "jagged" in the direction of the cutting axis (i.e. across slices). We propose to smooth those surfaces by evolving them under a mean curvature flow.

Mean curvature flow is a popular interface motion method, extensively used as an image smoothing and noise filtering technique (see [23] for a review). At a glance, it consists in moving each point on the extracted surfaces (or fronts) along their normal direction, with speed proportional to their curvature. This helps smoothing away their various kinks and bumps. An attractive formulation to the mean curvature flow was proposed by Osher et al. where the front was modelled implicitly as the zero level set of an higher dimensional function, a signed distance map [24]. Formally, if $\Gamma(t = 0)$ denotes the extracted front, then the level set function is $\phi(x, t = 0) = \pm distance(x, \Gamma(t = 0))$. If we further constrain the gradient of the signed distance function to be one, the general equation of motion [25] for speed function F is:

$$\phi_t + F \bigtriangledown \phi = 0 \tag{1}$$

When the speed is proportional to the curvature κ at each point, the equation becomes: $\phi_t + F(\kappa) \mid \bigtriangledown\phi \mid = 0$.

For the purpose of our histological reconstruction application, we modified this classical formulation to take into account the fact that the cutting axis (the axis going across slices) plays a different role from the other two, as argued in [2]. Indeed, we do not want the flow to go across the planes in which the slices reside since we need to compute from it the independent transformations to be applied to the original sections.

Restricting the flow to the planes can be simply obtained by setting the component of the velocity along the z-axis to zero. The speed function then becomes:

$$F(\kappa) = -b\kappa \cdot (1, 1, 0) \cdot \left(\frac{\bigtriangledown\phi}{\mid \bigtriangledown\phi \mid}\right) \tag{2}$$

where b is a positive constant. Plugging the new speed into the level set equation (1), the motion under the mean curvature flow constrained to the 2-D planes is given by:

$$\phi_t = \left[(b\kappa, b\kappa, 0) \cdot \left(\frac{\bigtriangledown\phi}{\mid \bigtriangledown\phi \mid}\right)\right] \cdot \bigtriangledown\phi \tag{3}$$

Note that this formulation of the flow still allows for the curvature and gradient to be computed in 3-D. It also somewhat mitigates the tendency for classical mean curvature flows to shrink volumes, even though we cannot guarantee surface shrinkage within slices. In our study we used the Euclidean distance approximation for the signed distance map [26] and the derivatives in equation 3 are computed by means of second order centred differences[1].

2.4   Estimating Individual Slice Transformations

Finally, we need to compute the transformations corresponding to each individual slice. Once the equation of motion has been discretized, we can track, within each slice, the trajectory of the points on the evolving front and generate

---

[1] The described scheme was implemented on top of the LS Toolbox for matlab http://www.cs.ubc.ca/ mitchell/ToolboxLS/

a sparse displacement field. The transformation corresponding to each slice can then be estimated from this field.

However, since the original signed distance map does not remain a distance map throughout the entire time-period of the motion, finding an accurate set of displacement vectors from the points on initial front to the points on the final front is a difficult task. In [27] Gomes et al. recall that the characteristics of the level set function (the integral curves of its gradient) are straight lines since the embedding function is a distance map. They use a tracking approach to find the position of the front at each iteration. Inspired by this scheme, we too track the position of the front at each iteration by looking for zero-crossing of the distance map in the normal direction, starting at previous position of the front. The final displacement is obtained by composing the small displacement vectors at intermediary points between the old and new position of the front.

Fig. 1(c) shows the evolution of the front under our constrained mean curvature flow formulation and the computed sparse displacement field. Note how the displacement vectors are indeed aligned horizontally (i.e. the flow was restricted to the horizontal direction). Fig. 1(d) displays a magnified view of the trajectory, during the flow, of two points taken within the white square in (c).

Once a displacement field has been computed, we can estimate a variety of transformations, from globally rigid or affine ones to arbitrarily flexible ones. Following [1,28], we estimate global transformations with a robust least square regression algorithm (Least Trimmed Squares, [29]). This approach differs from standard least square methods in that it minimizes the sum of a certain percent of the smallest squared residuals in an iterative fashion, which reduces the influence of outliers. It proved particularly amenable to our application where only a sparse displacement field is computed. When more flexible transformations are desired, we use the rigidity adaptable approach of Pitiot et al. [28]. In this approach, both the geometry and topology of the individual slices are taken into account (in particular, image components on either side of a gap are treated independently). The flexibility of the regularized field is controlled by setting a single parameter, the rigidity radius, which determines the amount of local rigidity (the larger the radius, the more rigid the transformation). Finally, for maximal flexibility, we can extrapolate the sparse field to the entire image, where the extrapolation is done independently for each slice, and apply the displacement directly to the original slices.

Fig. 1(e) shows the dense displacement field interpolated along each line from the global rigid translation estimated from the sparse field shown in Fig. 1(c). Note that for this 2-D toy example, the global rigid translation of each line was obtained by averaging the displacement vectors computed on the line rather than by LTS since there were only two vectors. Fig. 1(f) shows the final 2-D image once the estimated translations were applied to the individual lines of Fig.1(b): the reconstructed image is visibly much smoother.

3   Results

3.1   Reconstructing a NISSL-Stained Volume of the C57BL/6 Mouse Brain

We applied our smooth reconstruction approach to a set of 350 Nissl-stained sections of the C57BL/6 mouse brain obtained from the LONI database[2]. The mouse brain was cut serially along the anterior/posterior axis in $50\mu m$ thick coronal sections.

Fig. 3(a) displays a sagittal (left) and transverse (right) view of the initial rigidly reconstructed volume (step 1 of our method). As mentioned above, we picked the middle section in the stack as reference for this pair-wise reconstruction. After the intensity homogenization step, we extracted the gray/white matter boundary as our surface of interest and subjected it to the modified mean curvature flow.

We show on Fig. 3(b to e) the reconstruction results obtained with increasingly more flexible transformation models. For all results, we used the same parameters for our mean curvature flow implementation: $b = 0.05$, 153 time steps in total.

The reconstruction obtained when global rigid transformations were estimated from our modified flow is shown in (b). Note how even though the transformations applied to the original sections were global rigid for both (a) and (b), the reconstructed volume appears much smoother with our approach. Without surprise, estimating a global affine transformation instead of a rigid one yielded a smoother volume (Fig. 3(c)).

Fig. 3(d) shows the reconstruction results obtained with the adaptive rigidity approach[28]. We chose a radius of the order of the cortical thickness in this area of the brain. The resulting volume compares favourably against that obtained when directly applying the displacement field computed from the flow (Fig. 3(e)). In both case we obtain a visually very smooth volume, but the regularization approach prevented the cortical ribbon from collapsing in the bottom left and top right corners of the image.

3.2   Elements of Robustness

In an attempt to evaluate the robustness of our smooth reconstruction method while circumventing the lack of ground truth associated with actual histological data, we propose to reconstruct a volume from the artificially perturbed slices of an initially smooth volume and compare the former with the latter. As surrogate for smooth histological volume, we use a high resolution 0.65mm isotropic in-vivo T1-weighted MR scan of the human brain of a volunteer. In a similar fashion to our toy 2-D example, we apply to each individual axial slice a rigid or affine transformation whose parameters are drawn from zero mean normal distributions of specifiable standard deviation σ.

Fig. 2 shows both coronal and sagittal views of the original, perturbed and smoothly reconstructed volumes for rotation drawn at random from a zero mean normal distribution of standard deviation $\sigma_{rotation} = 1$ degree (b) and

---

[2] http://map.loni.ucla.edu

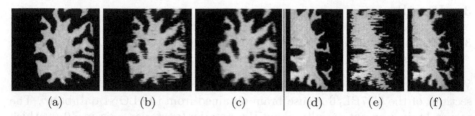

(a)   (b)   (c)   (d)   (e)   (f)

Fig. 2. Reconstructing a randomly perturbed MR image of the human brain: (a) coronal view of the original MRI; (b) coronal view of the perturbed MRI whose axial slices were randomly rotated ($\sigma_{rotation} = 1$ degree); (c) smooth reconstruction from slices rotated in (b); (d) sagittal view of the original MRI; (e) sagittal view of the perturbed MRI whose axial slices were randomly translated ($\sigma_{translation} = 2$ voxels); (f) smooth reconstruction from slices translated in (e).

translations drawn at random from a zero mean normal distribution of standard deviation $\sigma_{translation} = 2$ voxels (e). The reconstructed volumes (c and f) are indeed much smoother than the perturbed volumes and visually close to the original MRI. Note that because our reconstruction approach does not know about brain anatomy, there is no guarantee that the "smooth alignment" corresponds to the anatomically correct one. In particular, it could be smoother.

4   Conclusions

We have presented a reference-free image driven approach to volume reconstruction where smoothness is used as a means to drive the reconstruction process itself. A variant of the mean curvature flow constrained to 2-D planes is used to smooth the boundaries of structures of interest extracted from an initial reconstruction of the input histological sections. A displacement field is then computed from the resulting flow and arbitrarily flexible transformations are estimated and applied to the individual slices.

Preliminary results indicate that the reconstructed volumes are indeed visually smooth, even when the selected slice transformation model is globally rigid.

Note that our method is best suited for histological slices in which the discrepancy between boundaries of interest and texture is high enough to extract and smooth these boundaries. We are currently investigating the influence of noise and lack of contrast on the quality of the reconstruction and quantifying the robustness of our approach to random rotations and translations. We are evaluating volume preserving flows to further improve the quality of the reconstruction. Of particular interest are scale-dependent flows which would smooth out only those features artificially induced by the reconstruction, while leaving the overall shape of the structure intact.

Acknowledgements

This research is funded by the European Commission Fp6 Marie Curie Action Programme (MEST-CT-2005-021170).

References

1. Ourselin, S., Roche, A., Subsol, G., Pennec, X., Ayache, N.: Reconstructing a 3D structure from serial histological sections. Image and Vision Computing 19(1-2), 25–31 (2001)
2. Malandain, G., Bardinet, E., Nelissen, K., Vanduffel, W.: Fusion of autoradiographs with an MR volume using 2-D and 3-D linear transformations. NeuroImage 23(1), 111–127 (2004)
3. Deverell, M., Salisbury, J., Cookson, M., Holman, J., Dykes, E., Whimster, F.: Three-dimensional reconstruction: methods of improving image registration and interpretation. In: Analytical Cellular Pathology, vol. 5, pp. 253–263 (1993)
4. Toga, A., Goldkorn, A., Ambach, K., Chao, K., Quinn, B., Yao, P.: Postmortem cryosectioning as an anatomic reference for human brain mapping. Computerized Medical Imaging and Graphics 21(11), 131–141 (1997)
5. Guest, E., Berry, E., Baldock, R.A., Fidrich, M., Smith, M.A.: Robust point correspondence applied to two-and three-dimensional image registration. IEEE Trans. Pattern Anal. Mach. Intell. 23(2), 165–179 (2001)
6. Kim, B., Frey, K.A., Mukhopadhayay, S., Ross, B.D., Meyer, C.R.: Co-registration of MRI and autoradiography of rat brain in three-dimensions following automatic reconstruction of 2D data set. In: Ayache, N. (ed.) CVRMed 1995. LNCS, vol. 905, pp. 262–266. Springer, Heidelberg (1995)
7. Cohen, F., Yang, Z., Huang, Z., Nissanov, J.: Automatic matching of homologous histological sections. IEEE Transactions on Bio-medical Engineering 445(5), 642–649 (1998)
8. Ourselin, S., Bardinet, E., Dormont, D., Malandain, G., Roche, A., Ayache, N., Tande, D., Parain, K., Yelnik, J.: Fusion of histological sections and MR images: towards the construction of an atlas of the human basal ganglia. In: Niessen, W.J., Viergever, M.A. (eds.) MICCAI 2001. LNCS, vol. 2208, pp. 743–751. Springer, Heidelberg (2001)
9. Chakravarty, M.M., Bedell, B.J., Zehntner, S.P., Evans, A.C., Collins, D.L.: Three-dimensional reconstruction of serial histological mouse brain sections. In: ISBI, pp. 987–990 (2008)
10. Dauguet, J., Delzescaux, T., Condé, F., Mangin, J.F., Ayache, N., Hantraye, P., Frouin, V.: Three-dimensional reconstruction of stained histological slices and 3D non-linear registration with in-vivo MRI for whole baboon brain. Journal of Neuroscience Methods 164, 191–204 (2007)
11. Gefen, S., Tretiak, O., Nissanov, J.: Elastic 3D alignment of rat brain histological images. IEEE Transactions on Medical Imaging 22(11), 1480–1489 (2003)
12. Bardinet, E., Ourselin, S., Dormont, D., Malandain, G., Tandé, D., Parain, K., Ayache, N., Yelnik, J.: Co-registration of histological, optical and MR data of the human brain. In: Dohi, T., Kikinis, R. (eds.) MICCAI 2002. LNCS, vol. 2488, pp. 548–555. Springer, Heidelberg (2002)
13. Kim, B., Boes, J., Frey, K., Meyer, C.: Mutual information for automated unwarping of rat brain autoradiographs. NeuroImage 5(1), 31–40 (1997)
14. Wirtz, S., Fischer, B., Modersitzki, J., Schmitt, O.: Super–fast elastic registration of histologic images of a whole rat brain for three–dimensional reconstruction. In: Proceedings of SPIE 2004, Medical Imaging, vol. 5730, pp. 14–19 (2004)
15. Yushkevich, P.A., Avants, B.B., Ng, L., Hawrylycz, M., Burstein, P.D., Zhang, H., Gee, J.C.: 3D mouse brain reconstruction from histology using a coarse-to-fine approach. In: Pluim, J.P.W., Likar, B., Gerritsen, F.A. (eds.) WBIR 2006. LNCS, vol. 4057, pp. 230–237. Springer, Heidelberg (2006)

16. Guest, E., Baldock, R.: Automatic reconstruction of serial sections using the finite element method. BioImaging 3, 154–167 (1995)
17. Tan, Y., Hua, J., Dong, M.: Feature curve-guided volume reconstruction from 2D images. In: Proceedings of International Symposium on Biomedical Imaging, April 2007, pp. 716–719 (2007)
18. Ju, T., Warren, J., Carson, J., Bello, M., Kakadiaris, I., Chiu, W., Thaller, C., Eichele, G.: 3D volume reconstruction of a mouse brain from histological sections using warp filtering. Journal of Neuroscience Methods 156, 84–100 (2006)
19. Laissue, P., Kenwright, C., Hojjat, A., Colchester, A.C.F.: Using curve-fitting of curvilinear features for assessing registration of clinical neuropathology with in vivo MRI. In: Metaxas, D., Axel, L., Fichtinger, G., Székely, G. (eds.) MICCAI 2008, Part II. LNCS, vol. 5242, pp. 1050–1057. Springer, Heidelberg (2008)
20. Ourselin, S., Roche, A., Prima, S., Ayache, N.: Block matching: A general framework to improve robustness of rigid registration of medical images. In: Delp, S.L., DiGoia, A.M., Jaramaz, B. (eds.) MICCAI 2000. LNCS, vol. 1935, pp. 557–566. Springer, Heidelberg (2000)
21. Malandain, G., Bardinet, E.: Intensity Compensation within Series of Images. In: Ellis, R.E., Peters, T.M. (eds.) MICCAI 2003. LNCS, vol. 2879, pp. 41–49. Springer, Heidelberg (2003)
22. Dauguet, J., Mangin, J.F., Delzescaux, T., Frouin, V.: Robust inter-slice intensity normalization using histogram scale-space analysis. In: Barillot, C., Haynor, D.R., Hellier, P. (eds.) MICCAI 2004. LNCS, vol. 3216, pp. 242–249. Springer, Heidelberg (2004)
23. Suri, J.S., Liu, K., Singh, S., Laxminarayan, S., Zeng, X., Reden, L.: Shape recovery algorithms using level sets in 2-d/3-d medical imagery: a state-of-the-art review. IEEE Transactions on Information Technology in Biomedicine 6(1), 8–28 (2002)
24. Osher, S.J., Fedkiw, R.P.: Level Set Methods and Dynamic Implicit Surfaces. Springer, Heidelberg (2002)
25. Osher, S., Sethian, J.A.: Fronts propagating with curvature-dependent speed: Algorithms based on Hamilton-Jacobi formulations. Journal of Computational Physics 79, 12–49 (1988)
26. Borgefors, G.: On digital distance transforms in three dimensions. Computer Vision and Image Understanding 64(3), 368–376 (1996)
27. Gomes, J., Faugeras, O.D.: Level sets and distance functions. In: Vernon, D. (ed.) ECCV 2000. LNCS, vol. 1842, pp. 588–602. Springer, Heidelberg (2000)
28. Pitiot, A., Guimond, A.: Geometrical regularization of displacement fields for histological image registration. Medical Image Analysis 12(1), 16–25 (2008)
29. Rousseeuw, P.J.: Least median of squares regression. Journal of the American Statistical Association 79(388), 871–880 (1984)

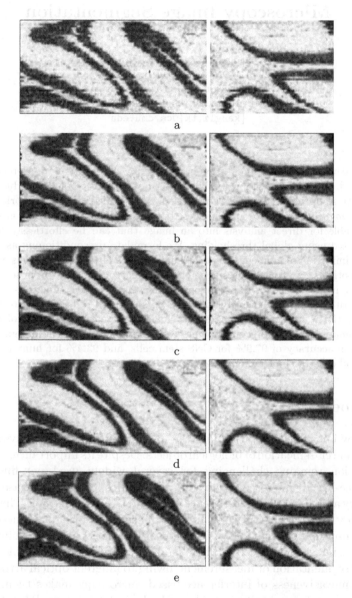

a

b

c

d

e

Fig. 3. Sagittal (left) and transversal (right) views of the LONI C57BL/6 mouse brain reconstructed from 2-D Nissl-stained sections using: (a) pair-wise globally rigid reconstruction; (b) smooth reconstruction approach with globally rigid transformations estimated at each slice. (c) same with globally *affine* transformations estimated at each slice. (d) same with rigidity adaptable regularization of the displacement field extracted from the flow; (e) same with direct application of the displacement field extracted from the flow.

Nonnegative Mixed-Norm Preconditioning for Microscopy Image Segmentation

Kang Li and Takeo Kanade

Carnegie Mellon University
5000 Forbes Ave, Pittsburgh, PA 15213, USA
{kangli,tk}@cs.cmu.edu

Abstract. Image segmentation in microscopy, especially in interference-based optical microscopy modalities, is notoriously challenging due to inherent optical artifacts. We propose a general algebraic framework for *preconditioning* microscopy images. It transforms an image that is unsuitable for direct analysis into an image that can be effortlessly segmented using global thresholding. We formulate preconditioning as the minimization of nonnegative-constrained convex objective functions with smoothness and sparseness-promoting regularization. We propose efficient numerical algorithms for optimizing the objective functions. The algorithms were extensively validated on simulated differential interference (DIC) microscopy images and challenging real DIC images of cell populations. With preconditioning, we achieved unprecedented segmentation accuracy of 97.9% for CNS stem cells, and 93.4% for human red blood cells in challenging images.

1 Introduction

Microscopy image segmentation lays the foundation for shape analysis, motion tracking, and classification of biological objects. Despite its importance, automated segmentation remains challenging for several widely used non-fluorescence, interference-based microscopy imaging modalities, such as phase contrast microscopy and differential interference contrast (DIC) microscopy. These modalities employ interference optics to convert phase shifts of light induced by otherwise transparent objects into visible intensity variations. While being visually contrastive, images generated by these modalities are often unsuitable for direct computer segmentation or measurement, owing to inherent optical artifacts.

The noninvasiveness of interference-based microscopy makes them uniquely suitable for long-term monitoring of living biological specimens. Recent advances in biology intensified the interest in using them for quantitative measurement of ongoing biological processes, e.g., for recognition and tracking of stem cell behaviors. These emerging applications call for novel algorithms that facilitate automated segmentation of interference-based optical microscopy images.

We propose in this paper a general algebraic framework for *preconditioning* interference-based microscopy images, which dramatically facilitates automated segmentation and analysis. Based on physical principles of microscopy image

J.L. Prince, D.L. Pham, and K.J. Myers (Eds.): IPMI 2009, LNCS 5636, pp. 362–373, 2009.

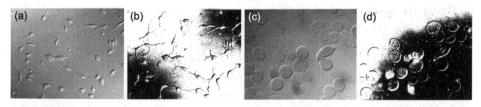

Fig. 1. DIC microscopy images of unstained cell populations. (a) CNS stem cells. (c) Human red blood cells. (b) and (d) are the thresholding outputs of (a) and (c), respectively, showing nonuniform background and unsymmetrical pixel intensity distribution in cells.

formation, we formulate preconditioning as the minimization of nonnegative-constrained convex objective functions with smoothness and sparseness-enhancing regularization. Taking advantage of recent advances in convex optimization [1, 2, 3], we propose efficient algorithms to solve the minimization problems.

The effectiveness of the proposed algorithms will be demonstrated for pre-conditioning DIC microscopy images. The dual-beam interference optics of DIC microscopes introduces nonuniform shadow-cast artifacts (Fig. 1), making direct segmentation notoriously difficult. Existing techniques for DIC image segmentation either are application-specific, relying on template matching and edge detection [4], or require *ad hoc* image preprocessing, e.g., line integration [5] or the Hilbert transform [6]. Attempts have also been made to derive exact imaging models, resulting in computationally expensive algorithms that are impractical for routine utilization [7, 8]. In contrast, our preconditioning algorithms efficiently reconstruct images according to well-defined optimality criteria, enabling high-quality segmentation using global thresholding. Moreover, our approach can be easily extended to other modalities (e.g., phase contrast microscopy) by incorporating appropriate imaging models, or to higher dimensions.

2   Algebraic Image Model

Our generic model for microscopy images consists of three components: 1) an *imaging* model $h(\cdot)$ that represents the image formation process of the microscope; 2) an additive *bias* $b(x, y)$ that compensates for a nonzero background level, nonuniform illumination, and spatial sensitivity variations of the detector; and 3) a *noise* model $n(\cdot)$ that accounts for imaging and detection noise. The model can be written as:

$$g(x, y) = n(h(f(x, y)) + b(x, y)), \tag{1}$$

with $g(x, y)$ being the *observed* image, and $f(x, y)$ being the ideal *object* image that we want to retrieve, which could represent the optical path length distribution in the object, fluorescence intensities, or an *phenomenological* image that simply facilitates object segmentation.

Under the assumption of additive noise, we can express our model succinctly in a linear algebraic framework, given by

$$g = \mathbf{H}f + b + n. \tag{2}$$

Here g denotes a vector representation of the observed image, which is formed by concatenating the image pixels in raster order. Specifically, given an image with $N = N_x \times N_y$ pixels $\{g_{x,y}\}^1$, where $x = 1, \ldots, N_x$ and $y = 1, \ldots, N_y$, the corresponding vector g is defined as:

$$g = (g_1, \ldots, g_i, \ldots, g_N)^T = (g_{x_1,y_1}, \ldots, g_{x_i,y_i}, \ldots, g_{x_N,y_N})^T, \tag{3}$$

where $(\cdot)^T$ denotes vector (or matrix) transposition, and (x_i, y_i) are the spatial coordinates of pixel g_{x_i,y_i}, or equivalently, of the ith element of vector g. The vectors f, b, n are defined likewise for the object, bias, and noise, respectively. The imaging model is expressed as a matrix-vector multiplication between the $N \times N$ transfer matrix $\mathbf{H}$ and f, which is adequate for representing a wide range of microscopy image formation processes. Since $\mathbf{H}$ can naturally represent shift-variant transfer functions, our expression is more flexible than the conventional convolution formulation in terms of a point spread function (PSF).

In the next section, we will elaborate on the preconditioning framework under the assumption of additive Gaussian noise. We will return to the discussion of alternative noise models in Section 6.

3   Nonnegative Mixed-Norm Preconditioning

With the image model specified in Eq. (2), we need to compute the ideal object image f given an observed image g. We tackle this inverse problem through a two-step process. First, we estimate and subsequently eliminate the bias from an observed image. Second, we reconstruct the object image f from the bias-corrected image by minimizing a constrained mix-norm objective function. Collectively, we refer to this two-step process as *preconditioning*, which transforms an observed image that is unfriendly for computer analysis into an image that facilitates automated object segmentation and measurement.

3.1   Bias Elimination

As the first step of preconditioning, we estimate the bias field from an image and obtain a bias-corrected image. This process is also known as flat-field correction or background subtraction. While many methods exist for this purpose, we present a simple approach that is sufficient for most microscopy images.

Under the assumption that the bias field is smooth and spatially slowly varying, we model it as a K-th order polynomial surface:

$$b(x,y) = \sum_{k=0}^{K} \sum_{j=0}^{k} p_{j+\frac{k(k+1)}{2}} x^{k-j} y^j = p_0 + p_1 x + p_2 y + p_3 x^2 + p_4 xy + p_5 y^2 + \cdots \tag{4}$$

---

[1] $g_{x,y}$ denotes the discrete value sampled from the continuous function $g(x,y)$ at (x,y).

Algebraically, we can express the polynomial as $b = \mathbf{X}p$, where $p = (p_0, p_1, p_2 \ldots)^T$ is the coefficient vector, and $\mathbf{X}$ is a matrix of N rows and $(K + 1)(K + 2)/2$ columns with the i-th row being $(1, x_i, y_i, x_i^2, x_i y_i, y_i^2, \ldots)$. To eliminate the bias, we first compute the optimal coefficients by solving the over-determined linear system $\mathbf{X}p = g$. This amounts to solving the least-squares problem $p^* = \arg\min_p \|\mathbf{X}p - g\|_2^2$, which has a closed-form solution $p^* = (\mathbf{X}^T\mathbf{X})^{-1}\mathbf{X}^Tg$. The bias-corrected image is then computed as $g^* = g - \mathbf{X}p^*$.

3.2 Object Reconstruction via Convex Optimization

The second step of preconditioning reconstructs the object from the bias-corrected image. Ideally, the background pixels of the reconstructed image should be uniformly zero while the foreground pixels are positive, facilitating foreground-background separation. This goal is achieved by minimizing:

$$\mathbf{O}(f) = \|g^* - \mathbf{H}f\|_2^2 + \gamma\text{Smoothness}(f) + \beta\text{Sparsity}(f), \quad \text{subject to } f \geq 0, \quad (5)$$

where $\|\cdot\|_2$ denotes a L_2 norm.

The objective function $\mathbf{O}(f)$ consists of three terms. Their relative importance is controlled by the positive coefficients γ and β. The first term penalizes the sum-of-squares difference between the reconstructed and observed images, promoting data *fidelity*. The second and third terms encourage the spatial *smoothness* and *sparseness* of the reconstructed image, respectively, which collectively provide *regularization*. Regularization ensures the well-posedness of the objective function, and is essential for high-quality reconstruction.

Next, we will introduce two specific formulations of the objective function and discuss the corresponding optimization algorithms.

Case 1: L_2 Smoothness + Weighted L_1 Sparsity. The first formulation employs an L_2 (Tikhonov) smoothness term and a weighted L_1 sparseness term:

$$\mathbf{O}_1(f) = \|g^* - \mathbf{H}f\|_2^2 + \gamma\|\mathbf{R}f\|_2^2 + \beta\|\mathbf{W}f\|_1, \quad \text{s.t. } f \geq 0. \quad (6)$$

The smoothness term penalizes the L_2 norm of the Laplacian of f, where the $N \times N$ matrix $\mathbf{R}$ represents an algebraic Laplacian operator with symmetric boundary condition. In particular, the i-th element of $\mathbf{R}f$ is computed as:

$$(\mathbf{R}f)_i = f_{x_i,y_i} - \sum_{j,k\in\{-1,1\}} \frac{f_{x_i+j,y_i+k}}{8}, \quad (7)$$

with $x_i + j = x_i - j$ if $x_i + j < 1$ or $> N_x$, and likewise for y_i. The sparseness term penalizes the weighted L_1 norm of f, where $\mathbf{W}$ is a diagonal matrix with positive weights $w_1, \ldots, w_N$ on the diagonal and zeros elsewhere.

By rewriting $\mathbf{O}_1(f)$ in terms of the symmetric positive definite matrix $\mathbf{Q} = \mathbf{H}^T\mathbf{H} + \gamma\mathbf{R}^T\mathbf{R}$ and the vector $l = -\mathbf{H}^Tg^*$, and letting w denote the weight vector $(w_1, \ldots, w_N)^T$, we can express the minimization problem as the following nonnegative-constrained quadratic program (NQP):

$$f^* = \arg\min_f \frac{1}{2}f^T\mathbf{Q}f + (l + \beta w)^Tf, \quad \text{s.t. } f \geq 0. \quad (8)$$

We propose a simple and efficient iterative algorithm, the *sparseness-enhanced multiplicative update* (**SEMU**) algorithm, which is well-tailored for the NQP. Our algorithm exploits a nonnegativity-preserving multiplicative update rule [2] and the sparseness-enhancing effect of an iteratively reweighted L_1 scheme. To introduce the algorithm, we express the matrix $\mathbf{Q}$ in Eq. (8) in terms of its positive and negative components. Specifically, we let $\mathbf{Q} = \mathbf{Q}^+ - \mathbf{Q}^-$, where $\mathbf{Q}^+$ and $\mathbf{Q}^-$ are *nonnegative* matrices given by:

$$Q_{i,j}^+ = \begin{cases} Q_{i,j}, & \text{if } Q_{i,j} > 0, \\ 0, & \text{otherwise,} \end{cases} \quad \text{and} \quad Q_{i,j}^- = \begin{cases} |Q_{i,j}|, & \text{if } Q_{i,j} < 0, \\ 0, & \text{otherwise.} \end{cases}$$

The algorithm, defined in terms of $\mathbf{Q}^+$ and $\mathbf{Q}^-$, alternates between updating $\boldsymbol{f}$ and (optionally) recomputing $\boldsymbol{w}$, as outlined below:

Initialize. Set iteration number $t = 0$, and $f_i^{(0)} = 1$, $w_i^{(0)} = 1$, $\forall i \in \{1, \dots, N\}$.
Repeat. Update $\boldsymbol{f}$ and $\boldsymbol{w}$ alternately according to:

$$f_i^{(t+1)} \leftarrow \left[\frac{-(l_i + \beta w_i^{(t)}) + \sqrt{(l_i + \beta w_i^{(t)})^2 + 4(\mathbf{Q}^+ \boldsymbol{f}^{(t)})_i (\mathbf{Q}^- \boldsymbol{f}^{(t)})_i}}{2(\mathbf{Q}^+ \boldsymbol{f}^{(t)})_i} \right] f_i^{(t)}, \quad (9)$$

$$(\text{optional}) \quad w_i^{(t+1)} \leftarrow \frac{1}{f_i^{(t+1)} + \alpha}, \quad \text{where } \alpha \text{ is a positive constant,} \quad (10)$$

Until. $\|\boldsymbol{f}^{(t+1)} - \boldsymbol{f}^{(t)}\|_2^2 \le \epsilon$, where ϵ is a small positive constant.

The multiplicative updates as given by Equations (9) and (10) are applied independently to each pixel, and can be trivially parallelized.

To understand the algorithm, we first exclude Eq. (10) and consider $\boldsymbol{w}$ being constant at unity. In this case, the sparseness term in $\mathbf{O}_1(\boldsymbol{f})$ is reduced to an ordinary L_1 norm. If we define $a_i = (\mathbf{Q}^+ \boldsymbol{f})_i$, $b_i = l_i + \beta w_i$, and $c_i = (\mathbf{Q}^- \boldsymbol{f})_i$, it is instantly recognizable that the multiplicative factor in Eq. (9) is the larger root of the quadratic equation $a_i \nu_i^2 + b_i \nu_i - c_i = 0$. This factor, which we denote as ν_i^+, is guaranteed to be real and nonnegative as long as $\boldsymbol{f}$ is nonnegative, which in return preserves the nonnegativity of $\boldsymbol{f}$. Moreover, using the fact that $\partial \mathbf{O}_1/\partial f_i = a_i + b_i - c_i$, we can verify that the update rule have fixed points at $f_i = 0$ and $\partial \mathbf{O}_1/\partial f_i = 0$ (i.e., $\nu_i^+ = 1$), which are consistent with the Karush-Kuhn-Tucker (KKT) condition for the NQP. While a rigorous convergence proof is nontrivial, it is evident that $\partial \mathbf{O}_1/\partial f_i < 0$ implies $\nu_i^+ > 1$, and $\partial \mathbf{O}_1/\partial f_i > 0$ implies $\nu_i^+ < 1$. Hence, the updates increase or decrease each f_i along the opposite direction of its partial derivative. Thanks to the convexity of $\mathbf{O}_1(\boldsymbol{f})$, the iterations convergence monotonically to the unique global minimum [2].

If we iteratively reweight $\boldsymbol{w}$ according to Eq. (10), the L_1 sparseness term in $\mathbf{O}_1(\boldsymbol{f})$ is in effect replaced with a *log-sum* penalty function $\sum_i \log(f_i + \alpha)$ [3]. The log-sum penalty is much more sparseness-encouraging than the L_1 norm, because it charges increasingly larger penalties for smaller nonzeros. Despite the change, $f_i = 0$ and $\partial \mathbf{O}_1/\partial f_i = 0$ remain as fixed points of the updates, and the monotonic convergence of the algorithm is not violated. However, since the log-sum penalty function is concave, we cannot expect the algorithm to always achieve a global minimum. Nevertheless, achieving global optimality is immaterial for preconditioning. In practice, iterative reweighting encourages background pixels to quickly converge to zero, achieving faster and superior reconstruction.

Case 2: Total Variation Smoothness + L_1 Sparsity. As an alternative to the L_2 smoothness term in Eq. (6), total variation (TV) regularization [9] can be incorporated into the objective function:

$$\mathbf{O}_2(\boldsymbol{f}) = \|\boldsymbol{g}^* - \mathbf{H}\boldsymbol{f}\|_2^2 + \gamma\|\boldsymbol{f}\|_{\mathrm{TV}} + \beta\|\boldsymbol{f}\|_1, \quad \text{subject to } \boldsymbol{f} \geq 0. \tag{11}$$

The TV norm, denoted as $\|\cdot\|_{\mathrm{TV}}$ in Eq. (11), is defined as:

$$\|\boldsymbol{f}\|_{\mathrm{TV}} = \sum_{i=1}^{N} \sqrt{(\mathbf{D}_x\boldsymbol{f})_i^2 + (\mathbf{D}_y\boldsymbol{f})_i^2}, \tag{12}$$

where $\mathbf{D}_x$ and $\mathbf{D}_y$ are matrix representations of the forward-difference operators with homogeneous Neumann boundary conditions, i.e.,

$$(\mathbf{D}_x\boldsymbol{f})_i = f_{x_i+1,y_i} - f_{x_i,y_i}, \quad \text{and} \quad (\mathbf{D}_y\boldsymbol{f})_i = f_{x_i,y_i+1} - f_{x_i,y_i}, \tag{13}$$

with the exception that $(\mathbf{D}_x\boldsymbol{f})_i = 0$ if $x_i \geq N_x$, and $(\mathbf{D}_y\boldsymbol{f})_i = 0$ if $y_i \geq N_y$. The TV norm is essentially the L_1 norm of the image gradient, which promotes the sparseness of gradients in the reconstructed image. It is well-known for its advantage in preserving discontinuities (i.e., sharp edges) in an image.

The minimization of $\mathbf{O}_2(\boldsymbol{f})$ can be solved as a second-order cone program (SOCP) [10]:

$$\boldsymbol{f}^* = \arg\min_{t,\boldsymbol{f}}(\mathbf{1}^T\boldsymbol{t} + \beta\mathbf{1}^T\boldsymbol{f}), \tag{14}$$

$$\text{s.t. } \mathbf{D}_x\boldsymbol{f} - \boldsymbol{u} = 0, \quad \mathbf{D}_y\boldsymbol{f} - \boldsymbol{v} = 0, \quad \mathbf{H}\boldsymbol{f} + \boldsymbol{w} = \boldsymbol{g}^*, \quad w_0 = \tau,$$

$$\text{and } \sqrt{u_i^2 + v_i^2} \leq t_i, \quad \sqrt{w_1^2 + \cdots + w_N^2} \leq w_0, \quad f_i \geq 0, \quad t_i \geq 0, \quad \forall i = 1,\ldots,N,$$

where $\boldsymbol{t}$, $\boldsymbol{u}$, $\boldsymbol{v}$, $\boldsymbol{w}$ and w_0 are slack variables; $\mathbf{1}$ and $\mathbf{0}$ denote N-dimensional vectors of ones and zeros, respectively; and τ is an adjustable noise-tolerance parameter. The SOCP as given in (14) can be solved robustly using interior-point methods (*a.k.a.* barrier methods) with general-purpose convex optimization software [10,11]. We will refer to this approach as "**TV-SOCP**". It alleviates the slow convergence and instability issues that plague traditional gradient-based algorithms [9], and allows easy incorporation of additional constraints.

4 Differential Interference Contrast Microscopy

DIC microscopy is widely used to provide contrast of unstained, transparent specimens, such as cells and microorganisms. Such specimens, known as *phase objects*, cause no detectable amplitude change to the light that passes through them. They are essentially invisible under an ordinary transmitted-light micro-scope. However, they diffract light due to the difference of their refractive indices with respect to the surrounding media, causing phase shifts to the incident light waves. DIC microscopy employs dual-beam interference optics to transform the invisible phase shifts into intensity variations in the observed image.

4.1   Physics of DIC Image Formation

The DIC image formation process can be summarized by the following equations. First, consider an illuminating light beam with amplitude A that is entering a DIC microscope parallel to its optical axis. Upon transiting through a polarizer, the wavefront of the light becomes coherent and plane-polarized, represented by:

$$u_0(\boldsymbol{x}) = A \exp(-i f_0(\boldsymbol{x})). \tag{15}$$

Here $\boldsymbol{x} = (x, y)$, and $f_0(\boldsymbol{x})$ represents the phase of the light field. A condenser prism splits the polarized light into two mutually coherent beams, spatially sep-arated by a minute shear $\boldsymbol{s} = (s\cos(\theta), s\sin(\theta))$, where s is the *shear distance* and θ is the *shear angle*. The two beams pass through the condenser and interact with the object, resulting in an altered phase $f(\boldsymbol{x})$ containing object information:

$$u_1(\boldsymbol{x}) = A \exp(-i f(\boldsymbol{x})), \tag{16}$$
$$u_2(\boldsymbol{x}) = A \exp(-i(f(\boldsymbol{x} + \boldsymbol{s}) + f_b)). \tag{17}$$

In the above equations, f_b is a constant relative phase shift between the two wavefronts, known as the *bias retardation*. After being focused by the objective lens, the two beams are recombined into a single beam by an objective prism in the objective back aperture. Finally, another polarizer, called the analyzer, transmits plane-polarized light from the objective that is able to interfere and generate an image $g(\boldsymbol{x})$. For ideal imaging, $g(\boldsymbol{x})$ can be expressed as:

$$g(\boldsymbol{x}) = 4A^2(1 - \cos(D_\theta f(\boldsymbol{x}) + f_b)), \tag{18}$$

where $D_\theta f(\boldsymbol{x}) = \nabla f(\boldsymbol{x}) \cdot \boldsymbol{s} \approx f(\boldsymbol{x} + \boldsymbol{s}) - f(\boldsymbol{x})$ is the first derivative of phase shift taken along the shear axis. Therefore, the intensity of a DIC image is a nonlinear function of the phase shift introduced by the object.

Linear Approximation. The phase shift introduced by an object is related to its optical path length distribution, which is the product of refractive index and thickness distributions of the object relative to the surrounding medium. Since most biological specimens have refractive indices that differ little from that of water (or the medium in which they are immersed), they introduce sufficiently small phase shift differences. If a microscope is properly adjusted such that $f_b = 90°$, the image that it produces can be approximated by

$$g(\boldsymbol{x}) \approx 4A^2(1 + D_\theta f(\boldsymbol{x})), \tag{19}$$

which is a linear function of the phase shift derivative.

4.2   Algebraic Imaging Model

Based on the previous derivation, we define the DIC imaging model as the first derivative of the phase shift distribution $f(x, y)$ along the shear angle θ. Specifically, we define $h(f(x, y)) = D_\theta f(x, y) \approx f(x, y) * \text{epsf}(x, y)$, where $\text{epsf}(x, y)$ is an *effective* PSF, defined as a steerable first-derivative-of-Gaussian kernel:

$$\text{epsf}(x, y) \propto -xe^{-\frac{x^2+y^2}{\sigma^2}} \cos(\theta) - ye^{-\frac{x^2+y^2}{\sigma^2}} \sin(\theta). \tag{20}$$

Rather than assuming fixed shear angles [5, 6], our definition can be adapted to arbitrary angles according to particular microscopes. In practice, $\text{epsf}(x, y)$ is discretized as an $M \times M$ matrix. We define the transfer matrix $\mathbf{H}$ such that

$$(\mathbf{H}f)_i = \sum_{j=1}^{M} \sum_{k=1}^{M} \text{epsf}(i - \frac{M}{2}, j - \frac{M}{2}) f_{x_i+j-\frac{M}{2}, y_i+k-\frac{M}{2}}. \tag{21}$$

5   Experiments

The proposed algorithms were implemented in ISO C++. Experiments were carried out on a computer with a 2.53GHz Intel®Core™2 Duo processor and 8 gigabytes of memory, running 64-bit Ubuntu Linux. The large-scale optimization library MOSEK [11] was utilized as an SOCP solver.

5.1   Data

Our method has been validated on three different types of data:

1. *Computer-simulated DIC images*, including 12 simulated images of block structures with sizes ranging from 16^2 to 1024^2. The images were generated according to the model given in Section 4.2, and were corrupted with randomly-generated nonuniform bias and additive Gaussian noise.

2. *Real DIC images of CNS stem cell populations*, consisting of a sequence of 1795 images of central nervous system (CNS) stem cells. The images are 640×512 pixels each, captured every 5 minutes using a 12-bit Orca ER (Hamamatsu) CCD camera mounted on a Zeiss Axiovert 135TV microscope with a 40×, 1.3 NA oil-immersion DIC objective. 51 images were manually segmented by an expert biologist, and utilized as the ground truth.

3. *Real DIC images of human red blood cells*, including three extremely challenging images from the Broad bioimage benchmark collection[2], for which ground-truth segmentations are available. The images are of size 800×600.

---

[2] Available online at http://www.broad.mit.edu/bbbc

5.2   Parameter Settings

Our algorithms involve up to seven parameters. The common ones include the bias order K, sparseness coefficient β, DIC shear angle θ, and the DIC kernel standard deviation σ (Eq. 20). Parameters specific for SEMU include the smoothness coefficient γ, the reweighting coefficient α, and the stopping threshold ϵ. TV-SOCP requires the noise factor τ instead of γ.

We set $K = 2$, $\sigma = 1$, and $\epsilon = 10^{-6}$ for all experiments. The shear angle θ is defined to be zero along the three-o'clock direction, increasing clockwise. It is usually multiples of $45°$, and can be easily estimated by observation. Specifically, we set $\theta = 225°$ for the simulated DIC images and the images of red blood cells, and we set $\theta = 45°$ for the images of CNS stem cells. The parameters α, β, γ, and τ were manually adjusted for the simulated images. For each dataset of cell populations, the optimal parameters were determined using grid search based on the receiver operating characteristic (ROC) of one image. The specific values will be reported in the next section along with the results.

5.3   Results

Fig. 2 shows the preconditioning results for one of the simulated DIC images. The pixel values of the input images was normalized to the range of $[0, 1]$, and was superposed with severe bias and zero-mean Gaussian noise of standard deviation 10^{-4}. The figure shows that the image was effectively corrected for bias, and the object was reconstructed with high fidelity. In particular, the TV-SOCP algorithm, which is well-suited for regularizing "blocky" structures, reconstructed the object near perfectly. The overall mean squared error (MSE) of the reconstructed images in the dataset using SEMU and TV-SOCP are $1.95 \times 10^{-3} \pm 1.02 \times 10^{-4} \text{SD}^3$ and $4.48 \times 10^{-5} \pm 3.40 \times 10^{-6} \text{SD}$, respectively. The running times of both algorithms are roughly linear with respect to the number of pixels, as depicted in Fig. 2(f).

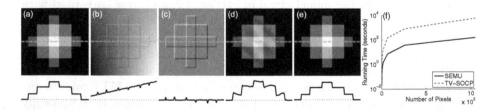

Fig. 2. Preconditioning of simulated DIC images. (a) Ground truth. (b) Observed image. (c) Bias-corrected image. (d) Preconditioned image with SEMU. (e) Preconditioned image with TV-SOCP. (f) Running time of the preconditioning algorithms in logarithmic scale.

---

[3] SD stands for (one) standard deviation.

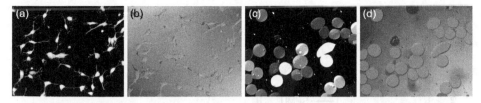

Fig. 3. Preconditioned images of cell populations. (a) CNS stem cells (brightness in decibel scale). (c) Human red blood cells. (b) and (d) are color-coded thresholding outputs of (a) and (c). Green stands for true positive, red for false positive, and blue for false negative.

Next, we present the results for the two datasets of living cell populations. Each of the datasets possesses unique challenges. The CNS stems cells have long, thin processes that extend from the cell body, which sometimes interconnect different cells (see Fig. 1(a)). Segmenting the processes is of significant biological value, and yet extremely challenging. The images of the red blood cells are of very low contrast, and contain various visual contaminations (see Fig. 1(c)).

Despite the various artifacts in the DIC images, the preconditioned images became dramatically clean-cut. In particular, Fig. 3(a) shows an image of CNS stem cells corresponding to Fig. 1(a), which was preconditioned using the SEMU algorithm with parameters $\alpha = 0.2$, $\beta = 0.0005$, and $\gamma = 0.5$. The pixel intensities are displayed in decibel scale to increase the visibility of thin structures. The average processing time was 32.5 seconds/image. Preconditioning preserved the fine details in the original images, especially the thin processes. Fig. 3(c) shows an image of red blood cells corresponding to Fig. 1(c), which was preconditioned using TV-SOCP with $\beta = 0.05$ and $\tau = 9$. The average processing time was 102.9 minutes/image. Preconditioning removed the nonuniformity in the original image, while preserving details of the internal structures of cells.

The preconditioned images enabled us to achieve high-quality cell segmentation using global thresholding. To evaluate the performance of preconditioning and not the separate problem of thresholding, we plotted the ROC curves for each dataset in Fig. 4 by trying every possible threshold on the preconditioned images. We use "positive" (or P) to refer to the set of pixels belonging to cells according to the ground truth, and "negative" (or N) for the background pixels. For pixels that are labeled as cells by thresholding, the subset that indeed belongs to cells is *true positive* (or TP), and the remaining subset is *false positive* (or FP). True positive rate and false positive rate are defined, respectively, as $TPR = |TP|/|P|$, and $FPR = |FP|/|N|$. In addition, we define *accuracy* as $ACC = (|TP| + |TN|)/(|P| + |N|)$, where $TN = N - FP$ is the *true negative*.

As shown in Fig. 4(a), both SEMU and TV-SOCP achieved excellent performances for preconditioning the images of CNS stem cells. The areas under the ROC curves (AUC) for SEMU and TV-SOCP are 96.3% and 93.6%, respectively. By visual inspection, we found that TV-SOCP was less capable in preserving long, thin processes of CNS stem cells. It was also slightly more sensitive to parameter settings, i.e., the optimal settings vary according to cell density. Since

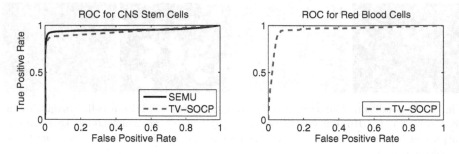

Fig. 4. ROC curves for the proposed preconditioning algorithms

we used identical parameters to process all images, the performance was suboptimal for some. Contrarily, SEMU was relatively insensitive to cell density changes, which contributed to its superior performance. Excellent performance was also achieved for images of red blood cells, for which we tested TV-SOCP only. The ROC curve is shown in Fig. 4(b), and the corresponding AUC is 95.4%.

Finally, we segmented each image using the threshold value that maximizes the segmentation accuracy for that image. The results that correspond to the images shown in Fig. 1 are presented in Fig. 3 (b) and (d). Overall, we achieved a 97.9% accuracy for segmenting CNS stem cells, and 93.4% for red blood cells.

6   Discussions and Conclusion

Alternative Noise Models. The long-tailed *Laplacian* distribution is often used for modeling impulsive noise. This model can be imposed by replacing the relevant L_2 norms in the objective functions by L_1 norms. Another important noise model is the *Poisson* model, which is non-additive, and is well-suited for describing quantum-limited noise. The Poisson noise model can be imposed by using Csiszár's I-divergence [12] as the data fidelity measure. A well-known minimizer for the I-divergence is the Richardson-Lucy (RL) algorithm [13]. The algorithm is nonnegativity-preserving under the assumption that all elements of the transfer matrix and input images are nonnegative, which does not hold for DIC microscopy. In contrast, the SEMU and TV-SOCP algorithms preserve nonnegativity for arbitrary matrices and inputs.

7   Conclusion

We proposed a general framework for preconditioning microscopy images for facilitating segmentation. The approach reconstructs the intensities of an image utilizing principles of microscopy image formation under realistic assumptions. The reconstruction is performed by minimizing convex objective functions with nonnegativity constraints. Two specific objective functions were proposed and corresponding efficient algorithms, namely SEMU and TV-SOCP, were presented. SEMU is well suited for images of small, smooth objects, while TV-SOCP is better for relatively large, flat, and blocky objects. The preconditioned images can be effortlessly segmented using thresholding. The algorithm achieved excellent performance on both simulated and real DIC images. It can be straightforwardly extended to other imaging modalities or higher dimensions.

Acknowledgements

We would like to thank Drs. Rea Ravin and Daniel J. Hoeppner (NINDS) for providing DIC images of CNS stem cells with ground truth. This work was supported partially by NIH grants R01 EB007369-01, R01 EB0004343-01, and a fellowship from Intel Research Pittsburgh. Special thanks also goes to Drs. Mei Chen, Lee E. Weiss, and Phil G. Campbell for their selfless support, and to Steven Kang for his help. This work would not have been accomplished without the computing resources provided freely by Intel Research.

References

1. Goldfarb, D., Yin, W.: Second-order cone programming methods for total variation-based image restoration. SIAM J. Sci. Comput. 27(2), 622–645 (2005)
2. Sha, F., Lin, Y., Saul, L.K., Lee, D.D.: Multiplicative updates for nonnegative quadratic programming. Neural Computation 19, 2004–2031 (2007)
3. Candes, E.J., Wakin, M.B., Boyd, S.P.: Enhancing sparsity by reweighted l1 minimization. J. Fourier Anal. Appl. 14(5), 877–905 (2008)
4. Young, D., Glasbey, C., Gray, A., Martin, N.: Identification and sizing of cells in microscope images by template matching and edge detection. In: Proc. IEEE Image Proc. App., July 1995, pp. 266–270 (1995)
5. Heise, B., Sonnleitner, A., Klement, E.P.: DIC image reconstruction on large cell scans. Microsc. Res. Tech. 66, 312–320 (2005)
6. Arnison, M.R., Cogswell, C.J., Smith, N.I., Fekete, P.W., Larkin, K.G.: Using the Hilbert transform for 3D visualization of differential interference contrast microscope images. J. Microsc. 199(1), 79–84 (2000)
7. Preza, C., Snyder, D.L., Conchello, J.A.: Theoretical development and experimental evaluation of imaging models for differential interference contrast microscopy. J. Opt. Soc. Am. A 16(9), 2185–2199 (1999)
8. Kagalwala, F., Kanade, T.: Reconstructing specimens using DIC microscope images. IEEE Trans. Syst., Man, Cybern. 33(5), 728–737 (2003)
9. Rudin, L.I., Osher, S., Fatemi, E.: Nonlinear total variation based noise removal algorithms. Physica D 60, 259–268 (1992)
10. Boyd, S., Vandenberghe, L.: Convex Optimization. Cambridge University Press, Cambridge (2004), http://www.stanford.edu/~boyd/cvxbook
11. The MOSEK optimization software, Mosek ApS, Copenhagen, Denmark, http://www.mosek.com/
12. Csiszár, I.: Why least squares and maximum entropy? An axiomatic approach to inference for linear inverse problems. Ann. Stat. 19(4), 2032–2066 (1991)
13. Dey, N., Blanc-Féraud, L., Zimmer, C., Roux, P., Kam, Z., Olivo-Marin, J.C., Zerubia, J.: Richardson-Lucy algorithm with total variation regularization for 3D confocal microscope deconvolution. Microsc. Res. Tech. 69, 260–266 (2006)

Coupled Minimum-Cost Flow Cell Tracking

Dirk Padfield[1,2], Jens Rittscher[1], and Badrinath Roysam[2]

[1] GE Global Research, One Research Circle, Niskayuna, NY 12309
[2] Rensselaer Polytechnic Institute, 110 8th St., Troy, NY 12180

Abstract. A growing number of screening applications require the automated monitoring of cell populations in a high-throughput, high-content environment. These applications depend on accurate cell tracking of individual cells that display various behaviors including mitosis, occlusion, rapid movement, and entering and leaving the field of view. We present a tracking approach that explicitly models each of these behaviors and represents the association costs in a graph-theoretic minimum-cost flow framework. We show how to extend the minimum-cost flow algorithm to account for mitosis and merging events by coupling particular edges. We applied the algorithm to nearly 6,000 images of 400,000 cells representing 32,000 tracks taken from five separate datasets, each composed of multiple wells.Our algorithm is able to track cells and detect different cell behaviors with an accuracy of over 99%.

Keywords: Tracking, minimum-cost flow, cell analysis, graph-theoretic, segmentation, wavelets, quantitative analysis.

1   Introduction

High-throughput automated screening of in-vitro systems is of great importance to biological research. For example, the measurement of cell motility and mitosis are useful for fluorescence microscopy applications in areas such as cancer research, immunology, and developmental biology. To enable such studies, automated microscopes allow researchers to run large numbers of experiments in a high-throughput and high-content fashion over extended periods of time. Quantitative time-lapse analysis on the single-cell level derived from segmentation and tracking algorithms can provide detailed insight into such experiments.

While each biological application has specific requirements, they share several core challenges. Each data set typically contains a large number of cells to be tracked. Events such as mitosis (cell division) need to be accurately captured. Furthermore, since the field of view of the microscope is limited, some cells will move in and out of the image. Limiting the potential for cytotoxicity induced by fluorescent labels is another important factor that influences the design of imaging protocols: Low concentrations of fluorescent dyes result in low signal-to-noise which makes the segmentation of the image data challenging. Also, in order to reduce photobleaching the experiments are only imaged occasionally; while some experiments may be imaged every 3 or 5 minutes, others may only be imaged every 30 minutes. Consequently, there is often no spatial overlap of the cells between adjacent frames.

J.L. Prince, D.L. Pham, and K.J. Myers (Eds.): IPMI 2009, LNCS 5636, pp. 374–385, 2009.

The focus of this work is the design of a tracking framework that addresses these challenges, which are summarized in Table 1.Our framework is composed of defocused image detection, stage shift measurement, wavelet-based object segmentation, and graph-theoretic tracking. The first three of these have been presented previously, so the focus of this paper is on the new tracking approach, which optimally matches objects across frames based on the features measured from the segmented objects.

This paper is organized as follows. A survey of previous approaches to cell tracking is given in Section 2. The details of our graph-theoretic tracking approach is given in Section 3. In Section 4, experimental results on five different data sets with multiple wells and different imaging conditions representing nearly 400,000 cells and nearly 32,000 tracks are presented. Our conclusions are given in Section 5.

2   State of the Art

Extensive research in the field of computer vision has resulted in powerful and versatile algorithms for visual tracking. The existing methods can roughly be divided into three groups: independent segmentation of individual frames followed by data association, model based contour evolution approaches [1], and stochastic filtering [2]. We here present a brief summary of the application of each of these methods to the problem of live cell monitoring as summarized in Table 1.

Contour evolution approaches, and in particular level-sets, offer some advantages as they can easily handle changes in topology. Yang *et al.* [3] and Padfield *et al.* [4] make use of this fact by evolving level sets on the spatio-temporal volume to effectively associate detections over time. In other approaches, such as that of Dufour *et al.* [5], levels sets are propagated over time by using the contour from the previous image as an initialization. While dealing effectively with topology changes, fast motion or the appearance and disappearance of new cells require the re-initialization of the level sets and additional heuristics

In general, probabilistic approaches rely on strong model assumptions. The necessary model parameters are typically learned from training data sets. Mean-shift tracking [6] can, for example, be used to track objects using a basic appearance model as in [7]. This approach depends heavily on the accuracy of the object localization, and the model tends to drift over time. Stochastic filters [8,9] can be extremely powerful if a object motion can be modeled, and such approaches are used for cell tracking in [10] and [11]. In [12], Kachouie *et al.* introduce a maximum *a posteriori* based probabilistic framework for tracking cells across all images at once, but the number of cells that the system can track is limited because of the large number of required hypotheses. The fact that cells can undergo mitosis and the temporal sampling may be very low make the application of stochastic filters less effective.

Segment and associate algorithms have also been shown to be effective for cell tracking. Al-Kofahi *et al.* [13] use linear programming on various matching hypotheses, but their approach does not capture cell occlusion and cells entering and leaving the field of view. Matching based on Euclidean distances is used by Dehauwer *et al.* [14] to associate targets across frames. Padfield *et al.* [15] associate cells in a spatio-temporal volume by training features from tracks of single cells and using them to split tracks

Table 1. Comparison of different approaches to cell tracking. This table summarizes how well three main approaches to visual tracking address particular cell tracking challenges. The "+" indicates that the method is effective at handling a particular challenge, and "-" indicates the method has difficulties. Several example references of the application of these approaches to cell tracking are also given. These references employ additional processing to address the limitations of the tracking approaches.

Challenge	Contour Evolution	Stochastic Filtering	Segment & Associate
Mitosis & Merging	+	-	-
Appearing & Disappearing	-	-	-
Low Temporal Resolution	-	+	+
Fast Motion	-	+	+
Tracking Drift	-	-	+
Accurate Segmentation	+	-	+
Selected References	[3,4,5]	[7,10,11,12]	[13,14,15,16,17]

consisting of multiple-cells. Zhang *et al.* [16] use a minimum-cost flow network for globally assigning a small number of detections over time in which the optimization is run multiple times as different hypotheses are tested; this is computationally expensive, and the large number of hypotheses limits its application to problems with a small number of tracks. Sbalzarini *et al.* [17] solve the matching problem using a particle matching algorithm that minimizes a cost functional that also includes "dummy particles" for objects entering and leaving. The failure modes that are typical for this category of algorithms suggest that standard matching techniques are not sufficient for associating entering and leaving cells and that mitosis and occlusion events need to be treated carefully.

Combining elements of these various approaches can lead to powerful tracking algorithms. While effective, such approaches often result in very complex systems which are difficult to maintain and implement. The focus of the present work is the development of a graph-theoretic framework for matching that not only effectively models mitosis and occlusion events but also models the appearance and disappearance of cells. Our results demonstrate that, combined with a suitable segmentation method, this tracking algorithm enables robust tracking of large high-throughput data sets.

3   Methods

In this section, we present our tracking approach, which follows the model of independent frame segmentation followed by cell association. Our approach models different cell behaviors including moving, splitting, merging, moving into the image, moving out of the image, appearing, and disappearing. We will show that modeling cells moving, entering, and leaving can be solved directly using an algorithm called minimum-cost flow by appropriately setting up a corresponding graph. The conditions of mitosis and merging, however, are challenging to model in the minimum-cost flow framework because one object is present on one frame and two on another. To solve this, we introduce a method we call "coupled minimum-cost flow" to enable coupling of graph edges so that if certain edges are chosen by the optimization step, the coupled edges are also chosen.

3.1 Coupled Minimum-Cost Flow

A flow network $G = (V, E)$ is a directed graph in which each edge $(u, v) \in E$ has a non-negative capacity $c(u, v) \geq 0$. For the purpose of matching M cells in a previous image to N cells in a current image, the set of vertices in G can be partitioned as $V = L \cup R \cup T_+ \cup T_-$, where L are the vertices corresponding to the cells on the previous image, R are the vertices corresponding to the cells on the current image, T_+ is a source vertex, and T_- is a target vertex. In this construction, edges of G are directed from L to R, along with $|L|$ edges from T_+ to each of the L vertices and $|R|$ edges from the R vertices to the T_- vertex.

Suppose that each edge (u, v) has, in addition to a capacity $c(u, v)$, a real-valued cost $a(u, v)$. If we send $f(u, v)$ units of flow over edge (u, v), we incur a cost of $a(u, v) f(u, v)$. We also specify a flow requirement d with the goal of sending d units of flow from T_+ to T_- in such a way that the total cost incurred by the flow, $\sum_{(u,v) \in E} a(u, v) f(u, v)$, is minimized. The problem of finding the cheapest possible way of sending this flow through a flow network is known as the minimum-cost flow problem [18] and can be described as:

$$\text{minimize} \quad \sum_{(u,v) \in E} a(u, v) f(u, v)$$

subject to

Capacity constraint:	$f(u, v) \leq c(u, v)$	for each $u, v \in V$
Skew symmetry:	$f(u, v) = -f(v, u)$	for each $u, v \in V$
Flow conservation:	$\sum_{v \in V} f(u, v) = 0$	for each $u \in V - \{T_1, T\}$
Flow requirement:	$\sum_{v \in V} f(T_+, v) = d$	

Simple matching of cells between two frames can be directly represented in the minimum-cost flow framework, but additional generalizations are required for more complex cell behaviors as described in the following paragraphs.

Appearance and Disappearance of Cells. Cells may enter or leave the image from the image border or from a different z-plane, so this behavior must be incorporated into the graph. This can be accomplished by adding A and D vertices to the graph as in the left graph of Figure 1, which shows an example for the case with two left vertices and three right vertices. With $M = |L|$ cells in the previous image and $N = |R|$ cells in the current image, the A vertex must have edges to all of the N right vertices, meaning that each cell in the current frame could potentially have moved into the frame. Analogously, the D vertex needs an edge from each of the M left vertices, meaning that each cell in the previous frame could potentially have moved out of the frame. If N is greater than M, then at least $N - M$ cells appeared in the current image. To observe the

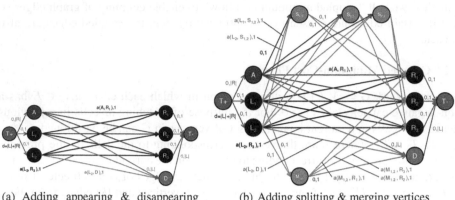

(a) Adding appearing & disappearing vertices

(b) Adding splitting & merging vertices

Fig. 1. Minimum-cost flow graphs. The graph on the left adds appearing and disappearing vertices to a standard bipartite graph. The graph on the right further adds splitting and merging vertices. In this simple example, two cells are present on the previous image and three on the current image. The cost and capacity, respectively, of the edges are marked explicitly.

flow conservation constraint in the extreme case where exactly $N - M$ cells appeared, the rest of the M units flowing into the A vertex must flow to the D vertex through an edge that must therefore have capacity M. Using this model, the required flow d is $M + N = |L| + |R|$, which ensures that all of the left and right vertices have exactly one entering and one leaving edge so that all of the cells on the previous and current image are accounted for.

Merging and Splitting of Cells. To fully generalize the graph to handle complex cell behaviors, models for splitting (mitotic) cells are needed as well as models for merging (occluding) cells. The complexity of these cases results from the fact that the number of edges entering a split or merge vertex is different from the number of edges leaving, which violates the flow conservation constraint of the graph. To observe the flow conservation constraint, an edge can be included from the appear vertex to each of the splitting vertices and from each of the merging vertices to the disappear vertex. Since the edges are connected to the appear and disappear vertices, the required flow constraint is still valid as exactly $M + N$ units still flow from the source vertex (and to the target vertex).

The graph on the right in Figure 1 shows an example of the graph resulting from adding splitting and merging events to the graph on the left. In this figure, $s_{j,k}$ represents that R_j and R_k in the current frame are daughters of one of the cells in the previous image. Analogously, $m_{i,j}$ represents that L_i and L_k in the previous frame were merged into one cell in the current image.

Given the cost and capacity constraints described in Figure 1 and the flow requirement $d = M + N$, the flow equations can be determined. The flow into each of the left vertices is exactly 1, which is used to define the flow equation for the "left" vertices. The flow requirement also causes the flow entering the appear vertex to be exactly N, which is used to define the "appear" flow equation. The "split" flow equation states that the flow entering the vertex must be equal to the flow exiting the vertex; this flow is either 2 if the vertex is part of the solution, or 0 if not. The flow equations for the target, right, disappear, and merge vertices are analogous to those of the source, left, appear, and split vertices, respectively.

$$\text{Source: } \sum_{i=1}^{M} f(T_+, L_i) + N \cdot f(T_+, A) = M + N = d$$

$$\text{Left: } \quad f(T_+, L_i) = 1 = \sum_{j=1}^{N} f(L_i, R_j) + f(L_i, D)$$

$$+ \sum_{j=1}^{N} \sum_{k=j+1}^{N} f(L_i, S_{j,k}) + \sum_{k=i+1}^{M} f(L_i, M_{i,k}) + \sum_{l=1}^{i-1} f(L_i, M_{l,j}) \qquad i = 1...M$$

$$\text{Appear: } f(T_+, A) = N = \sum_{j-1}^{N} f(A, R_j) + f(A, D) + \sum_{j=1}^{N} \sum_{k=j+1}^{N} f(A, S_{j,k})$$

$$\text{Split: } \quad \sum_{i=1}^{M} f(L_i, S_{j,k}) + f(A, S_{j,k}) = f(S_{j,k}, R_j) + f(S_{j,k}, R_k) \qquad j = 1...N$$

$$k = j+1...N$$

One problem remains, however: a constraint is needed to ensure that **exactly two or zero** units flow to and from splitting and merging vertices. Without such a constraint, it is possible that one unit would flow into and out of a splitting (merging) vertex, leading to a confusion of cell behavior. To enforce this constraint, we introduce the concept of coupling edges. This coupling ensures that if the edge from a left vertex to a splitting vertex is chosen, then the corresponding edge from the appear vertex to the splitting vertex is also chosen. Thus, if this edge is part of the solution, exactly two units enter the splitting vertex, and this forces exactly two units to exit the splitting vertex as well, leading to consistent hypotheses. The coupling constraint for the splitting vertices is as follows (merging is analogous).

$$\text{Split: } \sum_{i=1}^{M} f(L_i, S_{j,k}) = f(A, S_{j,k}) = f(S_{j,k}, R_j) = f(S_{j,k}, R_k) \ j = 1...N$$

$$k = j+1...N$$

We will show in Section 3.2 a simple way of realizing this coupling.

3.2 Solving the Coupled Minimum-Cost Flow Problem

To solve the coupled minimum-cost flow problem for the graph shown in Figure 1, an incidence matrix of size $|V| \times |E|$ can be used, where each column corresponds to an edge and each row corresponds to a vertex. In this matrix, shown on the left in Figure 2, all entries in each column are zero except those corresponding to the vertices that are connected by the edge corresponding to the column. The entry in a column corresponding to the start of an edge is set to -1, and the entry corresponding to the

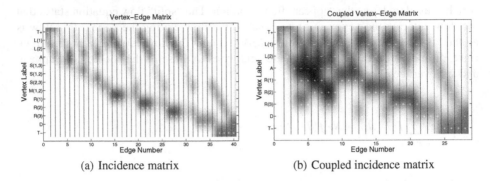

(a) Incidence matrix   (b) Coupled incidence matrix

Fig. 2. Incidence matrices corresponding to the graph in 1. In the incidence matrix on the left, each column corresponds to an edge in Figure 1 and is color-coded as in that figure. In the coupled incidence matrix on the right, the coupled matrix allows columns to account for more than one edge and thus have more than two entries. The vertex labels are indicated on the y-axis, and the columns correspond to the edges of the graph. For each column, the entries with negative signs indicate the source vertex of an edge and those with positive signs indicate the destination vertex of an edge.

end of an edge is set to 1. The $|E|$ columns consist of various sets of associations: those corresponding to moving cells, appearing cells, disappearing cells, splitting cells, and merging cells.

Enforcing the coupling constraint is straightforward using the incidence matrix. For each split and merge vertex, all of the columns (four) corresponding to edges entering and leaving the vertex are added to form a new column, and the four columns are removed. For each split and merge vertex, this yields a column that has more than two nonzero entries so that, in order for this column to be included in the solution, all edges included in this combined column must be chosen together. Combining the columns in this manner has the added benefit of reducing the number of edges and nodes in the incidence matrix, reducing the computational complexity. Because the edges entering and exiting the split and merge vertices are summed, these vertices are no longer needed and are not present in this matrix. The resulting coupled incidence matrix is shown on the right in Figure 2. Several columns of this matrix have four entries rather than two, indicating that edges are coupled. The optimal matches are then determined using linear programming by finding a subset of columns in this matrix such that the sum of the cost of these columns is minimized, under the constraint that no two columns share common nonzero entries.

3.3   Calculation of Association Costs

Incorporating data driven information into the model is the primary role of the association costs, $a(u,v)$. These costs are formulated differently according to whether an edge is associated with a cell splitting, merging, moving, appearing, or disappearing event. The formulation of $a(u,v)$ is based on a generalized distance function

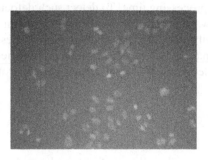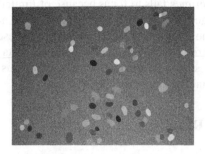

Fig. 3. Wavelet segmentation example. The figure on the left shows a typical low-dose stained image, and the figure on the right shows the segmentation using the wavelet approach. Despite the low contrast-to-noise, the segmentation result is very accurate.

$$a(u,v) = \sum_{i=0}^{K} w_i |\phi_i(u) - \phi_i(v)| \qquad (1)$$

where $\Phi(u) = \{\phi_i(u)\}$ is the feature vector of the cell that is associated to the vertex u, and K is the number of elements of the vector. Any number of features can be incorporated into this feature vector including the cell centroid, area, eccentricity, orientation, and features based on the wavelet coefficients. w acts as a linear weighting function.

In the case of cell splitting, the association cost represents features measured on combined objects, and is written as

$$a(u,(v_1,v_2)) = \sum_{i=0}^{K} w_i |\phi_i(u) - \phi_i(v_1,v_2)| \qquad (2)$$

where $\phi_i(v_1,v_2)$ represents features computed from the combined cells. Merging is analogous. For the edges associated with entering and leaving events, the distance to the image border is used to compute the association cost.

3.4   Additional Framework Components

Additional algorithms are required for the full tracking framework as follows. **Wavelet Segmentation.** We make use of the fact that the representation of the images in the wavelet domain enables de-noising and segmentation of the images in one step. The details are presented in [15], and the approach is similar to that taken in [11,19]. An example is given in Figure 3. The segmentation results yield the features used for measuring the association costs in Section 3.3. Under-segmentation errors are corrected implicitly by the tracking algorithm by splitting objects detected as having merged; over-segmentation errors will result in detection of false mitosis events by the tracker. **Stage Shift Measurement.** In time-lapse high-throughput experiments, the microscope may drift over time leading to tracking errors and biased measurements. To correct this stage shift effect, we register each pair of images by correlating the images in the Fourier domain. This yields a transform that is used to offset the centroid features of the cells in the tracking step. **Defocus Detection**. In high-throughput applications, the microscope sometimes fails to focus because of limited processing time. To detect such defocused images, we decompose the images using a wavelet transform and compare the energy of the coefficients at various levels as described in [20]. These defocused images are then removed and tracked over. The results in Section 4 demonstrate that the segmentation, stage shift measurement, and defocus detection algorithms are sufficiently robust so that tracking errors rarely occur.

4 Results

In this section, we present results of the tracking algorithm on five time-lapse datasets with varying conditions and biological hypotheses and multiple wells as outlined in Table 2. Each of the datasets consists of images taken from different wells with many of the wells containing different doses of various treatments. In total, nearly 400,000 cells were segmented and tracked representing nearly 32,000 tracks.

For each of the datasets, 25% of the wells were chosen at random and validated for segmentation and tracking accuracy, representing a validation of over 104,000 cells and nearly 8,000 tracks as indicated in Table 3. To enable such large-scale validation, it was carried out in an edit-based validation framework wherein the automatic results were presented to the user whose corrections were recorded and tabulated. The results in Table 3 were carried out by the authors, and a subset of 809 tracks (not all tracks because of time constraints) were further validated by two expert biologists from different institutions who identified a number of additional errors. However, these additional errors reduced the overall accuracy by less than 0.5%.

Our results indicate that the accuracy of the algorithms to correctly detect mitosis, move, and appear/disappear events is 97.8%, 100%, and 99.8% overall, respectively. For each track, if any event is incorrect, the track is considered invalid. Despite this stringent requirement, the percentage of correct tracks is 99.2%, indicating the accuracy and robustness of the algorithms. The robustness of the algorithms is further demonstrated by their ability to track through defocused images and large stage shift. Datasets 1, 2, and 5 contained wells with defocused images, all of which were detected by the defocus detection algorithm resulting in a total of 0 missed detections and 5 false positives

Table 2. Dataset Descriptions. This table gives a brief overview of the different data sets. The pixel spacing for datasets 1, 2, 3, 5 is 0.323 μm in x and y; for dataset 4 it is 0.645 μm. The acquisition time spacing for datasets 1-4 is 15 minutes; for dataset 5 it is 6 minutes.

Dataset	Wells	Time Points	Images	Total Cells	Total Tracks	Mitosis	Appear	Disappear
1	96	41	3,936	168,589	10,151	467	5,499	5,037
2	24	41	984	116,041	13,359	521	9,487	9,699
3	4	112	448	28,570	558	71	168	211
4	1	88	88	12,301	258	20	83	89
5	36	12	432	68,270	7,517	205	1,501	1,518
Total	161	294	11,776	393,771	31,843	1,284	16,738	16,554

Table 3. Summary of tracking results for all datasets. Overall tracks, mitosis events, move events, and appear/disappear events are shown separately. A mitosis error occurs if a cell splitting event is missed. Two move errors occur if two cell tracks switch identities. Two appear/disappear errors occur if a cell moves close to the boundary of the image and is detected as leaving and then entering as a new cell. Any of these errors will invalidate the track so that the number of correct tracks in the first column includes only tracks with no errors.

	Tracks		Mitosis		Move		Appear/Disappear	
	Ratio	%	Ratio	%	Ratio	%	Ratio	%
1	2,157 / 2,177	99.1	95 / 96	99.0	35,170 / 35,183	100.0	2,182 / 2,188	99.7
2	3,454 / 3,471	99.5	132 / 135	97.8	26,607 / 26,619	100.0	4,949 / 4,951	100.0
3	166 / 171	97.1	33 / 33	100.0	8,375 / 8,379	100.0	72 / 73	98.6
4	244 / 258	94.6	20 / 20	100.0	12,032 / 12,043	99.9	169 / 172	98.3
5	1,733 / 1,737	99.8	34 / 37	91.9	14,008 / 14,008	100.0	747 / 748	99.9
Total	7,754 / 7,814	99.2	314 / 321	97.8	96,192 / 96,232	100.0	8,119 / 8,132	99.8

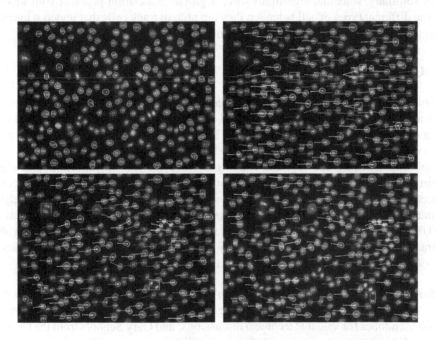

Fig. 4. Tracking results in the presence of large stage shift. Four consecutive frames from one sequence are shown from left to right and top to bottom. The motion vectors indicate the motion of each individual cell. Blue boxes indicate cells entering, red boxes indicate cells leaving, and green boxes indicate cells splitting.

out of nearly 6,000 images. Furthermore, the stage shift was correctly estimated for all of the images, leading to correct tracking results even when the actual cell movement was many times smaller than the movement of the stage.

The time required by each of the algorithms is as follows. Tracking: 0.17 seconds/cell; segmentation: 11.9 seconds/image; stage shift correction: 9.7 seconds/image; defocus detection: 1.1 seconds/image. For an average image with 50 cells, this leads to a processing time of 31.2 seconds. This timing was calculated on a dual-core 2.6GHz Dell laptop with 3.5GB of RAM. The algorithms were implemented in Matlab, and it is expected that the processing time will decrease by a factor of 5 for a C/C++ implementation.

Several example tracking results are given in Figure 4. The track tails indicate the location of the cell in the previous image, demonstrating that there is often no overlap of the cells between adjacent images. The blue boxes indicate cells entering the image, red boxes indicate cells leaving, and green boxes indicate mitosis events. Although the cells move in clusters, touch one another, and undergo mitosis, the algorithms are able to successfully separate the cells into individual tracks. Because of the accurate cell segmentation, the algorithms can extract not only the tracks, but also the shape of the cells over time as shown in the figure.

In summary, since the algorithms solve a global association problem with models for the different types of cell behavior, they are able to track cells that undergo mitosis, merge, move in and out of the image, and move quickly and erratically.

5   Conclusions

We have presented a tracking approach based on the minimum-cost flow algorithm that embeds the association costs in a weighted directed graph. We have presented an efficient edge coupling approach for handling splitting and merging events, and we have shown how to appropriately set the costs and capacities to represent cell behaviors such as splitting, merging, moving, and entering and leaving the field of view. This algorithm is supported by wavelet segmentation, stage shift measurement, and defocused detection algorithms, all of which combine to form an effective quantitative analysis framework. These algorithms have been applied to nearly 6,000 images representing 400,000 cells and 32,000 tracks. The validation indicates that the algorithms are able to track the cells with an accuracy of 99.2% under the strict requirement that a track is considered failed if any errors are present in the track.

Acknowledgments. We would like to thank Elizabeth Roquemore, Angela Williams, and Alla Zaltsman for generating the image sets and assisting with result validation; Paulo Mendonça for valuable technical discussions; and Gary Schools from the Ordway Research Institute for assisting with the result validation.

References

1. Paragios, N., Deriche, R.: Geodesic active regions for motion estimation and tracking. In: ICCV, vol. 1, pp. 688–694 (1999)
2. Blake, A., Isard, M.: Active Contours. Springer, Heidelberg (1998)
3. Yang, F., Mackey, M., Ianzini, F., Gallardo, G., Sonka, M.: Cell segmentation, tracking, and mitosis detection using temporal context. In: Duncan, J.S., Gerig, G. (eds.) MICCAI 2005. LNCS, vol. 3749, pp. 302–309. Springer, Heidelberg (2005)

4. Padfield, D., Rittscher, J., Thomas, N., Roysam, B.: Spatio-temporal cell cycle phase analysis using level sets and fast marching methods. Med. I.A (2008)
5. Dufour, A., Shinin, V., Tajbakhsh, S., Guillen-Aghion, N., Olivo-Marin, J., Zimmer, C.: Segmenting and tracking fluorescent cells in dynamic 3-D microscopy with coupled active surfaces. TIP 14(9) (2005)
6. Comaniciu, D., Ramesh, V., Meer, P.: Real-time tracking of non-rigid objects using mean shift. In: CVPR, vol. 2, pp. 142–149 (2000)
7. Debeir, O., Van Ham, P., Kiss, R., Decaestecker, C.: Tracking of migrating cells under phase-contrast video microscopy with combined mean-shift processes. TMI 24(6), 697–711 (2005)
8. Gelb, A. (ed.): Applied Optimal Estimation. MIT Press, Cambridge (1979)
9. Blake, A., Isard, M.: Condensation – conditional density propagation for visual tracking. IJCV 28(1), 5–28 (1998)
10. Li, K., Miller, E., Chen, M., Kanade, T., Weiss, L., Campbell, P.: Cell population tracking and lineage construction with spatiotemporal context. Med. I.A. 12(5), 546–566 (2008)
11. Genovesio, A., Liedl, T., Emiliani, V., Parak, W.J., Coppey-Moisan, M., Olivo-Marin, J.: Multiple particle tracking in 3-d+t microscopy: method and application to the tracking of endocytosed quantum dots. TIP 15(5), 1062–1070 (2006)
12. Kachouie, N., Fieguth, P., Ramunas, J., Jervis, E.: Probabilistic model-based cell tracking. International Journal of Biomedical Imaging, 1–10 (2006)
13. Al-Kofahi, O., Radke, R.J., Goderie, S.K., Shen, Q., Temple, S., Roysam, B.: Automated cell lineage construction: a rapid method to analyze clonal development established with murine neural progenitor cells. Cell Cycle 5(3), 327–335 (2006)
14. De Hauwer, C., Darro, F., Camby, I., Kiss, R., Van Ham, P., Decaesteker, C.: In vitro motility evaluation of aggregated cancer cells by means of automatic image processing. Cytometry 36(1), 1–10 (1999)
15. Padfield, D., Rittscher, J., Roysam, B.: Spatio-temporal cell segmentation and tracking for automated screening. In: IEEE ISBI (2008)
16. Zhang, L., Li, Y., Nevatia, R.: Global data association for multi-object tracking using network flows. In: CVPR (2008)
17. Sbalzarini, I.F., Koumoutsakos, P.: Feature point tracking and trajectory analysis for video imaging in cell biology. Journal of Structural Biology 151(2), 182–195 (2005)
18. Cormen, T., Leiserson, C., Rivest, R., Stein, C.: Introduction to Algorithms, 2nd edn. MIT Press, Cambridge (2001)
19. Olivo-Marin, J.: Automatic detection of spots in biological images by a wavelet-based selective filtering technique. In: ICIP, pp. I: 311–314 (1996)
20. Padfield, D., Rittscher, J., Roysam, B.: Defocus and low CNR detection for cell tracking applications. In: MICCAI MIAAB Workshop (2008)

Persistence Diagrams of Cortical Surface Data

Moo K. Chung[1,2], Peter Bubenik[3], and Peter T. Kim[4]

[1] Department of Biostatistics and Medical Informatics
[2] Waisman Laboratory for Brain Imaging and Behavior
University of Wisconsin, Madison, WI 53706, USA
[3] Department of Mathematics
Cleveland State University, Cleveland, Ohio 44115, USA
[4] Department of Mathematics and Statistics
University of Guelph, Guelph, Ontario N1G 2W1, Canada
mkchung@wisc.edu

Abstract. We present a novel framework for characterizing signals in images using techniques from computational algebraic topology. This technique is general enough for dealing with noisy multivariate data including geometric noise. The main tool is persistent homology which can be encoded in persistence diagrams. These diagrams visually show how the number of connected components of the sublevel sets of the signal changes. The use of local critical values of a function differs from the usual statistical parametric mapping framework, which mainly uses the mean signal in quantifying imaging data. Our proposed method uses all the local critical values in characterizing the signal and by doing so offers a completely new data reduction and analysis framework for quantifying the signal. As an illustration, we apply this method to a 1D simulated signal and 2D cortical thickness data. In case of the latter, extra homological structures are evident in an control group over the autistic group.

1 Introduction

In neuroimaging, it is usually assumed that measurements f in images follow the familiar signal plus noise framework

$$f(x) = \mu(x) + \epsilon(x), \; x \in \mathbb{M} \subset \mathbb{R}^d, \tag{1}$$

where μ is the unknown mean signal, to be estimated, and ϵ is noise [3] [15] [18] [19] [25] [36]. The unknown signal is usually estimated by various spatial image smoothing over $\mathbb{M}$. The most widely used smoothing technique is kernel smoothing and its variants because of their simplicity, and because they provide the theoretical context for scale spaces and Gaussian random field theory [32] [36].

In the usual statistical parametric mapping framework [15] [19] [36], inference on the model (1) proceeds as follows. If we denote an estimate of the signal by $\hat{\mu}$, the residual $f - \hat{\mu}$ gives an estimate of the noise. One then constructs a test statistic $T(x)$, corresponding to a given hypothesis about the signal. As a way to account for spatial correlation of the statistic $T(x)$, the global maximum

J.L. Prince, D.L. Pham, and K.J. Myers (Eds.): IPMI 2009, LNCS 5636, pp. 386–397, 2009.

of the test statistic over the search space $\mathbb{M}$ is taken as the subsequent test statistic. Hence a great deal of the neuroimaging and statistical literature, have been devoted to determining the distribution of $\sup_{x \in \mathbb{M}} T(x)$ using random field theory [34] [36], permutation tests [30] and the Hotelling–Weyl volume of tubes calculation [29].

The use of the mean signal is one way of performing data reduction, however, this may not necessarily be the best way to characterize complex multivariate imaging data. Thus instead of using the mean signal, in this paper we propose to use what is known as persistent homology, which pairs local critical values [12] [13] [39]. It is intuitive that local critical values of $\hat{\mu}$ approximately characterizes the shape of the continuous signal μ using only a finite number of scalar values. By pairing these local critical values in a nonlinear fashion and plotting them, one constructs the persistence diagram [7] [12] [28] [38].

Persistent homology is popular in computational algebraic topology with applications in protein structure analysis [31], gene expression [11], and sensor networks [9]. As far as the authors are aware, there is no such applications in medical image analysis even though this technique is well suited for it. This is the first paper that applies the concept of persistent homology to medical imaging data. The proposed method is illustrated using both simulated and real neuroimaging data. For the simulation, we use 1D Gaussian noise in (1) mainly for illustration. The 2D neuroimaging data comes from an MRI autism study [4] where the interest is in quantifying the abnormal cortical thickness pattern in autistic subjects if there is any. It is shown that certain persistent homology patterns unique to the autism group is evident.

2   Persistence Diagrams

A function is called a Morse function if all critical values are unique and non-degenerate, i.e. the Hessian does not vanish [27]. We note that for integer valued digital images, critical values of intensity may not be all unique; however, the underlying continuous signal μ in (1) is likely and assumed to be a Morse function. We estimate the signal using a kernel function and obtain a smooth estimate.

For illustrative purposes, we will show how to construct the persistence diagram for a 1D Morse function. Assuming μ is a Morse function with a finite number of critical values, define a sublevel set $R(y) = \mu^{-1}(-\infty, y]$. The sublevel set is the subset of $\mathbb{R}$ that satisfies $\mu(x) \leq y$. The sublevel set can have many disjoint components. Let $\#R(y)$ be the number of connected components in the sublevel set. Let us denote the local minimums as $g_1, \cdots, g_m$ and the local maximums as $h_1, \cdots, h_n$. Since the critical values of the Morse function are all unique, we can strictly order the local minimums from the smallest to the largest as

$$g_{(1)} < g_{(2)} < \cdots < g_{(m)}$$

and similarly for the local maximums as

$$h_{(1)} < h_{(2)} < \cdots < h_{(n)}.$$

We further collect all the critical values,

$$z_1 = g_1, \ldots, z_m = g_m, z_{m+1} = h_1, \ldots, z_{m+n} = h_n$$

and order them as

$$z_{(1)} < z_{(2)} < \cdots < z_{(m+n)}.$$

At each minimum, we have the birth of a new component, i.e.

$$\#R(g_i) = \#R(g_i - \varepsilon) + 1$$

for sufficiently small ε. The new component is identified with the local minimum g_i. Similarly at each maximum, we have the death of a component, i.e.

$$\#R(h_i) = \#R(h_i - \varepsilon) - 1,$$

and two components will merge as one. The number of connected components will only change if we pass through critical points and we can iteratively compute $\#R$ at each critical value as

$$\#R(z_{(i+1)}) = \#R(z_{(i)}) \pm 1.$$

The sign depends on whether $z_{(i+1)}$ is a maximum (-1) or a minimum $(+1)$. This is the basis of Morse theory [27] that says the topological characteristics of a topological space is characterized by the local behavior at critical points of a Morse function on that space. Persistent homology produces pairs (h_i, g_j) of critical values so that a component is born at g_j and dies at h_i. Of course these are the (topological) parameters of interest which are unknown and to be statistically estimated with data generated according to (1).

As an example, the birth and death processes are illustrated in Figure 1, where the gray dots are simulated with Gaussian noise with mean 0 and variance 0.2^2 as

$$f(x) = \mu(x) + N(0, 0.2^2)$$

with signal $\mu(t) = 10(t - 1/2)^2 + \cos(7\pi t)/2$. The signal μ is estimated using heat kernel smoothing [3] and plotted as the red line. Now we increase y from $-\infty$ to ∞. When we hit the first critical value $y = a$, the sublevel set consists of a single point, i.e. $\widehat{\#R(a)} = 1$. When we hit the minimum at $y = b$, we have the birth of a new component at b, i.e. $\widehat{\#R(b)} = 2$. When we hit the maximum at $y = c$, the two components identified by a and b are merged together to form a single component, i.e. $\widehat{\#R(c)} = 1$.

When we pass through a maximum and merge two components, we pair the maximum with the higher of the two minimums of the two components [12]. Doing so we are pairing the birth of a component to its death. Obviously the paired extremes do not have to be adjacent to each other. If there is a boundary, the function value evaluated at the boundary is treated as a critical value. In our simulated example, we need to pair (b, c) and (d, e). Other critical values are paired similarly. The reduced persistence diagram is then the scatter plot of these pairings. For technical reasons, the persistence diagram also include all of the points (a, a), where $a \in \mathbb{R}$.

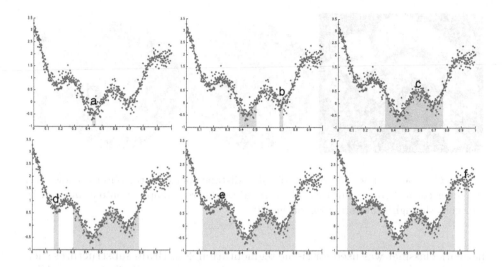

Fig. 1. The births and deaths of components in sublevel sets. We have critical values a, b, c, d, e, f, where $a < b < d < f$ are minimums and $c < e$ are maximums. At $y = a$, we have a single component marked by a single gray area. When we increase the level to $y = b$, we have the birth of a new component in addition to the existing component born at a. At the maximum $y = c$, the two components merge together to form a single component. Following the pairing rule [12], we pair (c, b) and (e, d). Other critical values are paired similarly.

2.1   Persistence Diagram for Cortical Data

For a 2D Morse function defined on a cortical manifold $\mathbb{M} \subset \mathbb{R}^3$, we need to also consider saddle points so the situation is more complicated. At a saddle point, we can have two possible pairings corresponding to either birth or death. A saddle point may join two components. This case is analogous to the local maximum in the 1D case. In this case, persistent homology pairs the value of the saddle point with the larger of the minimums of the two components. This pair is recorded as the *persistence diagram of degree* 0 (Figure 4). If the saddle point does not join two disconnected components, then a hole is born in the sublevel set. Persistent homology pairs the value at this saddle point with the value of the local maximum where this hole disappears. This pair is recorded as *the persistence diagram of degree* 1 (Figure 4). A more precise definition is given in Section 4.

Among various cortical measures, in this paper we consider cortical thickness, which has been used in characterizing various clinical populations [4] [14] [22] [23] [26] [37]. High resolution magnetic resonance images of age-matched right-handed males (16 high functioning autistic and 11 normal controls) were obtained using a 3-Tesla GE SIGNA scanner. The collected images went through intensity nonuniformity correction [33] and were spatially normalized into the MNI stereotaxic space *via* a global affine transformation [8]. Subsequently a supervised neural

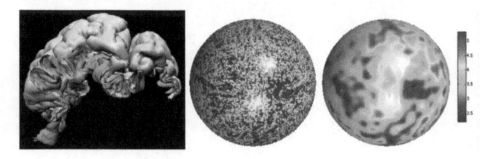

Fig. 2. Cortical thickness is computed as the distance between the outer (yellow) and the inner cortical (blue) surfaces. The cortical thickness is mapped onto a unit sphere and goes through heat kernel smoothing [3].

network classifier was used for tissue segmentation [21]. Brain substructures such as the brain stem were removed to make both the outer and the inner surfaces to be topologically equivalent to a sphere. A deformable surface algorithm [24] was used to obtain the inner cortical surface by deforming from a spherical mesh (Figure 2). Then the outer surface was obtained by deforming the inner surface. The deformation process establishes the structural correspondence between the two surfaces. The cortical thickness f is then defined as the distance between the corresponding vertices along the cortical mesh $\mathbb{M}$.

Since the deformable surface algorithm starts with a spherical mesh, there is no need to use other available surface flattening algorithms [5] [6] [16] [17] [35]

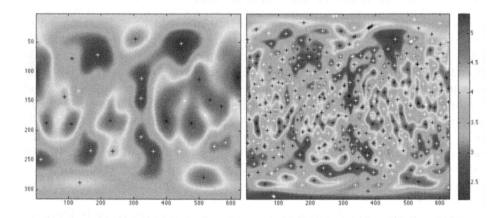

Fig. 3. The flat maps of cortical thickness at different smoothing scales. The maximums and minimums are denoted with black and white crosses respectively. The smoothing is done along the unit sphere and flattened using the angles θ (zenith angle) and φ (azimuth angle) associated with the 2-sphere. Smoother thickness produces less number of critical points and, in turn, less number of pairings.

for mapping thickness to the unit 2–sphere S^2. Let $\zeta : \mathbb{M} \to S^2$ be a sufficiently smooth surface flattening obtained from the deformable surface algorithm. Then the pullback $(\zeta^{-1})^*\widehat{\mu} = \widehat{\mu} \circ \zeta^{-1}$ projects the cortical thickness from the cortical surface $\mathbb{M}$ to the unit sphere. Figure 2 shows the pull back and the corresponding heat kernel smoothing on S^2. Note that in the process of flattening, the critical values do not change so the persistence diagram should be identical for $\widehat{\mu}$ and its pullback $(\zeta^{-1})^*\widehat{\mu}$. Therefore, we will construct the persistence diagram on the unit 2–sphere by projecting the cortical data to the sphere.

3 Kernel Smoothing

As described in Section 2.1, after the application of a deformable surface algorithm, our data is on the unit 2– sphere, S^2. So our measurement, $f : S^2 \to \mathbb{R}$ is given by the nonparametric regression formula (1), where μ is the unknown signal and ϵ is the noise. In this section, we estimate the persistent homology of the sublevel sets of $\widehat{\mu}$, an estimator of μ.

We begin by smoothing the data using the kernel,

$$K_{x_0}(x) = \max(1 - \kappa \arccos(x_0' x), 0),$$

where κ is given in [20] and $\arccos(x'y)$ gives the geodesic distance between x and y on the unit sphere. We smooth the data using the usual kernel function estimator

$$\widehat{\mu}(x) = \frac{\sum_i f(x_i) K_{x_i}(x)}{\sum_i K_{x_i}(x)}. \tag{2}$$

To implement this we need to choose the corresponding design points which we do in the following way. We start by choosing a triangulation, $\mathcal{T}$, of the sphere whose number of vertices satisfies the conditions in [1]. For our data, we start with an icosahedron and iteratively subdivide it three times, obtaining a triangulation with 1280 faces and 642 vertices.

For a sample of size n, define the estimator $\widehat{\mu}_n$ in the following way. For each vertex v in our triangulation, we define $\widehat{\mu}_n(v) = \widehat{\mu}(v)$ according to (2). For each face in our triangulation, we define $\widehat{\mu}_n$ on the face by affine interpolation from the values on the vertices. This construction is well defined on the edges, and defines a function on the sphere.

3.1 The Persistence Diagrams of $\widehat{\mu}_n$

It remains to calculate the persistence diagrams of the sublevel sets of $\widehat{\mu}_n$. We will see that because of the way $\widehat{\mu}_n$ is constructed, we can calculate its persistence diagrams using our triangulation, $\mathcal{T}$.

We filter $\mathcal{T}$ using $\widehat{\mu}_n$ as follows. Let $r_1 \leq r_2 \leq \ldots \leq r_m$ be the ordered list of values of $\widehat{\mu}_n$ on the vertices of the triangulation. For $1 \leq i \leq m$, let $\mathcal{T}_i$ be the subcomplex of $\mathcal{T}$ containing all vertices v with $\widehat{\mu}_n(v) \leq r_i$ and all edges whose

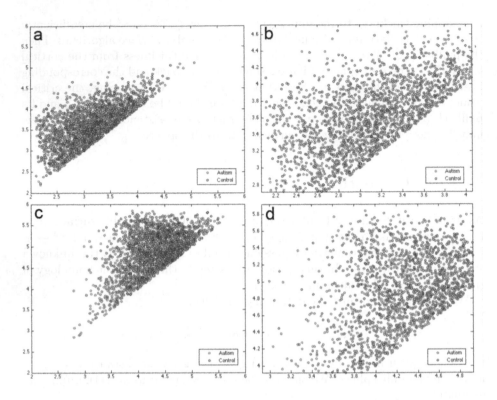

Fig. 4. The persistence diagrams for 11 control (blue) and 16 autistic (red) subjects in degree 0, (a) and (b), and degree 1, (c) and (d). One notices an additional layer of structure in the autistic group in both persistence diagrams. The figures clearly demonstrate the feasibility of using persistence diagrams for discriminating populations.

boundaries are in T_i and all faces whose boundaries are in T_i. We obtain the following filtration of T,

$$\phi = T_0 \subset T_1 \subset T_2 \subset \cdots \subset T_m = T.$$

The end result is that the topological properties of the sublevel sets of $\widehat{\mu}_n$ will equal the topological properties of the above filtration of T.

Using the software Plex, [10], we calculate the persistent homology, in degrees 0, 1 and 2 of the triangulation T filtered according to the estimator for each of the 27 subjects. Since the data is two–dimensional, we do not expect any interesting homology in higher degrees. In degree two, the persistent homology consists of a single persistence pair (a, ∞), where a is the maximum of $\widehat{\mu}_n$.

To compare the autistic subjects and control subjects, we take the union of the persistence diagrams of the subjects (Figure 4).

4   Statistical Properties of Persistence Diagram

In this section we will make more precise the definition of a persistence diagram [7] and present results that compare the topological parameters and their estimators [1] [2].

The persistent homology of the signal, μ, is encoded in its reduced persistence diagram, $\bar{D}(\mu)$, which is a multiset of points each corresponding to the persistence of one topological feature, as in the examples above. In order to define a metric for such diagrams, it is convenient to add the ordered pairs (a, a) for all $a \in \mathbb{R}$, each with infinite multiplicity. Call this multiset the *persistence diagram* of μ, denoted $D(\mu)$. We now give the precise definition.

Let k be a nonnegative integer. Given $\mu : S^2 \to \mathbb{R}$ and $a \leq b \in \mathbb{R}$ the inclusion of sublevel sets $i_a^b : S_{\mu \leq a}^2 \hookrightarrow S_{\mu \leq b}^2$ induces a map on homology

$$H_k(i_a^b) : H_k(S_{f \leq a}^2) \to H_k(S_{f \leq b}^2).$$

The image of $H_k(i_a^b)$ is the persistent homology group from a to b and $S_{f \leq c}^2 = \{f(x) \leq c\}$. Let β_a^b be its dimension. This counts the independent homology classes which are born by time a and die after time b.

Call a real number a a *homological critical value* of μ if for all sufficiently small $\varepsilon > 0$ the map $H_k(i_{a-\varepsilon}^{a+\varepsilon})$ is not an isomorphism. Call μ *tame* if it has finitely many homological critical values, and for each $a \in \mathbb{R}$, $H_k(S_{\mu \leq a}^2)$ is finite dimensional. In particular, any Morse function on a compact manifold is tame.

Assume that μ is tame. Choose ε smaller than the distance between any two homological critical values. For each pair of homological critical values $a < b$, we define their *multiplicity* μ_a^b which we interpret as the number of independent homology classes that are born at a and die at b. We count the homology classes born by time $a + \varepsilon$ that die after time $b - \varepsilon$. Among these subtract those born by $a - \varepsilon$ and subtract those that die after $b + \varepsilon$. This double counts those born by $a - \varepsilon$ that die after $b + \varepsilon$, so we add them back. That is,

$$\mu_a^b = \beta_{a+\varepsilon}^{b-\varepsilon} - \beta_{a-\varepsilon}^{b-\varepsilon} - \beta_{a+\varepsilon}^{b+\varepsilon} + \beta_{a-\varepsilon}^{b+\varepsilon}.$$

The *reduced persistence diagram* of μ, $\bar{D}(\mu)$, is the multiset of pairs (b, a) together with their multiplicities μ_a^b. We call this a diagram since it is convenient to plot these points on the plane. We will see that it is useful to add homology classes which are born and die at the same time. Let the *persistence diagram* of μ, $D(\mu)$, be given by the union of $\bar{D}(\mu)$ and $\{(a, a)\}_{a \in \mathbb{R}}$ where each (a, a) has infinite multiplicity.

A metric on the space of persistence diagrams is the bottleneck distance which bounds the Hausdorff distance [7]. It is given by

$$d_B(D(\mu), D(\nu)) = \inf_{\gamma} \sup_{p \in D(\mu)} \|p - \gamma(p)\|_{\infty}, \tag{3}$$

where the infimum is taken over all bijections $\gamma : D(\mu) \to D(\nu)$ and $\| \cdot \|_{\infty}$ is the sup-norm metric. In [7], the following result is proven:

$$d_B(D(\mu), D(\nu)) \leq \|\mu - \nu\|_{\infty} \tag{4}$$

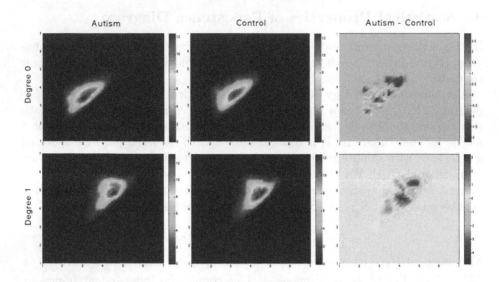

Fig. 5. The pairing concentration is computed by counting the number of pairings within a circle of fixed radius 0.2 at the point $x \in [1,7]^2$. The first (second) row is the mean concentration map for degree 0 (1) persistence. The first (second) column is the concentration map of autistic (control). The concentration difference (autism - control) is given in the last column which shows concentration difference between the groups.

where $\mu, \nu : \mathbb{M} \to \mathbb{R}$ are tame functions. As an immediate consequence of (4), we can apply it to the model (1). Let $\Lambda_t(\beta, L)$ denote the subset of tame functions in $\Lambda(\beta, L)$ the class of Hölder functions

$$\Lambda(\beta, L) = \{f : S^2 \to \mathbb{R} \mid |f(x) - f(z)| \leq L(\arccos(x'y))^\beta, x, z \in S^2\}, \quad (5)$$

where $0 < \beta \leq 1$ and $L > 0$.

If we assume $\mu \in \Lambda_t(\beta, L)$ for the model (1) ϵ is $N(0, \sigma^2)$, for the estimator $\widehat{\mu}_n$ with $0 < \beta \leq 1$ and $L > 0$,

$$\sup_{\mu \in \Lambda_t(\beta, L)} \mathbb{E} d_B \left(D(\hat{\mu}_n), D(\mu)\right) \leq L^{2/(2\beta+2)} \left(\frac{\sigma^2 \; (\beta+2)2^3}{\beta^2} \; \frac{\log n}{n}\right)^{\beta/(2\beta+2)} \quad (6)$$

as $n \to \infty$ [1], where expectation $\mathbb{E}$ is with respect to the model (1).

For typical brain images ($L = \beta = \sigma^2 = 1$) using (6), the order of accuracy per individual is $10^{-3/2}$. Consequently, Figure 4 is an accurate description of the population parameters.

5   Discussion

We have presented the concept of persistence diagrams and described the filtration based algorithm for constructing them. Since cortical thickness is highly noisy, kernel smoothing is applied to remove high frequency spatial noise before the filtration. At this point, it is unclear how one determines the possible statistical significance of persistent diagram difference. One may be tempted to use hypothesis-free classification frameworks for inference, however, Figure 4 shows that classification based on possibly discriminating spatial pattern is likely to be challenging. Note that the autistic scatter plots basically encompass the control scatter plots for the degree 0 and degree 1 persistence diagrams. Since there is considerable overlap, machine learning techniques would need to be adapted for this challenge. On the other hand, there seems to be spatial concentration difference in the pairings.

We have computed the pairing concentration by computing the number of parings within a circle of radius 0.2 at the point $x \in [1, 7]^2$. The average pairing concentration maps are shown in Figure 5, where we can see concentration difference for both the degree 0 and 1 persistence diagrams. The significance of the concentration map difference is determined using a permutation test. We first constructed the two sample t statistic map $T(p)$. The type-I error for correcting for multiple comparisons of a one-sided test is given by $\sup_{p \in [1,7]^2} T(p)$ [36]. The empirical distribution of $\sup_{p \in [1,7]^2} T(p)$ is then estimated from 5000 random permutations. For the degree-0 persistence, we obtain the maximum T-stat value of 3.51 corresponding to the corrected p-value of 0.078 at the position (2.3, 4.2). For the degree-1 persistence, the maximum T-stat value is 3.95 corresponding to the corrected p-value of 0.021 at the position (5.5, 5.8).

Our finding is consistent with previous neuroanatomical studies that show the abnormal neuroanatomical structures for autistic subjects [4]. Here we only presented a simple nonparametric approach for determining statistical significance based on the pairing concentration. Possibly a better statistical inference procedure is needed. It is hoped that this paper presents itself as a spring board for further investigation of persistence diagram based characterization of medical images. There are many methodological issues we have not discussed such as rigorous inferential procedures or the estimation of confidence regions around paired points possibly *via* the bootstrap. These are the next challenges in future works.

Acknowledgment

Authors wish to thank Vikas Singh of the University of Wisconsin-Madison for discussion on the persistence diagram. PK's research was supported in part by NSERC (Canada). Kim M. Dalton and Richard J. Davidson of the Waisman Laboratory for Brain Imaging and Behavior provided the MRI data used in the study.

References

1. Bubenik, P., Carlsson, G., Kim, P.T., Luo, Z.: Asymptotic minimax sup-norm risk on manifolds with application to topology (preprint, 2008)
2. Bubenik, P., Kim, P.T.: A statistical approach to persistent homology. Homology, Homotopy and Applications 9, 337–362 (2007)

3. Chung, M.K., Shen, L., Dalton, K.M., Evans, A.C., Davidson, R.J.: Weighted fourier representation and its application to quantifying the amount of gray matter. IEEE Transactions on Medical Imaging 26, 566–581 (2007)

4. Chung, M.K., Robbins, S., Davidson, R.J., Alexander, A.L., Dalton, K.M., Evans, A.C.: Cortical thickness analysis in autism with heat kernel smoothing. NeuroImage 25, 1256–1265 (2005)

5. Angenent, S., Hacker, S., Tannenbaum, A., Kikinis, R.: On the laplace-beltrami operator and brain surface flattening. IEEE Transactions on Medical Imaging 18, 700–711 (1999)

6. Brechbuhler, C., Gerig, G., Kubler, O.: Parametrization of closed surfaces for 3D shape description. Computer Vision and Image Understanding 61, 154–170 (1995)

7. Cohen-Steiner, D., Edelsbrunner, H., Harer, J.: Stability of persistence diagrams. Discrete and Computational Geometry 37 (2007)

8. Collins, D.L., Neelin, P., Peters, T.M., Evans, A.C.: Automatic 3d intersubject registration of MR volumetric data in standardized talairach space. J. Comput. Assisted Tomogr. 18, 192–205 (1994)

9. Ghrist, R., de Silva, V.: Homological sensor networks. Notic. Amer. Math. Soc. 54, 10–17 (2007)

10. de Silva, V., Perry, P.: Plex version 2.5 (2005), http://math.stanford.edu/comptop/programs/plex

11. Dequent, M.-L., Mileyko, Y., Edelsbrunner, H., Pourquie, O.: Assessing periodicity in gene expression as measured by microarray data (preprint, 2008)

12. Edelsbrunner, H., Harer, J.: Persistent homology - a survey. In: Twenty Years After, American Mathematical Society (2008) (in press)

13. Edelsbrunner, H., Letscher, D., Zomorodian, A.: Topological persistence and simplification. Discrete and Computational Geometry 28, 511–533 (2002)

14. Fischl, B., Dale, A.M.: Measuring the thickness of the human cerebral cortex from magnetic resonance images. PNAS 97, 11050–11055 (2000)

15. Friston, K.J.: A short history of statistical parametric mapping in functional neuroimaging. Technical Report Technical report, Wellcome Department of Imaging Neuroscience, ION, UCL., London, UK (2002)

16. Gu, X., Wang, Y.L., Chan, T.F., Thompson, T.M., Yau, S.T.: Genus zero surface conformal mapping and its application to brain surface mapping. IEEE Transactions on Medical Imaging 23, 1–10 (2004)

17. Hurdal, M.K., Stephenson, K.: Cortical cartography using the discrete conformal approach of circle packings. NeuroImage 23, S119–S128 (2004)

18. Joshi, S.C.: Large Deformation Diffeomorphisms and Gaussian Random Fields For Statistical Characterization of Brain Sub-manifolds. Ph.D. thesis. Washington University, St. Louis (1988)

19. Kiebel, S.J., Poline, J.-P., Friston, K.J., Holmes, A.P., Worsley, K.J.: Robust smoothness estimation in statistical parametric maps using standardized residuals from the general linear model. NeuroImage 10, 756–766 (1999)

20. Klemelä, J.: Asymptotic minimax risk for the white noise model on the sphere. Scand. J. Statist. 26, 465–473 (1999)

21. Kollakian, K.: Performance analysis of automatic techniques for tissue classification in magnetic resonance images of the human brain. Technical Report Master's thesis, Concordia University, Montreal, Quebec, Canada (1996)

22. Lerch, J.P., Evans, A.C.: Cortical thickness analysis examined through power analysis and a population simulation. NeuroImage 24, 163–173 (2005)

23. Luders, E., Narr, K.L., Thompson, P.M., Rex, D.E., Woods, R.P., Jancke, L., Toga, A.W., DeLuca, H.: Gender effects on cortical thickness and the influence of scaling. Human Brain Mapping 27, 314–324 (2006)
24. MacDonald, J.D., Kabani, N., Avis, D., Evans, A.C.: Automated 3-D extraction of inner and outer surfaces of cerebral cortex from MRI. NeuroImage 12, 340–356 (2000)
25. Miller, M.I., Banerjee, A., Christensen, G.E., Joshi, S.C., Khaneja, N., Grenander, U., Matejic, L.: Statistical methods in computational anatomy. Statistical Methods in Medical Research 6, 267–299 (1997)
26. Miller, M.I., Massie, A.B., Ratnanather, J.T., Botteron, K.N., Csernansky, J.G.: Bayesian construction of geometrically based cortical thickness metrics. NeuroImage 12, 676–687 (2000)
27. Milnor, J.: Morse Theory. Princeton University Press, Princeton (1973)
28. Morozov, D.: Homological Illusions of Persistence and Stability. Ph.D. thesis, Duke University (2008)
29. Naiman, D.Q.: Volumes for tubular neighborhoods of spherical polyhedra and statistical inference. Ann. Statist. 18, 685–716 (1990)
30. Nichols, T., Hayasaka, S.: Controlling the familywise error rate in functional neuroimaging: a comparative review. Stat. Methods Med. Res. 12, 419–446 (2003)
31. Ozturk, O., Ferhatosmanoglu, H., Sacan, A., Wang, Y.:
32. Siegmund, D.O., Worsley, K.J.: Testing for a signal with unknown location and scale in a stationary gaussian random field. Annals of Statistics 23, 608–639 (1996)
33. Sled, J.G., Zijdenbos, A.P., Evans, A.C.: A nonparametric method for automatic correction of intensity nonuniformity in MRI data. IEEE Transactions on Medical Imaging 17, 87–97 (1988)
34. Taylor, J.E., Worsley, K.J.: Random fields of multivariate test statistics, with applications to shape analysis. Annals of Statistics 36, 1–27 (2008)
35. Timsari, B., Leahy, R.: An optimization method for creating semi-isometric flat maps of the cerebral cortex. In: The Proceedings of SPIE, Medical Imaging (2000)
36. Worsley, K.J., Marrett, S., Neelin, P., Vandal, A.C., Friston, K.J., Evans, A.C.: A unified statistical approach for determining significant signals in images of cerebral activation. Human Brain Mapping 4, 58–73 (1996)
37. Yezzi, A., Prince, J.L.: An eulerian pde approach for computing tissue thickness. IEEE Transactions on Medical Imaging 22, 1332–1339 (2003)
38. Zomorodian, A.J.: Computing and Comprehending Topology: Persistence and Hierarchical Morse Complexes. Ph.D. Thesis, University of Illinois, Urbana-Champaign (2001)
39. Zomorodian, A.J., Carlsson, G.: Computing persistent homology. Discrete and Computational Geometry 33, 249–274 (2005)

Exploratory fMRI Analysis
without Spatial Normalization

Danial Lashkari and Polina Golland

Computer Science and Artificial Intelligence Laboratory, MIT, USA

Abstract. We present an exploratory method for simultaneous parcellation of multisubject fMRI data into functionally coherent areas. The method is based on a solely functional representation of the fMRI data and a hierarchical probabilistic model that accounts for both intersubject and intra-subject forms of variability in fMRI response. We employ a Variational Bayes approximation to fit the model to the data. The resulting algorithm finds a functional parcellation of the individual brains along with a set of population-level clusters, establishing correspondence between these two levels. The model eliminates the need for spatial normalization while still enabling us to fuse data from several subjects. We demonstrate the application of our method on a visual fMRI study.

1 Introduction

Analyzing data from multisubject neuroimaging studies is one of the challenging aspects of functional brain imaging. Presence of multiple sources of variability significantly complicates inference from the evidence provided by a group of individual fMRI scans [1]. First, the fMRI response in each subject varies from experiment to experiment giving rise to intra-subject variability. Moreover, two distinct sources contribute to inter-subject variability of fMRI signals. Since the brain structure is highly variable across subjects, establishing accurate correspondence among anatomical images of different subjects is intrinsically difficult. In addition to this anatomical variability, functional properties of the same anatomical structures are likely to vary somewhat across subjects.

The conventional localization approach to fMRI analysis constructs statistical parametric maps (SPM) [2] that indicate the significance of activation based on the hypotheses specified a priori. In order to perform group analysis, the method assumes all subjects are normalized into a common anatomical space where we can average the response across subjects. The performance of this approach is thus constrained by the limitations of spatial normalization techniques and the unknown relationship between function and anatomy. These issues are extensively discussed and studied in the literature, and different ways have been suggested to tackle them in the traditional localization framework [3,4,5,6].

The alternative approach employs unsupervised learning techniques to analyze fMRI data in an exploratory fashion. Most methods consider raw fMRI time courses and use clustering [7] or Independent Component Analysis (ICA)

J.L. Prince, D.L. Pham, and K.J. Myers (Eds.): IPMI 2009, LNCS 5636, pp. 398–410, 2009.

[8,9] to estimate a decomposition of the data into a set of distinct time courses and their corresponding spatial maps. Some variants use information from the experimental setup to define a measure of similarity between voxels, effectively projecting the original high-dimensional time courses to a low dimensional feature space, and then perform clustering in the new space [10,11]. Application of these exploratory methods to multisubject data has mainly relied on the same spatial mapping paradigm which requires spatial normalization [7]. More recently, a technique for exploratory group analysis was proposed that represents a voxel time course by a normalized profile of response to different experimental conditions [12]. The method clusters voxels from all the subjects together in the common functional space defined by these vectors. Although the results demonstrate the success of this approach in a multisubject experiment, such a model does not take any form of inter-subject variability into account.

Here, we present an exploratory method for simultaneous functional brain parcellation based on fMRI response in a cohort of subjects. The method also constructs cross-subject parcel correspondence through common functional labels. The parcellation procedure follows directly from a hierarchical probabilistic model that explicitly accounts for both intra-subject and inter-subject forms of variability in fMRI response. Similar to [12], our method takes advantage of a common functional space, rather than spatial normalization, to fuse data from different subjects. In effect, our results yield a parcel-level functional normalization of the data by associating groups of voxels from different subjects with the same population-level functional pattern.

Our method operates on vectors that represent the response of voxels to the experimental conditions. At the subject-level, we model the set of these response vectors as a mixture of several, distinct, functionally-defined parcels, each with a representative response vector. We assume that these subject-level representative vectors can be further clustered into a smaller set of population-level groups. The representative vector for each population level cluster defines a certain pattern of functionality. In the framework of hypothesis-based localization methods, a similar hierarchical structure is employed in random effects analysis (RFX) to model the two distinct types of variability [13]. In addition to offering the advantage of generating hypotheses from data, our method also eliminates the need for spatial normalization due to its fully functional representation of fMRI signals.

2   Method

We represent the group data by a set of response vectors $y_v^s \in I\!R^N$ where $s \in \{1, \cdots, S\}$ indexes the subject and $v \in \{1, \cdots, V\}$ denotes different voxels of the corresponding subject. These response vectors can be constructed from raw fMRI time courses based on the details of the experimental protocol [10]. In our work, we use the estimated GLM regression coefficients [2] for different experimental conditions as the vector components.

2.1   Model

Our hierarchical model is comprised of two clustering layers, each accounting for one type of variability in the data. We call the subject-level groupings of voxels in each subject *parcels* and refer to the population-level groupings of such parcels as *clusters*. In what follows, we use lower case Latin letters for random variables and Greek letters for distribution parameters. To facilitate notation, we sometimes define meta-variables composed of a group of vector variables, in which case we denote them with bold font.

Subject-Level Model. We assume that each response vector belongs to one of K parcels. We let the hidden variable $c_v^s = [c_{v,1}^s, \cdots, c_{v,K}^s]$ be a binary indicator vector such that $c_{v,k}^s = 1$ if y_v^s belongs to parcel k, and $c_{v,k}^s = 0$ otherwise. In our generative model, we assume a likelihood model for the response vectors

$$f(y; m, \lambda) = e^{-\lambda\, D(y,m) + Z(\lambda)} \tag{1}$$

parameterized by the mean parameter m and the variance-related parameter λ. Here, $D(\cdot, \cdot)$ defines a distance between y and m, and $Z(\cdot)$ is the log-partition function. For the subject s, we assume a common parameter λ^s for all parcels and allow K possible mean parameters $\boldsymbol{m} = [m_k^s]$ defining the functional centers (representative response vectors) of the parcels. Given parcel centers $\boldsymbol{m}$ and memberships $\boldsymbol{c} = [c_v^s]$, different response vectors are independent:

$$p_{\boldsymbol{y}|\boldsymbol{cm}}(\boldsymbol{y}|\boldsymbol{c}, \boldsymbol{m}; \lambda) = \prod_{s,v} \left[\prod_k \left(f(y_v^s; m_k^s, \lambda^s) \right)^{c_{v,k}^s} \right], \tag{2}$$

where $\boldsymbol{y} = [y_v^s]$ is the set of combined response vectors. We do not put any prior on the assignment variables $\boldsymbol{c}$, which is equivalent to assuming that all voxels within a subject are equally likely a priori to be from any parcel.

To eliminate irrelevant effects of the response magnitude and normalize response vectors across subjects, we scale the response vectors to have unit length, i.e., $\|y\| = \sqrt{\langle y, y \rangle} = 1$ where $\langle \cdot, \cdot \rangle$ is the inner product in $\mathbb{R}^N$. Since these normalized vectors lie on the unit hyper-sphere S^{N-1}, an appropriate likelihood model is the directional *von Mises-Fisher distribution* [14]

$$f_{\mathrm{V}}(y; m, \lambda) = \left(\tfrac{\lambda}{2\pi}\right)^{N/2} \frac{1}{\lambda\, I_{N/2-1}(\lambda)} e^{\lambda\langle y, m \rangle}, \tag{3}$$

where $I_\gamma(\cdot)$ is the γ-th order modified Bessel function of the first kind. The parameter λ controls the concentration of the distribution around the mean direction m in a way similar to the precision (reciprocal of variance) parameter of a Gaussian distribution. The model could be expressed based on (1) as:

$$D_{\mathrm{V}}(y, m) = 1 - \langle y, m \rangle, \qquad Z_{\mathrm{V}}(\lambda) = \tfrac{N}{2} \log \tfrac{\lambda}{2\pi} - \log \lambda - \lambda - \log I_{N/2-1}(\lambda). \tag{4}$$

In Appendix B, we provide another instantiation of our derivations for a Gaussian likelihood.

Population-Level Model. Conventional mixture-model approach to clustering fMRI data uses model (2), where m is a set of parameters estimated separately for different subjects. In our hierarchical model, we treat the parcel centers as random variables generated from a higher-level distribution that characterizes the functional patterns shared among all subjects. More specifically, we assume that the vectors m_k^s in each subject are generated from a mixture of L components. The mixture components are centered around representative vectors $\mu = [\mu_l]_{l=1}^L$ and have subject-specific mixture weights $w^s = [w_l^s]_{l=1}^L$. We let z_k^s be the L-dimensional binary vector that indicates the cluster membership of m_k^s (similar to c_v^s in the subject-level model). Weights w^s serve as the parameters of the multinomial distribution that generates cluster membership vectors z_k^s:

$$p_{z|w}(z|w) = \prod_{s,k}\left[\prod_l (w_l^s)^{z_{k,l}^s}\right]. \tag{5}$$

We can now form the likelihood model for the parcel centers

$$p_{m|z}(m|z;\mu,\sigma) = \prod_{s,k}\left[\prod_l \left(f(m_k^s;\mu_l,\sigma_l)\right)^{z_{k,l}^s}\right], \tag{6}$$

where f is consistent with the likelihood model for response vector y. Finally, we set the common prior over the set of weights w^s to be a Dirichlet distribution over an $(L-1)$-simplex of multinomial probability weights, parameterized by positive-valued vector $\alpha \in \mathbb{R}^L$:

$$p_w(w;\alpha) = \prod_s \mathrm{Dir}(w^s;\alpha) = \prod_s \left[\frac{\Gamma(\alpha_o)}{\prod_{l'=1}^L \Gamma(\alpha_{l'})}\prod_{l=1}^L (w_l^s)^{\alpha_l - 1}\right], \tag{7}$$

where $\alpha_o = \sum_{l'}\alpha_{l'}$ and $\Gamma(\cdot)$ is the Gamma function. Concentration of the distribution around the expected value $Ew_l^s = \frac{\alpha_l}{\alpha_o}$ is controlled by α_o.

Joint Model. Fig. 1(a) illustrates our model. We denote the set of all hidden variables by $h = \{c, m, z, w\}$ and the set of all model parameters by $\theta = \{\mu, \sigma, \alpha, \lambda\}$. We can now form the joint model:

$$\log p(y, h; \theta) = -\sum_{s,v,k} c_{v,k}^s \left[\lambda^s D(y_v^s, m_k^s) - Z(\lambda^s)\right] + \sum_{s,k,l} z_{k,l}^s \log w_l^s \tag{8}$$

$$-\sum_{s,k,l} z_{k,l}^s \left[\sigma_l D(m_k^s, \mu_l) - Z(\sigma_l)\right] + \sum_s \left[\sum_l \alpha_l \log w_l^s + B(\alpha)\right],$$

where $B(\alpha) = \log\Gamma(\alpha_o) - \sum_{l'}\log\Gamma(\alpha_{l'})$ and the constant prior over c is dropped.

Fitting this model to the data could be cast as the maximum likelihood (ML) parameter estimation for the observed data:

$$\theta^* = \underset{\theta}{\mathrm{argmax}}\ \log p_y(y;\theta) = \underset{\theta}{\mathrm{argmax}}\ \log \int_h p(y, h; \theta). \tag{9}$$

Solving this problem requires integrating the joint distribution over all possible states of the hidden variables h. Because of the first three terms in (8) that involve interaction between hidden variables, the integration in (9) is hard.

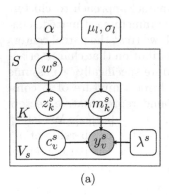
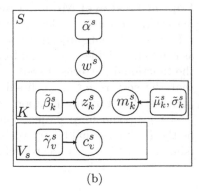

(a)   (b)

Fig. 1. Graphical model showing the structure of (a) the model $p(\boldsymbol{y}, \boldsymbol{h}; \boldsymbol{\theta})$, and (b) distribution $q(\boldsymbol{h}; \tilde{\boldsymbol{\theta}})$ that approximates the posterior $p(\boldsymbol{h}|\boldsymbol{y}; \boldsymbol{\theta})$ over the hidden variables. Parameters and random variables are illustrated by squares and circles, respectively.

Variational Bayes. We employ a Variational Bayes approach to solve the problem [15]. Accordingly, we define a parameterized distribution $q(\boldsymbol{h}; \tilde{\boldsymbol{\theta}})$ on the hidden variables to approximate the posterior $p(\boldsymbol{h}|\boldsymbol{y}; \boldsymbol{\theta})$. As illustrated in Fig. 1(b), we assume a fully factorable model q whose components are compatible with the original model, that is, multinomial for parcel/cluster memberships $\boldsymbol{c}$ and $\boldsymbol{z}$, f for parcel centers $\boldsymbol{m}$, and Dirichlet for the weights $\boldsymbol{w}$:

$$q(\boldsymbol{h}; \tilde{\boldsymbol{\theta}}) = q_c(\boldsymbol{c}; \tilde{\gamma}) \, q_m(\boldsymbol{m}; \tilde{\boldsymbol{\mu}}, \tilde{\boldsymbol{\sigma}}) \, q_z(\boldsymbol{z}; \tilde{\boldsymbol{\beta}}) \, q_w(\boldsymbol{w}; \tilde{\boldsymbol{\alpha}})$$
$$= \prod_{s,v} \left(\prod_k (\tilde{\gamma}_{v,k}^s)^{c_{v,k}^s} \right) \cdot \prod_{s,k} f(m_k^s; \tilde{\mu}_k^s, \tilde{\sigma}_k^s) \cdot \prod_{s,k} \left(\prod_l (\tilde{\beta}_{k,l}^s)^{z_{k,l}^s} \right) \cdot \prod_s \mathrm{Dir}(w^s; \tilde{\alpha}^s), \tag{10}$$

where $\tilde{\boldsymbol{\theta}} = \{\tilde{\gamma}, \tilde{\boldsymbol{\mu}}, \tilde{\boldsymbol{\sigma}}, \tilde{\boldsymbol{\beta}}, \tilde{\boldsymbol{\alpha}}\}$ is the combined set of parameters. With our choice of von Mises model f_{v}, we find the expression for the Variational Bayes cost function, also called the free energy:

$$\mathcal{F}(\tilde{\boldsymbol{\theta}}; \boldsymbol{\theta}) \triangleq E_q \log q(\boldsymbol{h}) - E_q \log p(\boldsymbol{y}, \boldsymbol{h}; \boldsymbol{\theta})$$
$$= \sum_{s,k} Z(\tilde{\sigma}_k^s) + \sum_{s,v,k} \tilde{\gamma}_{v,k}^s \left[\log \tilde{\gamma}_{v,k}^s + \lambda^s D_{\mathrm{v}}(y_v^s, \tilde{\mu}_k^s) - Z(\lambda^s) \right]$$
$$+ \sum_{s,k,l} \tilde{\beta}_{k,l}^s \left[\log \tilde{\beta}_{k,l}^s - (\Psi(\tilde{\alpha}_l^s) - \Psi(\tilde{\alpha}_o^s)) + \sigma_l D_{\mathrm{v}}(\tilde{\mu}_k^s, \mu_l) - Z(\sigma_l) \right]$$
$$+ \sum_s \left[\sum_l (\tilde{\alpha}_l^s - 1)(\Psi(\tilde{\alpha}_l^s) - \Psi(\tilde{\alpha}_o^s)) + B(\tilde{\alpha}^s) \right]$$
$$- S \left[\sum_l (\alpha_l - 1)\left(\frac{1}{S} \sum_s (\Psi(\tilde{\alpha}_l^s) - \Psi(\tilde{\alpha}_o^s)) \right) + B(\alpha) \right], \tag{11}$$

where $\Psi(x) = \frac{d}{dx} \log \Gamma(x)$ and $\tilde{\alpha}_o^s = \sum_l \tilde{\alpha}_l^s$. Appendix A provides the details of the derivation.

2.2   Algorithm

We alternate between minimizing the free energy over posterior and model parameters $\tilde{\theta}$ and θ similar to the basic Expectation-Maximization algorithm. For a fixed θ, minimizing $\mathcal{F}$ over $\tilde{\theta}$ corresponds to finding the approximate posterior distribution, i.e., making *inference* using the given set of model parameters. Minimization of the free energy with respect to θ corresponds to *learning* the model parameters for a particular posterior distribution.

Inference. We can split the posterior parameters in (11) into two sets of non-interacting parameters, $(\tilde{\gamma}, \tilde{\beta})$ and $(\tilde{\mu}, \tilde{\sigma}, \tilde{\alpha})$. Fixing the values of either set, the optimization problem leads to a closed form solution for the parameters in the other set. Hence, we choose to use a coordinate descent approach which simplifies the update rules and significantly improves the overall speed of the algorithm. The efficiency of this approximation allows us to repeat the algorithm with numerous different initializations to better search the space of solutions.

For fixed $(\tilde{\mu}, \tilde{\sigma}, \tilde{\alpha})$, the cost function for $\tilde{\gamma}$ involves only the second term of (11); the third term is only relevant for $\tilde{\beta}$. We find

$$\tilde{\gamma}^s_{v,k} \propto e^{-\lambda^s D_V(y^s_v, \tilde{\mu}^s_k)} , \qquad \tilde{\beta}^s_{k,l} \propto e^{\Psi(\tilde{\alpha}^s_l)} \, e^{-\sigma_l D_V(\tilde{\mu}^s_k, \mu_l) + Z_V(\sigma_l)} . \tag{12}$$

The update rules for the parcel/cluster assignments are quite similar to the standard cluster assignment update rules. The term $e^{\Psi(\tilde{\alpha}^s_l)}$ acts as a prior weight for cluster l in subject s.

For fixed parameters $(\tilde{\gamma}, \tilde{\beta})$, the parameter $\tilde{\alpha}$ becomes fully decoupled from $(\tilde{\mu}, \tilde{\sigma})$. The solution takes the form:

$$\tilde{\alpha}^s_l = \alpha_l + \sum_k \tilde{\beta}^s_{k,l} , \qquad \tilde{\mu}^s_k \propto \sum_l \tilde{\beta}^s_{k,l} \sigma_l \mu_l + \lambda^s \sum_v \tilde{\gamma}^s_{v,k} y^s_v . \tag{13}$$

The update for $\tilde{\alpha}^s_l$ combines current values of cluster weight α_l with the sum of multinomial weights $\tilde{\beta}$ assigned to cluster l. The update for $\tilde{\mu}^s_k$, which is further normalized to unit length, linearly combines the cluster centers and the response vectors, each with corresponding weights $\tilde{\beta}^s_{k,l}$ and $\tilde{\gamma}^s_{v,k}$. We note that $\tilde{\sigma}$ only appears in the first term of (11); the minimum is achieved when $\tilde{\sigma}^s_k \to \infty$. However, since $\tilde{\sigma}$ does not appear in the learning stage, this does not affect the rest of the derivations.

Learning. The von Mises parameters are found as

$$\mu_l \propto \sum_{s,k} \tilde{\beta}^s_{k,l} \tilde{\mu}^s_k , \qquad \sigma_l = A_N^{-1} \left(\frac{\| \sum_{s,k} \tilde{\beta}^s_{k,l} \tilde{\mu}^s_k \|}{\sum_{s,k} \tilde{\beta}^s_{k,l}} \right),$$

$$\lambda^s = A_N^{-1} \left(\frac{1}{V_s} \sum_{v,k} \tilde{\gamma}^s_{v,k} \langle \tilde{\mu}^s_k, y^s_v \rangle \right), \tag{14}$$

where $A_N(\lambda) = I_{N/2}(\lambda) / I_{N/2-1}(\lambda)$, and μ_l vectors are normalized to unit length. The update rules are similar to the parameter estimation steps of the ordinary single level clustering models. The last term of (11) is simply the Dirichlet log-likelihood function with the observed statistics $\frac{1}{S}\sum_s(\Psi(\tilde{\alpha}_l^s) - \Psi(\tilde{\alpha}_o^s))$. Estimation of the Dirichlet parameters α and computing the inverse of $A_N(\cdot)$ involve solving nonlinear equations. We employ standard zero-finding algorithms to solve both problems [16,17].

Implementation. It is not hard to show that our algorithm always converges to a local minimum of the free energy function. This implies that, similar to most clustering algorithms, the solution depends on the initialization and selecting reasonable initializations can substantially improve the results. To initialize the values of parameters $(\tilde{\theta}, \theta)$, we first run a simple mixture model clustering into L components on a group data pooled from all subjects. We use the resulting cluster centers and weights as initial values for cluster centers μ and weights α. Then we cluster individual data sets separately to find K clusters for each subject. We use the corresponding centers and assignment probabilities as the initialization of posterior parcel center and weight parameters $\tilde{\mu}$ and $\tilde{\gamma}$. The rest of the parameters are initialized to one or appropriate random numbers. For the results presented in the next section, we used between 40 to 70 initializations depending on the number of cluster/parcels.

We empirically observed that the following order of update rules, in each iteration, yields better results: $(\tilde{\gamma}, \tilde{\beta})$, (μ, σ), $(\tilde{\mu}, \tilde{\alpha})$, and $(\mu, \sigma, \lambda, \alpha)$, respectively. We terminate the algorithm for each initialization when the relative change in the free energy between successive iterations falls bellow 10^{-9}.

Similar to all other exploratory methods, we face the challenge of determining the right number of components. In our method, the question becomes more important due to the hierarchical structure of the model where we need to determine both L and K. We use a heuristic method to select these numbers but, as we will see, the results show robustness to changing cluster and parcel numbers. When we incrementally increase the number of clusters L, the value of the cost function monotonically decreases. If we interpret the value of the drop $\Delta\mathcal{F} = \mathcal{F}_{L-1} - \mathcal{F}_L$ in the free energy as the gain achieved by reaching L from $L-1$, a *good* number of clusters is the one for which this gain is locally optimal. We use the same heuristic in selecting the parcel number K as well.

3   Experimental Results

We demonstrate application of our method in an fMRI study of category selectivity in the visual cortex. Prior hypothesis-based studies have localized selective regions in the ventral visual pathway for a few categories of visual stimuli such as bodies, faces, and places [18]. Here, we aim to employ our method to *discover* modules shared across all subjects that show distinct profiles of response to the variety of images presented during an fMRI experiment [12]. In our analysis, a cluster center μ_l represents the selectivity profile of a shared module and the corresponding cluster assignments $\tilde{\beta}_{k,l}^s$ establish functional correspondence among the parcels $\tilde{\mu}_k^s$ found with a similar type of selectivity in different subjects. Agreement of the discovered selectivity profiles with the prior results in the

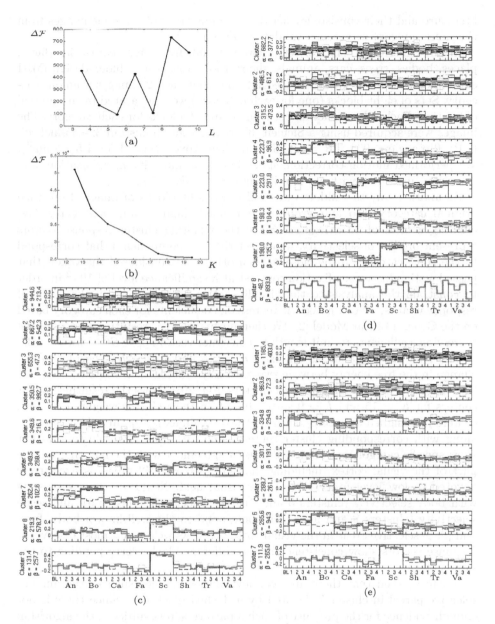

Fig. 2. Improvement in the final value of free energy achieved by incrementally increasing (a) L for $K = 15$, and (b) K for $L = 8$. Each data point in these plots shows the change in $\mathcal{F}$ between the two neighboring numbers of clusters or parcels. (c)-(e) Components of the individual and population-level cluster centers for $(K, L) = (9, 15), (8, 16)$, and $(7, 15)$, respectively. For each cluster center μ_l (thick red line), the parcel centers $\tilde{\mu}_k^s$ assigned to this cluster based on weights $\tilde{\beta}_{k,l}^s$ are shown for all the 6 subjects (thin lines). The labels denote the baseline (BL) and the four coefficients for each category of images: Animals, Bodies, Cars, Faces, Scenes, Shoes, Trees, Vases.

literature and their consistency across representations of different images from the same category serves as a validations of our method.

In our experiment, six subjects viewed stimuli from eight categories (faces, places, bodies, trees, cars, animals, shoes, tools, vases) in a block-design fMRI experiment. Each block lasted 16 seconds and contained 20 images from one category. Sets of eight blocks (one for each category) were separated by an interval of fixation. Each subject viewed between 16 and 29 blocks for each category. The images were acquired using a Siemens 3T scanner and a custom 32-channel coil (EPI, flip angle $= 90^o$, TR $= 2$s, 28 axial slices, voxel size $= 1.5 \times 1.5 \times 2$mm^3). We performed motion correction, spike detection, intensity normalization, and Gaussian smoothing with a 3 mm kernel using FsFast [19].

As another way to validate our results, we split blocks of images from each original category into four groups and labeled them as four *new* categories, creating a total of 32 categories. Since the resulting cluster response vectors represent profiles of selectivity, we expect the four components that correspond to the same category to be close to each other. We considered the voxels that passed a stimulus-versus-fixation contrast at a significance level of 10^{-2} in order to constrain the analysis to the visually active cortex. To form the space of response vectors, we estimated the regression coefficients for each category based on the General Linear Model [2]. We then normalized the resulting vectors of the regression coefficients to unit length to construct vectors $y_v^s \in S^{N-1}$ for $N = 32$.

First, we ran the analysis for fixed $K = 15$ and varied L. The plot of the change in the free energy between two successive values of L, Fig 2(a), suggests the choice of 7 or 9 population-level clusters. Fig. 2(c) shows the resulting cluster centers for $K = 15$ and $L = 9$ sorted based on their cluster weights α. Parcel centers $\tilde{\mu}_k^s$ assigned to each μ_l, such that $l = \text{argmax}_{l'} \tilde{\beta}_{k,l'}^s$, are also presented along with corresponding cluster centers. The first four large clusters do not show specific category selectivity. This is in agreement with the fact that a large part of the visual cortex, including the early V1 and V2 areas, is exclusively devoted to low level processing of the visual field. Next, we observe clusters with body selectivity (clusters 5 and 7), face selectivity (cluster 6), and scene selectivity (clusters 8 and 9), which correspond to the well-known body, face, and place selective areas in the visual cortex [18]. As we expect, most discovered response vectors show consistency across different blocks corresponding to the same category.

It can be seen that there are very few outlier parcels, such as the animal-selective parcel in cluster 7 denoted by a dashed black line. Since there is not enough evidence for the presence of such a pattern across subjects, the algorithm assigns the parcel to the closest cluster. All other subject parcels closely follow the selectivity profile of their population clusters. We can interpret the deviations of parcel centers $\tilde{\mu}_k^s$ around each cluster center μ_l as the inter-subject variability. For instance, as we expect, parcels assigned to the non-selective clusters show highly variable patterns while the variability is lower for the highly selective clusters. Fig. 2(e) shows the estimated clusters for $K = 15$ and $L = 7$. These

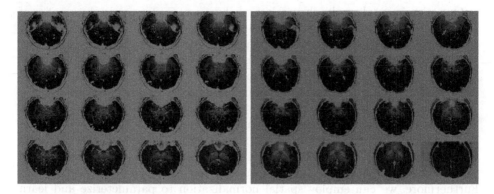

Fig. 3. Spatial maps of the parcels assigned to the scene selective cluster 7 in Fig. 2(d) in two different subjects

results are similar and confirm our observations above. We conclude that the algorithm successfully matched functionally similar parcels across subjects.

To investigate the effect of changing the number of subject parcels, we let $L = 8$ and change K. Fig 2(b) shows the incremental difference $\Delta\mathcal{F}$ for K which behaves much more smoothly compared to the one of L. Selecting $K = 16$, a value which is slightly higher than its local trend, the results are shown in Fig. 2(d). Most clusters are almost the same as those of $L = 7$ and $K = 15$, except cluster 8 that is comprised solely of parcels from a single subject and does not represent a trend shared across all subjects. This explains why the improvement achieved by changing the number of clusters from 7 to 8 is much smaller than that of 6 to 7, or 8 to 9 in Fig. 2(a). Overall, these results demonstrate a relative robustness in the estimation of cluster centers to changes in the number of population and subject-level clusters and parcels.

We also examine the spatial maps of voxels assigned to the identified parcels. Based on our model, the posterior probability that voxel v in subject s belongs to cluster l equals $\sum_k \tilde{\gamma}^s_{v,k} \tilde{\beta}^s_{k,l}$. In our results, most of these probabilities are very close to 0 or 1 yielding almost binary spatial maps for the clusters. Fig. 3 shows the spatial map for the scene-selective cluster 7 in Fig. 2(d) in two different subjects. The maps clearly exhibit similarities in several regions in spite of their sparsity. We emphasize that the algorithm uses no spatial information other than the Gaussian smoothing performed in the pre-processing stage.

4   Discussion and Conclusions

In this paper, we presented a probabilistic model for unsupervised parcellation of the brain based on multisubject fMRI data. Applying this method to data from a vision experiment on a cohort of 6 subjects, we were able to discover several types of category selectivity in the visual cortex that have been previously reported using hypothesis-driven methods. The discovered profiles show consistency across different image representations from the same category.

Our experimental results show relative robustness to changes in the number of parcels and clusters. However, it is hard to analyze all possible settings in order to find the best combination of component numbers. It is therefore interesting to set for discovery of the natural number of parcels as suggested by the data. We plan to study possible generalizations of the current model to include the number of components as an unknown using nonparametric approaches.

Another direction for extending the current model is the choice of a prior for parcel memberships c. The current model assumes uniform prior on the assignment variables. Since we expect the subject-level parcels to be also spatially clustered, we can assume a prior for c with spatial smoothness properties as a rigorous modeling replacement for the Gaussian smoothing in the pre-processing. Furthermore, we can employ spatial normalization to parameterize and learn a specific inter-subject spatial prior for c, merging our method with the conventional approach to the population analysis. We aim to investigate ways for designing such models.

Acknowledgements. We thank Ed Vul and Nancy Kanwisher for providing us with the fMRI data. This research was supported in part by the MIT McGovern Institute Neurotechnology Program, the NSF CAREER grant 0642971, and the NIH grants NIBIB NAMIC U54-EB005149, and NCRR NAC P41-RR13218.

References

1. Brett, M., et al.: The problem of functional localization in the human brain. Nat. Rev. Neurosci. 3, 243–249 (2002)
2. Friston, K.J., et al. (eds.): Statistical Parametric Mapping. Academic Press, London (2007)
3. Gee, J.C., et al.: Effect of spatial normalization on analysis of functional data. In: Proc. SPIE Med. Imaging, vol. 3034, pp. 550–560 (1997)
4. Thirion, B., et al.: Dealing with the shortcomings of spatial normalization: multi-subject parcellation of fMRI datasets. Hum. Brain Mapp. 27, 678–693 (2006)
5. Thirion, B., et al.: Analysis of a large fMRI cohort: statistical and methodological issues for group analyses. NeuroImage 35, 105–120 (2007)
6. Thirion, B., et al.: Structural analysis of fMRI data revisited: improving the sensitivity and reliability of fMRI group studies. TMI 26, 1256–1269 (2007)
7. Golland, P., et al.: Detection of spatial activation patterns as unsupervised segmentation of fMRI data. In: Ayache, N., Ourselin, S., Maeder, A. (eds.) MICCAI 2007, Part I. LNCS, vol. 4791, pp. 110–118. Springer, Heidelberg (2007)
8. McKeown, J.M., et al.: Analysis of fMRI data by blind separation into independent spatial components. Hum. Brain Mapp. 10, 160–178 (1998)
9. Beckmann, C.F., Smith, S.M.: Tensorial extensions of independent component analysis for group fMRI data analysis. NeuroImage 25(1), 294–311 (2005)
10. Goutte, C., et al.: On clustering fMRI time series. NeuroImage 9, 298–310 (1999)
11. Thirion, B., Faugeras, O.: Feature detection in fMRI data: the information bottleneck approach. In: Ellis, R.E., Peters, T.M. (eds.) MICCAI 2003. LNCS, vol. 2879, pp. 83–91. Springer, Heidelberg (2003)

12. Lashkari, D., et al.: Discovering structure in the space of activation profiles in fMRI. In: Metaxas, D., Axel, L., Fichtinger, G., Székely, G. (eds.) MICCAI 2008, Part I. LNCS, vol. 5241, pp. 1015–1024. Springer, Heidelberg (2008)
13. Penny, W.D., Holmes, A.: Random effects analysis. In: Frackowiak, R.S.J., Friston, K.J., Frith, C.D. (eds.) Human brain function II. Elsevier, Oxford (2003)
14. Mardia, K.V.: Statistics of directional data. J. R. Statist. Soc. Series B 37, 349–393 (1975)
15. Jordan, M.I., et al.: An introduction to variational methods for graphical models. Mach. Learn. 37, 183–233 (1999)
16. Blei, D.M., et al.: Latent Dirichlet allocation. J. Mach. Learn. Res. 3, 993–1022 (2003)
17. Banerjee, A., et al.: Clustering on the unit hypersphere using von Mises-Fisher distribution. J. Mach. Learn. Res. 6, 1345–1382 (2005)
18. Kanwisher, N.G.: The ventral visual object pathway in humans: evidence from fMRI. In: Chalupa, L., Werner, J. (eds.) The Visual Neurosciences. MIT Press, Cambridge (2003)
19. http://surfer.nmr.mgh.harvard.edu/fswiki/FsFast

A   Variational Inference

For a distribution q on the hidden variables h, the free energy functional

$$\mathcal{F}[q, p(\theta)] \triangleq E_q \log q(h) - E_q \log p(y, h; \theta) = E_q \log \frac{q(h)}{p(h|y; \theta)} - \log p(y; \theta)$$

serves as a lower bound for $-\log p(y; \theta)$ since the first term is $\mathcal{D}_{KL}(q\|p_{h|y}) \geq 0$.

With the distribution $q(h; \tilde{\theta})$ defined in (10), the free energy $\mathcal{F}(\tilde{\theta}; \theta)$ is now a function of both sets of posterior and model parameters. Using the expansion of $\log p(y, h; \theta)$ in (8), we obtain

$$\begin{aligned}
\mathcal{F} = {} & \sum_{s,v,k} E_q[c_{v,k}^s] \log \tilde{\gamma}_{v,k}^s - \sum_{s,k}\left[\tilde{\sigma}_k^s E_q\left[D(m_k^s, \tilde{\mu}_k^s)\right] - Z(\tilde{\sigma}_k^s)\right] \\
& + \sum_{s,k,l} E_q[z_{k,l}^s] \log \tilde{\beta}_{k,l}^s + \sum_s\left[\sum_l(\tilde{\alpha}_l^s - 1)E_q[\log w_l^s] + B(\tilde{\alpha}^s)\right] \quad (15)\\
& + \sum_{s,v,k} E_q[c_{v,k}^s]\left[\lambda^s E_q[D(y_v^s, m_k^s)] - Z(\lambda^s)\right] - \sum_{s,k,l} E_q[z_{k,l}^s]\, E_q[\log w_l^s] \\
& + \sum_{s,k,l} E_q[z_{k,l}^s]\left[\sigma_l E_q[D(m_k^s, \mu_l)] - Z(\sigma_l)\right] - \sum_{s,l}(\alpha_l - 1)E_q[\log w_l^s] - S\,B(\alpha).
\end{aligned}$$

The factored structure of q and properties of the Dirichlet distribution imply

$$E_q[c_{v,k}^s] = \tilde{\gamma}_{v,k}^s\,, \qquad E_q[z_{k,l}^s] = \tilde{\beta}_{k,l}^s\,, \qquad E_{q_w}[\log w_l^s] = \Psi(\tilde{\alpha}_l^s) - \Psi(\tilde{\alpha}_o^s), \quad (16)$$

where $\Psi(x) = \frac{d}{dx}\log \Gamma(x)$ and $\tilde{\alpha}_o^s = \sum_l \tilde{\alpha}_l^s$. From (4), the distance D_V is linear in the case of von Mises distribution. Thus, the value of a term $E_q[D_V(m, \eta)]$ under the distribution $q(m) = f_V(m; \tilde{\mu}_k^s, \tilde{\sigma}_k^s)$ is simply equal to $D_V(\eta, \tilde{\mu}_V^s)$. Substituting these expressions in (15) completes the computation of the free energy cost function in (11).

B Gaussian Model

We show the derivation for the case when the likelihood model f is the commonly used Gaussian distribution. Based on the general expression (1), $f_G(y; m, \lambda)$ is defined by $D_G(y, m) = \frac{1}{2}\|y - m\|^2$ and $Z_G(\lambda) = \frac{N}{2}\log\frac{\lambda}{2\pi}$. The interesting technical distinction between Gaussian and von Mises distributions appears in the computation of the free energy (15). The quadratic expression $E_q[D_G(m, \eta)]$ under the distribution $q(m) = f_G(m; \tilde{\mu}_k^s, \tilde{\sigma}_k^s)$ is equal to $D_G(\eta, \tilde{\mu}_k^s) + \frac{N}{2\tilde{\sigma}_k^s}$.

In the inference stage, we find the cluster and parcel assignment update rules:

$$\tilde{\gamma}_{v,k}^s \propto e^{-\lambda^s D_G(y_v^s, \tilde{\mu}_k^s) - \frac{N\lambda^s}{2\tilde{\sigma}_k^s}} \ , \quad \tilde{\beta}_{k,l}^s \propto e^{\Psi(\tilde{\alpha}_l^s)} \ e^{-\sigma_l D_G(\tilde{\mu}_k^s, \mu_l) + Z_G(\sigma_l) - \frac{N\sigma_l}{2\tilde{\sigma}_k^s}}. \quad (17)$$

Comparing these rules with (12), we interpret the last terms in the exponents of (17) as a correction that accounts for the uncertainty in cluster center estimates $\tilde{\mu}$, reflected by the values of $\tilde{\sigma}$. While the update for $\tilde{\alpha}$ remains the same, the mean and precision of parcel centers are updated as

$$\tilde{\mu}_k^s = \frac{\sum_l \tilde{\beta}_{k,l}^s \sigma_l \mu_l + \lambda^s \sum_v \tilde{\gamma}_{v,k}^s y_v^s}{\sum_l \tilde{\beta}_{k,l}^s \sigma_l + \lambda^s \sum_v \tilde{\gamma}_{v,k}^s} \ , \quad \tilde{\sigma}_k^s = V_s \lambda^s + \sum_l \tilde{\beta}_{k,l}^s \sigma_l. \quad (18)$$

Here, in contrast to the von Mises case, the finite values of $\tilde{\sigma}_k^s$ propagate the effects of our posterior uncertainty about m to the estimates of the other variables. In the learning stage, the Gaussian parameters are computed according to the update rules

$$\mu_l = \frac{1}{\sum_{s,k} \tilde{\beta}_{k,l}^s} \sum_{s,k} \tilde{\beta}_{k,l}^s \tilde{\mu}_k^s \ , \quad (\sigma_l)^{-1} = \frac{1}{\sum_{s,k} \tilde{\beta}_{k,l}^s} \sum_{s,k} \tilde{\beta}_{k,l}^s \left[(\tilde{\sigma}_k^s)^{-1} + \frac{1}{N}\|\tilde{\mu}_k^s - \mu_l\|^2 \right],$$

$$(\lambda^s)^{-1} = \frac{1}{V_s} \sum_{v,k} \tilde{\gamma}_{v,k}^s \left[(\tilde{\sigma}_k^s)^{-1} + \frac{1}{N}\|y_v^s - \tilde{\mu}_k^s\|^2 \right], \quad (19)$$

that again look quite similar to the conventional clustering update rules accompanied with the correction terms involving $\tilde{\sigma}$.

Marginal Space Learning for Efficient Detection of 2D/3D Anatomical Structures in Medical Images

Yefeng Zheng, Bogdan Georgescu, and Dorin Comaniciu

Integrated Data Systems Department, Siemens Corporate Research, USA
{yefeng.zheng, bogdan.georgescu, dorin.comaniciu}@siemens.com

Abstract. Recently, marginal space learning (MSL) was proposed as a generic approach for automatic detection of 3D anatomical structures in many medical imaging modalities [1]. To accurately localize a 3D object, we need to estimate nine pose parameters (three for position, three for orientation, and three for anisotropic scaling). Instead of exhaustively searching the original nine-dimensional pose parameter space, only low-dimensional marginal spaces are searched in MSL to improve the detection speed. In this paper, we apply MSL to 2D object detection and perform a thorough comparison between MSL and the alternative full space learning (FSL) approach. Experiments on left ventricle detection in 2D MRI images show MSL outperforms FSL in both speed and accuracy. In addition, we propose two novel techniques, constrained MSL and nonrigid MSL, to further improve the efficiency and accuracy. In many real applications, a strong correlation may exist among pose parameters in the same marginal spaces. For example, a large object may have large scaling values along all directions. Constrained MSL exploits this correlation for further speed-up. The original MSL only estimates the rigid transformation of an object in the image, therefore cannot accurately localize a nonrigid object under a large deformation. The proposed nonrigid MSL directly estimates the nonrigid deformation parameters to improve the localization accuracy. The comparison experiments on liver detection in 226 abdominal CT volumes demonstrate the effectiveness of the proposed methods. Our system takes less than a second to accurately detect the liver in a volume.

1 Introduction

Efficiently detecting an anatomical structure (e.g., heart, liver, and kidney) in medical images is often a prerequisite for the subsequent procedures, e.g., segmentation, measuring, and classification. Albeit important, automatic object detection is largely ignored in previous work. Most existing 3D segmentation methods focus on boundary delineation using active shape models (ASM) [2], active appearance models (AAM) [3], and deformable models [4] by assuming that a rough pose estimate of the object is available. Sometimes, heuristic methods may be used for automatic object localization by exploiting the domain specific knowledge [5]. As a more generic approach, the discriminative learning based method has been proved to be efficient and robust for many 2D object detection problems [6]. In this method, object detection is formulated as a classification problem: whether an image block contains the target object or not. To build a robust system, a classifier only tolerates limited variation in object pose. The object

J.L. Prince, D.L. Pham, and K.J. Myers (Eds.): IPMI 2009, LNCS 5636, pp. 411–422, 2009.
© Springer-Verlag Berlin Heidelberg 2009

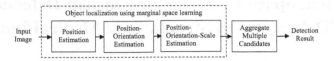

Fig. 1. Object localization using marginal space learning [1]

is found by scanning the classifier exhaustively over all possible combinations of position, orientation, and scale. Since both learning and searching are performed in the full pose parameter space, we call this method full space learning (FSL). This search strategy is different from other parameter estimation approaches, such as deformable models [4], where an initial estimate is adjusted (e.g., using the gradient descent technique) to optimize a predefined objective function. Exhaustive search makes the learning based system [6] robust under local minima. However, the number of testing hypotheses increases exponentially with respect to the dimension of the parameter space. We cannot directly apply FSL to 3D object detection since the pose parameter space for a 3D object has nine dimensions: three for position, three for orientation, and three for anisotropic scaling. Recently, we proposed an efficient learning-based technique, marginal space learning (MSL), for 3D object detection [1]. MSL performs parameter estimation in a series of marginal spaces with increasing dimensionality. To be specific, the task is split into three steps: object position estimation, position-orientation estimation, and position-orientation-scale estimation (as shown in Fig. 1). Instead of exhaustively searching the original nine-dimensional parameter space, only low-dimensional marginal spaces are searched in MSL. Mathematical analysis shows that MSL can reduce the number of testing hypotheses by about six orders of magnitude [1], compared to a naive implementation of FSL.

MSL was originally proposed for efficient 3D object detection. Due to the huge number of hypotheses, FSL does not work for a 3D object detection problem. Therefore, there is no direct comparison experiment between MSL and FSL. The comparison on computation time of MSL and FSL in [1] was based on mathematical analysis. In this paper, we apply MSL to 2D object detection to estimate five object pose parameters (two for translation, one for orientation, and two for anisotropic scaling). In this low-dimensional space, it is possible to apply FSL with a coarse-to-fine strategy to achieve a reasonable detection speed. FSL is currently the state-of-the-art for 2D object detection [6]. There is a wide interest for a direct comparison between FSL and MSL. As a contribution of this paper, we perform a thorough comparison experiment on left ventricle (LV) detection in 2D magnetic resonance images (MRI). The experiment shows that MSL significantly outperforms FSL on both speed and accuracy.

In terms of computational efficiency, MSL outperforms a brute-force full space search by a significant margin on 3D object detection. However, it still has much room for improvement since the pose subspaces are exhaustively searched, though in a lower dimension. The variations of the object orientation and its physical size are normally bounded. The distribution range of a pose parameter can be estimated from the training set. During searching, each parameter is independently sampled within its own range to generate testing hypotheses [1]. Each of the three subspaces (the translation, orientation, and scale spaces) is exhaustively sampled without considering the correlation among parameters in the same space. However, in many real applications, the pose parameters are unlikely to be independent. For example, a large object (e.g., the liver of an adult) is likely to have larger scales than a small object (e.g., the liver of a baby) in all three directions. Independent sampling of each parameter results in much more testing hypotheses than necessary. Because the detection speed is roughly proportional to the number of testing hypotheses, reducing the hypotheses can speed up the system. In this paper, we propose to further constrain the search space using an example-based strategy to exploit the correlation among object pose parameters. Using constrained marginal space learning, we can further improve the detection speed by an order of magnitude. Besides speed-up, constraining the search to a small valid region can reduce the likelihood of detection outliers, therefore improve the detection accuracy.

The original MSL was proposed to estimate the rigid transformation (translation, rotation, and scaling) of an object [1]. To better localize a nonrigid object, we may need to further estimate its nonrigid deformation. In this paper, we apply the marginal space learning principle to directly estimate the nonrigid deformation parameters. Within the steerable feature framework [1], we propose a new sampling pattern to efficiently incorporate nonrigid deformation parameters into the image feature set. These image features are used to train a classifier to distinguish a correct estimate of the deformation parameters from the wrong estimates.

In summary, we make three major contributions in this paper.

1. We perform a thorough comparison experiment between MSL and FSL on 2D object detection. The experiment shows that MSL outperforms FSL on both speed and accuracy.
2. We propose constrained MSL to further reduce the search spaces in MSL, therefore improve the detection speed by an order of magnitude.
3. We propose nonrigid MSL to directly estimate nonrigid deformation parameters of an object to improve the localization accuracy.

2 Full Space Learning vs. Marginal Space Learning

2.1 Full Space Learning

Object detection is equivalent to estimating the object pose parameters in an image. As a straightforward application of a learning-based approach [6], we can train a discriminative classifier that assigns a high score to a hypothesis that is close to the true object pose and a low score to those far away. During testing, we need to exhaustively search the full parameter space (i.e., all possible combinations of position, orientation, and scale) to generate testing hypotheses. Suppose there are P pose parameters and parameter i is discretized to H_i values, the total number of testing hypotheses is $H_1 \times H_2 \ldots \times H_P$. Each hypothesis is then tested by the trained classifier to get a score and the hypothesis with the highest score is the best estimate of the pose parameters. (Please refer to Fig. 9 of [1] for an illustration of the basic idea). Since both learning and searching are performed in the full parameter space, we call it full space learning (FSL).

Due to the exponential increase of hypotheses w.r.t. the dimension of the parameter space, the computation demand of this naive implementation of FSL for 3D object detection is well beyond the current personal computers. For 2D object detection, we

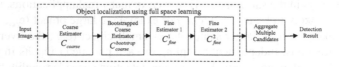

Fig. 2. Object localization using full space learning with a coarse-to-fine strategy

only need to estimate five object pose parameters, (X, Y, θ, S_x, S_y), with (X, Y) for the object position, θ for orientation, and (S_x, S_y) for anisotropic scaling. (Alternatively, we can use the aspect ratio $a = S_y/S_x$ to replace S_y as the last parameter.) A coarse-to-fine strategy can be exploited to accelerate the detection speed. The system diagram for left ventricle (LV) detection in 2D MRI images is shown in Fig. 2. In this particular implementation, in total, we train four classifiers.

At the coarse level, we use large search steps to reduce the total number of testing hypotheses. For example, the search step for position is set to eight pixels and the orientation search step is set to 20 degrees to generate 18 hypotheses for the whole orientation range. Even with these coarse search steps, the total number of hypotheses can easily exceed one million. As shown by the row labeled "C_{coarse}" in Table 1, in total, we search $36 \times 23 \times 18 \times 15 \times 6 = 1,341,360$ hypotheses at the coarse level. A classifier is trained to distinguish the hypotheses close to the ground truth from those far away. Interested readers are referred to [6, 1] for more details about the training of a classifier. Each hypothesis is then tested using the trained C_{coarse} classifier and the top 10,000 candidates are preserved. A bootstrapped classifier $C_{coarse}^{bootstrap}$ can be further exploited to reduce the number of candidates to 200.

As shown in Fig. 2, we use two iterations of fine level search to improve the estimation accuracy. In each iteration, the search step for each parameter is reduced by half. Around a candidate, we search three hypotheses for each parameter. In total, we search $3^5 = 243$ hypotheses around each candidate. Therefore, for the first fine classifier C_{fine}^1, in total we need to test $200 \times 243 = 48,600$ hypotheses. We preserve the top 100 candidates after the first fine-search step. After that, we reduce the search step by half again to start the second round refinement. The number of hypotheses and search step sizes for each classifier are listed in Table 1. In total, we test $1,341,360 + 10,000 + 46,800 + 23,400 = 1,424,260$ hypotheses.

2.2 Marginal Space Learning

Instead of exhaustively searching the full parameter space directly, MSL splits the task into three steps: object position estimation, position-orientation estimation, and position-orientation-scale estimation (as shown in Fig. 1). For each step, we train a classifier to assign a high score to a correct hypothesis. After each step, only a limited number of hypotheses are obtained for the following processing. Please refer to [1] for more details about MSL.

Following is an analysis on the number of testing hypotheses for MSL on LV detection in 2D MRI images. First all pixels are tested using the trained position classifier and the top 1000 candidates, (X_i, Y_i), $i = 1, \ldots, 1000$, are kept. Next, the whole

Table 1. Parameters for full space learning. The "# Hyph" columns show the number of hypotheses for each parameter. The "Step" columns show the search step size for each parameter. The "# Total Hyph" column lists the total number of hypotheses tested by each classifier. The "# Preserve" column lists the number of candidates preserved after each step.

	X		Y		θ		S_x		a		# Total Hyph	# Preserve
	# Hyph	Step	# Hyph	Step	# Hyph	Step	# Hyph	Step	# Hyph	Step		
C_{coarse}	36	8	23	8	18	$20°$	15	16	6	0.2	1,341,360	10,000
$C_{coarse}^{bootstrap}$	1	8	1	8	1	$20°$	1	16	1	0.2	$10,000 \times 1$	200
C_{fine}^1	3	4	3	4	3	$10°$	3	8	3	0.1	200×243	100
C_{fine}^2	3	2	3	2	3	$5°$	3	4	3	0.05	100×243	100

orientation space is discretized under the resolution of five degrees, resulting in 72 orientation hypotheses. Each position candidate is augmented with all orientation hypotheses, (X_i, Y_i, θ_j), $j = 1, \ldots, 72$. The trained position-orientation classifier is used to prune these $1000 \times 72 = 72,000$ hypotheses and the top 100 candidates are retained, $(\hat{X}_i, \hat{Y}_i, \hat{\theta}_i)$, $i = 1, \ldots, 100$. Similarly, we augment each position-orientation candidate with a set of hypotheses about scaling. For LV detection, we have 182 scale combinations, resulting in a total of $100 \times 182 = 18,200$ hypotheses. The position-orientation-scale classifier is then used to pick the best hypothesis. For a typical image of 300×200 pixels, in total, we test $300 \times 200 + 1000 \times 72 + 100 \times 182 = 150,200$ hypotheses. For comparison, a total of 1,424,260 hypotheses need to be tested in FSL. Since the speed of the system is roughly proportional to the number of hypotheses, MSL is about an order of magnitude faster than FSL.

3   Constrained Marginal Space Learning

In this section, we present our approach to effectively constraining the search of MSL in all three subspaces (i.e., translation, orientation, and scale spaces) for further speed-up in 3D object detection.

Due to the heterogeneity in scanning protocol, the position of an object may vary significantly in a volume. As shown in Fig. 6, the first volume focuses on the liver, while the second volume captures almost the full torso. A learning based object detection system [6, 1] normally tests all voxels as hypotheses of the object center. Therefore, for a big volume, the number of hypotheses is quite large. It is preferable to constrain the search to a smaller region. The challenge is that the scheme should be generic and works for different application scenarios. In this paper, we propose a generic way to constrain the search space. Our basic assumption is that, to study an organ, normally we need to capture the whole organ in the volume. Therefore, the center of the organ cannot be arbitrarily close to the volume border. As shown in Fig. 3a, for each training volume, we can measure the distance of the object center (e.g., the liver in this case) to the volume border in six directions (e.g., X^l for the distance to the left volume border, X^r for right, Y^t for top, Y^b for bottom, Z^f for front, and Z^b for back). The minimum value (e.g., X_{min}^l for the left margin) for each direction can be easily calculated from a training set. These minimum margins define a region (the white box in Fig. 3b) and we only need to test voxels inside the region for the object center. Using the proposed

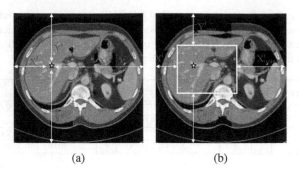

(a)   (b)

Fig. 3. Constraining the search for object center in a volume, illustrated for liver detection in a CT volume. (a) Distances of the object center to the volume borders. (b) Constrained search space (the region enclosed by the white box) based on the minimum distances to the volume borders.

method, on average, we get rid of 91% of voxels for liver detection (see Section 5.2), resulting in a speed-up in position estimation about 10 times.

In many applications, the orientation of an object is also constrained. Three Euler angles were used to represent the 3D orientation in [1]. The distribution range for an Euler angle can be calculated on a training set. Each Euler angle is then sampled independently within its own range to generate testing hypotheses. However, since the Euler angles are unlikely to be independent in a real application, sampling each Euler angle independently generates far more hypotheses than necessary. To constrain the search space, we should estimate the joint distribution of orientation parameters using the training set. We then generate hypotheses only in the region with a large probability. However, it is not trivial to estimate the joint probability distribution reliably since, usually, only a limited number of training samples (a couple of hundreds or even less) are available. In this paper, we propose to use an example-based strategy to generate testing hypotheses. The procedure is as follows (also illustrated in Fig. 4),

1. Uniformly sample the parameter space with a certain resolution r to generate S_u.
2. Set the selected hypothesis set S_t to empty.
3. For each training sample, its neighboring samples in S_u (with a distance no more than d to it) are added into S_t. Here, neighborhood size d should be large enough, otherwise, there may be no sample satisfying the condition. In our experiments, we set $d = r$.
4. Remove redundant elements in S_t to get the final testing hypothesis set S_t.

Using a discretization resolution of 9.72 degrees, we get S_u of 7416 samples uniformly distributed in the whole orientation space [7]. On a dataset of 226 abdominal computed tomography (CT) volumes, S_t of the liver orientation has only 42 unique orientations, which is much smaller than S_u (7416) and also smaller than the number of the training volumes (226). For comparison, if we sample each Euler angle independently under the same resolution, we get 2,686 hypotheses for orientation.

A big object normally has large scaling values along all three directions. Therefore, the same technique can also be applied to constrain the scale space by exploiting the

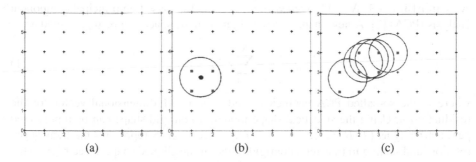

(a)   (b)   (c)

Fig. 4. Example-based selection of testing hypotheses. (a) Uniformly sampled hypotheses, shown as black '+'s. (b) After processing the first training sample. The blue dot shows the ground truth and the circle shows the neighborhood range. All hypotheses inside the circle (represented as red squares) are added to the testing hypothesis set. (c) The testing hypothesis set after processing five training samples.

strong correlation among three scaling parameters. On the same liver dataset, if we uniformly sample each scale independently using a resolution of 6 mm, we get 1,664 hypotheses. Using our example-based strategy, we only need 303 hypotheses to cover the whole training set.

4   Nonrigid Marginal Space Learning

The original MSL [1] only estimates the rigid transformation for object localization. In many cases, we want to delineate the nonrigid boundary of an organ. For this purpose, the mean shape was aligned with the estimated object pose as an initial rough estimate of the shape in [1]. The active shape model (ASM) was then exploited to deform the initial shape to achieve the final boundary delineation. Since ASM only converges to a local optimum, the initial shape needs to be close to the true object boundary. Otherwise, the deformation is likely to get stuck in a wrong configuration. This problem is manifest in liver segmentation since the liver is the largest organ in human body and it is cluttered with several other organs (e.g., heart, kidney, stomach, and diaphragm). As a soft organ, it deforms significantly under the pressure from the neighboring organs. As noted in [8], for a highly deformable shape, the pose estimation can be improved by further initialization. In this paper, we propose *nonrigid MSL* to directly estimate the nonrigid deformation of an object for better shape initialization.

There are many ways to represent a nonrigid deformation. We use the statistical shape model [2] since it can capture the major deformation modes with a few parameters. To build a statistical shape model, we need N shapes and each is represented by M points with correspondence in anatomy. Stacking the 3D coordinates of these M points, we get a $3M$ dimensional vector $X_i, i = 1, 2, \ldots, N$, to represent a shape. To remove the relative translation, orientation, and scaling, we first jointly align all shapes using generalized Procrustes analysis [2] to get the aligned shapes $x_i, i = 1, 2, \ldots, N$. The mean shape $\bar{x}$ is calculated as the simple average of the aligned shapes, $\bar{x} = \frac{1}{N} \sum_{i=1}^{N} x_i$. The shape space spanned by these N aligned shapes can be represented as a linear space with

$K = \min\{3M - 1, N - 1\}$ eigen vectors, $V_1, \ldots, V_K$, based on principal component analysis (PCA) [2]. A new shape y in the aligned shape space can be represented as

$$y = \bar{x} + \sum_{i=1}^{K} c_i V_i + e, \tag{1}$$

where c_i the so-called PCA coefficient, and e is a $3M$ dimensional vector for the residual error. Using the statistical shape model, a nonrigid shape can be represented parametrically as $(T, R, S, c_1, \ldots, c_K, \bar{x}, e)$, where T, R, S represents the translation, rotation, and scaling to transfer a nonrigid shape in the aligned shape space back to the world coordinate system.

With this representation, we can convert the segmentation (or boundary delineation) problem to a parameter estimation problem. Among all these parameters, $\bar{x}$ is fixed and e is sufficiently small if K is large enough (e.g., with enough training shapes). The original MSL only estimates the rigid part (T, R, S) of the transformation. Here, we extend MSL to directly estimate the parameters for nonrigid deformation $(c_1, \ldots, c_K)$. Given a hypothesis $(T, R, S, c_1, \ldots, c_K)$, we train a classifier based on a set of image features F to distinguish a correct hypothesis from a wrong one. The image features should be a function of the hypothesis, $F = F(T, R, S, c_1, \ldots, c_K)$, to incorporate sufficient information for classification. Steerable features were proposed in [1] to efficiently embed the object pose information into the feature set. The basic idea of steerable features is to steer (translate, rotate, and scale) a sampling pattern w.r.t. the testing hypothesis. On each sampling point, 24 local image features (e.g., intensity and gradient) are extracted. A regular sampling pattern was used in [1] to embed the object pose parameters (T, R, S). Here, we need to embed the nonrigid shape parameters $c_i, i = 1, \ldots, K$, into the sampling pattern too. For this purpose, we propose a new sampling pattern based on the synthesized nonrigid shape. Each hypothesis $(T, R, S, c_1, \ldots, c_K)$ corresponds to a nonrigid shape using the statistical shape model (see Eq. (1)). We use this synthesized shape as the sampling pattern and extract the local image features on its M points, resulting in a feature pool with $24 \times M$ features. If the hypothesis is close to the ground truth, the sampling points should be close to the true object boundary. The image features (e.g., gradient of the image intensity) extracted on these sampling points can help us to distinguish it from a wrong hypothesis where the sampling points are far from the object boundary and likely to lie in a smooth region. Similar to [1], we use the boosting technique to learn the classifier.

Due to the exponential increase of testing hypotheses, we cannot train a monolithic classifier to estimate all nonrigid deformation parameters simultaneously. Using the marginal space learning principle, we split the nonrigid deformation parameters into groups and estimate them sequentially. To be specific, we train a classifier in the marginal space of (T, R, S, c_1, c_2, c_3), where (c_1, c_2, c_3) correspond to the top three deformation modes. Given a small set of candidates after position-orientation-scale estimation, we augment them with all possible combinations of (c_1, c_2, c_3) and use the trained nonrigid MSL classifier to prune these hypotheses to a manageable number. In theory, we can apply the MSL principle to estimate more and more nonrigid deformation parameters sequentially. In practice, we find that with the increase of the dimensionality of the marginal spaces, the classifier is more likely to over-fit the data due to

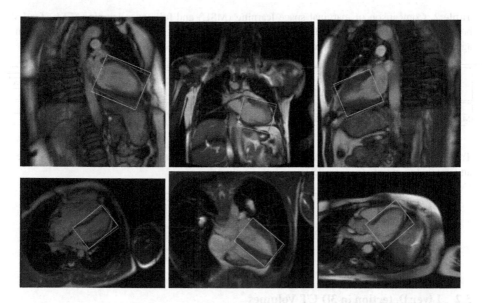

Fig. 5. Left ventricle detection results on 2D MRI images. Red boxes show the ground truth, while cyan boxes show the detection results.

the limited number of training samples. No significant improvement has been achieved by estimating more than three nonrigid deformation parameters.

5   Experiments

5.1   Left Ventricle Detection in 2D MRI Images

In this experiment, we quantitatively evaluate the performance of marginal space learning (MSL) and full space learning (FSL) for left ventricle (LV) detection in 2D MRI images. We collect 795 images of the LV long-axis view. Among them, 400 images are randomly selected for training and the remaining 395 images are reserved for testing. Two error measurements are used for quantitative evaluation, the center-center distance and the vertex-vertex distance (which is defined as the mean Euclidean distance between the corresponding vertices of the box). Table 2 shows detection errors of the LV bounding box obtained by MSL and FSL. It is quite clear that MSL achieves much better results than FSL. The mean center-center and vertex-vertex errors on the test set are 13.49 mm and 21.39 mm for MSL, respectively, which are about one third of the corresponding errors of FSL. MSL was originally proposed to accelerate 3D object detection [1]. In this comparison experiment, we find it also significantly improves the accuracy for 2D object detection.

MSL is faster than FSL since much fewer hypotheses need to be tested. On a computer with a 3.2 GHz processor and 3 GB memory, the detection speed of MSL is about 1.49 seconds/image, while FSL takes about 13.12 seconds to process one image.

Table 2. Comparison of marginal space learning (MSL) and full space learning (FSL) for LV bounding box detection in 2D MRI images on both the training (400 images) and test (395 images) sets. The errors are measured in millimeters.

	Training Set				Test Set			
	Center-Center Distance		Vertex-Vertex Distance		Center-Center Distance		Vertex-Vertex Distance	
	Mean	Median	Mean	Median	Mean	Median	Mean	Median
Full Space Learning	9.73	1.79	17.31	5.07	43.88	21.01	63.26	46.49
Marginal Space Learning	**1.31**	**1.15**	**3.09**	**2.82**	**13.49**	**5.77**	**21.39**	**10.19**

Table 3. Comparison of unconstrained and constrained MSL on the number of testing hypotheses and computation time for liver detection in CT volumes

	Unconstrained MSL [1]		Constrained MSL	
	#Hypotheses	Speed	#Hypotheses	Speed
Position	∼403,000	2088.7 ms	∼38,000	167.1 ms
Orientation	2686	2090.0 ms	42	59.5 ms
Scale	1664	1082.8 ms	303	243.7 ms
Overall		6590.8 ms		470.3 ms

5.2 Liver Detection in 3D CT Volumes

In this experiment, we compare constrained MSL and nonrigid MSL against the baseline version [1] on liver detection in 226 3D CT volumes. Our dataset is very challenging (including both contrasted and non-contrasted scans) because the volumes come from diverse sources. After object localization, we align the mean shape (a surface mesh) with the estimated transformation. Similar to [1], the accuracy of the initial shape estimate is measured with the symmetric point-to-mesh distance E_{p2m}. We can then deform the mesh to fit the image boundary to further reduce the error. In this paper, we focus on object localization. Therefore, in the following we only measure the error of the initialized shapes for comparison purpose.

The detection speed of MSL is roughly proportional to the number of testing hypotheses. The analysis presented in Section 3 shows that constrained MSL significantly reduces the number of testing hypotheses. Table 3 shows the break-down computation time for all three steps in MSL (see Fig. 1). Overall, constrained MSL uses only 470.3 ms to process one volume, while unconstrained MSL uses 6590.8 ms. Using constrained MSL, we achieve a speed-up by a factor of 14. Constrained MSL also improves detection accuracy marginally. Since we constrain the search to a smaller but more meaningful region, the likelihood of detection outliers is reduced. As shown in

Table 4. Comparison of constrained MSL and nonrigid MSL against the baseline version [1] on liver detection in 226 CT volumes. "Constrained + Nonrigid MSL" is the version combining both constrained MSL and nonrigid MSL. Average point-to-mesh error E_{p2m} (in millimeters) of the initialized shape is used for evaluation.

	Mean	Standard Deviation	Median
Unconstrained MSL [1]	7.44	2.26	6.99
Constrained MSL	7.12	2.15	6.73
Constrained + Nonrigid MSL	6.65	1.96	6.25

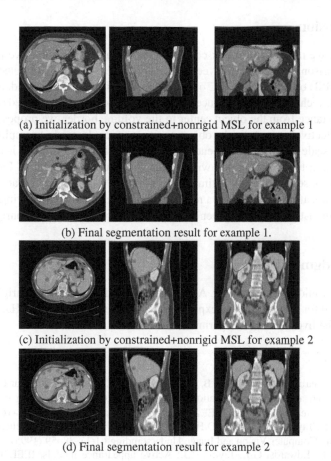

(a) Initialization by constrained+nonrigid MSL for example 1

(b) Final segmentation result for example 1.

(c) Initialization by constrained+nonrigid MSL for example 2

(d) Final segmentation result for example 2

Fig. 6. Typical liver segmentation results on two CT volumes. From left to right: transversal, sagittal, and coronal views.

Table 4, constrained MSL reduces the mean E_{p2m} error from 7.44 mm to 7.12 mm, and the median error from 6.99 mm to 6.73 mm, in a three-fold cross-validation.

To further reduce the initialization error, we estimate three more nonrigid deformation parameters (top three PCA coefficients) to improve the object localization accuracy. As shown in the last row of Table 4, combining nonrigid MSL with constrained MSL, we can further reduce the average E_{p2m} to 6.65 mm (about 11% improvement compared to the original error of 7.44 mm).

Fig. 6 shows typical liver segmentation results on two volumes. Accurate boundary delineation is achieved starting from the good initial estimate of the shape achieved by the proposed method. After applying the learning-based non-rigid deformation estimation method [1], we achieve a final E_{p2m} error of 1.45 mm on 226 CT volumes (based on a three-fold cross-validation), which compares favorably with the state-of-the-art [9]. Our overall system runs as fast as ten seconds per volume (1 s for object localization using constrained+nonrigid MSL and 9 s for boundary delineation), while the state-of-the-art solutions take at least one minute [10], often up to 15 minutes [11,8], to process a volume.

6   Conclusion

In summary, we made three major contributions in this paper. First, we performed a direct comparison experiment between MSL and FSL on 2D object detection, which shows that MSL outperformed FSL on both speed and accuracy. Second, a novel constrained MSL technique was introduced to reduce the search space. Based on the statistics of the distance from the object center to the volume border, we proposed a generic method to effectively constrain the object position space. Instead of sampling each orientation and scale parameter independently, an example-based strategy is used to constrain the search to a small region with a high distribution probability. Last, nonrigid MSL was proposed to directly estimate the nonrigid deformation parameters to improve the localization accuracy for a nonrigid object. Comparison experiments on liver detection demonstrated the effectiveness of both the constrained and nonrigid versions of MSL.

Acknowledgments

The authors would like to thank Dr. Adrian Barbu for discussion on nonrigid MSL, Dr. Xiaoguang Lu for the comparison experiment on LV detection, and Dr. Haibin Ling for the help on the liver detection experiment.

References

1. Zheng, Y., Barbu, A., Georgescu, B., Scheuering, M., Comaniciu, D.: Four-chamber heart modeling and automatic segmentation for 3D cardiac CT volumes using marginal space learning and steerable features. IEEE Trans. Medical Imaging 27(11), 1668–1681 (2008)
2. Cootes, T.F., Taylor, C.J., Cooper, D.H., Graham, J.: Active shape models—their training and application. Computer Vision and Image Understanding 61(1), 38–59 (1995)
3. Cootes, T.F., Edwards, G.J., Taylor, C.J.: Active appearance models. IEEE Trans. Pattern Anal. Machine Intell. 23(6), 681–685 (2001)
4. Kass, M., Witkin, A., Terzopoulos, D.: Snakes: Active contour models. Int. J. Computer Vision 1(4), 321–331 (1988)
5. Ecabert, O., Peters, J., Schramm, H., et al.: Automatic model-based segmentation of the heart in CT images. IEEE Trans. Medical Imaging 27(9), 1189–1201 (2008)
6. Viola, P., Jones, M.: Rapid object detection using a boosted cascade of simple features. In: Proc. IEEE Conf. Computer Vision and Pattern Recognition, pp. 511–518 (2001)
7. Karney, C.F.F.: Quaternions in molecular modeling. Journal of Molecular Graphics and Modeling 25(5), 595–604 (2007)
8. Heimann, T., Münzing, S., Meinzer, H.P., Wolf, I.: A shape-guided deformable model with evolutionary algorithm initialization for 3D soft tissue segmentation. In: Karssemeijer, N., Lelieveldt, B. (eds.) IPMI 2007. LNCS, vol. 4584, pp. 1–12. Springer, Heidelberg (2007)
9. van Ginneken, B., Heimann, T., Styner, M.: 3D segmentation in the clinic: A grand challenge. In: MICCAI Workshop on 3D Segmentation in the Clinic: A Grand Challenge (2007)
10. Ruskó, L., Bekes, G., Németh, G., Fidrichf, M.: Fully automatic liver segmentation for contrast-enhanced CT images. In: MICCAI Workshop on 3D Segmentation in the Clinic: A Grand Challenge (2007)
11. Kainmueller, D., Lange, T., Lamecker, H.: Shape constrained automatic segmentation of the liver based on a heuristic intensity model. In: MICCAI Workshop on 3D Segmentation in the Clinic: A Grand Challenge (2007)

A General and Unifying Framework for Feature Construction, in Image-Based Pattern Classification

Nematollah Batmanghelich[1], Ben Taskar[2], and Christos Davatzikos[1]

[1] Section of Biomedical Image Analysis, Raddiology Department, University of
Pennsylvania, Philadelphia PA 19014, USA
[2] Computer and Information Department, University of Pennsylvania, Philadelphia
PA 19104, USA
{batmangh@seas,taskar@cis,christos@rad}.upenn.edu

Abstract. This paper presents a general and unifying optimization
framework for the problem of feature extraction and reduction for high-
dimensional pattern classification of medical images. Feature extraction
is often an ad hoc and case-specific task. Herein, we formulate it as a
problem of sparse decomposition of images into a basis that is desired to
possess several properties: 1) Sparsity and local spatial support, which
usually provides good generalization ability on new samples, and lends
itself to anatomically intuitive interpretations; 2) good discrimination
ability, so that projection of images onto the optimal basis yields discriminant features to be used in a machine learning paradigm; 3) spatial smoothness and contiguity of the estimated basis functions. Our
method yields a parts-based representation, which warranties that the
image is decomposed into a number of positive regional projections. A
non-negative matrix factorization scheme is used, and a numerical solution with proven convergence is used for solution. Results in classification
of Alzheimers patients from the ADNI study are presented.

1 Introduction

Voxel-based analysis (VBA) has been widely used in the medical imaging community. It typically consists of mapping image data to a standard template space,
and then applying voxel-wise linear statistical tests on a Jacobian determinant
[1], [2], transformation-residuals [3], or tissue density maps [4], [5] or directly on
voxel intensity (e.g. diffusion imaging [6]). It therefore identifies regions in which
two groups differ (e.g. patients and controls [2]), or regions in which other variables (e.g. disease severity [7]) correlate with imaging measurements. However,
this method has limited ability to identify complex population differences, because it does not take into account the multivariate relationships in data [8], [9].
Moreover, since typically no single anatomical region offers sufficient sensitivity
and specificity in identifying pathologies that span multiple anatomical regions,
it has very limited diagnostic power on an individual basis. In other words, values of voxels or ROIs showing significant group difference are not necessarily
good discriminants when one wants to classify individuals into groups.

J.L. Prince, D.L. Pham, and K.J. Myers (Eds.): IPMI 2009, LNCS 5636, pp. 423–434, 2009.
© Springer-Verlag Berlin Heidelberg 2009

In order to overcome the limitations, high-dimensional pattern classification methods have been proposed in the relatively recent literature [9,10,11,12,13], which capture multi-variate nonlinear relationships in the data, and aim to achieve high classification accuracy of individual scans. A fundamental difficulty in these methods has been the availability of enough training samples, relative to the high dimensionality of the data. A critical problem has therefore persisted in these methods, namely how to optimally perform feature extraction and selection, i.e. to find a parsimonious set of image features that best differentiate between two or more groups, and which generalize well to new samples.

Feature reduction methods can be categorized into two general families: 1) feature selection and 2) feature construction [14]. Feature selection methods (e.g. SVM-RFE [15]) have two problems: first, they do not scale up for medical images; second, they do not consider domain knowledge (in our case: the fact that data is coming from images) thus they may end up selecting a subset of features which is not biologically interpretable. Another family of feature reduction methods includes feature construction like PCA, LDA or other linear or nonlinear transformations. These methods can take into account domain knowledge but they are challenged by two issues: first, constructed features do not have local support, but are typically extracted from spatially extensive and overlapping regions; moreover, they use both positive and negative weights, which render difficult anatomical interpretability. Finally, the number of basis vectors is usually bounded by the number of samples, which is usually less than the dimensionality of features.

In this paper, we propose a novel method which falls into the feature construction category. Finding optimal linear construction can be viewed as finding a linear transformation, i.e. basis matrix, which is to be estimated from data according to some desired properties that are discussed next. 1) The basis must be biologically meaningful: this means that a constructed basis vector should correspond to contiguous anatomical regions preferably in areas which are biologically related to a pathology of interest. Having local spatial support can be viewed mathematically as sparsity of a basis vector in combining voxel values. 2) The basis must be discriminant: we are interested in finding features, i.e. projection onto the basis, that construct spatial patterns that best differentiate between groups, e.g. patients and controls. 3) The basis must be representative of the data: in order to represent data, we derive a basis matrix with aforementioned properties and corresponding loadings. Matrix factorization has been adopted as a framework. Having simultaneously representative and parsimonious representation of an image is usually referred to parts-based representation in the literature. A specific variant of Matrix Factorization (MF) which is confined to be nonnegative (NMF) has been shown experimentally [16], and under some conditions mathematically [17], to yield parts-based representations of an image. Since general NMF does not consider that underlying data is an image, we have introduced a Markovian prior to address this issue. Furthermore, we have an extra prior to enforce sparsity (parts-based representation) of an image. 4) Generalization: the proposed method is general and can be applied to a wide variety of problems and data sets without significant adjustments. In this paper, we have formulated our problem as an optimization problem that seeks to satisfy the four criteria above. Moreover, we proposed a novel numerical solution with a proof of convergence to solve it. Unlike LDA and PCA, the number of basis vectors are not confined with number of samples in our method thus we are able to have more basis vectors than samples.

In the Methods section, we first discuss the idea of matrix factorization in general and NMF in particular (Sect.2.1). In the subsequent sections, a likelihood term (Sect.2.2) and proper regularization terms are introduced (Sect.2.3,2.4). In Sect. 2.5, the final optimization problem is formed and a proper method is suggested to solve it. In the Results section (Sect.3), we apply our method to the problem of classification of Alzheimer's disease patients and healthy controls.

2 Methods

2.1 General Formulation

Let's assume that we collect data into a matrix, $X \in \mathbb{R}^{+D \times N}$, such that each column x_i represents one image. This can be done by lexicographical ordering of voxels. D is number of voxels and N is number of samples. For this case, we assume that x_i's reside in positive quadrant which is a reasonable assumption for medical images. The goal is to decompose data matrix, X, into a positive matrix, B, which is a matrix whose columns are constructed basis vectors, and a loadings matrix , C, which holds corresponding loadings of the basis, namely $X \approx BC$. The elements of C will form the features extracted from the data via projection on B; they will be subsequently used for classification. In the literature, this decomposition is called Non-Negative Matrix Factorization (NMF). It is straightforward to verify that this is an ill-posed problem. Hence, a regularization is necessary. We formulate the problem as a MAP (Maximum a Posteriori) estimation problem as follows:

$$p(B,C|X) = \frac{p(X|B,C)p(B,C)}{p(X)} = \frac{p(X|B,C)p(B)p(C)}{p(X)} \tag{1}$$

Here, we assumed that B and C are independent. Therefore, the MAP estimation problem is formulated as an optimization problem as follows:

$$\max_{B,C} \log p(B,C|X) \equiv \max_{B,C} \log p(X|B,C) + \log p(B) + \log p(C) \tag{2}$$

in which the first term on the right hand side is a likelihood term and the second and third terms are priors for B and C respectively. Thus, we need to choose proper priors and likelihood function according to our problem. In general, NMF can be written as the following optimization problem:

$$\min_{B,C>0} D(X;BC) + \alpha(B) + \beta(C) \tag{3}$$

where $D(X;BC)$ is a negative likelihood function and measures the goodness of fit, and where the second ($\alpha(B)$) and third ($\beta(C)$) terms form negative log priors on B and C. Next, we discuss different choices for $D(.,.)$, $\alpha(.)$, and $\beta(.)$.

2.2   Likelihood Term: $D(X; BC)$

As it is discussed in [18], given a convex function $\varphi : S \subseteq \mathbb{R} \to \mathbb{R}$, Bregman divergence is a family of $D(.,.)$ functions which are defined as follows $D_\varphi : S \times \text{int}(S) \to \mathbb{R}_+$:

$$D_\varphi(x; y) := \varphi(x) - \varphi(y) - \varphi'(y)(x - y) \tag{4}$$

where $\text{int}(S)$ is the interior of set S. For cases in which x and y are matrices, it can be augmented as summation over all elements of a matrix:

$$D_\varphi(X; Y) := \sum_{ij} D_\varphi(x_{ij}, y_{ij}) \tag{5}$$

In this paper, we used $\varphi(x) = x \log x$ which readily converts (5) to the KL-Divergence:

$$D_\varphi(X; BC) = \sum_{ij} x_{ij} \log \frac{x_{ij}}{\sum_k b_{ik} c_{kj}} - \sum_{ij} x_{ij} + \sum_{ijk} b_{ik} c_{kj} \tag{6}$$

It is worth mentioning that other choices for φ are also possible (e.g. $\frac{1}{2}x^2$) and they yield other distance measures (e.g. Frobenius distance between matrices).

2.3   Regularizing the Basis: $\alpha(B)$

The regularization term can be broken down into two terms according to respective criteria that will be discussed in more detail in this section:

$$\alpha(B) = \alpha_1(B) + \alpha_2(B) \tag{7}$$

In our implementation, each regularization term has a weighting term which determines its contribution, however, we have omitted the weighting terms for the sake of simplicity in the notation.

It is reasonable to assume that anatomical regions are expected to display similar structural and functional characteristics, hence voxels should be grouped together into regional features. As discussed in the Introduction, local support and sparsity are two desirable properties which both can be achieved using the following terms:

$$\alpha_1(B) = \mathbf{1}^T B^T B \mathbf{1}, \quad \|b_i\|_1 = 1 \tag{8}$$

In order to see why this regularization enforces part-based representation, we should interpret it mathematically. Part-based representation means that we do not want our basis vectors, b_i, to have a lot of overlap with each other. Considering the fact that the basis are positive (hence, bounded below), having the least overlap could be translated to orthogonality. Mathematically speaking, $< b_i, b_j > \approx 0$ if $i \neq j$ which means that off-diagonal elements of $B^T B$ should be minimized.

It is also worth mentioning that it has been shown empirically [16] and under some mild conditions mathematically [17] that NMF yields sparse basis. Nevertheless, equality constraint in (8) in addition to the non-negativity constraint enforces sparsity even further. This ends the justification of the terms introduced in (8).

This is the first criterion for the prior over B and was mentioned earlier in [19]; nevertheless this is not enough when one deals with image data. Diseases typically affect anatomy and function in a somewhat continuous way. Therefore, we would prefer that b_i represents smooth and contiguous anatomical regions. Although smoothing can be applied as post processing after optimization and deriving B, it is preferable to add a smoothness penalty term to the prior of B. Similar to [20], we exploit the widely used Markov Random Field (MRF) model. In this model, voxels within a neighborhood interact with each other and smoothness of an image is modeled as in the Gibbs distribution as follows:

$$p(I) = \frac{1}{Z} \exp\left(-c\alpha_2(B)\right) \quad \Rightarrow \quad -\log p(I) = c\alpha_2(B) - \log Z \tag{9}$$

where I is a vector made by concatenating image voxels (e.g. lexicographically) and Z is a normalization constant called partition function and c is a constant. $\alpha_2(.)$ is a nonlinear energy function measuring non-smoothness of an image. For basis matrix B, we can write $\alpha_2(B)$ as follows:

$$\alpha_2(B) = \sum_{j=1}^{r} \sum_{i=1}^{D} \sum_{l \in U_i} w_{il} \psi(b_{ji} - b_{jl}, \delta) \tag{10}$$

where r is the number of basis vectors and D is dimensionality of the images and U_i is a set containing the neighborhood indices of the i'th voxel and $\psi(., \delta)$ is a potential function and δ is a free parameter and w_{kl} are weighting factors. There are plenty of choices for the potential function. We adopt a simple quadratic function that has all desired properties, including nonnegativity, strictly increasing, unboundedness and more importantly convexity in addition to the fact that it can be simply represented in a matrix form which will help us to derive an appropriate auxiliary function:

$$\psi(x, \delta) = \left(\frac{x}{\delta}\right)^2 \tag{11}$$

Adding both terms, α_1 and α_2, for basis, total regularization penalty would become:

$$\alpha(B) = \mathbf{1}^T B^T B \mathbf{1} + \sum_{j=1}^{r} \sum_{i=1}^{D} \sum_{l \in U_i} w_{il} \psi(b_{ji} - b_{jl}, \delta) \tag{12}$$

2.4   Regularizing Coefficients: $\beta(C)$

In this section, we will discuss the regularization term for the coefficient matrix. The main goal of these regularization terms is to boost bases that produce discriminant features, but also are found consistently across all training samples. We decompose the regularization terms for the C matrix into two terms and describe each one in detail:

$$\beta(C) = \beta_1(C) + \beta_2(C) \tag{13}$$

In our implementation, each regularization term has a weighting term which determines its contribution, however, we have omitted the weighting terms for the sake of simplicity in the notation.

Given the basis matrix, B, the coefficient matrix, C represents new features. If the final goal is classification, discriminative features are preferred. Similar to [21], we use Fisher linear discriminative analysis which is the largest generalized eigen value between within- and between- class matrices when c_{ij} coefficients are considered as new features:

$$\begin{aligned} S_i &= \frac{1}{N_i} \sum_{k \in \mathcal{I}_i} (c_k - \bar{c}_i)(c_k - \bar{c}_i)^T \\ S_W &= \frac{1}{2}(S_1 + S_2) \qquad i = 1, 2 \\ S_B &= \frac{1}{2}(\bar{c}_1 - \bar{c}_2)(\bar{c}_1 - \bar{c}_2)^T \end{aligned} \tag{14}$$

where $\mathcal{I}_i$ is a set containing indices of instances in the i'th class and and c_k is k'th column of matrix C and $\bar{c}_i$ is the mean of new features over i'th class ($\bar{c}_i = 1/N_i \sum_{k \in \mathcal{I}_i} c_k$). S_i is the within-class matrix for the i'th class and S_B is the between-class matrix. Here, we have assumed that we have two classes but the formulation can be easily extended. We would like to maximize the largest generalized eigen value between S_B and S_W, however there is no closed form formulation for that. Instead, we use an approximation as follows [21]:

$$p(C) \propto \exp(\beta_1(C)) \propto \frac{\exp(tr(S_B))}{\exp(tr(S_W))} \Rightarrow -\log p(C) \propto -\beta_1(C) \propto tr(S_B) - tr(S_W) \tag{15}$$

Trace of S_W which is summation of eigen values approximately measures how skewed the classes are, and trace of S_B roughly evaluates how far apart the two classes are. Hence, the more separable the classes are, the lower $\beta_1(C)$ is.

The second criterion for the C matrix is to seek bases which carry maximum image energy. Total *activity* of retained components, i.e. total squared projection coefficients summed over all training images, should be maximized [19]. Effectively, this constraint favors bases that represent components that tend to be present in all samples, and therefore reflect anatomically consistent regions that are likely to generate new samples. Energy of each retained basis is measured by the l_2 norm of c_i^T in which c_i^T is the i'th row of matrix C:

$$\beta_2(C) = -\sum_i \|c_i^T\|_2 \tag{16}$$

Adding up $\beta_1(.)$ and $\beta_2(.)$, yields the final regularization term on C matrix:

$$\beta(C) = \beta_1(C) + \beta_2(C) = tr(S_W) - tr(S_B) - \sum_i \|c_i^T\|_2 \tag{17}$$

2.5 Optimization

We have derived all necessary terms and constraints to form an optimization problem. Given the likelihood function, $D(.,.)$ in (6) and equations for regularization functions on B and C, $\alpha(.)$ in (12) and $\beta(.)$ in (17) and corresponding constraints, the optimization problem is as follows:

$$
\begin{aligned}
\min \quad & D_\varphi(X; BC) + \alpha(B) + \beta(C) \\
\text{subject to} \quad & \|b_i\|_1 = 1 \\
& [B]_{ij}, [C]_{ij} \geq 0
\end{aligned}
\tag{18}
$$

This formulation is not a convex optimization problem. Therefore, we seek a local minimum. A typical strategy to solve this kind of problem is to fix a block of parameters (e.g. C) and optimize other blocks (e.g. B) and alternate until convergence. If C is fixed, optimization over B is a convex problem. Although norm equality constraints for b_i's are not convex constraints in general, they become linear constraints due to the non-negativity of B. However, by fixing B, we do not have a convex optimization problem in C because in (17), $\sum_i \|c_i\|_2$ (a convex term) has to be maximized, not minimized.

Due to the dimensionality of the problem, we use a first order method to solve it. Similar to Lee et al. [16], we prefer a Multiplicative Update (MU). Multiplicative methods have two advantages: first, if initialization starts inside of a feasible set, as long as the current value of a variable is multiplied by a positive value, the new value of that variable is also positive; hence maintaining positivity constraints is trivial. Second, although MU is derived from gradient descent, it has no parameter like the step size of gradient descent. This makes the MU very easy to implement, except one has to make sure that in each iteration the value of cost function decreases. A common approach for optimization in NMF literature is to propose an *auxiliary* function.

Definition 1. $Z(B, \hat{B})$ is called auxiliary function of cost function $J(B)$, if it satisfies the following conditions:

$$
Z(B, \hat{B}) \geq J(B), \quad Z(B, B) = J(B)
\tag{19}
$$

In each iteration t, we optimize over the first parameter:

$$
B^{(t+1)} = \arg\min_B Z(B, B^{(t)})
\tag{20}
$$

By the definition of auxiliary function and minimum, we have $J(B^{(t)}) = Z(B^{(t)}, B^{(t)}) \geq Z(B^{(t+1)}, B^{(t)}) \geq J(B^{(t+1)})$. This method was applied earlier in Expectation Maximization [22] and widely used in NMF literature [16], [19], etc. Due to the lack of space, we have omitted the closed form for our proposed auxiliary function but the following theorems show update rules for B and C variables.

Theorem 1. *The following equations are the multiplicative updates for B variable:*

$$b_{ik} = \hat{b}_{ik}\sqrt{\frac{T_{ik}}{T'_{ik}}},$$
$$T_{ik} = 2(K^-\hat{B})_{ik} + \sum_j x_{ij}\frac{c_{kj}}{\sum_{k'}\hat{b}_{ik'}c_{k'j}}, \; (K = \mathcal{Q}(\Gamma^T)) \tag{21}$$
$$T'_{ik} = Q_{ik} + 2(H\hat{B}^T)_{ki} + 2(K^+\hat{B})_{ik}, \; (Q = \mathbf{1}_D\mathbf{1}_N^T C^T, H = \mathcal{Q}(\mathbf{1}_r))$$

where $\hat{B}$ denotes previous iteration of B variable and notation $[.]^+$ ($[.]^-$) indicates positive (negative) part of a matrix. $\mathbf{1}_D$ denotes a vector of all ones with length D. $\mathcal{Q}(.)$ is a squared function of the argument matrix defined as $\mathcal{Q}(A) = AA^T$. We can introduce the new matrix $\Gamma \in \mathbb{R}^{|U|D \times D}$ in which $|U|$ is neighborhood size and D is number of voxels. Γ is a matrix constituted of the following blocks:

$$\Gamma^T = [\Gamma_1^T, \Gamma_2^T, ..., \Gamma_D^T] \quad where \; \Gamma_i \in R^{|U| \times D}$$
$$where \; [\Gamma_i]_{jl} = \sqrt{\frac{w_{il}}{\delta}} \; if \; k = i \; and \; [\Gamma_i]_{jl} = -\sqrt{\frac{w_{il}}{\delta}} \; if \; l \in U_i(j) \tag{22}$$

Proof. Derivation of auxiliary function and multiplicative updates are omitted due to lack of space. For more information, please see our technical support. [1]

Theorem 2. *Following equations are multiplicative updates for C variable:*

$$c_{ik} = \hat{c}_{ik}\sqrt{\frac{T_{ik}}{T'_{ik}}},$$
$$T_{ik} = 2(\hat{C}\Lambda_1^{-T})_{ik} + 2(\hat{C}\Lambda_2^{+T})_{ik} + 2\sum_l(E^l\hat{C})_{ik} + \sum_j x_{ji}\frac{b_{jk}}{\sum_{k'}b_{jk'}\hat{c}_{k'i}}, \tag{23}$$
$$T'_{ik} = 2(\hat{C}\Lambda_1^{+T})_{ki} + 2(\hat{C}\Lambda_2^{-T})_{ki} + M_{ik}, \quad (M = \mathbf{1}_N\mathbf{1}_D^T B)$$

Here, N_1 and N_2 are numbers of samples for the first and the second classes respectively and we have assumed that samples from the first class constitute the first N_1 columns of X, and $E^l = e_l e_l^T$ in which e_l is l'th unit vector, $\Lambda_1 = \mathcal{Q}([(I_{N_1} - \frac{1}{N_1}\mathbf{1}\mathbf{1}^T); 0]) + \mathcal{Q}([0; (I_{N_2} - \frac{1}{N_2}\mathbf{1}\mathbf{1}^T)])$ and I_{N_1} is an identity matrix of size N_1 and $\Lambda_2 = \mathcal{Q}([\frac{1}{N_1}I_{N_1}; \frac{-1}{N_2}I_{N_2}])$ and $\mathcal{Q}(.)$ was described earlier.

Proof. Derivation of auxiliary function and multiplicative updates are omitted due to lack of space. For more information, please see our technical support.

3 Results

We tested our approach on MR images of Alzheimer's patients and healthy controls from the ADNI study [2]. The dataset we used for this paper included 60 Normal Control (NC) individuals, 60 individuals with Mild Cognitive Impairment (MCI), and 56 Alzheimer's (AD) disease, whose structural MR scans were analyzed. The data sets included standard T1-weighted MR images acquired sagittally using volumetric 3D MPRAGE with 1.25×1.25 mm in-plane spatial resolution and 1.2 mm thick sagittal slices (8 flip angle). Most of the images were obtained using 1.5 T scanners, while a few were obtained using 3T scanners.

---

[1] http://www.4shared.com/file/81316860/e2be6088/TechSupport.html
[2] http://www.loni.ucla.edu/ADNI/Data

Images were pre-processed similar to other VBA studies; i.e. AC-PC alignment, skull-removal; and non-rigid registration with a standard coordinate system using a non-rigid registration method [23]. Given deformation field for each individual, a map quantifying the regional distribution of gray matter (GM) was formed for each individual. The map quantifies an expansion (or contraction) to the tissue applied by the transformation to transform the image from the original space to the template space. Consequently, map values in the templates space are directly proportional to the volume of the respective structures in the original brain scan. Although this map can be formed for cerebral fluid (CSF), white matter (WM), and GM, we only used maps corresponding to the GM tissue type.

Ten images were chosen randomly from each group (AD, NC, and MCI) to form the matrix X. Entries of B and C matrices were initialized randomly using uniform random generator on the unit interval. After deriving the basis vectors, columns of B, we can rank them. A ranked basis helps to interpret the result by highlighting the most important features. To get robust results, we applied four different feature ranking methods including: (1) SVM Attribute Selection [15] ;(2) Information Gain Ranking [24] ; (3) Symmetrical Uncertainty [24] ; (4) χ^2 [24]; and then, found consensus (voting) on their results. Fig. 1 shows the top three important basis vectors. Interestingly, the most representative basis for group difference between the AD vs. NC groups is exactly localized at hippocampus which is known to be affected by Alzheimer's disease. Other areas are also very localized in the areas that are either associated with memory or known to be affected by AD.

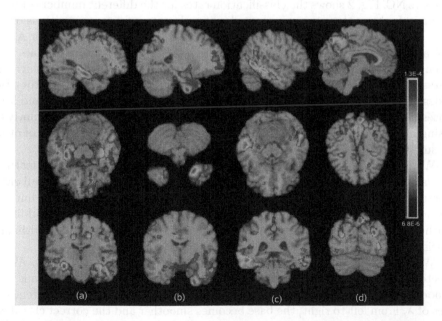

Fig. 1. Three top ranked bases for $r = 50$ and $\lambda = 10^3$: (a) the top ranked basis is localized in hippocampus (b) the second top ranked basis in localized in inferior medial temporal cortex (c) and (d) shows the third top ranked basis being localized in Precuneus and Occipito-parietal association cortex respectively

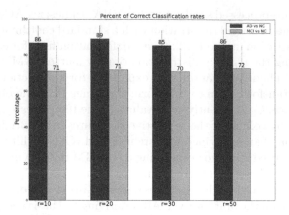

Fig. 2. Comparison of percentages of correct classification rates for the two classification cases when number of bases changes

In order to assess the separability of the new features, we used them for classification. Weka [24] was used to find the best classification strategy in two classification cases: AD vs NC and MCI vs NC. On average, the highest classification rates were obtained when a SVM classifier boosted by the Bagging method is used for AD vs NC and a simple Logistic boosted by Adaboost outperformed other methods for MCI vs NC. Fig. 2 shows the classification rates for the different numbers of basis vectors. It shows the average correct classification rates for ten repetitions of 10-fold cross validations. Classifiers yielded reasonable classification rates for AD vs NC and MCI vs NC cases It is worth mentioning that we used only ten samples from each group (30 samples in total) to build the B matrix. Nevertheless, classification rates are very robust with respect to the changing number of the basis vectors. Besides the fact that there is a narrow difference between definition of AD and MCI cases even for clinicians, we speculate that we can boost this result significantly by using more samples to build the B matrix and using the tissue densities of other tissue types (WM and CSF).

We have also compared the features extracted by our method with features extracted by projecting the data on the principal components (keeping all eigen vectors). The average classification rate with PCA was around %79 but the principal basis vectors were not sparse and hence hard to interpret. In addition, without the Fisher term (15) classification rates droped below %80 although basis vectors were sparse.

We also evaluated the effect of the MRF term introduced in Sect.2.3. As expected, increasing the weight of the MRF term (here we called it λ) leads to a smoother base. Fig.3 depicts the highest ranked basis image for three different values of λ. From left to right, the base becomes smoother and the correct classification rate (for AD vs NC) decreases monotically but not significantly. Eventually in Fig.3(c), the MRF term dominates the other terms and oversmoothes the image however λ was set to a very high value ($\approx 10^4$) to yield such result. This figure shows that our method is robust with regard to choice of weight for the MRF parameter.

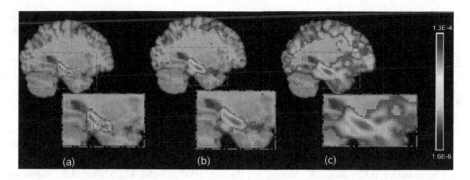

Fig. 3. Effect of the MRF term: (a) for $\lambda = 10$ classification rate was 88.4% $\pm$ 8.6, (b) for $\lambda = 10^3$ classification rate was 86.0% $\pm$ 8.4, (c) for $\lambda = 10^4$ classification rate was 84.7% $\pm$ 9.3

4   Discussion

In this paper, we proposed a novel method based on the NMF framework. Our method is able to produce bases which are simultaneously discriminative and representative of group differences. Moreover, the sparsity of the estimated basis is likely to lead to good generalization of new samples, and to better interpretability of the results via locally-extracted features. The method produces reasonable classification rates between AD patients and normal controls, as well as between normal controls and MCI individuals We plan to improve our results with the current dataset by amending implementation and using tissue density of white matter and CSF. We also plan to apply our method on other datasets and augment it for a vectorial dataset by extending our framework from matrix factorization to tensor factorization.

References

1. Teipel, S.J., Born, C., Ewers, M., Bokde, A.L., Reiser, M.F., Müller, H.J., Hampel, H.: Multivariate deformation-based analysis of brain atrophy to predict alzheimer's disease in mild cognitive impairment. NeuroImage 38(1), 13–24 (2007)
2. Hua, X., et al.: 3D characterization of brain atrophy in alzheimer's disease and mild cognitive impairment using tensor-based morphometry. NeuroImage 41(1), 19–34 (2008)
3. Davatzikos, C., Genc, A., Xu, D., Resnick, S.M.: Voxel-based morphometry using the ravens maps: Methods and validation using simulated longitudinal atrophy. NeuroImage 14(6), 1361–1369 (2001)
4. Wright, I.C., McGuire, P.K., Poline, J.B., Travere, J.M., Murray, R.M., Frith, C.D., Frackowiak, R.S.J., Friston, K.J.: A voxel-based method for the statistical analysis of gray and white matter density applied to schizophrenia. Neuroimage 2(4), 244–252 (1995)
5. Ashburner, J., Friston, K.J.: Voxel-based morphometry-the methods. NeuroImage 11(6), 805–821 (2000)

6. Snook, L., Plewesa, C., Beaulieu, C.: Voxel based versus region of interest analysis in diffusion tensor imaging of neurodevelopment. NeuroImage 34(1), 243–252 (2007)
7. Salmon, E., Collette, F., Degueldre, C., Lemaire, C., Franck, G.: Voxel-based analysis of confounding effects of age and dementia severity on cerebral metabolism in alzheimer's disease. Human Brain Mapping 10(1), 39–48 (2000)
8. Davatzikos, C.: Why voxel-based morphometric analysis should be used with great caution when characterizing group differences. NeuroImage 23, 17–20 (2004)
9. Fan, Y., Shen, D., Gur, R.C., Gur, R.E., Davatzikos, C.: Compare: Classification of morphological patterns using adaptive regional elements. IEEE Trans. on Med. Imag. 26(1), 93–105 (2007)
10. Csernansky, J.G., Joshi, S., Wang, L., Haller, J.W., Gado, M., Miller, J.P., Grenander, U., Miller, M.I.: Hippocampal morphometry in schizophrenia by high dimensional brain mapping. Proceedings of the National Academy of Sciences 95(19), 11406–11411 (1998)
11. Thomaz, C., Boardman, J., Counsell, S., Hill, D., Hajnal, J., Edwards, A., Rutherford, M., Gillies, D., Rueckert, D.: A multivariate statistical analysis of the developing human brain in preterm infants. Image and Vision Computing 25(6), 981–994 (2007)
12. Lashkari, D., Vul, E., Kanwisher, N., Golland, P.: Discovering structure in the space of activation profiles in fMRI. In: Metaxas, D., Axel, L., Fichtinger, G., Székely, G. (eds.) MICCAI 2008, Part I. LNCS, vol. 5241, pp. 1015–1024. Springer, Heidelberg (2008)
13. Terriberry, T.B., Joshi, S.C., Gerig, G.: Hypothesis testing with nonlinear shape models. Inf. Process. Med. Imaging 3565(19), 15–26 (2005)
14. Guyon, I., Elisseeff, A.: An introduction to variable and feature selection. Journal of Machine Learning Research 3, 1157–1182 (2003)
15. Guyon, I., Weston, J., Barnhill, S., Vapnik, V.: Gene selection for cancer classification using support vector machines. Machine Learning 46, 389–422 (2002)
16. Lee, D.D., Seung, H.S.: Algorithms for non-negative matrix factorization, 556–562 (2000)
17. Donoho, D., Stodden, V.: When does non-negative matrix factorization give a correct decomposition into parts? In: NIPS, vol. 16, pp. 1141–1148 (2004)
18. Sra, S., Dhillon, I.S.: Technical report, Dept. Computer Science, University of Texas at Austin, Austin, TX 78712, USA (June)
19. Feng, T., Li, S., Shum, H.Y., Zhang, H.: Local non-negative matrix factorization as a visual representation. In: The 2nd International Conference on Development and Learning (2002)
20. Zdunek, R., Cichocki, A.: Blind image separation using nonnegative matrix factorization with gibbs smoothing. In: Ishikawa, M., Doya, K., Miyamoto, H., Yamakawa, T. (eds.) ICONIP 2007, Part II. LNCS, vol. 4985, pp. 519–528. Springer, Heidelberg (2008)
21. Wang, Y., Jia, Y., Hu, C., Turk, M.: Fisher non-negative matrix factorization for learning local features. In: Proc. Asian Conf. on Comp. Vision (2004)
22. Dempster, A.P., Laird, N.M., Rubin, D.B.: Maximum likelihood from incomplete data via the em algorithm. Journal of the Royal Statistical Society, Series B 39(1), 1–38 (1977)
23. Shen, D., Davatzikos, C.: Very high resolution morphometry using mass-preserving deformations and hammer elastic registration. NeuroImage 18, 28–41 (2003)
24. Witten, I.H., Frank, E.: Data Mining: Practical Machine Learning Tools and Techniques, 2nd edn. Elsevier, Amsterdam (2005)

Bayesian Registration via Local Image Regions: Information, Selection and Marginalization

Matthew Toews and William M. Wells III

Brigham and Women's Hospital
Harvard Medical School
{mt,sw}@bwh.harvard.edu

Abstract. We propose a novel Bayesian registration formulation in which image location is represented as a latent random variable. Location is marginalized to determine the maximum a priori (MAP) transform between images, which results in registration that is more robust than the alternatives of omitting locality (i.e. global registration) or jointly maximizing locality and transform (i.e. iconic registration). A mathematical link is established between the Bayesian registration formulation and the mutual information (MI) similarity measure. This leads to a novel technique for selecting informative image regions for registration, based on the MI of image intensity and spatial location. Experimental results demonstrate the effectiveness of the marginalization formulation and the MI-based region selection technique for ultrasound (US) to magnetic resonance (MR) registration in an image-guided neurosurgical application.

1 Introduction

The task of image registration is central to many medical image analysis applications, and involves determining a geometrical mapping or transform relating different images. Registration is often formulated as determining a transform in the form of a smooth one-to-one mapping between images [1]. However, in a number of medical imaging contexts, a smooth one-to-one mapping may not exist or may be difficult to identify. Consider the context of image-guided surgery, for instance, in which intra-operative ultrasound (US) imagery is to be registered to pre-operative magnetic resonance (MR) imagery for the purpose of surgical guidance. In the case of resection, anatomical tissues present prior to surgery may be severely deformed or removed over the course of the procedure, and a valid one-to-one mapping between pre- and intra-operative images will not exist [2]. Furthermore, the intensity characteristic of US is spatially-varying [3], and certain tissues may be absent or incorrectly represented in the image due to tissue echogenicity or to artifacts relating to sensor gain, acoustic shadowing, reverberation, etc., further compounding the difficulty in estimating a transform.

A body of research focuses on registration based on local image regions [2, 4, 5, 7–9] in order to address the situation where a smooth one-to-one mapping is difficult to estimate. Working with local regions improves the ability to identify and cope with missing or altered tissue in images, and simplifies the modeling

J.L. Prince, D.L. Pham, and K.J. Myers (Eds.): IPMI 2009, LNCS 5636, pp. 435–446, 2009.

of geometrical and intensity relationships between images, which can be approximated as locally smooth and stationary. This paper makes three contributions to this line of research. First, a Bayesian registration formulation is proposed, in which image location is incorporated as a latent random variable. The key insight is that, while location is important in describing image content and the registration process, it is ultimately incidental, and should thus be marginalized in order to obtain the maximum a posteriori (MAP) transform relating images. Marginalization provides a principled means of leveraging local regional information for registration, in contrast to omitting location information or maximizing a joint distribution over locations and the transform. Second, a novel mathematical link is established between Bayesian registration and the mutual information (MI) similarity measure, motivating the use of MI in a Bayesian setting. Third, a new strategy is proposed for selecting informative local image regions for registration, based on the MI of image intensity and location within image regions. This strategy generalizes previous work advocating the selection of high-entropy image regions [10], by imposing the additional constraint that the intensity be informative with respect to image location.

The remainder of this paper is organized as follows. Section 2 outlines related work in the literature. Section 3 presents our Bayesian framework for location marginalization and informative region selection. Section 4 presents experiments involving registration of intra-operative US slices to pre-operative MR imagery in an image-guided neurosurgical (IGNS) application. In this challenging registration scenario, location marginalization is shown to outperform standard registration. Furthermore, mutual information-based selection of image regions is shown to outperform both uniform sampling and entropy-based region selection. A discussion follows in Section 5.

2   Previous Work

2.1   Incorporating Local Regions

The task of image registration, or determining a spatial mapping T between images I and J, is a cornerstone of medical image analysis. Cachier et al. propose two classes of techniques by which local image regions X are incorporated into image registration formulations [4]: geometrical feature-based and iconic feature-based. Geometrical feature-based techniques involve the segmentation of localized geometrical structures from image data, e.g. points or shapes, which are then aligned between different images to estimate T. In contrast, iconic feature-based techniques generally determine correspondences between images based on local image patches or blocks, after which these correspondences are used to improve estimation of T. Our work is most closely related to iconic feature-based techniques, which do not impose hard geometrical feature segmentations in both images to be registered.

A number of authors propose registration based on local regions which capture locally stable relationships. Hellier et al. present a technique which combines local constraints in the form of segmented anatomical structures into a deformable registration framework [11]. Clatz et al. describe a robust hierarchical block matching technique [2], where a fraction of blocks are iteratively rejected based on their displacement error with respect to the current transform. Toews et al. [5] and Loeckx et al. [8] propose computing the MI similarity measure locally to overcome spatially-varying multi-modal intensity relationships. Zhang et al. refine cardiological registration by considering locally affine deformations [7]. Wein et al. [9] propose a similarity measure based on a linear relationship between imaging parameters extracted in local windows.

Most work to date has advocated optimizing a function $E(X, T)$ over the joint space of the transform T and local regions X. In contrast, we note that while X may be important in modeling the image and the registration process, it is ultimately a nuisance parameter that should not be optimized but rather marginalized in order to obtain the optimal transform T.

2.2 Local Region Selection

Using local image information requires a sampling strategy in order to define the specific local regions to be used (e.g. their location, size, distribution). A simple and commonly used strategy is to consider a uniform sampling of regions over the image [2, 4, 7, 9]. In general, however, certain regions are more informative than others, in terms of the image patterns they contain, and registration can be improved by considering a subset of highly informative regions. Domain-specific regions or structures can be defined by experts, e.g. sulci for registering cortical imagery [11]. Fully automatic region selection methods can be used when the structures most useful for registration are not known a priori. In the medical imaging literature, Rohr et al. investigate automatic selection of landmarks for registration based on derivative operators [12]. A popular body of computer vision literature has focused on automatically identifying salient or informative regions in general imagery, typically via a search for image regions which maximize a particular saliency criterion. Examples of saliency criteria include the magnitude of image derivatives in scale-spaces [13, 14] and image entropy [10].

2.3 Multi-modal US Registration

Although the formulation we propose in this paper is generally applicable in many different contexts, experiments focus on the registration of intra-operative US imagery to pre-operative modalities. US is an attractive imaging modality due primarily to the low cost and portability of US sensors. The major drawback of US is the poor image quality, due to the shift-variant nature of the sensor [3] and numerous modality related artifacts. The US image formation process is the result of acoustic backscattering or echoing off of boundaries between tissues of differing acoustic impedance. Specular echoing occurs in the presence of smooth tissue boundaries which are significantly larger than the US wavelength, and results in hyperintense image measurements. Scattered echoing occurs in the presence of poorly reflective or irregularly-shaped microstructures of size equal to or smaller than the US wavelength, and results in the formation of US speckle [15]. While speckle can be treated as noise to be removed [16], speckle brightness patterns do reflect the echogenic properties of the underlying tissues, and have been shown to be useful for segmentation, classification and registration of anatomical tissues [9, 15, 17, 18].

Modeling the image intensity relationship is a key focus of inter-modality US registration, and the wide variety of techniques in the literature speak to the difficulty of modeling. Roche et al. [19] propose an information-based similarity measure combining MR intensity and gradient information. Wein et al. [9] simulate US imagery from CT, then compute similarity using a specialized correlation measure accounting for both specular and scattered US echoing. Arbel et al. [20] register the US image to a pseudo US image, generated from gradients in segmented MR imagery. Toews et al. [5] register MR and US imagery using MI coupled with Bayesian estimation of image intensity distributions. Brooks et al. compute MI based on image gradients alone [6]. Reinertsen et al. [21] propose MR-US registration of brain images based on vasculature trees extracted in both modalities, using doppler US imagery to highlight blood vessels. Zhang et al. register MR-US cardiological imagery using the MI of local phase information [7]. Penney et al. propose estimating vasculature images independently from both US and MR modalities, which are then registered [22]. Letteboer et al. report registration success using standard MI between MR and US images, however suggest that incorporation of gradient information may be beneficial [23].

3   Registration via Location Marginalization

The Bayesian registration formulation presented in this section is based on the observation that although local image regions X are helpful in describing image content and the registration process, identifying meaningful regions or their correspondences between images is incidental to computing T. In probabilistic terms, local regions can thus be considered as nuisance variables. While the majority of techniques in the literature advocate maximizing a joint function of X and T, this approach does not generally result in the most probable T given the data. Intuitively, the most probable pair X, T may be determined by noisy, spurious instantiations of X which coincide with potentially incorrect or suboptimal values of T. Bayesian theory suggests X should instead be marginalized, in order to determine the most probable T given the images to be registered [24].

3.1   Bayesian Formulation

Image registration is the task of determining a geometrical mapping T between images I and J. Bayesian techniques typically pose registration as the posterior probability of T conditional on the image data to be registered [25]. Registration can then be computed by searching for the MAP transform T_{MAP} maximizing the posterior:

$$T_{MAP} = \operatorname*{argmax}_{T} \left\{ p(T|I, J) \right\}. \tag{1}$$

While the Bayesian posterior provides a principled probabilistic basis for registration, there are other variables which, although not specifically required for registration, may offer important sources of information. Local anatomical structures produce distinct, spatially localized intensity patterns which drive registration, e.g. sulci in brain imagery [11], and information regarding image location can be incorporated in order to improve registration. Here, we propose a random variable of spatial location X, defined over a set of discrete spatial regions within one of the images to be registered I. The posterior in Equation (1) can then be expressed as the marginalization of the joint posterior distribution of X and T given images I and J:

$$T_{MAP} = \operatorname*{argmax}_{T} \left\{ \int p(X, T | I, J) dX \right\}. \tag{2}$$

By marginalizing over X as in Equation (2), T_{MAP} can be obtained while leveraging important information regarding spatial location. The joint posterior in Equation (2) can be expressed as:

$$p(X, T | I, J) = \frac{p(I, J | X, T)}{p(I | X, J) p(J | X, T)} p(T | X, J) p(X | I, J), \tag{3}$$

$$= \frac{p(I, J | X, T)}{p(I | X) p(J | X, T)} p(T | X) p(X). \tag{4}$$

Here, Equation (3) results from standard definitions of conditional probability and Equation (4) results from the assumptions of conditional independence of T and J given X, independence of X and images I and J, and conditional independence of I and J given X. The factor $\frac{p(I, J | X, T)}{p(I | X) p(J | X, T)}$ contains all expressions relating to image data, and expresses the ratio of the joint probability of images associated with region X vs. their marginal probabilities. $p(X)$ is a prior probability over image regions, which can generally be defined according to relative sizes or overlap of regions X. $p(T | X)$, the conditional probability of T given X, can be defined to reflect the nature of the relationship between the specific transform and set of regions used.

3.2   Informative Region Selection

Utilizing local image regions requires a sampling scheme to determine X, and an ideal region sampling would represent a set of informative image patterns which can be localized with certainty in new images. Here, we develop a criterion to quantify both the informativeness and the localizability of image regions within a single image prior to registration. A mathematical link between Bayesian registration and the MI similarity measure motivates our MI-based selection criterion.

Bayesian Registration and Mutual Information: Although Bayesian techniques and the MI similarity measure [26, 27] are both widely used in medical image registration, their relationship is not immediately obvious. Maximum likelihood has been linked to joint entropy minimization [28] and MI maximization [29], here we provide a novel connection between Bayesian registration and MI maximization. To begin, recall the ratio $\frac{p(I,J|X,T)}{p(I|X)p(J|X,T)}$ in Equation (4) contains all factors relating to image intensity data. Discrete distributions of either marginal or joint pixel intensity events are naturally parameterized as multinomial distributions; let $m_1, \ldots, m_n$ represent counts for a set of n discrete events, obtained from an experiment resulting in M independent intensity samples. Furthermore, let $f_1, \ldots, f_n$ represent model parameters of a prior distribution associated with corresponding intensity events. The probability of observing a set of event *counts* is:

$$P = \frac{m_1! \ldots m_n!}{M!} \prod_i^n f_i^{m_i}, \tag{5}$$

where $\prod_i^n f_i^{m_i}$ represents the probability of a specific event sequence and $\frac{m_1! \ldots m_n!}{M!}$ is the multinomial coefficient. When parameters f_i are known with certainty, Equation (5) can be used directly to maximize the ratio $\frac{p(I,J|X,T)}{p(I|X)p(J|X,T)}$ with respect to T. Usually, however, f_i are unknown a priori. In this case, a maximum entropy prior can be specified such that $f_i = f_k, \forall (i, k)$, and the probability P in Equation (5) becomes solely a function of the event counts as specified by the multinomial coefficient. One can maximize this probability or a suitable monotonically increasing function thereof. In particular, as $M \to \infty$, the Sterling approximation of $M^{-1} \log P$ converges to the negative entropy of the empirical distribution over event counts [30]:

$$M^{-1} \log \frac{m_1! \ldots m_n!}{M!} \to \sum_i^n \frac{m_i}{M} \log \frac{m_i}{M} = -H. \tag{6}$$

The data term $\frac{p(I,J|X,T)}{p(I|X)p(J|X,T)}$ in Equation (4) can be approximated in a similar manner, leading to the standard expression for MI:

$$M \log \left\{ \frac{p(I, J|X, T)}{p(I|X)p(J|X, T)} \right\} \to H(I|X) + H(J|X, T) - H(I, J|X, T). \tag{7}$$

Mutual Information-based Region Selection: The previous section showed how the data term of a Bayesian registration formulation is tied to the mutual informativeness of regions to be matched. As the MI of images I and J is upper-bounded by the marginal entropy of individual images,

$$0 \leq MI(I, J) = H(I) + H(J) - H(I, J) \leq min\{H(I), H(J)\}, \tag{8}$$

intuition would suggest that selecting regions with high image entropy $H(I)$ would be beneficial for registration. This technique is proposed by Kadir et al. [10], who use the Shannon entropy of the intensity distribution within an image region as a measure of informativeness. While $H(I)$ measures the informativenss of the intensity distribution within an image region, it does not necessarily reflect the ability to register or localize the region in new images, as illustrated in Figure 1.

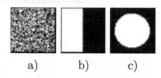

a)   b)   c)

Fig. 1. Images a), b) and c) represent three different binary images for which $H(I)$ is maximal. Image a) represents a region of homogenous image texture which may be unlocalizable. Image b) represents a boundary between two tissues, which may only be localizable in the direction normal to the boundary. Image c) represents a pattern whose localization can be constrained in all directions.

In particular, image intensity must be mutually informative with respect to image location, in order to correctly localize homologous regions in different images. We propose instead to quantify region informativeness in terms of the MI between image intensity I and spatial location S:

$$MI(I, S) = H(I) - H(I|S), \qquad (9)$$

where $H(I|S)$ represents the conditional entropy of I given spatial location:

$$H(I|S) = \sum_{i}^{n} p(S_i)H(I|S_i). \qquad (10)$$

In Equations (9) and (10), S represents a random variable of spatial location at sub-region image scale, defined over a set of n discrete spatial labels. As conditioning reduces entropy, $0 \leq H(I|S) \leq H(I)$ and thus $0 \leq MI(I, S) \leq H(I)$. Note that like the $H(I)$ criterion, the $MI(I, S)$ criterion in Equation (9) favors high entropy intensity distributions, however it imposes the additional constraint that the entropy of intensity conditioned on spatial location be low. The two criteria are thus equivalent when $H(I|S) = 0$, i.e. when the intensity distribution is perfectly predicted by spatial location.

An important implementation detail is to choose a suitable sub-region sampling scheme S. A generally useful sampling scheme would favor patterns which can be localized in space in an unbiased manner. We experiment with a two-class binary sampling scheme, where $p(S_1)$ and $p(S_2)$ are defined by Gaussian densities of differing variance $G(0, \sigma_1)$ and $G(0, \sigma_2)$. As Gaussian densities are rotationally symmetric, they are consistent with an uncommitted visual front-end feature extractor exhibiting no specific bias as to the orientation of image patterns [31]. Figure 2 illustrates the result of applying both criteria on a US image.

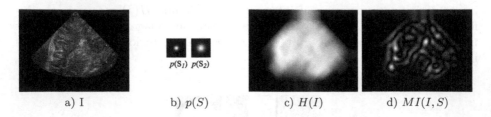

a) I b) $p(S)$ c) $H(I)$ d) $MI(I,S)$

Fig. 2. Image a) represents a transdural B-mode US slice of the brain. b) represents the distributions associated with the binary spatial variable S defined within a local region, where light regions indicate high $p(S)$. Images c) and d) represent the entropy $H(I)$ and $MI(I,S)$ criteria calculated at square regions of size 39 pixels in the US image. Note that most regions within the US fan in b) are of high $H(I)$, while a smaller number of US regions corresponding to distinctive image patterns in a) result in high $M(I,S)$.

4 Experiments

The context for experiments is an IGNS application, in which pre-operative anatomical MR imagery has been acquired and used as the basis for surgical planning. The brain may shift and deform over the course of surgery, invalidating the pre-operative MR imagery as a basis for guidance. The goal is thus to register intra-operative US imagery to the pre-operative MR, and thereby update the pre-operative MR imagery to correctly reflect changes due to brain shift. Brain shift correction and US-MR registration remain significant research challenges, due to the impoverished nature of the US modality.

The goals of the experiments are two-fold. First, location marginalization of X is compared with the alternative of registration in the absence of local regions. Second, region selection based on the $MI(I,S)$ criterion is compared with the alternatives of uniform sampling and selection based on the $H(I)$ criterion. Experiments involve registration trials aligning B-mode US slices acquired during surgery with a pre-operative MR image. The 3D position and orientation of US the probe are tracked externally and calibrated geometrically with respect to the pre-operative MRI within a neuronavigation system. The approximate geometry of the US slice relative to the MR volume can thus be established and used to evaluate registration accuracy with respect to ground truth. Experiments use a sequence of ten (320×240)-pixel US images acquired after skull removal but prior to opening the dura, in which brain deformation is relatively minor and ground truth can be considered reliable. Registration remains challenging, however, due the difficulty in modeling the US/MR intensity relationship, see Figure 3. As deformation is minimal, registration aims to recover T in the form of a global translation between the US image and the MR slice corresponding to the tracked position of the US probe. The data term $\frac{p(I,J|X,T)}{p(I|X)p(J|X,T)}$ is represented by the MI measure as in Equation (7). Factor $p(X)$ reflects the prior probability of image regions, which can generally be defined according to the relative sizes or overlap of regions. A set of regions of equal size is used here and $p(X)$ is thus taken to

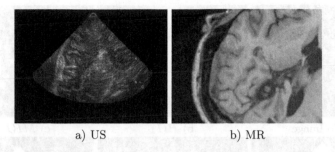

a) US   b) MR

Fig. 3. Images a) and b) illustrate an example of an US-MR image pair used in registration trials. Note the generally poor image quality of the US imagery.

be uniform. Finally, as T does not depend X in an obvious manner and we have no particular prior assumptions regarding T, and so $p(T|X) = p(T)$ is taken to be a uniform distribution.

To cope with the issue of data sparsity when calculating MI at a local scale, image intensities are first transformed into a mixture model over a small set of tissue classes as in [32]. Briefly, let $C = \{C_1, \ldots, C_K\}$ represent a discrete random variable over K tissue classes. Mixture modeling and expectation-maximization [33] can be used to estimate a set of class labels and associated parameters that maximize the likelihood of the image data I:

$$p(I) = \sum_i^K p(I|C_i)p(C_i). \tag{11}$$

Once the parameters of mixture components in (11) are estimated, a conditional probability distribution over class labels can be associated with each image intensity I:

$$p(C|I) \propto p(I|C)p(C). \tag{12}$$

Here, the K-means algorithm [33] is used to estimate Gaussian class-conditional densities $p(I|C_i)$. $K = 3$ tissue classes are used in experiments, and thus the size of the joint intensity histogram is $3 \times 3 = 9$. Varying K between 2-5 labels does not significantly affect registration accuracy, larger numbers of labels result in higher computational complexity however.

For each trial, local regions X are first defined in the US image as shown in Figure 4. The posterior is then calculated at all discrete pixel displacements T between the US image and its corresponding slice in the 3D MR volume, as determined by the geometry of the tracked US probe. In the case of the marginalized posterior, Equation (2) is evaluated by integrating over X for each displacement T. The results of registration based on various registration formulations and selection strategies are listed in Table 1. Note that MI-based region selection and localization marginalization results in both the highest number of successes (9 out of 10) and the lowest mean error. Incorporating no local regions resulted the fewest successes and high mean error. On this data, entropy-based region selection results in fewer successes and higher mean error than uniform sampling.

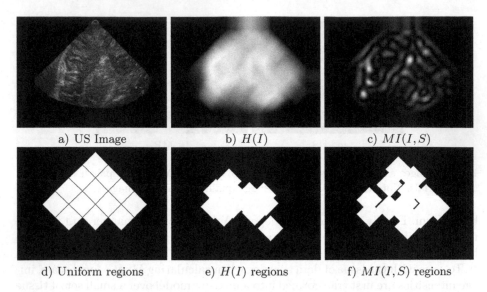

a) US Image   b) $H(I)$ c) $MI(I, S)$

d) Uniform regions   e) $H(I)$ regions f) $MI(I, S)$ regions

Fig. 4. a) is a US image, images b) and c) are entropy and MI region selection criteria evaluated at all pixel locations in image a). Images d)-f) illustrate the three region sampling/selection strategies applied to the US image. For each strategy, 13 diamond-shaped regions of size 39×39 are chosen in the US image. Region size is determined empirically, smaller regions tend to result in spurious matching and larger regions tend to be poorly localized. 13 regions are used to uniformly sample the US image in c), and automatic selection identifies the 13 image regions with the highest value of the particular criterion in d) and e). A minimum distance of 20 pixels is enforced between automatically selected regions to ensure even distribution throughout the image.

Table 1. Results for registration trials. A trial is considered successful if T_{MAP} is a global maximum, i.e. corresponds to the peak of the posterior closest to the known ground truth displacement. The mean and standard deviation are calculated for successfully identified T_{MAP} solutions.

Selection Technique	Registration Formulation	Successes (out of 10)	Error Mean (pix)	Error Stdev (pix)
$MI(I\|S)$	$\underset{T}{\operatorname{argmax}}\left\{\int p(T, X\|I, J)dX\right\}$	9	2.5	1.7
Uniform	$\underset{T}{\operatorname{argmax}}\left\{\int p(T, X\|I, J)dX\right\}$	9	3.3	1.9
$H(I)$	$\underset{T}{\operatorname{argmax}}\left\{\int p(T, X\|I, J)dX\right\}$	8	4.1	2.6
-	$\underset{T}{\operatorname{argmax}}\left\{p(T\|I, J)\right\}$	6	3.9	2.9

5   Discussion

This paper investigates a framework for the use of local image regions in registration, based on probability and information theory. Local regions are incorporated into a Bayesian registration framework in order to improve the ability to cope with missing tissue and non-stationary image intensity characteristics. Local region information is represented as a nuisance random variable, which is marginalized in order to obtain the MAP transform relating images. A novel link between a Bayesian registration formulation and the MI similarity measure is outlined, showing how MI results from the Bayesian data factor when the distribution of intensity events is modeled by a maximum entropy prior. This in turn motivates a new criterion for identifying a set of informative and localizable image regions for registration, the MI of intensity and location, which generalizes the entropy-based criterion of Kadir et al. [10].

A challenge of marginalizing location is computing the integral over local regions. Experiments here recover global translation via efficient numerical integration, where computation time is linear in the image size and in the number of regions used. Efficient marginalization with more complicated transforms could be addressed via coarse-to-fine methods or Monte Carlo integration, depending on the class of transforms used. The MI-based feature selection criterion is currently evaluated at a fixed image window size, but could be used to automatically determine more elaborate descriptions of local region geometry, including region size or shape, in order identify a wider variety of local image structures.

Acknowledgements

This work was funded in part by NIH grants U41 RR019703 and P41 RR13218, and by an NSERC postdoctoral fellowship. Image data was provided by D. Louis Collins of the Montreal Neurological Institute. Catherine Laporte was involved in helpful discussions regarding ultrasound.

References

1. Hajnal, et al. (eds.): Medical Image Registration. CRC Press, Boca Raton (2003)
2. Clatz, O., et al.: Robust nonrigid registration to capture brain shift from intraoperative MRI. IEEE TMI 24(11) (2005)
3. Ng, J., et al.: Modelling ultrasound imaging as a linear, shift-variant system. IEEE Trans. on Ultrasonics, Ferroelectrics and Frequency Control 53(3), 549–563 (2006)
4. Cachier, P., et al.: Iconic feature based nonrigid registration: the PASHA algorithm. CVIU 89(2-3), 272–298 (2003)
5. Toews, M., et al.: Maximum a posteriori local histogram estimation for image registration. In: Duncan, J.S., Gerig, G. (eds.) MICCAI 2005. LNCS, vol. 3750, pp. 163–170. Springer, Heidelberg (2005)
6. Brooks, R., et al.: Deformable Ultrasound Registration without Reconstruction. In: MICCAI, pp. 1023–1031 (2008)
7. Zhang, W., et al.: Adaptive non-rigid registration of real time 3D ultrasound to cardiovascular MR images. In: Karssemeijer, N., Lelieveldt, B. (eds.) IPMI 2007. LNCS, vol. 4584, pp. 50–61. Springer, Heidelberg (2007)
8. Loeckx, D., et al.: Nonrigid image registration using conditional mutual information. In: Karssemeijer, N., Lelieveldt, B. (eds.) IPMI 2007. LNCS, vol. 4584, pp. 725–737. Springer, Heidelberg (2007)

9. Wein, W., et al.: Automatic CT-ultrasound registration for diagnostic imaging and image-guided intervention. Medical Image Analysis 12, 577–585 (2008)
10. Kadir, T., et al.: Saliency, scale and image description. IJCV 45(2), 83–105 (2001)
11. Hellier, P., et al.: Coupling dense and landmark-based approaches for non rigid registration. IEEE TMI 22(2), 217–227 (2003)
12. Rohr, K., et al.: Landmark-based elastic registration using approximating thin-plate splines. IEEE TMI 20(6), 526–534 (2001)
13. Lowe, D.G.: Distinctive image features from scale-invariant keypoints. IJCV 60(2), 91–110 (2004)
14. Mikolajczyk, K., et al.: Scale and affine invariant interest point detectors. IJCV 60(1), 63–86 (2004)
15. Wagner, R.F., et al.: Statistics of speckle in ultrasound B-scans. IEEE Transactions on Sonics and Ultrasonics 30(3), 156–163 (1983)
16. Coupe, P., et al.: Bayesian non local means-based speckle filtering. In: ISBI, pp. 1291–1294 (2008)
17. Thijssen, J.M.: Ultrasonic speckle formation, analysis and processing applied to tissue characterization. Pattern Recognition Letters 24(4-5), 659–675 (2003)
18. Milko, S., et al.: Segmentation of the liver in ultrasound: a dynamic texture approach. Int. J. of Computer Assisted Radiology and Surgery 3(1-2), 143–150 (2008)
19. Roche, A., et al.: Rigid registration of 3D ultrasound with MR images: a new approach combining intensity and gradient information. IEEE TMI 20(10), 1038–1049 (2001)
20. Arbel, T., et al.: Automatic non-linear MRI-ultrasound registration for the correction of intra-operative brain deformations. Comput. Aided Surg. 9(4), 123–136 (2004)
21. Reinertsen, I., et al.: Validation of vessel-based registration for correction of brain shift. Medical Image Analysis 11(4), 374–388 (2007)
22. Penney, G., et al.: Registration of freehand 3D ultrasound and magnetic resonance liver images. Medical Image Analysis (8), 81–91 (2004)
23. Letteboer, M., et al.: Brain shift estimation in image-guided neurosurgery using 3-D ultrasound. IEEE Transactions on Biomedical Engineering 52(2), 268–276 (2005)
24. Gelman, A., et al.: Bayesian Data Analysis. Chapman & Hall/CRC, Boca Raton (2000)
25. Gee, J., et al.: Probabilistic matching of brain images. In: IPMI (1995)
26. Wells, W., et al.: Multi-modal volume registration by maximization of mutual information. MIA 1, 35–52 (1996)
27. Maes, F., et al.: Multimodality image registration by maximization of mutual information. IEEE TMI 16(2), 187–198 (1997)
28. Zollei, L., et al.: A marginalized map approach and em optimization for pair-wise registration. In: Karssemeijer, N., Lelieveldt, B. (eds.) IPMI 2007. LNCS, vol. 4584, pp. 662–674. Springer, Heidelberg (2007)
29. Roche, A., et al.: Unifying maximum likelihood approaches in medical image registration. IJIST 11, 71–80 (2000)
30. Jaynes, E.: Prior probabilities. IEEE Transactions on systems, science, and cybernetics SSC-4(3), 227–241 (1968)
31. Romeny, B.t.H.: Front-End Vision and Multi-Scale Image Analysis. Kluwer Academic Publisher, Dordrecht (2003)
32. D'Agostino, E., et al.: An information theoretic approach for non-rigid image registration using voxel class probabilities. In: Ellis, R.E., Peters, T.M. (eds.) MICCAI 2003. LNCS, vol. 2879, pp. 812–820. Springer, Heidelberg (2003)
33. Duda, R.O., et al.: Pattern classification, 2nd edn. Wiley, Chichester (2001)

A Non-rigid Registration Framework That Accommodates Resection and Retraction

Petter Risholm[1,2], Eigil Samset[1], Ion-Florin Talos[2], and William Wells[2]

[1] Center of Mathematics for Applications, University of Oslo
pettri@bwh.harvard.edu
[2] Harvard Medical School, Brigham and Womens Hospital

Abstract. Traditional non-rigid registration algorithms are incapable of accurately registering intra-operative with pre-operative images whenever tissue has been resected or retracted. In this work we present methods for detecting and handling retraction and resection. The registration framework is based on the bijective Demons algorithm using an anisotropic diffusion smoother. Retraction is detected at areas of the deformation field with high internal strain and the estimated retraction boundary is integrated as a diffusion boundary in the smoother to allow discontinuities to develop across the resection boundary. Resection is detected by a level set method evolving in the space where image intensities disagree. The estimated resection is integrated into the smoother as a diffusion sink to restrict image forces originating inside the resection from being diffused to surrounding areas. In addition, the deformation field is continuous across the diffusion sink boundary which allow us to move the boundary of the diffusion sink without changing values in the deformation field (no interpolation or extrapolation is needed). We present preliminary results on both synthetic and clinical data which clearly shows the added value of explicitly modeling these processes in a registration framework.

1 Introduction

The most common approach to image guided neurosurgery is the integration of pre-operative anatomical and functional images, as well as planned retraction and resection boundaries, with a neurosurgical navigation system which guides the surgeon during surgery. However, considerable brain-shifts due to various factors such as gravity, edema, tumor mass effect and cerebrospinal fluid leakage have been reported after the craniotomy and opening of the dura[1]. This decreases the intra-operative accuracy of these navigation systems significantly. Secondly, as a result of resection and retraction, additional morphological changes occur which render the pre-operative images obsolete with respect to the real intra-operative anatomy. The introduction of intra-operative MR scanners has provided the surgeon with anatomically correct images intra-operatively which facilitates a more aggressive resection. Unfortunately, intra-operative MR scanners are not typically capable of providing accurate functional information

J.L. Prince, D.L. Pham, and K.J. Myers (Eds.): IPMI 2009, LNCS 5636, pp. 447–458, 2009.

during a procedure. Hence, mapping the pre-operative image data to reflect intra-operative anatomy will increase the accuracy of the neurosurgical navigation system and hopefully improve the outcome of the neurosurgical procedure. Numerous nonrigid registration algorithms have been proposed to handle brain shifts. However, there are only a limited number of methods proposed to handle retraction and resection. Retraction and resection pose two different challenges – retraction requires the algorithm to facilitate development of discontinuities in the deformation field along the retraction boundary while resection necessitates the algorithm to handle data which is present in the pre-operative image but missing in the intra-operative image.

In [2] Periaswamy et al proposed a registration framework which handles missing data by applying the expectation maximization method to iteratively estimate the missing data and the registration parameters. However, their missing data model does not constrain the localization of the missing data in any way. For modeling of resection one can assume that data is not sporadically missing throughout the image, but confined to a single area. Miga et al proposed in [3] to use a bio-mechanical model to handle resection and retraction. They applied no automatic means of detecting the missing data due to resection or the retracted areas; they manually delineated the resected area and used a calibrated microscope to determine the position of the retractor during surgery. Bio-mechanical models are frequently simulated with finite element methods (FEM) which require a tessellation of the image domain. FEM based methods with automatic detection of retraction and resection require retessellation during the registration procedure which is a non-trivial and time consuming process and thus may not be very practical for intra-operative registration.

The demons algorithm[4] has over the last decade proven to be a fast, accurate and robust monomodal non-rigid registration algorithm[5]. It can be viewed as a two-stage energy minimization technique[6]. First it finds an unconstrained dense deformation field which matches the images whereupon it regularizes the deformation field to an elastic or fluid deformation by smoothing it with a Gaussian low-pass filter. In his original paper, Thirion pointed out that Gaussian smoothing can be interpreted as a diffusion process. In [7] Perona and Malik proposed a smoothing filter modeled by a non-linear anisotropic diffusion process where diffusion can be restricted across boundaries. We will show how the flexibility of this diffusion based smoother can be exploited to handle resection and retraction. In particular, we will model resection by what we have termed a *diffusion sink* and retraction with a *diffusion boundary*. Some of the ideas we have applied in our work are influenced by developments in the vision literature on handling occlusions and discontinuities in the estimation of optical flow[8].

2   Methods

2.1   Registration

Demons Registration. We wish to register two monomodal images, a preoperative image $P(x), x \in \Omega_P$ with an intra-operative image $I(x), x \in \Omega_I$ where

Ω_P and Ω_I are the pre-operative and intra-operative image domains respectively. By posing the registration as a diffusion process, the demons algorithm[4] is effective at finding the deformation $U_{IP}(x) = x + u_{IP}(x)$, where u_{IP} is a displacement field, which puts P into agreement with I. It is a two-step iterative method where the first step consist of finding an unconstrained velocity field with an optical flow computation followed by a smoothing step to regularize the deformation. The velocity field is computed by

$$v_{IP}^n(x) = \frac{(P \circ U_{IP}^{n-1}(x) - I(x))\nabla I(x)}{(P \circ U_{IP}^{n-1}(x) - I(x))^2 + |\nabla I(x)|^2} , \qquad (1)$$

where $\circ$ denotes composition. The regularization step, consisting of the application of a smoothing filter S can either be applied to the updated deformation field to achieve an elastic deformation $U_{IP}^n(x) = S(v_{IP}^n(x) + U_{IP}^{n-1}(x))$, or directly to the update which will result in a fluid deformation:

$$U_{IP}^n(x) = U_{IP}^{n-1}(x) + S(v_{IP}^n(x)) . \qquad (2)$$

In the traditional Demons algorithm, the smoother S is typically a Gaussian low-pass filter. This two-stage process proceeds until a convergence criterion is reached. The fluid version of the demons algorithm was applied for this work because of its ability to handle large deformations. In the following, whenever it is clear from the context, we will drop the dependence on x.

Bijective Demons. Because of the asymmetry in Eq. (1), there is no guarantee the final deformation field will be bijective. That is, if we compute U_{IP} and U_{PI} then there is no guarantee that $U_{IP} \circ U_{PI} = Id_{\Omega_I}$ or $U_{PI} \circ U_{IP} = Id_{\Omega_P}$ where Id_{Ω_i} denotes the identity over the domain Ω_i. A general way of enforcing bijectivity of a deformation field is to put the constraint $|J| > 0$ on the Jacobian matrix of the deformation field. However, it is computationally intensive to enforce this constraint[9]. Thirion[4] suggested a simpler solution where U_{IP}^*, U_{PI}^* and the residual $r_{PI} = u_{PI}^* + u_{IP}^* \circ U_{PI}^*$ are all calculated at each iteration. By subtracting half the residual from both deformation fields one can constrain them to be bijective: $U_{PI}^n = U_{PI}^{n,*} - \frac{1}{2}r_{PI}^n$ and $U_{IP}^n = U_{IP}^{n,*} - \frac{1}{2}r_{PI}^n \circ U_{IP}^{n,*}$.

Not only does this enforce bijectivity, it also provides us with the inverse deformation fields $U_{PI} = U_{IP}^{-1}$ and $U_{IP} = U_{PI}^{-1}$ for little extra computational cost. We will model retraction by allowing discontinuities to develop at certain areas of the deformation fields in such a way that r_{PI} will be close to zero while r_{IP} will have large residuals around the area of the discontinuity (see Fig. 1). Hence, we can guarantee that $U_{IP} \circ U_{PI} = Id_{\Omega_I}$, but conversely we will have $U_{PI} \circ U_{IP} \neq Id_{\Omega_P}$ around this area.

Directional Diffusion as a Smoothing Process. Mathematically the diffusion process can be formulated as $\frac{\partial}{\partial t}q(x, t) = \nabla \cdot (C(x)\nabla q(x, t))$, where C controls the diffusion strength. Let us discretize this equation in 1D:

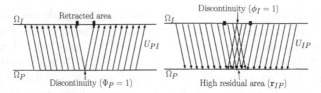

Fig. 1. Whenever an area in Ω_P is found where the strain in the deformation field exceeds a certain threshold, this point is added as boundary in the smoother to enable a discontinuity to develop in Ω_P. This can be seen in the *left* figure. At the same time, the corresponding boundary is placed in Ω_I which is shown in the *right* figure. Notice that the residual r_{IP} will be very large at the areas of retraction, something which can be effectively used to approximate the width of the retracted area.

$$\frac{\partial}{\partial t}q(x,t) = \nabla \cdot [C(x)\nabla q(x,t)] \tag{3}$$

$$= \frac{1}{\Delta x^2}\left[C\left(x+\frac{\Delta x}{2}\right)(q(x+\Delta x,t) - q(x,t))\right.$$

$$\left. - C\left(x-\frac{\Delta x}{2}\right)(q(x,t) - q(x-\Delta x,t))\right] . \tag{4}$$

At each point we calculate directional differences (East and West). We generalize the traditional diffusion model in Eq. (4) by introducing a separate conductance function for each direction:

$$\frac{1}{\Delta x^2}(C_E(x+\frac{\Delta x}{2})(q(x+\Delta x,t) - q(x,t))$$

$$- C_W(x-\frac{\Delta x}{2})(q(x,t) - q(x-\Delta x,t))) . \tag{5}$$

To ease readability we rewrite Eq. (5) as $\frac{1}{\Delta x^2}(\Lambda_E(x,t) - \Lambda_W(x,t))$. By using upwind differencing on the left hand side the update equation becomes $q(x,t+1) = q(x,t) + \mu(\Lambda_E(x,t) - \Lambda_W(x,t))$, where $\mu = \frac{\Delta t}{\Delta x^2}$. It becomes evident from Eq. (5) that a directional difference eastwards is analogous to diffusion in the opposite direction. We will operate with a separate conductance map for each diffusion direction. For the 2D case we will have C_E, C_W, C_N and C_S (due to space constraints we will refer to them collectively as $C_{E|W|N|S}$) which provides flexibility in restricting diffusion. One can for instance allow diffusion in one direction while restricting diffusion in the opposite direction which will prove useful for modeling a diffusion sink. The conductance term can be modeled in different ways[7]. We model the conductance in a certain direction at point x through the relation $C_{E|W|N|S}(x) = 1 - B_{E|W|N|S}(x)$, where $B_{E|W|N|S}$ are binary directional boundary maps specifying whether a diffusion boundary should occur at position x. Update Eq. (2) can thereby be rewritten as

$$U_{IP}^n = U_{IP}^{n-1} + S\left(v_{IP}^n; \mu, \eta, B_{E|W|N|S}\right) , \tag{6}$$

where η defines the number of diffusion iterations.

Diffusion Boundary. To accommodate for the development of discontinuities along a retraction path, the tear due to retraction will be modeled as a diffusion boundary. Let us define a label map

$$\Phi(\boldsymbol{p}) = \begin{cases} 1, \text{ if } \boldsymbol{p} \text{ is located on the tear.} \\ 0, \text{ otherwise.} \end{cases} \qquad (7)$$

for $\boldsymbol{p}$ on the lattice $(1 + m\frac{\Delta x}{2}, 1 + n\frac{\Delta y}{2}), m = 1 \ldots M - 1, n = 1 \ldots N - 1$ in Ω_P. To restrict diffusion across the tear and thereby allow a discontinuity to develop, values in Φ are incorporated into the directional boundary maps as follows:

$$B_{E|W}\left(x + \frac{\Delta x}{2}, y\right) = \begin{cases} 1, \text{ if } \Phi(x + \frac{\Delta x}{2}, y - \frac{\Delta y}{2}) + \Phi(x + \frac{\Delta x}{2}, y + \frac{\Delta y}{2}) = 2 \\ 0, \text{ otherwise} \end{cases} \quad (8)$$

$$B_{N|S}\left(x, y + \frac{\Delta y}{2}\right) = \begin{cases} 1, \text{ if } \Phi(x + \frac{\Delta x}{2}, y + \frac{\Delta y}{2}) + \Phi(x - \frac{\Delta x}{2}, y + \frac{\Delta y}{2}) = 2 \\ 0, \text{ otherwise} \end{cases} \quad (9)$$

Diffusion Sink. Another diffusion restriction which will prove useful for modeling resection is what we have termed a diffusion sink. A diffusion sink is basically an area $\Omega_{R_I} \in \Omega_I$ (resected area) where diffusion is allowed into the area and not out of it. This diffusion sink provides us with a number of nice properties 1) the deformation field will be continuous across the boundary of Ω_{R_I} denoted by $\partial \Omega_{R_I}$, 2) even though a pixel is initially labeled as resected it might change label to non-resected later in the registration procedure. Because the deformation field is continuous across $\partial \Omega_{R_I}$ we can move the boundary of the diffusion sink without changing values in the deformation field (no interpolation from the deformations on $\partial \Omega_{R_I}$ to the areas which changed label from resected to non-resected) and 3) unwanted demon forces occurring within Ω_{R_I} will not affect areas outside. Let us define a label map, Ψ, on the lattice $(m\Delta x, n\Delta y), m = 1 \ldots M, n = 1 \ldots N$ which takes on values 1 at locations assumed to be resected and 0 at locations outside the resection. A diffusion sink can then be incorporated in the anisotropic diffusion by using the following directional boundaries for the x-direction:

$$B_E\left(x + \frac{\Delta x}{2}, y\right) = |\Psi(x, y) - \Psi(x + \Delta x, y)|(1 - \Psi(x, y)) \qquad (10)$$

$$B_W\left(x - \frac{\Delta x}{2}, y\right) = |\Psi(x, y) - \Psi(x - \Delta x, y)|(1 - \Psi(x, y)), \qquad (11)$$

and the boundaries, B_N and B_S, for the y-direction are derived similarly. Figure 2 provides examples of applying diffusion boundaries and a diffusion sink to a smoothing problem.

2.2 Modeling Retraction

Tearing of tissue has been modeled in surgical simulators where tissue tears whenever the strain/stress of the deformation applied to the tissue exceeds a certain threshold[10]. We apply a similar model – around the area of retraction,

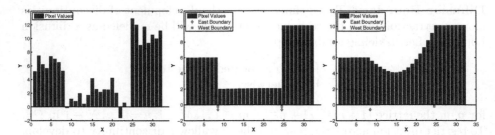

Fig. 2. The *left* plot shows three different compartments, each having a mean value of $y = 6, 2, 10$ with uniform noise added to it. One approach for modeling diffusion here would be to add diffusion boundaries between the compartments. The *middle* plot includes the results from running this through the diffusion filter ($\eta = 100, \mu = 0.2$). Notice that values have effectively been confined to their respective compartments which has resulted in discontinuities at the boundaries. We will use this concept for modeling retraction. Another approach is to model the middle compartment as a diffusion sink which allows diffusion into the compartment but not out of it. The *right* figure shows results from running the diffusion filter on this case. Notice the continuous values across the boundaries between the compartments and that none of the information from the middle compartment has diffused into the two neighboring compartments.

where there are discontinuities in the movement of tissue, our assumption is that a considerable strain will build up in the deformation field as the registration algorithm proceeds to match the images (see Fig. 1). The general idea is to let the registration proceed until a location in Ω_P is found where the strain exceeds a certain threshold. From this location the tear is propagated along the direction normal to the direction of maximal strain until the strain drops below the threshold. The algorithm proceeds by iterating between registering the images and estimating the tear.

Detecting Tearing of Deformation Field. For in-plane problems the strain tensor can be expressed as

$$\varepsilon(\boldsymbol{x}) = \begin{bmatrix} \varepsilon_{xx}\ \varepsilon_{xy} \\ \varepsilon_{xy}\ \varepsilon_{yy} \end{bmatrix} = \begin{bmatrix} \dfrac{\partial \boldsymbol{u}_x}{\partial x} & \dfrac{\partial \boldsymbol{u}_x}{\partial y} + \dfrac{\partial \boldsymbol{u}_y}{\partial x} \\ \dfrac{\partial \boldsymbol{u}_x}{\partial y} + \dfrac{\partial \boldsymbol{u}_y}{\partial x} & \dfrac{\partial \boldsymbol{u}_y}{\partial y} \end{bmatrix}. \tag{12}$$

At an area of retraction in Ω_P, deformation vectors on different sides of the retraction in $\boldsymbol{U}_{PI}$ will point towards each other. Hence, the minimum eigenvalue and the corresponding eigenvector, $\lambda(\boldsymbol{x})$ and $\boldsymbol{v}(\boldsymbol{x})$, of the strain tensor in Ω_P determines the direction and magnitude of maximum strain. At each iteration of the registration procedure we compute the minimum eigenvalue $\lambda(\boldsymbol{p})$ and the corresponding eigenvector $\boldsymbol{v}(\boldsymbol{p})$ of the strain at interpixel locations $(1+m\frac{\Delta x}{2}, 1+ n\frac{\Delta y}{2})$, $m = 1 \ldots M-1$ and $n = 1 \ldots N-1$. Should the minimum eigenvalue over the whole image, $\lambda_{\min} = \min_{\boldsymbol{p} \in \Omega_P}(\lambda(\boldsymbol{p}))$ be less than the strain threshold τ, $\boldsymbol{p}$ and the corresponding displacement $\boldsymbol{u}_{PI}(\boldsymbol{p})$ are added to the lists ι_p and ι_d respectively. The data in these lists will be used to transfer the estimated tear to Ω_I. From this point of maximum strain, the tear is propagated along the two directions, n and $-n$, normal to the direction of maximum strain v to a new point p'. If $\lambda(p') < \tau$ the lists ι_p and ι_d are updated and the next step will be in the corresponding new direction n'. When a point is reached where $\lambda \geq \tau$ the tear tracking process stops.

If we expect negligible deformations around the tear due to brain shift (for instance when registering images taken after craniotomy with images acquired after resection/retraction) this estimation of the tear will be quite reliable. Whenever there is a considerable brainshift as well, the tear estimation is more likely to be stuck in a local minimum or diverge from the real tear. To add some robustness to the detection of the tear and to reduce the importance of choosing a suitable τ we incorporate some a-priori information in the retraction estimation. A line originating from the tumor center t_c in the pre-operative image is fitted to the points in ι_p weighted by the amount of strain (minimum eigenvalue) at this point. Assuming we have a model of the tumor in Ω_P and may know the length of the retractor, the part of the line which is represented by the retractor can easily be estimated.

Because the tearing is calculated in Ω_P, it is also necessary to estimate the tear in Ω_I to enable calculations of U_{IP} using the bijective demons algorithm. We estimate the corresponding tear in Ω_I by fitting a line going through $u_{PI}(t_c) + t_c$ to the points $\iota_p(k) + \iota_d(k), k = 1 \ldots K$, where K denotes the number of points along the tear. The part of the lines which are estimated to be representing the retraction is embedded in the boundary map Φ and transferred into directional boundaries by applying Eqs. (8)-(9). The algorithm then proceeds by alternating between registering the images and estimating the tear.

Determining the Retracted Area. Once a tear has been detected and added as a diffusion boundary, discontinuities will occur in both U_{PI} and U_{IP}. As the residuals, r_{PI}, in the bijective demons algorithm are computed in the pre-operative image domain, we will not see large residuals around the area of the tear (see Fig. 1). However, if the residual is computed in Ω_I, large residuals will appear in the area where tissue has been retracted. A simple thresholding scheme provides a good approximation of the area of retraction in the intra operative image.

$$\Gamma_I(x) = \begin{cases} 1, \text{ if } r_{IP}(x) > \frac{1}{N} \sum_{p \in \Omega_I} |r_{IP}^2(p)| \\ 0, \text{ otherwise} \end{cases} \tag{13}$$

2.3   Modeling Resection

We wish to register a pre-operative image, P, with an intra-operative image, I, under the assumption that an area (volume in 3D) of tissue, $\Omega_{R_P} \subset \Omega_P$ is present in P but is missing in I. The corresponding resected area in I will be denoted by $\Omega_{R_I} \subset \Omega_I$. One can make a few assumptions about the areas Ω_{R_I} and Ω_{R_P}: 1) we will in general have large intensity disagreements $(I(x) - (P \circ U_{IP})(x)), x \in \Omega_{R_I}$ in the area of resected tissue, 2) large image gradients, ∇I, will be present along $\partial \Omega_{R_I}$, the boundary of the resected tissue, 3) there might be some smaller image gradients inside Ω_{R_I} due to blood or other fluids in the resected cavity, 4) image gradients in and around Ω_{RP} can be substantial due to a contrast enhanced tumor. These assumptions lead to unwanted forces being generated in and around Ω_{RI} and Ω_{RP} which will most likely lead the algorithm to converge to an incorrect result. Large image intensity disagreements are expected to be present inside the resected area which enables us to capture this area using a level set approach evolving in the space of image intensity disagreements. We incorporate Ω_{RI} and Ω_{RP} as diffusion sinks in the bijective demons approach. The general idea is to alternate between performing the registration under the constraint of the diffusion sinks and approximating the area of resected tissue with a level set formulation.

Determining the Resected Area. We are interested in propagating a front $\eta(t) \subset \Omega_I$ in time along its normal direction $\mathbf{n}$ until it embeds Ω_{RI}. In the level set formulation [11] this is achieved by embedding the front, η, as a zero level set of a time varying higher dimensional function

$$\phi(\mathbf{x}, t) = dist(\mathbf{x}, \eta(t)), \mathbf{x} \in \Omega_I \tag{14}$$

where the function $dist$ computes the signed distance d from $\mathbf{x}$ to the front η. If $\mathbf{x}$ is inside the front then $d < 0$ and if $\mathbf{x}$ is outside the front, $d > 0$. Let us define the label map

$$\Psi_I^k(\mathbf{x}, t) = \begin{cases} 1, & \phi(\mathbf{x}, t) \leq k, \mathbf{x} \in \Omega_I \\ 0, & \phi(\mathbf{x}, t) > k, \mathbf{x} \in \Omega_I \end{cases} \tag{15}$$

where Ψ_I^0 labels all pixels within the front as 1 (resected) and all pixels outside the front as 0 (non-resected) at time t. We will denote the area where $\Psi_I^k(\mathbf{x}, t) = 1$ by $\Omega_{\eta(t)}^k$. The level set function evolves according to the partial differential equation

$$\phi_t = b\kappa|\nabla\phi| - a|\nabla\phi| . \tag{16}$$

On the right hand side we have two terms. The first term moves the front proportional to its curvature while the second term moves the front in the normal direction with a speed and direction determined by a. To maintain the property of ϕ being a distance function, it is necessary to reinitialize the levelset function using Eq. (14) at regular time intervals. We are interested in $\Omega_{\eta(t)}^k$ being the best possible approximation of the resected area, Ω_{RI}, at every step of the algorithm. To achieve this we model the normal velocity of the front as

$$a(\mathbf{x}) = (1 - \Gamma_I(\mathbf{x}))|\mathbf{I}(\mathbf{x}) - (\mathbf{P} \circ \mathbf{U}_{IP})(\mathbf{x})|e^{-|\nabla\mathbf{I}|/\sigma} - \rho, \mathbf{x} \in \Omega_I . \tag{17}$$

The middle term makes the interface expand fast where there is a large intensity disagreement, the exponential will effectively stop the propagation of the front at large gradients (such as at $\partial\Omega_{RI}$). Due to the exponential, the evolution of the front will stop right before reaching $\partial\Omega_{RI}$ hence Ψ_I^0 will consistently underestimate the real resection. We use Ψ_I^1 as the estimate of Ω_{RI}. After the levelset evolution converges for the first time we will most likely have $\Omega_{\eta(t)}^1 \supset \Omega_{RI}$. As the algorithm progresses, more and more of $\Omega_{\eta(t)}^1 \setminus \Omega_{RI}$ will find its corresponding area in the pre-operative image and result in a good image intensity agreement.

This requires the front to shrink in this area to relabel it as non-resected which is modeled by ρ. The first term becomes zero in the area of retraction where we want the front to contract. It is important to balance the magnitude of ρ versus the magnitude of the intensity difference term such that a large intensity disagreement results in a positive a, while a good agreement results in a negative a.

Registration Constrained by a Diffusion Sink. In the classical demons method, the computed forces are diffused over the whole image domain. Whenever unwanted or incorrect image forces occur due to for instance resection, they will be propagated throughout the image by the Gaussian filter which will result in an incorrect deformation field. To prevent the forces occurring on and within $\partial \Omega_{R_I}$ from being diffused into the non-resected areas we use an over-estimation of the resected area, Ψ_I^3, as a diffusion sink in the smoothing component of the registration.

Because of the dual nature of the bijective demons method, the label map $\Psi_I^k(\boldsymbol{x})$ also needs to be defined in Ω_P:

$$\Psi_P^k(\boldsymbol{x}) = (\Psi_I^k \circ \boldsymbol{U}_{PI})(\boldsymbol{x}) \ . \tag{18}$$

The directional diffusion boundaries in both image domains are computed by Eqs. (10)-(11).

2.4 Algorithm

To capture large deformations and speed up the algorithm, the registration method was integrated in a 3-level multi-resolution pyramid with a subsampling factor of 2. Modeling of retraction and resection was only applied on the lowest level of the pyramid while the two higher levels were used to get a good initial non-rigid deformation field. The algorithm applied to the lowest level of the pyramid can be summarized as follows:

Initialize the levelset function with Eq. (14) and the initial front $\eta(0)$.

while $\sum_{\boldsymbol{x}}(\boldsymbol{I}(\boldsymbol{x}) - \boldsymbol{P} \circ \boldsymbol{U}_{IP}(\boldsymbol{x}))^2 >$ SSDThreshold **do**
    Propagate tear as explained in Sec. 2.2.
    Evolve the levelsets using Eqs. (16) and (17).
    Extract resected area using Eqs. (15) and (18).
    Compute $B_{E|W|N|S}$ according to Eqs. (8)-(11).
    Calculate $\boldsymbol{U}_{PI}^i$ and $\boldsymbol{U}_{IP}^i$ using the bijective demons and Eq. (6).
end while

3 Results

In this section we present preliminary results from applying the algorithm on 2D image data. All images used to generate results had a resolution of 256x256 with pixel intensities in the interval $[0, 1]$. The level set parameters, $b = 0.2, \rho = 0.1$ and $\sigma = 0.01$, diffusion filter parameters, $\mu = 0.2$, and $\eta = 170$ and strain threshold, $\tau = -0.4$, were applied for all experiments.

3.1 Experiments on Synthetic Data

To facilitate quantitative evaluation of how the algorithm handles both resection and retraction an artificial data set with a known deformation field was generated. The deformation field U_{IP} was generated by defining the displacements occurring on $\partial \Omega_{R_I}$ and $\partial \Omega_{T_I}$, where Ω_{T_I} is the area of tearing in Ω_I, and then applying the smoothing filter with diffusion boundaries preventing diffusion into Ω_{R_I} and Ω_{T_I}. A displacement of magnitude 4 in the direction of the retracted area was defined on $\partial \Omega_{T_I}$ while the displacement on $\partial \Omega_{R_I}$ was set to 3 in the direction normal to the boundary. In addition, a displacement of about 6 pixels due to brain shift was also simulated. Fig. 3 shows both the resulting dataset as well as the qualitative results of the registration. We computed the dice coefficient between the estimated labelmaps Ψ_P, Ψ_I and Γ_I and the real labelmaps used to generate the synthetic dataset which resulted in the values $0.93, 0.94$ and 0.91 respectively.

3.2 Experiments on Clinical Data

The algorithm was also tested on a set of clinical T1 MRI data acquired from a neurosurgical procedure where retraction was necessary to perform the resection. First the pre-operative and intra-operative datasets were rigidly registered. Two corresponding slices were extracted along the retraction line and a manual skull stripping procedure was performed. The two slices can be seen in Fig. 4 together with the qualitative results which were achieved.

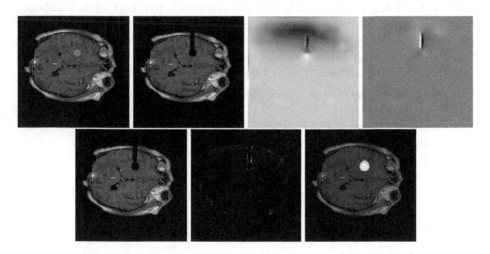

Fig. 3. [a b c d; e f g]: The top row shows [a] the pre-operative image, [b] the synthetically deformed image and [c]-[d] the estimated x- and y-components of the deformation field. [e] shows the deformed pre-operative image (with the estimated Ψ_I and Γ_I zeroed out), [f] the difference image in Ω_I and [g] the pre-operative image with the estimated resected area highlighted.

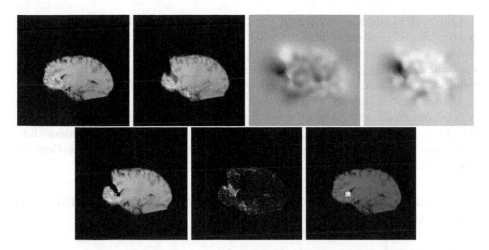

Fig. 4. [a b c d; e f g]: In [a] we have pre-operative image, [b] the intra-operative image, [c]-[d] the estimated x- and y- components of the deformation field U_{IP}, [e] the deformed pre-operative image $P \circ U_{IP}$ after masking out the estimated resected and retracted areas, [f] the difference image $|I - P \circ U_{IP}|$ after masking out the estimated retracted and resected areas and [g] the pre-operative image with the estimated resected area highlighted. From these qualitative results we can see that the algorithm provides fairly good estimates of both the retracted and resected areas.

4   Discussion

In this paper we have proposed a registration framework which can handle retraction and resection. The main contributions are the detection of tearing of the deformation field due to retraction, and detection of missing tissue due to resection as well as how to model these in the demons algorithm. We have shown the framework's applicability on both synthetic and clinical image data.

A few parameters need to be specified for the algorithm to work properly. Two parameters are exposed by the smoother, but none of them are directly data-dependent. The number of diffusion iterations mimics the standard deviation of the Gaussian filter applied in the traditional Demons method. To achieve more smoothing one needs to increase the number of diffusion iterations, or equivalently increase the standard deviation of the Gaussian smoothing filter. To achieve a stable solution of the diffusion equation the step length should be $\mu < 0.25$. Both the detection of retraction and resection exposes data-dependent parameters. In the case of retraction, the algorithm is quite sensitive to the specific value of τ. If it is too low, no retraction line is detected but if it is set too high a too long retraction line is detected. However, with the inclusion of the a-priori information regarding the tumor center and the length of the retractor the algorithm is considerably less sensitive to the specific value of τ. In the specification of the normal velocity of the front for the level set formulation, one has to specify the parameter ρ. This parameter defines what intensity difference is acceptable and has to be balanced according to the magnitude of the intensity differences which can occur.

Our current implementation of the framework is limited to 2D, but we see no big obstacles in extending it to 3D. Because of the current dimensionality constraint we had to extract two corresponding slices from two 3D data sets to construct the clinical data. We acknowledge that there might be out of plane deformations which we have not accounted for in the slice extraction process.

Using a Matlab implementation and a Dual Core 2.16 GHz processor, about 20 min of computational time was required to run 100 iterations on each level. Solving the anisotropic diffusion equation is by far the slowest part of the algorithm, but considerable speedups can be achieved by parallelizing the computations by utilizing GPGPU methods or multi-core processors.

Acknowledgments. This work was supported by NIH grants U41RR019703 and P41RR13218.

References

1. Hartkens, T., Hill, D.L.G., Castellano-Smith, A.D., Hawkes, D.J., Maurer, C.R., Martin, A.J., Hall, W.A., Liu, H., Truwit, C.L.: Measurement and analysis of brain deformation during neurosurgery. IEEE Transactions on Medical Imaging 22(1), 82–92 (2003)
2. Periaswamy, S., Farid, H.: Medical image registration with partial data. Medical Image Analysis 10, 452–464 (2006)
3. Miga, M.I., Roberts, D.W., Kennedy, F.E., Platenik, L.A., Hartov, A., Lunn, K.E., Paulsen, K.D.: Modeling of retraction and resection for intraoperative updating of images. Neurosurgery 1(1), 75–85 (2001)
4. Thirion, J.P.: Image matching as a diffusion process: an analogy with Maxwell's demons. Medical Image Analysis 2(3), 243–260 (1998)
5. Hellier, P., Barillot, C., Corouge, I., Gibaud, B., Le Goualher, G., Collins, D.L., Evans, A., Malandain, G., Ayache, N., Christensen, G.E., Johnson, H.J.: Retrospective evaluation of intersubject brain registration. IEEE Trans. Med. Imaging 22(9), 1120–1130 (2003)
6. Cachier, P., Bardinet, E., Dormont, D., Pennec, X., Ayache, N.: Iconic feature based nonrigid registration: the pasha algorithm. Comput. Vis. Image Underst. 89(2-3), 272–298 (2003)
7. Perona, P., Malik, J.: Scale-space and edge detection using anisotropic diffusion. IEEE Trans. Pattern Anal. Mach. Intell. 12(7), 629–639 (1990)
8. Alvarez, L., Deriche, R., Papadopoulo, T., Sánchez, J.: Symmetrical dense optical flow estimation with occlusions detection. Int. J. Comput. Vision 75(3), 371–385 (2007)
9. Noblet, V., Heinrich, C., Heitz, F., Armspach, J.P.: 3-D deformable image registration: a topology preservation scheme based on hierarchical deformation models and interval analysis optimization. IEEE Transactions on Image Processing 14(5), 553–566 (2005)
10. Müller, M., McMillan, L., Dorsey, J., Jagnow, R.: Real-time simulation of deformation and fracture of stiff materials. In: Proceedings of the Eurographic workshop on Computer animation and simulation, pp. 113–124. Springer, New York (2001)
11. Osher, S.J., Fedkiw, R.P.: Level Set Methods and Dynamic Implicit Surfaces. Springer, Heidelberg (2002)

Discriminative Shape Alignment

Marco Loog[1,3] and Marleen de Bruijne[2,3]

[1] Pattern Recognition Group, Faculty of Electrical Engineering, Mathematics, and Computer Science, Delft University of Technology, Delft, The Netherlands
m.loog@tudelft.nl

[2] Biomedical Imaging Group Rotterdam, Departments of Radiology and Medical Informatics, Erasmus Medical Center, Rotterdam, The Netherlands

[3] The Image Group, Department of Computer Science, University of Copenhagen, Copenhagen, Denmark

Abstract. The alignment of shape data to a common mean before its subsequent processing is an ubiquitous step within the area shape analysis. Current approaches to shape analysis or, as more specifically considered in this work, shape classification perform the alignment in a fully unsupervised way, not taking into account that eventually the shapes are to be assigned to two or more different classes. This work introduces a discriminative variation to well-known Procrustes alignment and demonstrates its benefit over this classical method in shape classification tasks. The focus is on two-dimensional shapes from a two-class recognition problem.

1 Introduction

Medical shape analysis can aid differential diagnosis and monitoring and can be employed in predicting disease progression or status. Many applications involve the shape analysis of neuro-anatomical structures in the brain—typically hippocampi or corpora callosa [1, 2], but for instance also the classification of facial [3] and mandible [4] morphology, gait recognition [5], and risk analysis of vertebral fractures [6] are tackled by means of shape information.

The typical approach is based on landmarked shapes that are in correspondence, aligned using a Procrustes analysis [1, 7–9], and subsequently subjected to further analyses like a classification in the shape space obtained [10]. It is this approach that is also of interest to us and in this paper a discriminative alignment method is proposed that potentially improves supervised shape analysis approaches like the ones mentioned above. What we do not consider is obtaining increased performance from improved shape representations or shape modeling, although it can of course not be denied that also on that side various advances are possible [11–13].

Our basic idea is illustrated by the observation that the well-known dimensionality reduction technique called linear discriminant analysis (LDA, or Fisher's linear discriminant, see [14–16]) can be considered an extension of unsupervised principal component analysis (PCA) to the supervised setting in which not only feature vectors (e.g. landmark locations) are available but each feature vector has been assigned to one of two or more classes. Now, in this contribution the unsupervised alignment procedure

J.L. Prince, D.L. Pham, and K.J. Myers (Eds.): IPMI 2009, LNCS 5636, pp. 459–466, 2009.

Procrustes analysis [8, 9] is extended in a way similar to the extension from PCA to LDA, incorporating labels in the alignment process with the aim to improve subsequent classification performance. In other words we still search for a single reference shape to align all other shapes to, but this shape is chosen with the goal of discriminating between shapes of different classes, i.e., only the optimality criterion that this shape fulfills is altered.

More specifically, landmarks in two dimensions from two-class problems are considered and the common reference to which all shapes are registered is obtained in a discriminative way, trying to pull apart both classes as well as possible before any further analysis is performed.

1.1   Outline

The next section, Section 2, starts out with a detailed description of our discriminative approach to the alignment problem, after which Section 3 introduces the data sets on which the new procedure is tested together with the rest of the experimental setup, including the choice of classifiers. Section 4 then provides the results coming from the experiments and, finally, Section 5 rounds up the paper and provides a discussion and conclusion.

2   Theory

The discriminative part of our method relies on a linear regression formulation of LDA [16–18] in which the predictor variables, i.e., the landmark coordinates, are regressed onto a numerical representation of the corresponding categorical class labels, e.g., an indicator matrix or, in our case, simply a $(+1, -1)$-vector the length of the number of shapes. In other terms, given that the multi-dimensional input variables are N vectors $x_i \in \mathbb{R}^n$, and given the corresponding numerical labels denoted by y_i, the LDA solution is obtained by finding the $a \in \mathbb{R}^n$ that minimizes

$$\sum_{i=1}^{N} \left(a^{\mathrm{T}} x_i - y_i \right)^2 . \tag{1}$$

2.1   Discriminative Alignment Criterion

To get to our precise optimality criterion for discriminative shape alignment let $w_i \in \mathbb{C}^n$ represent a two-dimensional shape consisting of n landmarks given as points in the complex plane. Additionally, assume we have N shapes, w_1 to w_N, for which landmark correspondence has been established. Assume moreover that all of the shapes have been centered such that the center of mass is at 0 and normalized such that $w_i^{\mathrm{H}} w_i = 1$. Now, given another shape $m \in \mathbb{C}^n$, all shapes w_i can be optimally aligned to m — in a least square sense — by the following operation [7]:

$$w_i' = w_i w_i^{\mathrm{H}} m, \tag{2}$$

where $w_i' \in \mathbb{C}^n$ are the aligned shapes.

The aim is to determine a reference shape m such that the two shape classes are as far apart as possible. We propose to measure this separability by means of a criterion similar to the one in Equation (1) and one may guess that this is simply a matter of substituting $a^T w_i' = a^T w_i w_i^H m$ for $a^T x_i$ in that equation. The problem in this case is that the regression should be done using real numbers while $w_i w_i^H m$ is not necessarily real — one cannot straightforwardly use complex numbers in this setting. In fact, a should have twice the dimensionality of w_i' and act separately on the latter's real and imaginary part. That is, we should solve

$$\sum_{i=1}^{N} \left(a^T \begin{pmatrix} \operatorname{Im} w_i' \\ \operatorname{Re} w_i' \end{pmatrix} - y_i \right)^2 , \tag{3}$$

with $a \in \mathbb{R}^{2n}$ and y_i equal to $+1$ or -1, depending on which class the ith shape belongs to. In addition, as normally done in linear regression, an overall bias term $c \in \mathbb{R}$ is included, which leads to our discriminative Procrustes criterion

$$\sum_{i=1}^{N} \left(a^T \begin{pmatrix} \operatorname{Im} w_i' \\ \operatorname{Re} w_i' \end{pmatrix} + c - y_i \right)^2 . \tag{4}$$

2.2 Optimization

It should first of all be noted that in Equation (4) both a and m (which is hidden in the w_i's) should be minimized over. The former takes care of the optimal discrimination, while the latter provides the optimal alignment "mean" for our goal. Now, in order to find a way to minimize this criterion, we proceed by a further manipulation of the above expression. Choosing the vector $\mu \in \mathbb{R}^{2n}$ as

$$\mu = \begin{pmatrix} \operatorname{Im} m \\ \operatorname{Re} m \end{pmatrix} \tag{5}$$

and taking the $2n \times 2n$-matrices W_i to equal

$$W_i = \begin{pmatrix} \operatorname{Re} w_i w_i^H & -\operatorname{Im} w_i w_i^H \\ \operatorname{Im} w_i w_i^H & \operatorname{Re} w_i w_i^H \end{pmatrix} , \tag{6}$$

Equation 4 can be rewritten as follows:

$$\sum_{i=1}^{N} \left(a^T W_i \mu + c - y_i \right)^2 . \tag{7}$$

For the overall optimization, we cannot find a closed-form solution. However, the above criterion can be seen as two intertwined linear regression problems: given a, $a^T W_i$ is a fixed vector of the same size and one can solve for μ by means of standard linear least squares regression. Similarly, given μ, one can easily get a hold of a using the same procedure. This suggests to perform the minimization by alternately solving the afore-mentioned linear regression problems in which every time either a or μ is kept fixed. In the first iteration a is the free variables to be optimized and μ is set to the real and imaginary parts of the original (unsupervised) Procrustes mean, which can be obtained in the regular way [7, 8]. Note that the final reference shape in complex notation m can be recovered straightforwardly from the optimal solution for μ if necessary.

We should also remark that in relatively high dimensional problems, with many landmarks compared to the number of shapes, it may be beneficial to perform both regression steps in a regularized way. In our experiments in the following section, we use a simple ridge regression [16, 18].

3   Experimental Setup

A set of leave-one-out experiments was conducted to compare the classification accuracy obtained after standard Procrustes and discriminative Procrustes alignment.

3.1   Data

The experiments involve two data sets: Bookstein's schizophrenia data set [1, 2] and a collection of vertebrae from the spine database used in the study reported on in [6].

Bookstein's data set consists of 14 landmarked corpora callosa extracted from the midsagittal planes of brain MRI data of 14 people suffering from schizophrenia. In addition, 14 controls were included in the database. All shapes are represented using 13 mutually corresponding landmarks and were originally used in a study of the structural neuropathology of schizophrenics [2].

The second data set is selected from a cohort of post-menopausal women who were screened for osteoporosis and atherosclerosis using X-rays[19]. We selected 109 women who had no fracture at baseline and who developed at least one vertebral fracture in the course of the five years between baseline and follow-up imaging. Landmarks were place on the vertebra corners and on the midpoints of the vertebral endplates. In [6], the same 109 women were matched with 109 controls who maintained skeletal integrity during the course of the study, and shape characteristics of the full spine were learned based on the longitudinal training data, providing an estimate of the risk of future vertebral fractures. In our work, the classification of individual vertebrae in (predicted to become) fractured or not fractured is considered. For this, two data sets are constructed, one from the baseline data (therefore concerned with prediction) and one from follow-up (resulting in a simpler detection task).

1. In the original data set 156 fractured vertebrae occur at follow-up. We take these 156 vertebra shapes and choose 156 non-fractured shapes to complete the first data set. The set of non-fractures were randomly taken from the spines that had one or more fractures and balanced such that the distribution over the location in the spine was the same for both fractures and non-fractures. Both measures make sure that the classification performance is not positively biased and good performance may be hard to obtain.
2. From the baseline data set, we take the vertebrae corresponding to the ones in the first data collection. So they also are taken only from women who developed a fracture, the main difference of course being that now none of the shapes really

shows a fracture. This is probably the most interesting setting, as this allows one, potentially, to estimate the risk of future vertebral fractures. This was also the main goal pursued in [6].

Finally, we note that the task of fracture prediction in spines is a rather challenging task and the original work using the same dataset reports an accuracy of merely 0.67 (i.e., an error of 0.33). For more details, the reader is referred to [6].

3.2 Classification

To measure the discrimination ability after alignment, three rather differently behaving classifiers [20] are employed in the $2n$-dimensional feature space. The first classifier is Fisher's linear discriminant analysis (LDA) (now indeed as a classifier and not as dimensionality reduction technique), the second one is the first nearest neighbor approach (1NN), a nonlinear method [14–16], and the third is the more general k nearest neighbor approach (kNN) in which k is optimized on the training data.

In addition, we note that the experimental results are based on leave-one-out estimates, including the optimization of the alignment shape, and that the number of iterations to train the discriminative Procrustes was set to 1000, which ensured sufficient convergence in all cases. Finally, we conducted discriminative Procrustes based with and without regularized regression and report both the former nonregularized result and the optimal result for the latter.

4   Results

The results are summarized in Tables 1 and 2. The first table reports the error rates on the schizophrenia data set both for standard and discriminative Procrustes and for LDA, 1NN, and kNN. Note the high errors in some of the entries—higher even than 0.5. These are due to the large unfavorable bias of the leave-one-out estimation [18], especially in the case of (relatively) high-dimensional data (see also [21] for instance). Though disturbing, they do not necessarily hamper a relative comparison of the alignment techniques.

Table 1. Estimated classification errors on the schizophrenia data based on leave-one-out. Unsupervised and supervised alignment are used, as well as three different classifiers.

	LDA	1NN	kNN
Procrustes analysis	0.57	0.36	0.46
discriminative Procrustes	0.64	0.46	0.46
... + regularization	0.36	0.32	0.25

The second table also reports errors for all nine possible combinations of classifiers and alignment methods, but does so for the vertebra data set at follow-up in (a) and for the baseline set in (b).

Table 2. Estimated classification errors on the two vertebra data sets based on leave-one-out. Table (a) provides the errors on the follow-up data where Table (b) concerns the baseline set. Unsupervised and supervised alignment are used in combination with three different classifiers.

(a)	LDA	1NN	kNN
Procrustes analysis	0.13	0.14	0.10
discriminative Procrustes	0.10	0.27	0.23
...+ regularization	0.10	0.12	0.08

(b)	LDA	1NN	kNN
Procrustes analysis	0.37	0.43	0.39
discriminative Procrustes	0.32	0.43	0.31
...+ regularization	0.32	0.43	0.31

5 Discussion and Conclusion

First of all, the most notable result that can be derived from the previous experiments is that the proposed discriminative Procrustes analysis improves, or performs at least equal to, standard, unsupervised Procrustes analysis in half of the cases and even in all cases when the appropriate regularization is performed. Concerning the latter, it should be pointed out that in several settings a regularization is indeed indispensable. This is especially the case for the corpora callosa. This is basically a small sample problem on which direct discriminative Procrustes probably overtrains and therefore performs poorly. Considerable improvements are however possible as shown. All in all, it does indeed illustrate that if classification, detection, or prediction is the goal, early-on application of discriminative techniques may be beneficial, leading to better separability and reduced error rates. This situation is also commonly observed when comparing PCA to LDA in classification tasks.

What is particularly promising is the improvement obtained when predicting future vertebra fractures from baseline data. This is a difficult task and although 1NN's performance is very poor, when using LDA or kNN as classifier and discriminative alignment instead of standard alignment, the error rates drop from 0.37 to 0.32 and from 0.39 to 0.31, respectively. These are relative improvements of over 13% and 20%, respectively, which is significant in practice.

We note that one may expect that LDA should naturally outperform the nearest neighbor methods, because discriminative Procrustes is closely related to LDA as a classifier. The results, however, clearly show that this is not always the case. From the pattern recognition literature it is indeed known that linear dimensionality reduction methods can also improve the performance of nonlinear, even nonparametric, classification procedures [15, 16, 22, 23] cf. [24].

Two of the principle variations of the current method that we like to consider in forthcoming research are the extensions to multi-class data and the extension from two-dimensional to three-dimensional shapes. Where the former can probably be accommodated relatively easy given the current setup (cf. [16–18]), the latter extension may prove to be more difficult. The main problem in this seems to boil down to the issue of whether or not we can find similar expressions for the matrices W_i in Equation (6) and the alignment operation in Equation (2). There is a good chance that such is possible (see for example [25]), but also in the absence of such expressions, the formulation of a criterion similar to Equation (7) may still be possible. Nonetheless, in the latter case, its optimization probably becomes much more intricate and involved as one cannot resort to the simple, alternating regression scheme employed in this work. Finally, extending the framework even further to, for instance, the situation in which landmark correspondence is unknown would certainly also be of interest. Works like [26] may provide the necessary inspiration to tackle this problem.

Regarding the current method, we think a point that needs further investigations is the optimization of Equation (7), our principal objective function. The main issue is that our optimization procedure seems to converge, but we do not have a clear idea of how close the actual solution is to the (global) optimum. Surely, having a better understanding of this will enable us to devise more efficient algorithms to optimize the discriminative Procrustes. A first direction to look into seems the work that has been done in parallel factor analysis in which an objective function resembling ours plays a role [27].

For two-dimensional shapes with corresponding landmarks, however, the potential advantage of our approach has been illustrated and our discriminative version of classical Procrustes will hopefully prove to increase performance in many other shape analysis problems.

Acknowledgments

We sincerely thank Nordic Bioscience Imaging, and specifically Mads Nielsen (also with the University of Copenhagen), for allowing us to use the spine data derived from the Prospective Epidemiological Risk Factors (PERF) study [19]. ML and MdB were partly funded by the Innovational Research Incentives Scheme of the Netherlands Research Organization (NWO).

References

1. Bookstein, F.: Shape and the information in medical images: A decade of the morphometric synthesis. Computer Vision and Image Understanding 66(2), 97–118 (1997)
2. DeQuardo, J., Bookstein, F., Green, W., Brundberg, J., Tandon, R.: Spatial relationships of neuroanatomic landmarks in schizophrenia. Psychiatry Research: Neuroimaging 67(1), 81–95 (1996)
3. Hammond, P., Hutton, T., Allanson, J., Campbell, L., Hennekam, R., Holden, S., Patton, M., Shaw, A., Temple, I., Trotter, M., Murphy, K., Winter, R.: 3D analysis of facial morphology. American Journal of Medical Genetics 126(4), 339–348 (2004)
4. Nicholson, E., Harvati, K.: Quantitative analysis of human mandibular shape using three-dimensional geometric morphometrics. American Journal of Physical Anthropology 131(3), 368 (2006)
5. Wang, L., Tan, T., Hu, W., Ning, H.: Automatic gait recognition based on statistical shape analysis. IEEE Transactions on Image Processing 12(9), 1120–1131 (2003)
6. de Bruijne, M., Pettersen, P.: Supervised shape analysis for risk assessment in osteoporosis. In: Fifth IEEE International Symposium on Biomedical Imaging, pp. 1581–1584 (2008)

7. Dryden, I., Mardia, K.: Statistical shape analysis. John Wiley & Sons, New York (1998)
8. Goodall, C.: Procrustes methods in the statistical analysis of shape. Journal of the Royal Statistical Society B 53, 285–339 (1991)
9. Kendall, D.: Shape manifolds, Procrustean metrics, and complex projective spaces. Bulletin of the London Mathematical Society 16(2), 81 (1984)
10. Golland, P., Grimson, W., Shenton, M., Kikinis, R.: Detection and analysis of statistical differences in anatomical shape. Medical Image Analysis 9, 69–86 (2005)
11. Davatzikos, C., Tao, X., Shen, D.: Applications of wavelets in morphometric analysis of medical images. In: Unser, M., Aldroubi, A., Laine, A. (eds.) Wavelets: Applications in Signal and Image Processing X, SPIE Conference, vol. 5207, pp. 435–444 (2003)
12. Davies, R., Twining, C., Allen, P., Cootes, T., Taylor, C.: Shape discrimination in the hippocampus using an MDL model. In: Taylor, C.J., Noble, J.A. (eds.) IPMI 2003. LNCS, vol. 2732, pp. 38–50. Springer, Heidelberg (2003)
13. Loog, M.: Localized maximum entropy shape modelling. In: Karssemeijer, N., Lelieveldt, B. (eds.) IPMI 2007. LNCS, vol. 4584, pp. 619–629. Springer, Heidelberg (2007)
14. Devijver, P., Kittler, J.: Pattern Recognition: A Statistical Approach. Prentice-Hall, London (1982)
15. Fukunaga, K.: Introduction to Statistical Pattern Recognition. Academic Press, London (1990)
16. Hastie, T., Tibshirani, R., Friedman, J.: Elements of statistical learning: data mining, inference and prediction. Springer, Heidelberg (2001)
17. Hastie, T., Buja, A., Tibshirani, R.: Penalized discriminant analysis. Annals of statistics 23, 73–102 (1995)
18. Ripley, B.: Pattern Recognition and Neural Networks. Cambridge University Press, Cambridge (1996)
19. Bagger, Y., Tankó, L., Alexandersen, P., Hansen, H., Qin, G., Christiansen, C.: The long-term predictive value of bone mineral density measurements for fracture risk is independent of the site of measurement and the age at diagnosis: results from the prospective epidemiological risk factors study. Osteoporosis International 17, 471–477 (2006)
20. Mansilla, E., Ho, T.: On classifier domains of competence. In: Proceedings of the 17th International Conference on Pattern Recognition, pp. 136–139 (2004)
21. Schulerud, H.: Bias of error rates in linear discriminant analysis caused by feature selection and sample size. In: Proceedings of the 15th International Conference on Pattern Recognition, vol. 2 (2000)
22. Loog, M., Duin, R.: Linear dimensionality reduction via a heteroscedastic extension of LDA: the Chernoff criterion. IEEE Transactions on Pattern Analysis and Machine Intelligence 26(6), 732–739 (2004)
23. Loog, M., van Ginneken, B., Duin, R.: Dimensionality reduction of image features using the canonical contextual correlation projection. Pattern Recognition 38(12), 2409–2418 (2005)
24. Van der Maaten, L., Postma, E., Van den Herik, H.: Dimensionality reduction: A comparative review (preprint, 2007)
25. Dam, E., Koch, M., Lillholm, M.: Quaternions, interpolation and animation. Technical Report DIKU-98/5, Department of Computer Science, University of Copenhagen (1998)
26. Gold, S., Rangarajan, A., Mjolsness, E.: Learning with preknowledge: clustering with point and graph matching distance measures. Neural Computation 8(4), 787–804 (1996)
27. Harshman, R.: Foundations of the PARAFAC procedure: Models and conditions for an "explanatory" multi-modal factor analysis. UCLA working papers in phonetics 16(1-84), 246 (1970)

Inverse-Consistent Surface Mapping with Laplace-Beltrami Eigen-Features

Yonggang Shi, Jonathan H. Morra, Paul M. Thompson, and Arthur W. Toga

Lab of Neuro Imaging, UCLA School of Medicine, Los Angeles, CA, USA
yshi@loni.ucla.edu

Abstract. We propose in this work a novel variational method for computing maps between surfaces by combining informative geometric features and regularizing forces including inverse consistency and harmonic energy. To tackle the ambiguity in defining homologous points on smooth surfaces, we design feature functions in the data term based on the Reeb graph of the Laplace-Beltrami eigenfunctions to quantitatively describe the global geometry of elongated anatomical structures. For inverse consistency and robustness, our method computes simultaneously the forward and backward map by iteratively solving partial differential equations (PDEs) on the surfaces. In our experiments, we successfully mapped 890 hippocampal surfaces and report statistically significant maps of atrophy rates between normal controls and patients with mild cognitive impairment (MCI) and Alzheimer's disease (AD).

1 Introduction

Surface mapping is an important problem in medical image analysis with applications in population studies[1] and the creation of 3D shape prior models[2]. While significant progresses have been made with the development of various techniques[3–9], most of them focus heavily on the *regularization* part of the problem. The lack of informative *data terms* makes it still a challenging problem to resolve the ambiguity in defining homologous points on smooth surfaces. To this end we propose in this paper a novel variational framework to compute maps directly between surfaces. By combining data terms from Laplace-Beltrami eigen-features and regularizing forces from inverse consistency and harmonic energy, our method can generate robust and high quality maps for a class of subcortical structures with clinical significance.

Many interesting techniques have been proposed in previous work to solve various surface mapping problems. A popular approach is to first map the surface onto the sphere and then solve the registration problem in this canonical domain [5–7, 9]. By viewing the surface as a subset of $\mathbb{R}^3$, successful image registration techniques were applied to compute surface maps with possible landmark constraints [3, 4, 8]. Landmark curves detected by shape context features were used to guide the mapping of hippocampal surfaces[10]. The medial model provides a compact surface representation and is also very useful to construct maps between surfaces[11–13].

J.L. Prince, D.L. Pham, and K.J. Myers (Eds.): IPMI 2009, LNCS 5636, pp. 467–478, 2009.

We propose in this work a variational approach to automatically compute both the forward and backward maps between two surfaces with inverse consistency. An important feature of our method is that we use the Reeb graph of the Laplace-Beltrami eigenfunctions to define intrinsic features for the data fidelity term in our energy function. These features provide quantitative descriptions of the salient geometry shared by elongated structures such as the hippocampus and significantly remove the ambiguity in finding correspondences for such surfaces. Another interesting feature of our method is that we incorporate both inverse consistency[14] and harmonic energy [15] as the regularization term to improve the quality of maps. The harmonic energy encourages the smoothness in the maps and the inverse consistency term helps reduce area distortions. In our experiments, we perform extensive tests to demonstrate the quality of the maps generated by our method. We also demonstrate the robustness of our method with its successful mapping of 890 hippocampal surfaces and report statistically significant results.

The rest of the paper is organized as follows. In section 2, we develop the variational framework that combines data terms of intrinsic features and regularization terms including both inverse consistency and harmonic energy. We propose the Laplace-Beltrami eigen-features for the modeling of elongated structures such as hippocampus in section 3. Experimental results are presented in section 4 to demonstrate the quality and robustness of our mapping algorithm. Finally conclusions and future work are discussed in section 5.

2   A Variational Framework

In this section, we propose a variational framework for the direct mapping of surfaces. Let $(\mathcal{M}_1, g)$ and $(\mathcal{M}_2, h)$ be two Riemann surfaces with their metric tensor g and h. To obtain inverse consistency, we compute two maps jointly in our method. We denote $u_1 : \mathcal{M}_1 \to \mathcal{M}_2$ as the map from $\mathcal{M}_1$ to $\mathcal{M}_2$, and $u_2 : \mathcal{M}_2 \to \mathcal{M}_1$ the map from $\mathcal{M}_2$ to $\mathcal{M}_1$. We also assume there are L feature functions defined on each surface and denote $\xi_1^j : \mathcal{M}_1 \to \mathbb{R}$ and $\xi_2^j : \mathcal{M}_2 \to \mathbb{R}(1 \leq j \leq L)$ as the j-th feature function on $\mathcal{M}_1$ and $\mathcal{M}_2$, respectively.

In our variational framework, the maps are computed as the minimizer of the following energy function:

$$E = E_D + E_{IC} + E_H. \tag{1}$$

There are three terms in the energy function and all of them are symmetric with respect to $\mathcal{M}_1$ and $\mathcal{M}_2$. We call the first energy E_D as the data fidelity term and it is defined as:

$$E_D = \sum_{j=1}^{L} \alpha_D^j \left[\int_{\mathcal{M}_1} (\xi_1^j - \xi_2^j \circ u_1)^2 d\mathcal{M}_1 + \int_{\mathcal{M}_2} (\xi_2^j - \xi_1^j \circ u_2)^2 d\mathcal{M}_2 \right]. \tag{2}$$

This energy penalizes the mismatch of feature functions induced by the two maps, and the parameters α_D^j are used to assign proper weights for different feature functions.

The other two terms are for regularization, where E_{IC} encourages inverse consistency and E_H is the harmonic energy and it ensures the smoothness in the maps. Let I denote the identity function such that $I(\mathbf{x}) = \mathbf{x}$. We define the energy E_{IC} as:

$$E_{IC} = \alpha_{IC} \left[\int_{\mathcal{M}_1} (I - u_2 \circ u_1)^2 d\mathcal{M}_1 + \int_{\mathcal{M}_2} (I - u_1 \circ u_2)^2 d\mathcal{M}_2 \right] \tag{3}$$

where α_{IC} is a regularization parameter. For inverse consistency, this energy penalizes the difference between the identity map I and the composition of the two maps $u_2 \circ u_1$ and $u_1 \circ u_2$. The harmonic energy term E_H is defined as [15, 16]:

$$E_H = \alpha_H \left[\int_{\mathcal{M}_1} \| J_{u_1} \|^2 d\mathcal{M}_1 + \int_{\mathcal{M}_2} \| J_{u_2} \|^2 d\mathcal{M}_2 \right] \tag{4}$$

where J_{u_1} and J_{u_2} are the Jacobian of the two maps defined on the surfaces, and α_H is the regularization parameter for this term.

To minimize the energy function with respect to the maps u_1 and u_2, we derive their gradient flows and compute them iteratively via the solution of these partial differential equations(PDEs) on the two surfaces $\mathcal{M}_1$ and $\mathcal{M}_2$. For the energy E_D, the gradient flows of u_1 and u_2 are:

$$\frac{\partial E_D}{\partial u_1} = -2 \sum_{j=1}^{L} \alpha_D^j (\xi_1^j - \xi_2^j \circ u_1) \nabla_{\mathcal{M}_2} \xi_2^j(u_1)$$

$$\frac{\partial E_D}{\partial u_2} = -2 \sum_{j=1}^{L} \alpha_D^j (\xi_2^j - \xi_1^j \circ u_2) \nabla_{\mathcal{M}_1} \xi_1^j(u_2) \tag{5}$$

where $\nabla_{\mathcal{M}_1}$ and $\nabla_{\mathcal{M}_2}$ denote the intrinsic gradient on the surfaces. For the energy E_{IC}, the gradient flows are:

$$\frac{E_{IC}}{\partial u_1} = -2\alpha_{IC} \left[J_{u_2}^T (I - u_2 \circ u_1) + (u_2^{-1} - u_1) |J_{u_2^{-1}}| \right]$$

$$\frac{E_{IC}}{\partial u_2} = -2\alpha_{IC} \left[J_{u_1}^T (I - u_1 \circ u_2) + (u_1^{-1} - u_2) |J_{u_1^{-1}}| \right] \tag{6}$$

where u_1^{-1} and u_2^{-1} are the inverse maps of u_1 and u_2, and the determinant of their Jacobian are denoted as $|J_{u_2^{-1}}|$ and $|J_{u_2^{-1}}|$.

To derive the gradients of the harmonic energy, we denote (x^1, x^2) and (y^1, y^2) as the local coordinates of $\mathcal{M}_1$ and $\mathcal{M}_2$. In the local coordinates, the maps can be represented as $u_1 = (u_1^1, u_1^2)$ and $u_2 = (u_2^1, u_2^2)$. The gradient flow of u_1 can then be expressed in the form of Einstein's summation as [15]:

$$\frac{\partial E_H}{\partial u_1^r} = -\alpha_H \left[\Delta_{\mathcal{M}_1} u_1^r + g^{\alpha\beta} \Gamma_{2,pq}^r \frac{\partial u_1^p}{\partial x^\alpha} \frac{\partial u_1^q}{\partial x^\beta} \right] \quad (r = 1, 2) \tag{7}$$

where $\Delta_{\mathcal{M}_1}$ is the Laplace-Beltrami operator on $\mathcal{M}_1$, $g^{\alpha\beta} = (g_{\alpha\beta})^{-1}$, and $\Gamma^r_{2,pq}$ is the Christoffel symbol on the manifold $\mathcal{M}_2$. Similarly, the gradient flow of u_2 is:

$$\frac{\partial E_H}{\partial u_2^s} = -\alpha_H \left[\Delta_{\mathcal{M}_2} u_2^s + h^{pq} \Gamma^s_{1,\alpha\beta} \frac{\partial u_2^\alpha}{\partial y^p} \frac{\partial u_2^\beta}{\partial y^q} \right] \quad (s = 1, 2) \tag{8}$$

where $\Delta_{\mathcal{M}_2}$ is the Laplace-Beltrami operator on $\mathcal{M}_2$, $h^{pq} = (h_{pq})^{-1}$, and $\Gamma^s_{1,\alpha\beta}$ is the Christoffel symbol on the manifold $\mathcal{M}_1$.

By combining the above results, we have the gradient descent flows of u_1 and u_2 to minimize the energy:

$$\begin{cases} \dfrac{\partial u_1}{\partial t} = -\dfrac{\partial E_D}{\partial u_1} - \dfrac{\partial E_{IC}}{\partial u_1} - \dfrac{\partial E_H}{\partial u_1} \\ \dfrac{\partial u_2}{\partial t} = -\dfrac{\partial E_D}{\partial u_2} - \dfrac{\partial E_{IC}}{\partial u_2} - \dfrac{\partial E_H}{\partial u_2} \end{cases} \tag{9}$$

To numerically solve these two equations on $\mathcal{M}_1$ and $\mathcal{M}_2$, we use the approach of solving PDEs on implicit surfaces[16–18] and represent $\mathcal{M}_1$ and $\mathcal{M}_2$ as a signed distance function ϕ and ψ, respectively. With the implicit representation, we have a very simple formulation for the gradient flow of the harmonic energy. Using the signed distance function, we can express gradient operators on surfaces in terms of conventional gradient operators in $\mathbb{R}^3$. For example, the intrinsic gradient $\nabla_{\mathcal{M}_1} f$ of a function f on $\mathcal{M}_1$ can be expressed as $\Pi_{\nabla\phi}\nabla f$, where ∇f is the gradient of f in $\mathbb{R}^3$ and $\Pi_{\nabla\phi} = I - \nabla\phi\nabla\phi^T$ is the projection operator. By substituting the implicit form of gradient operators into (9), we can write the gradient descent flow of u_1 and u_2 as:

$$\begin{cases} \dfrac{\partial u_1}{\partial t} = 2\sum_{j=1}^{L} \alpha_D^j (\xi_1^j - \xi_2^j \circ u_1) \Pi_{\nabla\psi} \nabla \xi_2^j(u_1) \\ \quad + \alpha_{IC} \Pi_{\nabla\psi} \left[J_{u_2}^T (I - u_2 \circ u_1) + (u_2^{-1} - u_1)|\Pi_{\nabla\phi} J_{u_2}^{-1}| \right] + \alpha_H \Pi_{\nabla\psi} \nabla \cdot (\Pi_{\nabla\phi} J_{u_1}^T) \\ \dfrac{\partial u_2}{\partial t} = 2\sum_{j=1}^{L} \alpha_D^j (\xi_2^j - \xi_1^j \circ u_2) \Pi_{\nabla\phi} \nabla \xi_1^j(u_2) \\ \quad + \alpha_{IC} \Pi_{\nabla\phi} \left[J_{u_1}^T (I - u_1 \circ u_2) + (u_1^{-1} - u_2)|\Pi_{\nabla\psi} J_{u_1}^{-1}| \right] + \alpha_H \Pi_{\nabla\phi} \nabla \cdot (\Pi_{\nabla\psi} J_{u_2}^T) \end{cases} \tag{10}$$

For numerical efficiency, all computations are performed on narrow bands surrounding the surfaces. More details of the computational schemes can be found in [16].

3   Laplace-Beltrami Eigen-Features

To use the above variational framework, it is important to design proper features that can capture the common geometry across surfaces. This is generally a difficult problem and the solution is application dependent. In this section, we propose two feature functions to characterize the global geometry of elongated structures with neuroanatomical significance such as hippocampus and putamen. Both features are invariant to scale differences and natural pose variations. For a surface $\mathcal{M}$, the first feature function $\xi_1 : \mathcal{M} \to \mathbb{R}$ characterizes the tail-to-head trend of elongated structures, and the second feature $\xi_2 : \mathcal{M} \to \mathbb{R}$ describes the lateral profile of the surface. We next develop the algorithm to compute both features from the Laplace-Beltrami eigenfunction of $\mathcal{M}$.

For a surface $\mathcal{M}$, the eigenfunctions of its Laplace-Beltrami operator is defined as [19–23]:

$$\Delta_{\mathcal{M}} f = -\lambda f \tag{11}$$

The spectrum of $\Delta_{\mathcal{M}}$ is discrete and the eigenvalues can be ordered as $0 = \lambda_0 \leq \lambda_1 \leq \lambda_2 \leq \cdots$. For λ_i, the corresponding eigenfunction of λ_i is denoted as f_i. For the first eigenvalue $\lambda_0 = 0$, the eigenfunction f_0 is constant, so it is not useful to describe the shape. Among the rest eigenfunctions, the second eigenfunction f_1 is particularly interesting for modeling the global characteristics of elongated subcortical structures such as the hippocampus. If we view f_1 as a map from $\mathcal{M}$ to $\mathbb{R}$, it has the following property[24]:

$$f_1 = \arg \min_{f \perp f_0, ||f||=1} \int_{\mathcal{M}} |\nabla_{\mathcal{M}} f|^2 d\mathcal{M}. \tag{12}$$

with

$$\lambda_1 = \int_{\mathcal{M}} |\nabla_{\mathcal{M}} f|^2 d\mathcal{M}. \tag{13}$$

Thus this function f_1 can be viewed as the smoothest, non-constant map from $\mathcal{M}$ to $\mathbb{R}$ in the space orthogonal to f_0. To numerically compute the eigenfunction, we represent $\mathcal{M}$ as a triangular mesh $\mathcal{M} = (\mathcal{V}, \mathcal{T})$, where $\mathcal{V}$ is the set of vertices and $\mathcal{T}$ is the set of triangles. By using the weak form of (11) and the finite element method, we can compute the eigenfunction by solving a generalized matrix eigenvalue problem [22]:

$$Qf = \lambda U f \tag{14}$$

where Q and U are matrices derived with the finite element method.

To show how the eigenfunction f_1 can model the global shape of elongated structures, we construct its Reeb graph to obtain an explicit representation [25]. For a function f_1 defined on a manifold $\mathcal{M}$, its Reeb graph is defined as the quotient space with its topology defined via the equivalent relation $x \simeq y$ if $f_1(x) = f_1(y)$ for $x, y \in \mathcal{M}$. To numerically construct the Reeb graph, we trace a set of level contours of the eigenfunction f_1 on the triangular mesh representation of $\mathcal{M}$. To ensure the level contours distribute evenly over the entire surface, we use an adaptive sampling scheme developed in [23]. These level contours are used as the nodes of the Reeb graph and the connectivity of these nodes are established

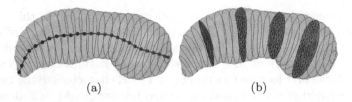

Fig. 1. The Reeb graph of a hippocampus. (a) The Reeb graph of the f_1. (b) The surface patches interpolating the level contours.

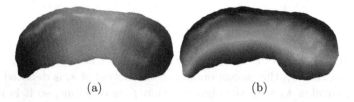

Fig. 2. The feature functions of a hippocampus. (a) The first feature function ξ_1. (b) The second feature function ξ_2.

according to the neighboring relations of level contours. As an example, we show in Fig. 1(a) the Reeb graph of a hippocampus. By representing each node of the Reeb graph as the centroid of the level contour, we can see this graph has a chain structure and provides a compact model of the essentially one dimensional, tail-to-head trend of the hippocampus.

Based on the Reeb graph of f_1, we define the first feature function ξ_1. Because the eigenfunction is generally a Moss function [26], its Reeb graph has a tree structure for genus zero surfaces. For hippocampus, the Reeb graph of f_1 typically has a chain structure as shown in Fig. 1. In the case there are branches in the Reeb graph, we prune the smaller branches according to the size of the associated level contour to ensure the pruned graph has a chain structure. We order the nodes on this chain with the increase of the function f_1 and denote the level contour at each node as $C_i (i = 1, \cdots, N)$. Each contour is digitized into K points $C_i = [C_{i,1}, C_{i,2}, \cdots, C_{i,K}]$. Because these points are obtained from the vertices of the mesh, we have the following relation

$$C = A\mathcal{V} \tag{15}$$

where $C = [C_1, C_2, \cdots, C_N]^T$ is the set of all the points on level contours, and the matrix A represents the linear interpolation operation that generates the level contours. To quantitatively describe the tail-to-head trend of the shape, we first define the feature function ξ_1 on the level contours as $\xi_1(C_{i,k}) = -1 + 2 * i/N$ for points on C_i. To define the function ξ_1 on the entire mesh, we solve the following regularized linear inverse problem:

$$\|\xi_1(C) - A\xi_1(\mathcal{V})\|^2 + \beta\xi_1(\mathcal{V})^T Q\xi_1(\mathcal{V}) \tag{16}$$

where $\xi_1(C)$ and $\xi_1(\mathcal{V})$ are vectors of the values of ξ_1 on the level contours and the vertices of the mesh, respectively. The matrix Q is the same as in (14) and the term $\xi_1(\mathcal{V})^T Q \xi_1(\mathcal{V})$ encourages smoothness of the function ξ_1. For this least square problem, we have the solution for $\xi_1(\mathcal{V})$ as

$$\xi_1(\mathcal{V}) = (A^T A + \beta Q)^{-1} A^T \xi_1(C). \tag{17}$$

We define the second feature function ξ_2 also based on the eigenfunction of the Laplace-Beltrami operator to characterize the lateral profile of elongated structures. For each level contour C_i, we generate a surface patch that approximates the minimal surface of C_i. This is achieved by first building a Delaunay triangulation of $C_{i,k}(k = 1, \cdots, K)$ using the software *triangle* [27] and then applying Laplacian smoothing to this mesh to obtain a smooth patch interpolating the interior of the boundary C_i as shown in Fig. 1(b). For this surface patch, we compute the second eigenfunction of its Laplace-Beltrami operator and denote it as γ_2^i. The Reeb graph of γ_2^i is then computed with N level contours D_i ordered with the increase of the function γ_2^i. For each level contour D_i, we assign a value $-1 + 2 * i/N$ to describe its lateral position on the surface. The value of the feature function ξ_2 on $C_{i,k}$ is defined using linear interpolation from the values of neighboring level contours. Once we define the feature function ξ_2 on the level contours, we can compute its value on the vertices of the entire mesh similarly as:

$$\xi_2(\mathcal{V}) = (A^T A + \beta Q)^{-1} A^T \xi_2(C) \tag{18}$$

where $\xi_2(C)$ and $\xi_2(\mathcal{V})$ are the vectors of values of ξ_2 on the level contours and the vertices, respectively.

As an illustration, we show the feature functions of a hippocampus in Fig. 2 (a) and (b) with the parameter $\beta = 10, N = 100, K = 100$, which clearly illustrates the power of the eigen-features in characterizing the relative locations of points on the surfaces.

4   Experimental Results

In this section we present experimental results to demonstrate our method. We will first illustrate our algorithm on the mapping of two types of surfaces: hippocampus and putamen. After that, we apply our method to a data set of 890 hippocampal surfaces and present statistically significant results.

4.1   Hippocampus Results

In the first experiment, we tested our algorithm on nine hippocampal surfaces. We chose one of them as the atlas and computed maps between this surface and the other eight surfaces. The parameters in the energy function are $\alpha_D^1 = 100, \alpha_D^2 = 50, \alpha_{IC} = 6, \alpha_H = 1$. To start the iterative algorithm, we use the same approach that we developed in [23] to automatically find an initial map. For all

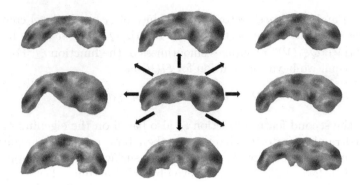

Fig. 3. A visualization of the hippocampal mapping results. The texture pattern on the atlas surface in the center is projected onto the other eight surfaces.

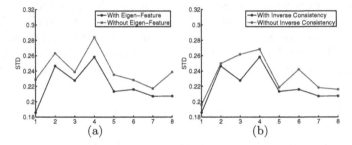

Fig. 4. The effect of eigen-features and inverse consistency on the quality of maps. (a) The standard deviation of the Jacobian with ($\alpha_D^1 = 100, \alpha_D^2 = 50$) and without ($\alpha_D^1 = 0, \alpha_D^2 = 0$) the eigen-features. (b) The standard deviation of the Jacobian with ($\alpha_{IC} = 6$) and without ($\alpha_{IC} = 0$) inverse consistency.

the surfaces, the mapping algorithm converged in less than 1500 iterations and the computational process took less than 10 minutes on a PC of 1.6GHz and 1.5GB memory. The mapping results between the atlas and the eight surfaces are visualized in Fig. 3 by projecting a texture pattern onto these surfaces with the correspondences established by the computed maps. While the surfaces vary quite significantly, we can see the corresponding parts are matched correctly and this shows the robustness of our method to structural variations across population.

To illustrate the importance of the Laplace-Beltrami eigen-features and inverse consistency, we turned off these terms separately and measured quantitatively their impact on the quality of maps. In our experiments, we computed the standard deviation of $|J_{u_1}|$ and $|J_{u_2}|$ as an indicator of the quality of maps because it measures the area distortion resulting from the maps. As shown in Fig. 4(a) and (b), smaller area distortions have been achieved for all the surfaces by incorporating both the eigen-features and inverse consistency.

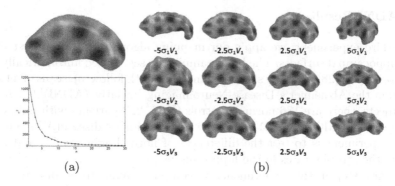

(a)   (b)

Fig. 5. The result of PCA on the 30 putamen surfaces. (a) Top: the mean shape. Bottom: the eigenvalues of PCA. (b) Shapes generated by varying the coefficients of the first three principal components.

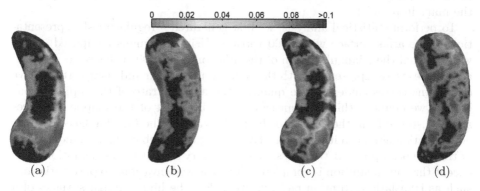

Fig. 6. The p-value map of atrophy rates. (a)(b) NC vs MCI. (c)(d) NC vs AD.

4.2   Putamen Results

In the second experiment, we tested our method on a group of 30 putamen surfaces. By choosing one of the surfaces as the atlas, we computed the maps from the other 29 surfaces to the atlas with the same parameters as in the first experiment. Using the correspondences across the 30 putamen surfaces that have been established by the maps, we can build a shape prior model for the putamen by performing a principal component analysis (PCA) [2]. The mean shape of the putamen is shown at the top of Fig. 5(a), where a texture pattern is also generated for visualization. The eigenvalues computed from the PCA process are plotted at the bottom of Fig. 5(a) where we can see most of the variations are captured by the first few components. As an illustration of the shape prior model, we plotted the shapes generated with the first three principle components. The texture pattern on the mean shape is also plotted on each synthesized surface in Fig. 5(b) to visualize correspondences across the shapes. From the results we can see the shape prior model is able to generate valid shapes with a quite large range ($\pm 5\sigma_i$) of coefficients for the principal components.

4.3   ADNI Results

In the third experiment, we apply our mapping algorithm to a data set of 890 right hippocampal surfaces. The hippocampi were segmented automatically with the algorithm in [28] from the screening and 12-month follow-up scans of 445 subjects from the Alzheimer's Disease Neuroimaging Initiative(ADNI)[29]. Among the subjects, there are 136 normal controls (NC), 228 patients with mild cognitive impairment(MCI), and 81 patients with Alzheimer's disease(AD). The goal of this experiment is to test the differences of normal aging, MCI, and AD in terms of the atrophy rates in the hippocampus.

As a first step in this experiment, we computed maps from all 890 surfaces to the atlas surface used in the first experiment as shown in the center of Fig. 3, and the same parameters as in the first experiment were used for all surfaces. In order to compute such a large amount of surface maps, we implemented our method on a grid of more than 1000 CPUs and this enables us to compute all the maps in parallel.

To perform statistical analysis, we first generated a regular mesh representation of the atlas surface with 2000 vertices. Using the maps computed above, we projected the triangular mesh of the atlas onto the 890 surfaces. As a result, all surfaces were represented with the same triangulation and their vertices have one-to-one correspondences. To quantify the atrophy rate of the hippocampus locally, we define a thickness measure at each vertex of the mapped surfaces as the distance from the vertex to the Reeb graph of the first Laplace-Beltrami eigenfunction as shown in Fig. 1 (a). By viewing this Reeb graph as a medial core of the hippocampus, our thickness measure is very similar to the definition in [1] except that our definition is completely intrinsic and invariant to pose variations such as translation, rotation and reflection. For the hippocampal surfaces of a subject, the atrophy rate at each corresponding vertex then equals the change of the thickness over the 12-month period as a percentage of the thickness at the screening scan.

Given the atrophy rates at corresponding vertices of all subjects, we performed two group analyses. In the first group study, we compared the NC group with the MCI group. At each vertex, a one-tailed t-test is applied to test the hypothesis that the MCI group has a higher atrophy rates than the NC group. The resulting p-value map is plotted onto the mean shape of the NC group in Fig. 6(a) and (b) in the top and bottom view. This map shows the significance level across different regions of the hippocampus. To correct for multiple comparisons, we performed 10,000 permutation tests and an overall statistically significance p-value 0.0063 was obtained. In the second group analysis, we compared the NC group with the AD group. Similarly, a one-tailed t-test was applied to test the hypothesis that the AD group has a higher atrophy rate than the NC group. The p-value map of this group analysis is plotted in Fig. 6(c) and (d). We also applied 10,000 permutation tests to correct for multiple comparisons and the overall p-value is 0.001, which shows the map is statistically significant. By comparing the maps in Fig. 6(c)(d) and Fig. 6(a)(b), we can clearly see the expansion of the regions with higher atrophy rates from the MCI to the AD group.

5 Conclusions and Future Work

We proposed a general framework for surface mapping with both eigen-feature-based data terms and regularizing terms for inverse consistency and smoothness. We successfully demonstrated its application in computing maps between elongated structures such as hippocampus and putamen. For future work, we will design new eigen-features and apply the current framework to other anatomical structures. We will also perform validations to compare our method with previous techniques.

Acknowledgment

This work was funded by the National Institutes of Health through the NIH Roadmap for Medical Research, Grant U54 RR021813 entitled Center for Computational Biology (CCB).

References

1. Thompson, P.M., Hayashi, K.M., de Zubicaray, G.I., Janke, A.L., Rose, S.E., Semple, J., Hong, M.S., Herman, D.H., Gravano, D., Doddrell, D.M., Toga, A.W.: Mapping hippocampal and ventricular change in Alzheimer disease. NeuroImage 22(4), 1754–1766 (2004)
2. Cootes, T., Taylor, C., Cooper, D., Graham, J.: Active shape models-their training and application. Computer Vision and Image Understanding 61(1), 38–59 (1995)
3. Christensen, G.E., Rabbitt, R.D., Miller, M.I.: Deformable templates using large deformation kinematics. IEEE Trans. Imag. Process. 5(10), 1435–1447 (1996)
4. Joshi, S., Miller, M.I.: Landmark matching via large deformation diffeomorphisms. IEEE Trans. Imag. Process. 9(8), 1357–1370 (2000)
5. Gerig, G., Styner, M., Jones, D., Weinberger, D., Lieberman, J.: Shape analysis of brain ventricles using SPHARM. In: Proc. Workshop on Mathematical Methods in Biomedical Image Analysis, pp. 171–178 (2001)
6. Davies, R.H., Twining, C.J., Allen, P.D., Cootes, T.F., Taylor, C.J.: Shape discrimination in the hippocampus using an MDL model. In: Taylor, C.J., Noble, J.A. (eds.) IPMI 2003. LNCS, vol. 2732, pp. 38–50. Springer, Heidelberg (2003)
7. Gu, X., Wang, Y., Chan, T.F., Thompson, P.M., Yau, S.T.: Genus zero surface conformal mapping and its application to brain surface mapping. IEEE Trans. Med. Imag. 23(8), 949–958 (2004)
8. Wang, L., Miller, J.P., Gado, M.H., McKeel, D.W., Rothermich, M., Miller, M.I., Morris, J.C., Csernansky, J.G.: Abnormalities of hippocampal surface structure in very mild dementia of the alzheimer type. NeuroImage 30(1), 52–60 (2006)
9. Yeo, B., Sabuncu, M., Vercauteren, T., Ayache, N., Fischl, B., Golland, P.: Spherical demons: Fast surface registration. In: Metaxas, D., Axel, L., Fichtinger, G., Székely, G. (eds.) MICCAI 2008, Part I. LNCS, vol. 5241, pp. 745–753. Springer, Heidelberg (2008)
10. Shi, Y., Thompson, P.M., de Zubicaray, G., Rose, S.E., Tu, Z., Dinov, I., Toga, A.W.: Direct mapping of hippocampal surfaces with intrinsic shape context. NeuroImage 37(3), 792–807 (2007)
11. Pizer, S.M., Fritsch, D.S., Yushkevich, P.A., Johnson, V.E., Chaney, E.L.: Segmentation, registration, and measurement of shape variation via image object shape. IEEE Trans. Med. Imag. 18(10), 851–865 (1999)

12. Styner, M., Gerig, G., Lieberman, J., Jones, D., Weinberger, D.: Statistical shape analysis of neuroanatomical structures based on medial models. Med. Image. Anal. 7(3), 207–220 (2003)
13. Yushkevich, P.A., Zhang, H., Gee, J.C.: Continuous medial representation for anatomical structures. IEEE Trans. Med. Imag. 25(12), 1547–1564 (2006)
14. Christensen, G., Johnson, H.: Consistent image registration. IEEE Trans. Med. Imag. 20(7), 568–582 (2001)
15. Eells, J., Lemaire, L.: Two reports on harmonic maps. World Scientific, Singapore (1995)
16. Mémoli, F., Sapiro, G., Osher, S.: Solving variational problems and partial differential equations mapping into general target manifolds. Journal of Computational Physics 195(1), 263–292 (2004)
17. Osher, S., Sethian, J.: Fronts propagation with curvature-dependent speed: algorithms based on Hamilton-Jacobi formulations. Journal of computational physics 79(1), 12–49 (1988)
18. Bertalmío, M., Cheng, L., Osher, S., Sapiro, G.: Variational problems and partial differential equations on implicit surfaces. Journal of Computational Physics 174(2), 759–780 (2001)
19. Reuter, M., Wolter, F., Peinecke, N.: Laplace-Beltrami spectra as Shape-DNA of surfaces and solids. Computer-Aided Design 38, 342–366 (2006)
20. Qiu, A., Bitouk, D., Miller, M.I.: Smooth functional and structural maps on the neocortex via orthonormal bases of the Laplace-Beltrami operator. IEEE Trans. Med. Imag. 25(10), 1296–1306 (2006)
21. Niethammer, M., Reuter, M., Wolter, F.E., Bouix, S., Koo, N.P.M.S., Shenton, M.: Global medical shape analysis using the laplace-beltrami spectrum. In: Ayache, N., Ourselin, S., Maeder, A. (eds.) MICCAI 2007, Part I. LNCS, vol. 4791, pp. 850–857. Springer, Heidelberg (2007)
22. Shi, Y., Lai, R., Krishna, S., Sicotte, N., Dinov, I., Toga, A.W.: Anisotropic Laplace-Beltrami eigenmaps: Bridging Reeb graphs and skeletons. In: Proc. MM-BIA, pp. 1–7 (2008)
23. Shi, Y., Lai, R., Kern, K., Sicotte, N., Dinov, I., Toga, A.W.: Harmonic surface mapping with Laplace-Beltrami eigenmaps. In: Metaxas, D., Axel, L., Fichtinger, G., Székely, G. (eds.) MICCAI 2008, Part II. LNCS, vol. 5242, pp. 147–154. Springer, Heidelberg (2008)
24. Belkin, M., Niyogi, P.: Laplacian eigenmaps for dimensionality reduction and data representation. Neural Computation 15(6), 1373–1396 (2003)
25. Reeb, G.: Sur les points singuliers d'une forme de Pfaff compla etement integrable ou d'une fonction nemérique. Comptes Rendus Acad. Sciences 222, 847–849 (1946)
26. Uhlenbeck, K.: Generic properties of eigenfunctions. Amer. J. of Math. 98(4), 1059–1078 (1976)
27. Shewchuk, J.R.: Delaunay refinement algorithms for triangular mesh generation. Comput. Geom. Theory & Applications 22(1–3), 21–74 (2002)
28. Morra, J., Tu, Z., Apostolova, L., Green, A., Avedissian, C., Madsen, S., Parikshak, N., Hua, N., Toga, A., Jack, C., Weiner, M., Weiner, M., Thompson, P.: The ADNI: Validation of a fully automated 3D hippocampal segmentation method using subjects with Alzheimer's disease, mild cognitive impairment, and elderly controls. NeuroImage (in press)
29. Mueller, S., Weiner, M., Thal, L., Petersen, R., Jack, C., Jagust, W., Trojanowski, J., Toga, A., Beckett, L.: The Alzheimer's disease neuroimaging initiative. Clin. North Am. 15, 869–877, xi–xii (2005)

Estimating Uncertainty in Brain Region Delineations

Karl R. Beutner III[1], Gautam Prasad[2], Evan Fletcher[1], Charles DeCarli[1], and Owen T. Carmichael[1]

[1] University of California at Davis, Davis CA 95616, USA
[2] University of California at Los Angeles, Los Angeles CA 90095, USA

Abstract. This paper presents a method for estimating uncertainty in MRI-based brain region delineations provided by fully-automated segmentation methods. In large data sets, the uncertainty estimates could be used to detect fully-automated method failures, identify low-quality imaging data, or endow downstream statistical analyses with per-subject uncertainty in derived morphometric measures. Region segmentation is formulated in a statistical inference framework; the probability that a given region-delineating surface accounts for observed image data is quantified by a distribution that takes into account a prior model of plausible region shape and a model of how the region appears in images. Region segmentation consists of finding the maximum *a posteriori* (MAP) parameters of the delineating surface under this distribution, and segmentation uncertainty is quantified in terms of how sharply peaked the distribution is in the vicinity of the maximum. Uncertainty measures are estimated through Markov Chain Monte Carlo (MCMC) sampling of the distribution in the vicinity of the MAP estimate. Experiments on real and synthetic data show that the uncertainty measures automatically detect when the delineating surface of the entire brain is unclear due to poor image quality or artifact; the experiments cover multiple appearance models to demonstrate the generality of the method. The approach is also general enough to accommodate a wide range of shape models and brain regions.

1 Uncertainty in Brain Region Delineations

1.1 Importance of Uncertainty Estimation in Brain Region Delineations

Structural magnetic resonance imaging (MRI) is a technology for measuring biological properties of the brain. A widespread methodology for large-scale epidemiological studies is to collect MRI scans of a cohort of subjects, delineate brain regions on those scans using manual or automated methods, and relate morphometric measures derived from those region delineations to clinical variables of interest. Studies of this sort have played an important role in clarifying the biological course of a range of neurological disorders, including multiple sclerosis and dementia [9] [7].

J.L. Prince, D.L. Pham, and K.J. Myers (Eds.): IPMI 2009, LNCS 5636, pp. 479–490, 2009.
© Springer-Verlag Berlin Heidelberg 2009

This paper provides a method for quantifying uncertainty in brain region delineations. Once the uncertainty in a brain region delineation is known, we can use this information to identify and possibly discard images whose region delineations have high uncertainty and therefore may have been segmented imprecisely. Our formulation of uncertainty is chiefly concerned with the precision, rather than the accuracy, of the delineating boundaries of brain regions. As with every measurement, both the accuracy and precision of the delineating surface determine the validity of inference made from their derived measures: accuracy is the degree to which the measurement is close to the true value of the quantity being measured, while precision is the degree to which repeated measurements provide similar values [8]. If a measurement is imprecise, we cannot be certain whether the measurement value arises from underlying biological phenomena or random fluctuations in the measurement process. Our approach is to use a statistical sampling procedure to simulate the repeated measurement of the same brain region boundary by an automated segmentation method, and assess whether the segmentation method tells us that a diverse, widely-scattered set of boundary surfaces delineate the region equally well.

The uncertainty in a brain region delineations obtained via automated methods can be affected by several factors. Poor image quality or low contrast between two brain regions can both lead to images that are hard to segment precisely. Further, measurement uncertainties are exacerbated when the models of brain appearance and shape used by an automated method are oversimplified or invalid. In these cases, a measurement can be imprecise; to our knowledge, there are currently no automated tools for quantifying measurement precision so these errors may be left undetected in the absence of time-consuming, tedious manual checking of segmentation results.

For example, imagine that the area of the ellipses in figure 1 are to be used to estimate the volume of the brain in the image. When making this derived measurement for the blurred image in figure 1, we could not be sure what size the ellipse should be in order to best approximate the brain contour since the image is blurry and the boundary between the skull and the brain is uncertain. This is an important concern because the size of the ellipse will determine the computed volume, which in turn will be used in a statistical analysis to test a hypothesis about relationships between brain volume and other clinical measures. Thus, uncertainty in derived measures give rise to errors in the data which in turn result in errors in the statistical analyses.

Most current fully automated segmentation methods cannot detect corrupted images or grossly incorrect delineations. Our hypothesis is that this is partly due to the fact that modern segmentation methods suffer from the inability to incorporate a quantitative estimate for the precision of reported measurements and that there is currently not a standard method for obtaining such estimates. Though the uncertainty in this example was synthetically produced, there are many real sources of uncertainty in image delineation. For example, blurry or "'ghosted"' images can lead to measurement uncertainty as well as images of

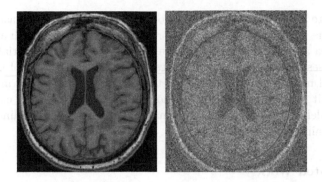

Fig. 1. The image on the right is the result of applying heavy white noise to the same image shown on the left. The ellipse on the left image is a region-delineation that partitions the image into brain region(inside the ellipse) and the non-brain region(outside of the ellipse). The ellipse on the right is the same as that on the left but due to the noise, it is no longer clear that the ellipse on the right truly does partitions the image correctly. Given the noisy image, different ellipses with different areas seem to fit the brain equally well.

brains with large pathologies which can sometimes deviate from the model assumptions of the segmentation method being used for the study.

1.2   Overview of Our Approach

A convenient way of formulating region-based delineation that encompasses many popular methods involves a Bayesian framework. The Bayesian approach seeks an answer to the question, 'what is the most probable delineating contour or surface of a desired region given the current image?' If we let I represent the image to be segmented and θ be a vector of parameters used to represent the shape of the delineating surface, then we can mathematically phrase this question by asking for a solution to the following conditional probability equation:

$$\hat{\theta} = \arg\max_{\theta} P(\theta|I) \tag{1}$$

$P(\theta|I)$ is the posterior probability of the parameters θ given the image, I. By Bayes Theorem equation 1 can be written as

$$\hat{\theta} = \arg\max_{\theta} L(I|\theta)q(\theta). \tag{2}$$

$L(I|\theta)$ is the *image model:* it is the likelihood of obtaining the image I given that the shape parameters are θ. The $q(\theta)$ term is known as the *shape model;* it is the prior probability that the region will take on the shape described by θ, regardless of the image I.

We estimate uncertainty in region delineation by using Markov Chain Monte Carlo (MCMC) to sample a series of θ from $P(\theta|I)$ and using the samples to approximate the solution to expectation integrals that give measures of uncertainty in the position of $\hat{\theta}$. Because morphometric measures such as volume and surface area are often derived from $\hat{\theta}$ and related to clinical variables in statistical analyses, the uncertainty measures can provide measures of uncertainty in the derived measures. We will demonstrate that the method is modular in the sense that it can be used in combination with a broad range of currently existing region delineation methods to estimate an optimal region-delineating surface and uncertainty in the surface.

1.3   Related Work

To our knowledge, the automated estimation of uncertainty in a single region delineation has not been addressed directly in the neuroimaging literature. The closest work to ours may be Simultaneous Truth and Performance Level Estimation (STAPLE) [12]. STAPLE formulates the region delineation problem in a probabilistic setting similar to ours, but is focused on using a statistical inference method to estimate variability across multiple manual delineations of the same region, along with the underlying ground-truth boundary surface. Here, in contrast, we are concerned with using statistical methods to estimate, for each input image and region, the delineating surface uncertainty that is inherent to a particular automated segmentation method. Uncertainty estimation differs from, and is more general than, segmentation validation method. Not only can uncertainty estimates be used to assess the quality of an image and/or segmentation, but it can also be used to enhance the statistical analysis that the segmentation was computed for in the first place. Outside of neuroimaging, estimating uncertainty in model parameters has been addressed in many fields. For example, [6] and [2] both use MCMC methods similar to the one presented here for estimating uncertainty in water catchment models and extra solar orbits respectively. Sampling methods such as MCMC have been used to represent uncertainty in time-varying variables being tracked by systems in computer vision and mobile robotics [3] [4]; and finally, some authors have used MCMC and related sampling methods as a means of finding extrema of complex probability distributions in computer vision problems, rather than for uncertainty estimation *per se* [1] [11].

2   Metropolis-Hastings and Markov Chain Monte Carlo

Monte Carlo integration is a numerical integration scheme used to estimate the expectation of a function $f(\theta)$ under a given distribution such as $P(\theta|I)$. Monte Carlo integration works by drawing sample θ values from $P(\theta|I)$. For example, let $\{\theta_0, \theta_1, ..., \theta_n\}$ be a sequence of independent identically distributed (i.i.d) random variables sampled from $P(\theta|I)$. Then the law of large numbers tells us that:

$$\frac{1}{n} \sum_{t=1}^{n} f(\theta_t) \rightarrow E_{P(\theta|I)}[\,f\,] = \int_{-\infty}^{\infty} f(\theta) P(\theta|I) d\theta \tag{3}$$

Thus, by evaluating the integrand at a sequence of points drawn from $P(\theta|I)$, Monte Carlo integration can approximate the population expectation for f under $P(\theta|I)$ to an arbitrary degree of precision by a sample mean computed from a sufficiently large sample.

The major assumption in Monte Carlo integration is that there exists a way to generate independent samples from an arbitrary distribution. This is not a trivial assumption because in many cases, $P(\theta|I)$ is highly non-standard and therefore difficult to sample from directly. The theory of Markov Chains and specifically the Metropolis-Hastings Algorithm helps to overcome this difficulty.

MCMC refers to a group of algorithms used to estimate $E_{P(\theta|I)}[f]$ by computing the mean of f over a set of samples drawn from a Markov chain whose stationary distribution is $P(\theta|I)$. The Metropolis-Hastings Algorithm is the most widely-used MCMC variant. Metropolis-Hastings simulates a Markov chain that transitions from a current state, θ_n, to a subsequent state θ_{n+1} based on a stochastically chosen candidate state, γ. γ is generated by sampling from a *proposal distribution*, $Q(\gamma|\theta_n)$ over the space of all possible states. γ is either *accepted*– $\theta_{n+1} = \gamma$– or *rejected*– $\theta_{n+1} = \theta_n$ depending on whether or not the following function passes a threshold:

$$\alpha(\theta_n, \gamma) = min(1, \frac{P(\gamma|I)Q(\theta_n|\gamma)}{P(\theta_n|I)Q(\gamma|\theta_n)}) \tag{4}$$

Hastings (1970) showed that the sequence of random variables that generated by this algorithm is a Markov chain whose states are eventually drawn from the distribution $P(\theta|I)$ after an appropriate number of initial states known as the *burn-in period*.

In practice, the three major design choices in MCMC are the selection of the proposal distribution, the criterion for determining that the burn-in period has ended, and the criterion for determining how many states to sample from the Markov chain after the burn-in period to estimate the required expectation. Once these design choices have been addressed, equation 3 tells us we can approximate $E_{P(\theta|I)}[f]$ in a Markov chain with an m-state burn-in period and n states required for expectation estimation as follows:

$$E_{P(\theta|I)}[f] \approx \frac{1}{(n-m)} \sum_{j=m+1}^{m+1+n} f(\theta_j). \tag{5}$$

3 Estimating Measurement Uncertainty with MCMC

3.1 The MCMC Approach

Given that a region-based delineation method as formulated in equation 2 provides an estimate $\hat{\theta}$ of the region delineating surface, we set $\hat{\theta}$ to be the initial state for a Markov chain, i.e. $\theta_0 = \hat{\theta}$, and use Metropolis-Hastings MCMC to construct the rest of the Markov chain. We approximate the expectations of two different functions. First we estimate $E[g(\theta)] = E[||\hat{\theta} - \theta||^2]$. This expectation is equal to the variance of $P(\theta|I)$ in the event that $\hat{\theta}$ is the mean of.

We also compute the expectation of the following characteristic function:

$$\chi_\rho(\theta) = \begin{cases} 1 \text{ if } \frac{|P(\hat{\theta}|I) - P(\theta|I)|}{P(\hat{\theta}|I)} \leq \rho \\ 0 \text{ otherwise.} \end{cases}$$

Geometrically, $E[\chi_\rho(\theta)]$ is the volume of the shape parameter space whose posterior probability is within a relative difference of ρ to the optimal delineating surface. Intuitively, this provides a sense of the uniqueness of $\hat{\theta}$. That is, if $E[\chi_\rho(\theta)]$ is large when ρ is small, then there are many diverse delineating surfaces that fit the image data just as well as the optimal surface; that is, there are many θ whose $P(\theta|I)$ is nearly equal to $P(\hat{\theta}|I)$. [1] We used a multivariate normal distribution, centered about the current state θ_n, as our proposal distribution.

4   Experiments

4.1   Overview

To demonstrate that this approach is modular with respect to image models, we test the method on two different methods for delineating the entire brain (a.k.a. "skull stripping"). Both use an ellipse shape model in which the size and rotation of the ellipse is fixed, and the two free parameters represent the x and y coordinates of the ellipse center. The first image model is the MeanSquaresPointSetToImageMetric (or MSPSM) model from the Insight Toolkit (ITK) software package. The MSPSM image model computes the average mean square difference between the pre-defined pixel values of a provided point set and intensity values of an image.

The second image model makes use of Intensity Profiles(IP, see Figure 2). It first computes the outward pointing unit normal vector to the surface at each point on the delineating surface. An array is constructed whose components are the image intensities of uniformly sampled points along the normal; a gaussian curve (whose peak represents the skull) and a logistic curve (whose low and high levels represent cerebrospinal fluid and parenchyma respectively) are fit to the array of intensities through maximum likelihood estimation. A new position of the brain-delineating surface along the surface normal is proposed based on the low points of the gaussian and logistic curves; the contribution of the surface point to the likelihood term is inversely proportional to the distance between the current position of the brain-delineating surface and the proposed one. Similar image models are used in [5] and [10].

---

[1] We note that $g(\theta)$ and $\chi_\rho(\theta)$ are just two examples of functions whose expectations can be estimated in this framework. As another example, $E_{P(\theta|I)}[||\theta - \hat{\theta}||^3]$ is the third moment of $P(\theta|I)$ about $\hat{\theta}$ and gives a measure of the skewness of $P(\theta|I)$ in the vicinity of $\hat{\theta}$.

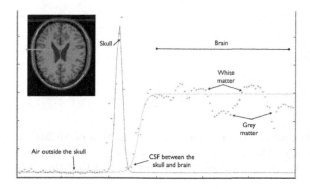

Fig. 2. An intensity profile going across the brain-skull interface has the general form of a Gaussian and logistic curve superimposed. From left to right, intensities along the profile correspond to air, skull, CSF, and parenchyma respectively

4.2   Data

The protocol for testing the MCMC uncertainty estimation method is as follows. First, the skull stripping of a 2D axial slice from a 3D T1 weighted MRI image is computed. Next, the output from the skull stripping, along with the 2D slice are given as input to the MCMC uncertainty estimation method and an uncertainty measure is computed. All images were axial-oblique 3D Fast Spoiled Gradient Recalled Echo (FSPGR) MRI scans of elderly individuals enrolled in the University of California, Davis Alzheimer's Disease Center (ADC). The 1.5-tesla GE Signal scanner parameters were: TE: 2.9 ms (min), TR: 9 ms (min), flip angle: 15 deg, slice thickness: 1.5 mm, slice spacing: 0.0 mm, number of slices: 128, NEX: 2, FOV: 25 cm x 25 cm, matrix: 256 x 256, bandwidth: 15.63 KHz, phase FOV: 1.00, frequency Direction: A/P. Because quantitative ground truth in region uncertainty is difficult to attain, the two experiments use simulated blurry images and real images with qualitative expert image ratings to assess the utility of the method.

4.3   Synthetic Data

The first test set, called the blurred test set, consists of a single test image along with 4 images that resulted from repetitively blurring the image with a gaussian kernel with an 8 pixel standard deviation. Because successive blurring increases the ambiguity of the brain-skull boundary, the blurred test set allows us to objectively test the strength of association between our uncertainty measures and increasing measurement uncertainty.

Figure 4 plots the 16,000 MCMC samples visited after burn-in for one, three, five, and seven iterations of blurring using the IP image model; samples for which $\chi_{0.01}(\cdot)$, $\chi_{0.05}(\cdot)$, and $\chi_{0.1}(\cdot)$ equal 1 are colored red, yellow, and blue respectively. A multivariate normal proposal distribution was used as our MCMC proposal distribution. Of the 20,000 iterations, approximately 4,000 were discarded as burn-in states. Visual inspection of the expectations as a function of

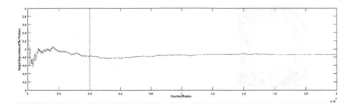

Fig. 3. The estimate of $E[g(\theta)]$ is plotted as a function of MCMC sample number for one example image. The green line shows the sample at which burn-in was stopped. The calm behavior of the chain after burn-in indicates that the chain has converged.

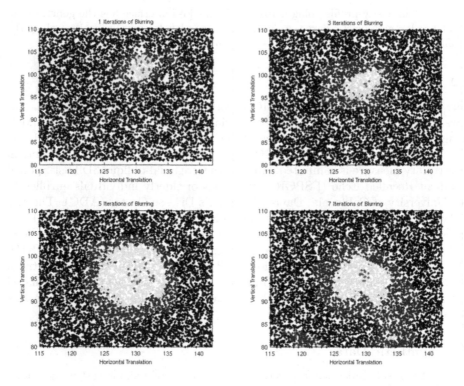

Fig. 4. These figures show how the regions where $\chi_{0.01}(.) = 1$ (red), $\chi_{0.05}(.) = 1$ (yellow) and $\chi_{0.1}(.) = 1$ (blue) grow as the image blurring increases. This example was made with the IP image model, and the ITK ellipse shape model.

sample number confirmed that the Markov chain appeared to reach the stationary distribution after the 4000th iteration (Figure 3).

Figure 4 shows that as the amount of blurring increases the regions in the parameter space for which $\chi_{0.05}(.) = 1$ and $\chi_{0.1}(.) = 1$ grow in size. This agrees with our intuitive understanding of how the brain-skull boundary is blurred by gaussian smoothing.

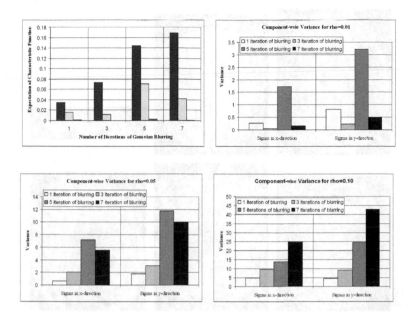

Fig. 5. Variance in the x- and y-directions for each of the colored regions shown in figure 4. Notice that the variance in the most blurred image is very large when $\rho = 0.10$, this implies a lack of precision.

The measure $E[\chi_\rho(.)]$ did not always increase with the amount of blurring due to its inadequacy as a simple volume measure. $E[\chi_\rho(.)]$ only gives information about the size of the region for which $\chi_\rho(.) = 1$, not its shape. For example, figure 5 reports a higher $E[\chi_{0.05}(.)]$ for 5 iterations of blurring than 7. However, the $\chi_{0.05}(.) = 1$ region for the 7 iteration case is more spatially elongated in the x direction than in the 5 iteration case. Because the range of plausible x values is higher in the 7 iteration case, the 7 iteration delineation could be considered more uncertain than its 5 iteration counterpart. To capture this behavior, we computed the component-wise variance of the parameter values over the samples in each of the regions of Figure 4. If we denote the jth component of the parameter vector θ by θ_j and the variance of a data set, S, by σ_S, then computing σ_{S_j} where $S_j = \{\theta_j | \chi_\rho(\theta_j) = 1\}$ for a pre-defined ρ will be a measure of the dispersion of the parameter values that are in the region defined by $\chi_\rho(\theta) = 1$.

The results from computing σ_{S_j} when ρ equals 0.01, 0.05 and 0.10 are given in figure 5. These plots capture the shape differences remarked on earlier. Thus, by combining the volumes and shapes of regions in the space of shape parameters, we detect the relative precision of the delineations.

4.4 Real 2D Data with Expert Uncertainty Ratings

The second test set consisted of 19 images selected out of the roughly 600 ADC images that have been analyzed to date by expert human raters who used

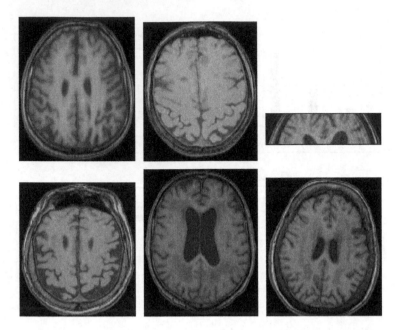

Fig. 6. The images shown in $a - e$ were all initially labeled as abnormal images. The image is subfigure c is truly just a fraction of an image; we added it to the abnormal test set to see if the method could detect such a problem in an image. It is unclear why image f was inaccurately segmented.

standardized protocols to manually trace the brain and hippocampus. Of these, 5 images were considered **normal** by the raters, 5 were annotated as **moderately poor**– having *either* moderately poor image quality or large pathological features present– and 9 were **extremely poor**, with either extremely low image quality, or simultaneous low image quality and large pathologies. These labels provide qualitative expert ground truth about image quality that should be reflected in the uncertainty measures. All expert annotations were made prior to the development of our method.

In the first stage of our analysis, we use the uncertainty measures to detect any brain delineations that are probably inaccurate. We do this by computing a quantity, β, which is the proportion of MCMC samples θ with $P(\theta|I) > P(\hat{\theta}|I)$ If β is large, the automated segmentation method must have failed because its θ do not even correspond to a local maximum of $P(\theta|I)$.

Of the 19 images, 11 had β values greater than 0.10 using the IP image model; only two had β values greater than 0.10 for the MSPSM image model. These were considered inaccurately segmented. Of the 11 removed by the IP image model, 5 were from the abnormal group. 6 of the excluded images are shown in figure 6.

Figure 7 shows the χ_ρ results for both segmentation methods tested. Expectations of $\chi_{0.01}(.)$ (red), $\chi_{0.05}(.)$ (yellow) and $\chi_{0.1}(.)$ (blue) are shown as colored

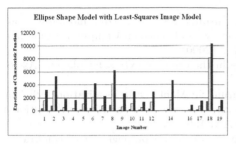
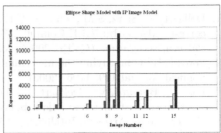

Fig. 7. Uncertainty estimations made on the back end of the MSPSM and IP segmentation methods. Missing data represents an image with $\beta > 0.10$.

bars. The first 4 images were labeled as normal; The next five were moderately poor; and the last four were extremely poor. Good and poor images provide similar uncertainty measures for MSPSM, suggesting that its image model is so over-simplified that it cannot to provide a precise delineation in any image; intuitively, the more complex IP model generally provided higher uncertainty estimates for the poor images (note, however, image 3). However, the IP model, with its more difficult task of optimizing more run-time parameters, is more prone to local minima as suggested by the larger number of discarded, high-β images. The high uncertainty of image 3 under the IP model may be due to an inadequacy in the expressive power of the IP model.

5   Discussion

In this paper we showed how MCMC methods can be used to sample the posterior distribution of an automated brain region delineation method for quantitative measurement of the uncertainty in a region-delineating surface. The method reported increasing brain region uncertainty as the blurring of a typical brain image increased; it also provided uncertainty measures that agreed well well qualitative expert ratings of image quality. By testing the method on a pair of image models we demonstrated that it is general enough to be used on the back end of a wide variety of current region delineation methods.

Future work will apply the method to other brain regions, including the hippocampus, and other automated segmentation methods. Methodologically, we will also explore novel modifications to the current method to increase sampling efficiency. Finally, we will explore the potential downstream uses of brain region uncertainty beyond detecting low-quality imaging data. For example, statistical analyses that relate brain region volume to clinical variables could use the uncertainty measures to down-weight region volumes derived from uncertain measurements.

References

1. Dellaert, F., Seitz, S.M., Thorpe, C.E., Thrun, S.: Structure from motion without correspondence. In: IEEE Computer Society Conference on Computer Vision and Pattern Recognition (CVPR 2000), vol. 2 (2000)
2. Ford, E.B.: Quantifying the uncertainty in the orbits of extrasolar planets. Astronomical Journal 129, 1706 (2005)
3. Fox, D., Burgard, W., Dellaert, F., Thrun, S.: Monte carlo localization: Efficient position estimation for mobile robots. In: Proceedings of the Sixteenth National Conference on Artificial Intelligence (AAAI 1999) (1999)
4. Isard, M., Blake, A.: Contour tracking by stochastic propagation of conditional density. In: Buxton, B.F., Cipolla, R. (eds.) ECCV 1996. LNCS, vol. 1064, pp. 343–356. Springer, Heidelberg (1996)
5. Kelemen, A., Szekely, G., Gerig, G.: Elastic model-based segmentation of 3-d neuroradiological data sets. IEEE Transactions on Medical Imaging 18(10), 828–839 (1999)
6. Kuczera, G., Parent, E.: Monte carlo assessment of parameter uncertainty in conceptual catchment models: the metropolis algortihm. Journal of Hydrology 211, 69–85 (1998)
7. Visser, S.P.J.: Medial temporal lobe atrophy and memory dysfunction as predictors for dementia in subjects with mild cognitive impairment. Journal of Neurology 246(6), 477–485 (1999)
8. Harper, B.R.R.: Reporting of precision of estimates for diagnostic accuracy: a review. BMJ 318(1), 1322–1323 (1999)
9. Schreiber, K., Sorensen, P.S., Koch-Henriksen, N., Wagner, A., Blinkenberg, M., Svarer, C., Petersen, H.C.: Correlations of brain MRI parameters to disability in multiple sclerosis 104(1), 24–30 (2001)
10. Smith, S.: Fast robust automated brain extraction. Human Brain Mapping 17(3), 143–155 (2002)
11. Tu, Z., Zhu, S.C.: Image segmentation by data-driven markov chain monte carlo. IEEE Transactions on Pattern Analysis and Machine Intelligence 24(5), 657–673 (2002)
12. Warfield, S.K., Zou, K.H., Wells, W.M.: Simultaneous truth and performance level estimation (staple): an algorithm for the validation of image segmentation. IEEE Medical Imaging 23, 903–921 (2004)

Unifying Encoding of Spatial Information in Mutual Information for Nonrigid Registration

Xiahai Zhuang, David J. Hawkes, and Sebastien Ourselin

Centre for Medical Image Computing, Medical Physics & Bioengineering
Department, University College London, WC1E 6BT, UK
x.zhuang@ucl.ac.uk

Abstract. As encoding spatial information into mutual information (MI) can improve the nonrigid registration against bias fields where the conventional MI is challenged, we propose to unify this encoding into the computation of the joint probability distribution function (PDF). The PDF is computed based on local volumes while the global intensity information is also incorporated to maintain the global intensity class linkage. We demonstrate this computation method can unify the PDF computation in regional MI, conditional MI, and the conventional MI. We then derive two categories of methods and apply them to different registration tasks. The experimental results demonstrate that both categories can significantly improve the registration.

Keywords: Spatial encoding, mutual information, free-form deformations, locally affine, registration.

1   Introduction

Mutual information (MI) has been a mostly investigated similarity measure in medical image registration since its invention independently by Viola and Wells [1] and Collignon et al. [2]:

$$\mathrm{MI}(I_r, I_f, T) = \sum_{r,f} p(r, f) \log \frac{p(r, f)}{p(r)p(f)}$$
$$= H(I_r) + H(T(I_f)) - H(I_r, T(I_f)) \, ,$$

(1)

where, $p(\circ)$ are the marginal and joint probability distribution functions (PDFs), and $H(\circ)$ are the marginal and joint entropies of the reference image I_r and floating image I_f.

Pluim et al. [3] had a survey on MI registration and summarized three different interpretations. One interpretation is based on the dispersion of the joint histogram table, meaning that the less dispersion of the joint histogram, the better the two image are assumed to be registered. Under this interpretation, the maximization of MI is related to the minimization of the dispersion of the joint histogram table, given the two images are initially well overlapped. Therefore, in MI registration, only the intensity class correspondence is assumed instead of the

J.L. Prince, D.L. Pham, and K.J. Myers (Eds.): IPMI 2009, LNCS 5636, pp. 491–502, 2009.

intensity correspondence of each pixel pair. The advantage of this assumption is the applicability of MI to images with different intensity distribution, including images from different imaging modalities where the image intensity classes reflect the tissue classes. However, there are three situations which can challenge the applicability of MI.

The first one is when one of the images (or both) are from imaging techniques that the imaged pixel intensity does not represent the tissue classes, then the assumption of intensity class correspondence can not be met. One example is from ultrasound imaging, where the intensity responds to the tissue boundaries instead of homogeneous tissues. Mellor and Brady [4] have proposed a feature based measure combined with MI, phase mutual information, for ultrasound registration. Therefore, we will not further discuss this situation in this paper.

The second situation arises when the images are with intensity non-uniformity (bias) and noise, which affects the estimation of the joint PDF in MI computation. This effect may not be so profound in rigid or affine registration, where the transformation parameters globally change the contribution of all pixel pairs to the joint histogram table. Therefore, the local effects from the bias can be either balanced out or reduced thanks to the basis of statistical estimation of the MI computation. However, in nonrigid registration with higher degree of freedom, the transformation parameters have more profound effects on local volumes, such as on their local support regions. As a result, the biased estimation of the joint probability distribution will generate false forces to misalign the local details. Figure 1 (left and middle) shows an example: the nonrigid MI registration of an identical brain T1 image pair [1] generates a small erroneous deformation field. However, when one of the image is contaminated with a bias field (intensity non-uniformity 40%), the same registration algorithm produces a much larger deformation field. This deformation field corresponds to the patten of the bias field.

The final situation happens when the intensity class correspondence is inhomogeneous. This happens more commonly in different modality registrations, such as the CT-MR registration discussed in [5]. But this inhomogeneity can also happen to images with different intensity distribution instead of strictly imaging modalities. Figure 1 gives an example of brain MR T1 and T2 image registration: a much larger deformation field is presented for T1 and T2 registration (bottom right) compared to that of same intensity distribution T1 and T1 (bottom left).

1.1 Related Work

Both of the last two challenges can be improved if the computation of information (entropy) in MI can consider the spatial difference of each message element. For example, the message *aabbaa* has the same information as that of *aabbbb* or *aaaabb*. However, in image registration, the message *112233* may be consider as more similar to *aabbaa* than the other two. To include this spatial information, one method is to use local mutual information (LMI) computed from a joint

---

[1] From BrainWeb: www.bic.mni.mcgill.ca/brainweb/

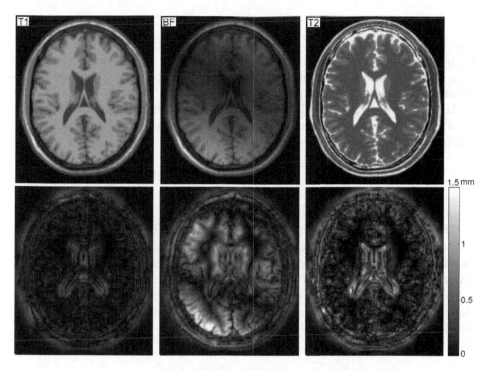

Fig. 1. Deformation fields of registering identical images using conventional mutual information. From left to right of top row are T1 brain image, 40% bias field, and T2 brain image; from left to right of bottom row are the deformation fields of the registration between non-bias T1 and T1, non-bias T1 and T1 with bias field, and non-bias T1 and T2. Red arrows are the displacement vectors.

histogram table estimated from sub-volumes of the images, such as computing the LMI between *aabb* of *aabbaa* and *1122* of *112233*.

However, estimating local joint histogram table from a small sample set reduces the statistical power of MI, thus it introduces extra local optima in the LMI functional [6,7]. Studholme *et al.* [8] proposed a regional mutual information (RMI) which regards the spatial information as an extra channel and computes the mutual information of the three channels. They also derived a simplified metric from RMI as the similarity measure, denoted as RMI′:

$$
\begin{aligned}
\mathrm{RMI}'(I_r, I_f, T) &= \sum_{\mathbf{x}} p(\mathbf{x}) \sum_r \sum_f p_{\mathbf{x}}(r, f) \log \left(\frac{p_{\mathbf{x}}(r, f)}{p_{\mathbf{x}}(r) p_{\mathbf{x}}(f)} \right) \\
&= \sum_{\mathbf{x}} p(\mathbf{x}) \mathrm{MI}'_{\mathbf{x}}(I_r, I_f, T) ,
\end{aligned}
\tag{2}
$$

which is the linearly weighted sum of LMI set $\{\mathrm{MI}'_{\mathbf{x}}\}$, where $\{\mathbf{x}\}$ are local regions. The LMIs are computed using local joint probability distribution $p_{\mathbf{x}}(r, f)$, based on local joint histogram table:

$$p_{\mathbf{X}}(r, f) = \mathcal{H}_{\mathbf{X}}(r, f)/N_{\mathbf{X}} , \tag{3}$$

where, $N_{\mathbf{X}} = \sum_{r.f} \mathcal{H}_{\mathbf{X}}(r, f)$ is the normalization factor. The weighted sum of LMIs from a set of overlapped sub-volume can improve registration performance compared to simply using single LMI. However, the local joint histogram tables are still constructed from the sub-volumes.

An alternative work from Loeckx et al. [5] regarded the spatial coordinates of pixels in the reference image as priorly known conditions and proposed to compute the conditional mutual information (cMI) of the two images:

$$\mathrm{cMI}(I_r, I_f, T | X) = \sum_{\mathbf{x}} p(\mathbf{x}) \sum_r \sum_f p(r, f | \mathbf{x}) \log \left(\frac{p(r, f | \mathbf{x})}{p(r | \mathbf{x}) p(f | \mathbf{x})} \right) . \tag{4}$$

Similarly to RMI, the conditional probability distribution is also based on $p(r, f, \mathbf{x})$ by extending the spatial dimension as an extra channel to construct the joint histogram table. Differently, the spatial binning in cMI uses a multi-dimensional cubic B-spline kernel function as the smoothing function in the Parzen window estimation (Parzen window function). The advantage is that the local joint probability is non-linearly weighted in the local cMI computation considering the distance of each pixel to the center of the spatial bin. If 0-order B-spline kernel function, the boxcar function in RMI [8] is used, the joint histogram becomes:

$$
\begin{aligned}
\mathcal{H}(r, f, \mathbf{x}) &= \sum_{\boldsymbol{x} \in \Omega} \omega_r(I_r(\boldsymbol{x})) \omega_f(I_f(\boldsymbol{x})) \omega_{\mathbf{x}}(\boldsymbol{x}) \\
&= \sum_{\boldsymbol{x} \in \Omega_{\mathbf{x}}} \omega_r(I_r(\boldsymbol{x})) \omega_f(I_f(\boldsymbol{x})) \cdot 1 = \mathcal{H}_{\mathbf{X}}(r, f) ,
\end{aligned} \tag{5}
$$

where, ω_r, ω_f, and $\omega_{\mathbf{x}}$ are Parzen window functions. Due to $p(\mathbf{x}) = N_{\mathbf{X}}/N$, where N is the normalization factor for $p(r, f, \mathbf{x})$ and $\sum_{\mathbf{x}} N_{\mathbf{X}} = N$, then,

$$
\begin{aligned}
p(r, f | \mathbf{x}) &= p(r, f, \mathbf{x})/p(\mathbf{x}) \\
&= \frac{\mathcal{H}_{\mathbf{X}}(r, f)/N}{N_{\mathbf{X}}/N} = p_{\mathbf{X}}(r, f) .
\end{aligned} \tag{6}
$$

Therefore, the derived conditional MI, denoted as cMI′, is identical to RMI′.

Another problem of LMI is the loss of global intensity class linkage due to the lack of maintaining a joint histogram table constructed from the global space, as discussed in [9]. Likar and Pernus [6] proposed to use the joint probability distribution from the histogram of the complementary volume of the local region, and regard it as *a priori* information to estimate the joint PDF using a mixture model:

$$p(r, f) = w\, p_{\mathbf{X}}(r, f) + (1 - w)\, p^*(r, f) . \tag{7}$$

The implementation in [6] used the portion of the sub-volume to the whole volume, $|\Omega_{\mathbf{X}}|/|\Omega|$, to value the weighting w for a local affine registration. This is equivalent to the implementation of the locally affine registration [9] using conventional MI under the assumption that the local support of the local affine transformation is within the sub-volume.

1.2   Contribution of This Work

From the discussion above, we summarize two points for improving MI against bias fields. One is that the local estimation of the joint probability distribution, which encodes spatial information and thus makes the MI more robust against bias, can provide important information for correcting local misalignment. The other is that to maintain the global intensity class linkage, the local estimation should be mixed with the global estimation under a weighting system that can encode spatial information.

In this paper, we propose an unified function to encode the spatial information into the computation of the joint PDF in nonrigid registration. This encoding is achieved by weighting the contribution of pixel pairs to the joint histogram table according to their spatial coordinates. We also derive two categories of methods for comparisons in the experiments, including applying them to free-form deformations (FFDs) registration and locally affine registration. The experiments and results are presented section 3, where the discussion are also provided. Section 4 draws the conclusion.

2   Method

2.1   A Mixture Model for Weighting Local and Global Information

Let I_r be the reference image, I_f be the source image, and θ be a parameter of a nonrigid transformation T, which has a local support region x. The conventional estimation of the joint PDF for MI is:

$$
\begin{aligned}
p(r,f) &= \frac{1}{N} \sum_{x \in \Omega} \omega_r(I_r(\boldsymbol{x}))\omega_f(I_f(\boldsymbol{x})) \\
&= \frac{N_{\mathbf{x}}}{N}\frac{1}{N_{\mathbf{x}}}\mathcal{H}_{\mathbf{x}}(r,f) + (1 - \frac{N_{\mathbf{x}}}{N})\frac{1}{N - N_{\mathbf{x}}}\mathcal{H}_{\bar{\mathbf{x}}}(r,f) \\
&= w\,p_{\mathbf{x}}(r,f) + (1-w)\,p_{\bar{\mathbf{x}}}(r,f)\,,
\end{aligned}
\tag{8}
$$

which is similar to eq. 7, regarding $p_{\bar{\mathbf{x}}}(r,f)$ as the prior probability $p^*(r,f)$.

In eq. 8, the joint histogram is separated into two: $\mathcal{H}_{\mathbf{x}}$ is constructed from the sub-volume $\Omega_{\mathbf{x}}$, regarded as local information of parameter θ, and $\mathcal{H}_{\bar{\mathbf{x}}}$ is built from the complementary volume $\bar{\Omega}_{\mathbf{x}}$, regarded as global information. By valuing $w = N_{\mathbf{x}}/N$, the pixel pairs from local or global information contribute the same influence to the estimation of $p(r,f)$. However, to optimize θ, we can estimate the PDF with more confidence on the pixel pairs from the local information, especially when the images are corrupted by bias fields. For example, valuing $w = 2N_{\mathbf{x}}/N$ gives more credits on the local information, thus the computed MI is expected to be able to more accurately optimize the registration within volume $\Omega_{\mathbf{x}}$. Based on this idea, we introduce a new parameter, $\lambda \in [0,1]$ indicating the trade-off between the local information and global (prior) information, to provide a general weighting scheme for them such that $w = w(\lambda)$. To interpolate $w(\lambda)$, three conditions are introduced:

1. When the global information has 100% confidence, $\lambda = 1$, which should correspond to a conventional mutual information situation:

$$w(\lambda) = w(1) = N_\mathbf{x}/N$$

2. When the global information has no confidence or is unavailable, $\lambda = 0$, meaning only LMI is applied:

$$w(\lambda) = w(0) = 1$$

$$w(\lambda) = w(0.5) = 0.5$$

Based on these conditions, a quadric polynomial function can be interpolated:

$$w(\lambda) = \frac{2N_\mathbf{x}}{N}\lambda^2 - (1 + \frac{N_\mathbf{x}}{N})\lambda + 1, \ \lambda \in [0,1] \ . \tag{9}$$

Note that the quadratic polynomial is one of the possible solutions for this interpolation.

In this scheme, the local information is discriminated from the global during the computation of the PDF for θ, thus it can encode the spatial difference between different regions.

2.2   Pixel-Wise Spatial Encoding

By valuing $w(\lambda)$, we can differentiate the importance of the local information from the global information. However, the PDF estimation still can not encode the fine detail of the spatial information within the local region. This means the pixel pairs from the same local region are always treated equally regardless their difference of spatial coordinates. Therefore, we further propose another function for weighting the contribution of each pixel pair to the histogram table:

$$\mathcal{H}(r, f) = \sum_\mathbf{x} \omega_r(I_r(\mathbf{x}))\omega_f(I_f(\mathbf{x})) \cdot \mathcal{E}(\mathbf{x}) \ , \tag{10}$$

where, $\mathcal{E}(\mathbf{x})$ is the weighting function, encoding spatial information at coordinate $\mathbf{x}$.

By using a constant value, $\mathcal{E}_\mathbf{x} = 1$, eq. 10 becomes the conventional estimation method; while by using the multi-dimensional cubic B-spline kernel function for $\mathcal{E}_\mathbf{x}$, it turns out to be the joint histogram table $\mathcal{H}(r, f, \mathbf{x})$ in conditional mutual information, where the spatial variable x corresponds to the FFDs control point.

Combining the local and global information weighting $w(\lambda)$ and the spatial coordinate weighting $\mathcal{E}(\mathbf{x})$, the estimation of joint probability distribution for a local support volume $\Omega_\mathbf{x}$ of a transformation parameter θ becomes:

$$p_\theta(\circ) = \frac{w(\lambda)}{N_\mathbf{x}} \sum_{x \in \Omega_\mathbf{x}} \omega(\circ)\mathcal{E}(\mathbf{x}) + \frac{1 - w(\lambda)}{N_{\bar{\mathbf{x}}}} \sum_{x \in \bar{\Omega}_\mathbf{x}} \omega(\circ)\mathcal{E}(\mathbf{x}) \ . \tag{11}$$

To maintain the global intensity class linkage, $\mathcal{E}$ should be a function which has non-zero value in global space Ω.

2.3 Implementation

Function for $\mathcal{E}(x)$. According to the different choice of function $\mathcal{E}$, we classify the methods into two categories. One is to choose a constant value for the function such that $\mathcal{E}(x) = 1$. Combining with different λ value in $\{0, 0.25, 0.5, 0.75, 1\}$, we derive five methods for experiments, denoted as $\mathcal{C}_0$, $\mathcal{C}_{.25}$, $\mathcal{C}_{.5}$, $\mathcal{C}_{.75}$, and $\mathcal{C}_1$ respectively. Note that $\mathcal{C}_1$ =MI is the conventional mutual information. The other is to use the multi-dimensional Gaussian function for $\mathcal{E}$. Combining with λ value 0.5 and 1, we derive two methods, denoted as $\mathcal{G}_{.5}$ and $\mathcal{G}_1$ respectively. The center of the Gaussian function is the center of the local support volume of the transformation parameter, and the standard deviation is set to the distance from the center to the local region boundary.

Cost function. Since we unify the computation of the joint PDF in nonrigid registration, the cost function can be either MI or its normalized measures such as the normalization mutual information in [10]. In experiment section, we use this normalized measure, though the results from the MI measure is similar to draw the same conclusion.

To construct the joint histogram table, two methods have been widely used for the interpolation, the partial volume interpolation [11] and the linear interpolation. In this paper, we use the latter to combine with the cubic B-spline kernel function as the Parzen Window function [12] and use 64 bins for intensity histogram.

Assuming $\Omega_{\mathbf{x}}$ is the local support volume of a transformation parameter θ or the approximate volume for force computation such as in fluid registration [8] or locally affine registration method [9], then the derivative of the PDF with respect to θ becomes:

$$\partial p_\theta(\circ)/\partial\theta = w(\lambda)\partial p_{\mathbf{x}}(\circ)/\partial\theta \ . \tag{12}$$

Transformations. Two transformation models will be investigated in the experiments.

One is the FFDs transformation model [14]. In this model, the center of the Gaussian function $\mathcal{G}_1$ and $\mathcal{G}_{0.5}$ is set to coordinate of each control point ϕ_θ when computing p_θ, and the standard deviation is set to twice spacing of the FFDs mesh. The other is the locally affine transformation model [9]. Due to irregular shape of local regions, the Gaussian center is set to the mass center of the pre-defined local region and the standard deviation is set to an average value of the distance from the boundary of the approximate local support volume to the Gaussian function center.

3 Experiments

3.1 FFDs Registration

This experiment uses brain MR T1 and T2 images, downloaded from BrainWeb. They are with 1% noise and of pixel size $1 \times 1 \times 1$ mm. Three different levels of

Table 1. The warping index (0.01 mm) of the FFDs registration results using different cost functions on the T1-T1 and T1-T2 images with 0%, 20%, 40% bias fields. Row T1-T1 and T1-T2 give the mean accuracy of the three different bias scales.

(0.01 mm)	$\mathcal{C}_0$	$\mathcal{C}_{.25}$	$\mathcal{C}_{.5}$	$\mathcal{C}_{.75}$	$\mathcal{C}_1$(MI)	$\mathcal{G}_{.5}$	$\mathcal{G}_1$
T1-T1(0%)	29 ± 28	21 ± 12	18 ± 8.3	18 ± 9.9	20 ± 16	23 ± 18	22 ± 15
T1-T1(20%)	32 ± 30	26 ± 21	24 ± 1.6	27 ± 1.8	42 ± 41	21 ± 6.3	21 ± 11
T1-T1(40%)	37 ± 34	28 ± 9.9	34 ± 11	44 ± 9.5	62 ± 29	22 ± 4.5	23 ± 8.7
T1-T1	33 ± 31	25 ± 15	25 ± 10	30 ± 13	41 ± 35	22 ± 11	22 ± 12
T1-T2(0%)	48 ± 45	34 ± 16	33 ± 10	35 ± 10	43 ± 17	40 ± 23	39 ± 20
T1-T2(20%)	56 ± 58	44 ± 32	46 ± 32	51 ± 27	60 ± 28	40 ± 18	40 ± 23
T1-T2(40%)	53 ± 49	49 ± 34	58 ± 36	71 ± 41	92 ± 53	46 ± 25	45 ± 28
T1-T2	53 ± 51	42 ± 29	46 ± 30	53 ± 32	65 ± 41	42 ± 22	42 ± 24

Table 2. The warping index (mm) of the locally affine registration results using different cost functions on cardiac MR image with 0%, 50%, 100% bias fields

(mm)	$\mathcal{C}_0$	$\mathcal{C}_{.25}$	$\mathcal{C}_{.5}$	$\mathcal{C}_{.75}$	$\mathcal{C}_1$(MI)	$\mathcal{G}_{.5}$
$\mathcal{B}\_0\%$	1.0 ± 1.2	0.27 ± 0.15	0.20 ± 0.02	0.22 ± 0.02	1.9 ± 2.7	0.20 ± 0.02
$\mathcal{B}\_50\%$	1.2 ± 1.1	1.1 ± 0.66	0.99 ± 0.29	1.0 ± 0.28	2.1 ± 2.4	0.89 ± 0.24
$\mathcal{B}\_100\%$	2.3 ± 1.3	2.3 ± 1.3	2.6 ± 1.6	3.2 ± 2.2	5.1 ± 3.3	2.2 ± 1.1
Total	1.5 ± 1.3	1.2 ± 1.2	1.3 ± 1.4	1.5 ± 1.8	3.0 ± 3.2	1.1 ± 1.1

bias fields are available, 0% (non-bias), 20%, and 40%. In the experiment, only 2D images from the central slice of the axial view are selected for registration due to the large number (1680) of registration tasks. Figure 1 top row shows the T1 image (left), a 40% bias field (middle), and the T2 image (right).

　　The initial transformations, regarded as ground truth for the registration accuracy assessment, are combinations of isotropic scalings and FFDs transformations with 45×54 mm mesh spacing. Ten scalings are chosen among [0.9, 1.10] and the FFDs transformations move the center control points either 15 mm or -15 mm at each direction, together generating 40 initial transformations. These initializations are applied to the T1 images of three different bias fields. The deformed images are then regarded as reference images, registering to the non-bias T1 and T2 images respectively using the seven methods: $\mathcal{C}_0$, $\mathcal{C}_{.25}$, $\mathcal{C}_{.5}$, $\mathcal{C}_{.75}$, $\mathcal{C}_1$ (MI), $\mathcal{G}_{.5}$, and $\mathcal{G}_1$. The warping index, root mean square, are calculated for brain surface pixels as the registration accuracy and the initial transformation fields, which range from 4.43 mm to 7.20 mm (4.64 ± 1.36 mm). The registration uses three-level FFDs (16mm, 8mm, 4mm on each dimension) and multiresolution [13] scheme for the gradient ascent optimization.

3.2　Locally Affine Registration

This section demonstrates the experiment of applying the two categories of methods to the locally affine registration of 3D cardiac MR images. For the locally affine transformation, four local regions are defined based on the four chambers, as the boundary line shown in figure 2 (top). The local support volume of each local affine is approximately defined to 10 mm dilation of its corresponding local region [9].

The cardiac MR image, shown in figure 2 (top), is an atlas image constructed from ten *in vivo* MR data which have been registered into a selected common space as described in [15]. The ten MR images were acquired with resolution $2 \times 2 \times 2$ mm, then all resampled into $1 \times 1 \times 1$ mm. By using the mean intensity from the ten aligned training images, the noise and bias in the resultant MR image can be significantly reduced.

The initial transformations are also local affine transformations, in which each local region randomly translates and rotates to provide a local displacement within 0 to 10 mm without overlapping each other. We generate twenty initial transformations, whose warping indexes range from 4.23 mm to 14.8 mm (8.23 ± 3.1 mm). Figure 2 (bottom) shows the deformed image with an initial transformation, whose warping index is 7.54mm.

Twenty bias fields are also simulated using the equation of $\mathcal{B} = a_1 x^2 + a_2 y^2 + a_3 z^3 + a_4 xy + a_5 xz + a_6 yz + a_7 x + a_8 y + a_9 z$, where $\boldsymbol{x} = [x, y, z]$ is the pixel coordinate, and $\{a_i\}$ are random values within $[-1, 1]$. The magnitudes of bias fields are normalized to 0% (non-bias), 50%, and 100% of the intensity range of the original image. Figure 2 (bottom) shows an image with a 100% bias field.

In the locally affine registration, the definition of the Gaussian function $\mathcal{G}$ is difficult to correspond to the irregular shape of the local regions. Hence, the center of the Gaussian function is defined to the mass center of the local region, and the standard deviation is simply set to isotropic 30 mm. Also, to lessen the influence of using a same standard deviation for the different sizes of local support volumes, λ is set to 0.5 to balance all w to 0.5. Again, the warping index of the endocardial surface of the heart are calculated to evaluate the registration accuracy.

3.3   Results and Discussion

Table 1 shows the results of the FFDs registration experiment. The registration using the constant $\mathcal{E}$ with λ from 0 to 1 perform the best when λ is around 0.25 to 0.75. Across different registration tasks, the ideal value for λ is not consistent. Smaller values of λ, corresponding to less confidence of the global information, tend to favor the registration tasks with stronger bias fields; and vice versa. But the registration with $\lambda = 0$ does not perform the best, even in 40% bias field, due to the less robustness of the registration without the global information. While the $\mathcal{C}_1$(MI) registration is sensitive to intensity bias, it is shown to be the worst choice for registering images with strong bias fields. In non-bias T1-T1 registration, where intensity class is assumed to be well corresponded, $\mathcal{C}_1$ (MI) performs no significantly worse than any other methods which encode spatial information. However, in non-bias T1-T2 registration, $\mathcal{C}_1$(MI) performs much worse compared to $\mathcal{C}_{0.5}$ which achieves the best result in this task. This confirms that the intensity class correspondence between T1 and T2 images is biased.

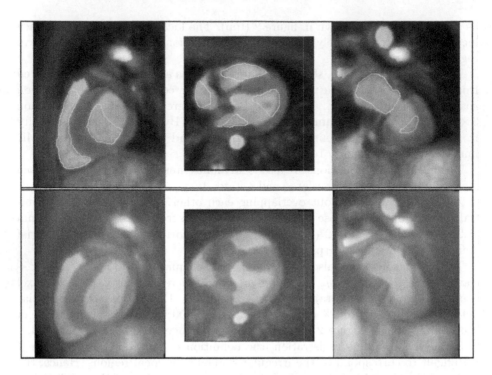

Fig. 2. The cardiac MR image for registration. Top is the MR image overlapping with the contour of the four chamber local regions, without bias field and initial deformation; bottom is the MR image with a 100% bias field and an initial transformation with warping index of 7.54 mm.

The results from the registration of $\mathcal{G}_{0.5}$ and $\mathcal{G}_1$ indicate that the spatial encoding in the construction of the joint histogram table achieves more robust registration, especially in strong bias fields. This is because the spatial encoding using $\mathcal{G}$ is pixel-wise; while using $\mathcal{C}$ and $w(\lambda)$, the spatial difference within local regions can not be differentiated in the derived measures. The other advantage of using $\mathcal{G}$ is the small differences between $\mathcal{G}_1$ and $\mathcal{G}_{0.5}$, which suggests the parameterization of λ can be simply set to 0.5. This is because using Gaussian weighting $\mathcal{G}$, the joint histogram table not only encodes the spatial information by non-linearly weighting the contribution of pixel pairs to the histogram, but also makes the distribution of function $w(\lambda)$ more flat. As shown in figure 3, the distribution of $w(\lambda)$ decreases much more sharply in $\mathcal{E} = 1$ than in $\mathcal{E} = \mathcal{G}$ due to the large difference between the two normalization factors $N_{\mathbf{x}}$ and $N_{\bar{\mathbf{x}}}$ in $\mathcal{E} = 1$.

The registration results for the locally affine registration are presented in table 2. Similar conclusion can be drawn from this experiment, but with two differences compared to the FFDs experiment. One is the more competitive of the $\mathcal{C}_0$ registration compared to its performance in the FFDs experiment. This is especially clear in the strong bias ($\mathcal{B}\_100\%$) registration, where the $\mathcal{C}_0$ achieves similar results as the other best methods, $\mathcal{C}_{.25}$ and $\mathcal{G}_{.5}$. The other is the much

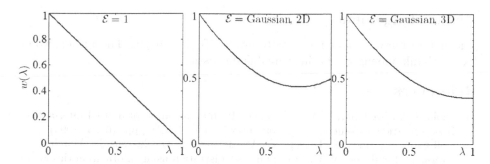

Fig. 3. The distribution of the weighting function $w(\lambda)$ under different choices of $\mathcal{E}$: constant value, $\mathcal{E} = 1$ (left), Gaussian function in two dimensions (middle), and Gaussian function in three dimensions. The distributions of $w(\lambda)$ using Gaussian are more flat between $[0.5, 1]$ for both two and three dimensions.

worse performance of the $\mathcal{C}_1(\text{MI})$ in the non-bias registration. Both these two are due to the factor that the cardiac MR image has large background tissues, such as abdomen and liver, which are not interests of the locally affine registration. Therefore, the information from the large volume of background does not provide much useful information for the registration of the endocardial surface. Instead, it introduces more bias for the estimation of the PDF. Therefore, paying too much credit to the global information actually diminishes the robustness of the locally affine registration in this situation. Furthermore, the approximate local support volume of each local affine includes both the blood pool and a similar volume size of either myocardium or background, hence $\mathcal{C}_0$ can perform better than $\mathcal{C}_1(\text{MI})$ registration, even without the global information.

4   Conclusion

In this paper, we have presented a framework, unifying the computation of the probability distribution function in mutual information, to encode spatial information for nonrigid registration. The encoding is achieved by weighting the contribution of pixel pairs to the joint histogram table according to their spatial coordinates. The constant weighting scheme for encoding pixel coordinate information, $\mathcal{C}$, combined with different λ to weight the credits of the global information, can significantly improve the registration accuracy against either non-bias or strong bias fields. However, the performance of this weighting scheme highly depends on the parameterization of λ for different registration tasks. While using the Gaussian weighting $\mathcal{G}$, where the spatial coordinates can be weighted pixel-wisely, the experiments have demonstrated two advantages: the better registration accuracy against strong bias and the more consistent performance with different valuing of λ. This makes it more promising and more applicable for different registration tasks.

Acknowledgement

The first author was funded by EPSRC grant GR/T11395/01. The authors would like to thank Yipeng Hu for his valuable discussion.

References

1. Viola, P.A., Wells III, W.M.: Alignment by maximization of mutual information. In: International Conference on Computer Vision (ICCV), pp. 16–23 (1995)
2. Collignon, A., Maes, F., Delaere, D., Vandermeulen, D., Suetens, P., Marchal, G.: Automated multimodality medical image registration using information theory. In: IPMI, Computational Imaging and Vision, vol. 3, pp. 263–274 (1995)
3. Pluim, J.P.W., Antoine Maintz, J.B., Viergever, M.A.: Mutual information based registration of medical images: A survey. IEEE Trans. Med. Imaging 22(8), 986–1004 (2003)
4. Mellor, M., Brady, M.: Phase mutual information as a similarity measure for registration. Medical Image Analysis 9, 330–343 (2005)
5. Loeckx, D., Slagmolen, P., Maes, F., Vandermeulen, D., Suetens, P.: Nonrigid image registration using conditional mutual information. In: Karssemeijer, N., Lelieveldt, B. (eds.) IPMI 2007. LNCS, vol. 4584, pp. 725–737. Springer, Heidelberg (2007)
6. Likar, B., Pernus, F.: A hierarchical approach to elastic registration based on mutual information. Image and Vision Computing 19, 33–44 (2001)
7. Pluim, J.P.W., Antoine Maintz, J.B., Viergever, M.A.: Interpolation artefacts in mutual information-based image registration. Computer Vision and Image Understanding 77(2), 211–232 (2000)
8. Studholme, C., Drapaca, C.S., Iordanova, B., Cardenas, B.: Deformation-based mapping of volume change from serial brain MRI in the presence of local tissue contrast change. IEEE Trans. Med. Imaging 25(5), 626–639 (2006)
9. Zhuang, X., Rhode, K., Arridge, S., Razavi, R., Hill, D., Hawkes, D.J., Ourselin, S.: An atlas-based segmentation propagation framework using locally affine registration – application to automatic whole heart segmentation. In: Metaxas, D., Axel, L., Fichtinger, G., Székely, G. (eds.) MICCAI 2008, Part II. LNCS, vol. 5242, pp. 425–433. Springer, Heidelberg (2008)
10. Studholme, C., Hill, D., Hawkes, D.J.: An overlap invariant entropy measure of 3D medical image alignment. Pattern Recognition 32(1), 71–86 (1999)
11. Maes, F., Collignon, A., Vandermeulen, D., Marchal, G., Suetens, P.: Multimodality image registration by maximization of mutual information. IEEE Trans. Med. Imaging 16(2), 187–198 (1997)
12. Loeckx, D., Maes, F., Vandermeulen, D., Suetens, P.: Comparison between parzen window interpolation and generalised partial volume estimation for nonrigid image registration using mutual information. In: Pluim, J.P.W., Likar, B., Gerritsen, F.A. (eds.) WBIR 2006. LNCS, vol. 4057, pp. 206–213. Springer, Heidelberg (2006)
13. Thévenaz, P., Unser, M.: Optimization of mutual information for multiresolution image registration. IEEE Transactions on Image Processing 9(12), 2083–2099 (2000)
14. Rueckert, D., Sonoda, L.I., Hayes, C., Hill, D.L.G., Leach, M.O., Hawkes, D.J.: Nonrigid registration using free-form deformations: Application to breast MR images. IEEE Trans. Med. Imaging 18, 712–721 (1999)
15. Zhuang, X., Rhode, K., Razavi, R., Hawkes, D.J., Ourselin, S.: Free-form deformations using adaptive control point status for whole heart MR segmentation. In: Ayache, N., Delingette, H., Sermesant, M. (eds.) FIMH 2009. LNCS, vol. 5528, pp. 303–311. Springer, Heidelberg (2009)

Projected Generalized Procrustes Alignment

Konstantin Chernoff[1] and Mads Nielsen[1,2]

[1] Department Of Computer Science, University of Copenhagen, Denmark
[2] Nordic Bioscience Imaging, Herlev, Denmark

Abstract. When observing the 3D world through a 2D projection, rigid 3D rotation will result in an apparent deformation not accounted for in traditional shape analysis methodologies, e.g. those based on Generalized Procrustes Alignment and Principal Component Analysis.

We propose using a 3D statistical model to infer relative depth to a 2D shape and consequently model the apparent deformation in a Procrustes alignment framework.

We test our approach on vertebra shapes and show that it leads to a more compact and generalizable shape model, as well as to improvement in vertebra fracture prediction.

1 Introduction

Many imaging devices, such as X-ray, dual energy X-ray absorptiometry (DXA), and various microscopy and optical images modalities, output 2D projections of the world. However, the scanned objects are usually 3D, and their 2D projections will generally be influenced by the relative orientation to the image plane.

Before performing shape analysis, the acquired shapes must be aligned in a global coordinate system. In this context, the alignment involves changing the scale, translation, and orientation. Traditionally, this type of alignment is achieved by performing Generalized Procrustes Alignment (GPA). However, GPA does not normalize for the 3D rotation out of the 2D projection plane. In some cases, such normalization can be performed by aligning the objects in 3D before performing any observations. However, this may be very tedious and sometimes impossible, i.e. when observing vertebrae in X-ray images taken from scoliosis affected subjects, the individual vertebra may have varying orientations, and a single X-ray cannot capture all vertebrae in standardized position.

We propose to normalize for the 3D orientation by modelling the apparent deformation of a set of 2D shapes. Each shape can consist of a finite number of landmarks and the apparent deformation can be interpreted as the 2D landmark displacement when the corresponding 3D landmarks, are rotated with respect to the projection plane. We represent the apparent deformation by using conditional normal densities of the relative depth of 2D shapes. In this paper, the apparent deformation is used to normalize a set of 2D vertebra shapes, and the relative depth is learned from an independent 3D data set. Two examples of apparent deformation are shown in Fig. 1.

J.L. Prince, D.L. Pham, and K.J. Myers (Eds.): IPMI 2009, LNCS 5636, pp. 503–514, 2009.

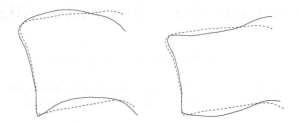

Fig. 1. Examples of apparent deformation. The dashed contour is deformed using positive (left) and negative (right) angle parameters.

The outline of the paper is as follows: Sect. 2 gives a overview of related work, Sect. 3 gives a short description of traditional shape models, Sect. 4 and Sect. 5 introduce linearization of 2D and 3D rotations and present our method, Sect. 6 presents the data which is used in Sect. 7 to perform an experimental evaluation involving shape reconstruction and vertebra fracture prediction.

2   Related Work

Generally, shape analysis consists of identifying and parametrizing the significant degrees of freedom in a collection of shapes [1]. This is accomplished by aligning the shapes according to some metric and possibly projecting them onto a low dimensional manifold. Traditionally, the shapes are represented by landmarks, Generalized Procrustes Alignment (GPA) is used to align the shapes, and Principal Component Analysis (PCA) is used to reduce the dimensionality. This approach is often referred to as a Point Distribution Model (PDM) [2].

Once constructed, the shape models can be combined with search algorithms and be used to extract semantic information from images. Some of the most popular applications of shape models include the Active Shape Model (ASM) and Active Appearance Model (AAM) [2]. Both of these methods are popular and have given rise to much progress in medical image processing [3].

Furthermore, both ASM and AAM have been the basic tools for modelling and segmenting the human vertebrae in X-rays and DXA images. Basic ASM [4], ASM with a non-parametric pixel classifier [5], a modified AAM constrained by neighboring vertebrae [6], and a similar model based only on shape information [7], have been successfully applied.

Several approaches have been introduced to improve the precision and the accuracy of the shape models. Most of these approaches are based on using other dimensionality reduction methods than PCA, modifying the GPA, or modifying the point matches [8].

Due to the large field of dimensionality reduction, it is natural to use other methods than PCA when modelling shape variation. This includes Kernel-PCA [9], Principal Geodesic Analysis [10], Independent Component Analysis (ICA) [11], and Locally Linear Embeddings [12]. In situations where outliers are present, robust dimensionality reductions methods can be utilized. Such an approach was taken in [13] where a robust version of PCA called Φ-PCA was used.

Several modifications of the traditional GPA are possible. According to Larsen et al. [14], Seigel et al. [15] made GPA robust by using medians when calculating the scale, translation, and orientation of objects. In [16], L1 norm was used when computing shape similarity. Furthermore, functional GPA [17] can be used on occasions where it is more appropriate to maximize the similarity between contours instead of landmarks.

Another logical step to improve the performance of GPA is to incorporate the 3D information that inherently existed when the 2D shapes were created. When several shapes of the same object are available, 3D reconstruction techniques can be used to reconstruct the 3D shapes [18]. The reconstructed 3D shapes could potentially be used to guide the alignment of the 2D shapes. In terms of medical image processing, this approach would require multiple overlapping X-rays or a CT scan, However, such data may be expensive when compared to the cost of a single X-ray.

Another approach that accounts the 3D orientation was introduced by Buxton et al. [19]. Their approach represented a set of shapes by using Centred Affine Trifocal Tensors (CATT) to calculate two sets of aligned basis shapes. However, since both 3D and 2D shapes must be inferred from the data set, much more data must be available when compared to approaches only inferring the 2D shape variations. Hence, we divide the methodology in two: first we infer 3D information in an independent 3D data set, then we infer the 2D apparent deformation based on the inferred 3D information.

3   Shape Model

A set of shapes can be represented by using a PDM. Thus, a single D-dimensional shape with N points can be represented by a $D \times N$ matrix, i.e. when $D = 3$, a shape is represented by:

$$
s = \begin{bmatrix} x_1 \ x_2 \ \dots \ x_N \\ y_1 \ y_2 \ \dots \ y_N \\ z_1 \ z_2 \ \dots \ z_N \end{bmatrix} \ . \tag{1}
$$

A set of shapes can be aligned by performing GPA. This consists of applying a similarity transformation to maximize the inter shape similarity. This is equivalent to minimizing the inter-landmark variances by using similarity transformations, and it can be formulated as a minimization problem with the following cost function:

$$
e = \sum_{i \neq j} \| A_i s_i - A_j s_j \| \ , \tag{2}
$$

where s_i is a shape and A_i is a similarity transformation. Solving for the optimal A_i is normally done in an iterative fashion [2].

The shape variation of a set of shapes is modelled using PCA by projecting the shapes onto the eigenvectors of the shape covariance matrix. Dimensionality is reduced by discarding eigenvectors with a small eigenvalue. The shape covariance matrix is computed using maximum likelihood estimates:

$$\mu = \frac{1}{n}\sum_{i=1}^{n} s_i \ , \quad \Sigma = \frac{1}{n-1}\sum_{i=1}^{n}(s_i - \mu)(s_i - \mu)^T \ , \tag{3}$$

where s_i has the same form as the vectorized transpose of (1).

4   3D Orientation

Before any sensible 3D information can be collected from the 3D shapes, they must be aligned. This is accomplished by performing GPA on 3D shapes. Thereafter, we assume that the 2D shapes are given as orthographic projections of the 3D shapes, and wish to model the apparent deformation. Generalizations to perspective projections are straight forward.

If we assume that the projection plane equals the $[x\ y]^T$ plane, then any rotation of the 3D shapes in the $[x\ y]^T$ plane will deform the 2D shapes consistently with a 2D rotation in this plane. Hence, the apparent deformation must only be learned for rotations in the $[x\ z]^T$ and $[y\ z]^T$ planes. These rotations can be described by the following rotation matrices:

$$R(\theta_1)_{[x\ z]^T} = \begin{bmatrix} 1 & 0 & 0 \\ 0 & \cos\theta_1 & -\sin\theta_1 \\ 0 & \sin\theta_1 & \cos\theta_1 \end{bmatrix} \ , \quad R(\theta_2)_{[y\ z]^T} = \begin{bmatrix} \cos\theta_2 & 0 & -\sin\theta_2 \\ 0 & 1 & 0 \\ \sin\theta_2 & 0 & \cos\theta_2 \end{bmatrix} . \tag{4}$$

The rotation can be linearized by using the first order Taylor expansion of the rotation operation around zero:

$$\begin{aligned} R(\theta) &\approx R(0) + \theta\frac{dR}{d\theta}(0) \\ &\approx (I + \theta\frac{dR}{d\theta}(0)) \ . \end{aligned} \tag{5}$$

A nice effect of the linearization is that the rotation in the $[x\ z]^T$ and $[y\ z]^T$ planes can be handled separately. Thus, after linearization 3D rotations commute. We see this as very expedient since, infinitesimally, the commutator of a $[x\ z]^T$ rotation and a $[y\ z]^T$ rotation is a $[x\ y]^T$ rotation, that is anyway handled separately in the GPA. Furthermore, it can be shown that $\frac{dR}{d\theta}(0)$ will be a skew symmetric matrix with zero diagonal values, which represents a Lie algebra of the 3D rotation matrices. Thus, direct exponentiation of $\frac{dR}{d\theta}(0)$ results in the original rotation matrix defined by θ, and (5) corresponds to the first two terms of the direct exponentiation. Hence, any other group of transformations to be discarded may likewise be handled based on its lie algebra formulation.

Without loss of generality, only rotation matrices that rotate in the $[y\ z]^T$ plane are considered. Given a 3D shape s_i and the 2D landmark displacement

D_i corresponding to a 3D rotation of s_i by the angle θ, the following relation can be formulated:

$$\theta D_i = PR_\theta s_i - P s_i \ , \qquad (6)$$

where P is an orthographic projection matrix. Equation (6) can be reduced by using (5) and rearranging the components:

$$\theta D_i = P\left(\theta \frac{dR}{d\theta}\right) s_i \ , \qquad (7)$$

By cancelling the rotation angle, the following is obtained:

$$D_i = P\left(\frac{dR}{d\theta}\right) s_i \ . \qquad (8)$$

Thus, for a given shape s_i, the linearized 2D displacement resulting from 3D rotation can be described by a scalar multiple of the projection of the differential rotation change in 3D. Furthermore, by inserting the projection and rotation matrices into (8), the following is obtained:

$$P\begin{bmatrix} 0 & 0 & 1 \\ 0 & 0 & 0 \\ -1 & 0 & 0 \end{bmatrix}\begin{bmatrix} x_1 & x_2 & \dots & x_N \\ y_1 & y_2 & \dots & y_N \\ z_1 & z_2 & \dots & z_N \end{bmatrix} = \begin{bmatrix} z_1 & z_2 & \dots & z_N \\ 0 & 0 & \dots & 0 \end{bmatrix} \ . \qquad (9)$$

Thus, the necessary information required to establish a linear model of the apparent deformation is, not surprisingly, the z-coordinates of the shapes. Furthermore, since θ was cancelled in (8), the apparent deformation is only dependent on the relative depth of the 2D shapes. In practice, this means that the degree of freedom resulting from the displacement of the z coordinates when a 3D rotation is performed can be discarded. The relative depths can be obtained by performing GPA on the 3D shapes.

5   Relative Depth Model

In the previous section, it is shown that the apparent deformation of a 2D shape is given by a scalar multiple of the relative depth. We employ a conditional Gaussian model to learn the relative depth given the spatial landmark coordinates. Thus, we are interested in the distribution of the relative depth d conditioned by the x and y coordinates:

$$P(d \mid x, y) \ . \qquad (10)$$

When it is assumed that the distribution of the x and y coordinates, and the relative depth are both Gaussian, the probability distribution function (10) is also Gaussian with a closed form solution [20].

Let Σ denote a $3n \times 3n$ covariance matrix. Then, it can be partitioned into four sub-matrices:

$$\Sigma = \begin{bmatrix} \Sigma_{11} & \Sigma_{12} \\ \Sigma_{21} & \Sigma_{22} \end{bmatrix} \ , \qquad (11)$$

where the sub-matrices Σ_{11} and Σ_{22} correspond to the covariance matrix of the depth and the covariance matrix of the spatial landmark coordinates, respectively.

The mean of $P(z)$ conditioned by $P(x, y)$ can be expressed as [20]:

$$\mu_{d|x,y} = \mu_z + \Sigma_{12}\Sigma_{22}^{-1}(s - \mu_{x,y}) \ . \tag{12}$$

However, due to the lack of data, Σ_{22} may be badly estimated and ill-conditioned or singular. In that case, ridge regression[20] can be used to regularize the co-variance matrix.

The covariance and mean matrices can be computed by using maximum likelihood methods analogous to (3). However, in practice, only a few shapes may be available, and each shape may consist of many points. Thus, to avoid the curse of dimensionality, some correlations must be removed from the model.

We propose to estimate the depth independently by having a separate depth model for each landmark. If the set of all landmark indexes is denoted by L, and a subset of these indexes is denoted by L_{sub}, the following model is constructed:

$$P(d_j \mid x_i, y_i) \ , \tag{13}$$

where d_j is the relative depth of the j'th landmark, $j \in L_{\text{sub}}$, $\forall i \in L_{\text{sub}} \in L$. Decreasing the subset L_{sub} decreases the number of correlations in Σ. Our implementation uses $1 + 2k$ landmarks for each depth model, where k is the number of neighboring points to each side of the j'th landmark.

This results in a globally consistent model that estimates the relative depth when given a set of landmarks. The apparent deformation is performed by adding the recovered relative depth to the shape coordinates. Furthermore, several depth models can be used to infer the relative depth. This may be necessary when the 3D and 2D shapes are not completely consistent with each other, as it is the case with the vertebrae shapes we use in this paper. In this case, the multiple estimates of the relative depth are weighted equally when being added with the landmark coordinates, and the sub-shapes are positioned correctly using similarity transformations. This transforms the apparent deformation to a nonlinear process.

Before evaluating (13) to obtain the depth, the x and y coordinates are aligned with the landmark coordinates used in the depth model. Furthermore, since a 3D rotation around the center not included in the 2D projection plane will generally also encompass an apparent translation, GPA is used to align shapes corrected for apparent deformation.

5.1 Projected Generalized Procrustes Alignment

By combining the descriptions from Sect. 5 with GPA, a set of shapes can be aligned. The Projected Generalized Procrustes Alignment (PGPA) procedure is outlined in the following steps:

1. Perform GPA and define the reference shape to be the mean shape.
2. For each shape s_i do:
   - infer the relative depth d_i using the model from Sect. 5.
   - perform apparent deformation by using the relative depth d_i to maximize the similarity between s_i and $s_{rotmean}$
3. Perform GPA to align the deformed 2D shapes.
4. Calculate a new mean shape, align it with the reference shape, and use it as a new reference shape
5. Terminate if the reference shape has changed less than some threshold ϵ, otherwise go to step 2.

The mean 2D shape can be used as an initial estimate of the shape $s_{rotmean}$. However, due to the linearity approximation of the 3D rotation, the 3D orientation alignment will break down for large angles. A simple approach is to constrain the θ parameter with an upper and a lower bound when calculating $s_{rotmean}$. Once $s_{rotmean}$ is calculated, the upper and lower bounds may be relaxed.

6 Data Sets

6.1 2D Data Set

A total of 76 subjects were selected from a cohort of Danish postmenopausal women who were followed for assessment of osteoporosis and atherosclerosis in the Prospective Epidemiological Risk Factors (PERF) study [21].

Lateral X-rays of the lumbar spine were obtained for each subject at a baseline and at a followup examination 7-10 years later. None of the selected subjects had any fractures at the baseline examination. A radiologist located visible fractures according to Genant's quantitative and semi-quantitative fracture scores [22] and annotated the full boundary contour of lumbar vertebrae L1-L4.

6.2 3D Data Set

The 3D data set was created by annotating 25 low-dose CT images of post-menopausal women. The CT scans were randomly selected from the Danish Lung Cancer Screening Trial (DLCST) [23]. The selected subjects were not related to the PERF study, and the risk of them obtaining a vertebrae fracture was not assessed.

The annotations were performed by placing four landmarks in coronal slices: starting at the posterior and progressing in the axial plane towards the anterior of the vertebra. This creates six connected 3D polylines. However, only a combination consisting of three polylines corresponds to the 2D vertebra shapes obtained from the PERF study. An example of the 3D annotation is shown in the left of Fig. 2.

To remove spurious shape variation, the annotated shapes were smoothed by minimizing an internal energy function. We have defined a simple energy function based on co-linearity of the shape points:

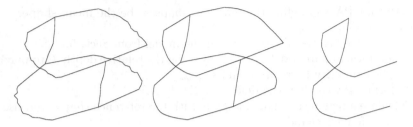

Fig. 2. Examples of 3D shapes. Left: raw annotated shapes. Middle: the same shape after smoothing. Right: subshape used to construct the relative depth model.

$$E(s) = \sum_{n=1}^{N-1} d(s_n, s_{n+1}) \; , \tag{14}$$

where s is a shape, N is the number of points in the shape, and $d(x_1, x_2)$ is the L_2 norm.

This energy function can be minimized iteratively by a gradient descent algorithm:

$$\nabla s = -\gamma \frac{\partial E(s)}{\partial s} \; , \tag{15}$$

where the constant $\gamma > 0$ is the learning rate.

By denoting the shapes at times t and $t+1$ by s^t and by s^{t+1}, respectively, and using a finite difference scheme, Equation (15) can be rewritten and solved for s^{t+1}:

$$s^{t+1} = s^t - \gamma \frac{\partial E(s)}{\partial s} \; . \tag{16}$$

To impose some degree of regularity, a fixed number of gradient descent steps based on the internal energy is performed (we have used $t^{\max} = 20$ with $\gamma = \frac{1}{2}$). However, a combined energy that also accounts for the deviation from the original data could have been used [24].

7   Results

Figure 1 shows the apparent deformation for a single 2D shape. It is seen that the vertebra shape appears to deform consistently with a rotation of the corresponding 3D shape.

Figure 3 shows an example of the PGPA and GPA applied to the whole 2D data set. Not surprisingly, since the shapes were deformed while maximizing the inter-shape similarity, the shapes in the PGPA aligned shapes have a smaller inter landmark variance than those aligned by GPA. The mean shape implied by PGPA appears less curved and more symmetric than the mean shape implied by the GPA. This suggests that the PGPA calculates plausible mean shapes.

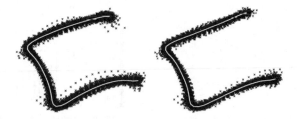

Fig. 3. Landmarks of the aligned shapes, the white line is the mean shape. Left: GPA alignment. Right: PGPA alignment. Note the smaller inter landmark variance and a simpler and more symmetric mean shape in the PGPA alignment.

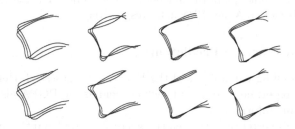

Fig. 4. Modes of variation. The first four modes of variation of the GPA and PGPA aligned data are shown. Top row: modes from GPA aligned data. Bottom row: modes from PGPA aligned data. Note the compactness of the lowest row, especially the difference between the second mode of variation in the top and bottom row: the former is more similar to the apparent deformation than the latter.

Figure 4 shows the first four modes of variation for the shapes aligned by GPA and PGPA. Generally, the modes of variation obtained from the shapes aligned by PGPA are more compact in terms of inter-landmark variance and encode more complex shape variations when compared to the modes obtained from the shapes aligned by GPA. The difference between the second mode of variation is especially noticeable: in the GPA aligned data, the second mode seems to be related to the apparent deformation due to a 3D rotation.

For further investigations of the shape variability of GPA and PGPA aligned data, eigenvalue decomposition of the shape covariance matrix was performed. The normalized, sorted, and accumulated eigenvalues are shown in the left part of Fig. 5. It is seen that the PGPA eigenvectors are able to capture more variation of the data when compared to the traditional GPA eigenvectors.

Leave-one-patient-out tests were performed to see how the GPA and PGPA generalize when combined with PCA. The right part of Fig. 5 shows the mean and the variance of the reconstruction errors when reconstructing unseen vertebrae shapes. The reconstruction errors were computed as the L2 norm of the residuals. It is seen that using PGPA improves both the mean and variance of the reconstruction errors by roughly 10 percent.

As a conclusion, PGPA implies a more compact model that generalizes better on this data set.

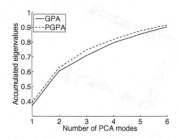 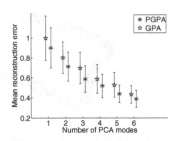

Fig. 5. Left: Accumulated eigenvalues of the shape covariance matrix, only the 6 largest eigenvalues were used. Right: means and variances of the reconstruction errors (L2 norm of the residual) as a function of the number of PCA modes. The dashed and the solid lines corresponds to PGPA and GPA data, respectively.

7.1 Vertebra Fracture Prediction

Above, the modelling capabilities of the PGPA were assessed. Here, we perform a fracture risk experiment to asses to which degree the PGPA also captures the clinically relevant information.

At baseline, all vertebrae were healthy according to Genant's quantitative and semi-quantitative fracture scores. We perform an experiment to see to which degree these healthy shapes can be classified into: those that fracture before followup and those that remain healthy.

As Osteopathis has both a systemic and localized component, we discard all vertebrae that remain healthy, but originates from subjects obtaining at least one fracture. This leaves 38 vertebrae that fractures and 160 vertebrae that remain healthy.

A quadratic Gaussian classifier is constructed based on these components. The receiver operating characteristic (ROC) curves and the corresponding area under ROC (AUROC) curves were calculated as a function of the number of principal components that were used when the dimensionality of the data was reduced. The results are shown in Fig. 6.

In our cases, the PGPA provides slightly superior predictive power. This shows that removing the apparent deformation does not only make the model more

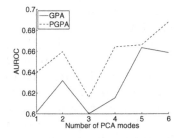

Fig. 6. AUROC as a function of the number of principal components. The dashed and the solid lines corresponds to PGPA and GPA data, respectively.

compact and generalize better, but it also improves the capability to capture the clinically relevant information.

8 Conclusions

We have proposed a method that aligns shapes by using a statistical model of the relative depth. Compared to GPA, out method gives a performance boost when performing vertebra shape modelling and when assessing vertebra fracture risk.

Visual inspection of the modes of variation of PGPA and the apparent deformation give intuitive results: the apparent deformation looks as originating from a 3D rotation and when compared to GPA, the modes of variation are more compact and have a superior generalization to unseen shapes.

Furthermore, the improvements obtained when predicting vertebra fractures suggest that PGPA does not introduce large modelling errors. On the contrary, it suggests that the resulting shape model captures the clinically relevant information better.

Acknowledgements

We thank CCBR-Synarc and Nordic Bioscience for providing facilities and data. This work was supported by the Danish research Foundation and the National Strategic Research Council under the grant "Learning Imaging Biomarkers".

References

1. Cootes, T.F., Cooper, D.H., Taylor, C.J., Graham, J.: Trainable method of parametric shape description. Image Vision Comput. 10, 10289–10294 (1992)
2. Cootes, T.F., Taylor, C.J.: Statistical models of appearance for computer vision, Technical report, University of Manchester, Wolfson Image Analysis Unit (1999)
3. Cootes, T.F., Hill, A., Taylor, C.J., Haslam, J.: The use of active shape models for locating structures in medical images. Image and Vision Computing 12(3), 355–366 (1994)
4. Smyth, P., Taylor, C., Adams, J.: Vertebral shape: Automatic measurement with active shape models. Radiology 2, 571–578 (1999)
5. de Bruijne, M., Nielsen, M.: Shape particle filtering for image segmentation. In: Barillot, C., Haynor, D.R., Hellier, P. (eds.) MICCAI 2004. LNCS, vol. 3216, pp. 168–175. Springer, Heidelberg (2004)
6. Roberts, M.G., Cootes, T., Adams, J.: Automatic segmentation of lumbar vertebrae on digitised radiographs using linked active appearance models. In: Proc. of MIUA Conference (2006)
7. de Bruijne, M., Lund, M.T., Tankób, L.B., Pettersen, P.C., Nielsen, M.: Quantitative vertebral morphometry using neighbor-conditional shape models. Medical Image Analysis 11, 503–512 (2007)
8. Davies, R.H., Cootes, T.F., Taylor, C.J.: A minimum description length approach to statistical shape modelling. In: Insana, M.F., Leahy, R.M. (eds.) IPMI 2001. LNCS, vol. 2082, pp. 50–63. Springer, Heidelberg (2001)

9. Romdhani, S., Gong, S., Psarrou, R.: A multi-view nonlinear active shape model using kernel pca. In: British Machine Vision Conference, pp. 483–492 (1999)
10. Dam, E., Fletcher, P.T., Pizer, S.M., Tracton, G., Rosenman, J.: Prostate shape modeling based on principal geodesic analysis bootstrapping. In: Barillot, C., Haynor, D.R., Hellier, P. (eds.) MICCAI 2004. LNCS, vol. 3217, pp. 1008–1016. Springer, Heidelberg (2004)
11. Üzümcü, M., Frangi, A.F., Reiber, J.H., Lelieveldt, B.P.: Independent component analysis in statistical shape models. In: Proceedings of SPIE, vol. 5032, pp. 375–383 (2003)
12. Elgammal, A.: Nonlinear generative models for dynamic shape and dynamic appearance. In: Computer Vision and Pattern Recognition Workshop, vol. 27, pp. 182–182 (2004)
13. Iglesias, J.E., de Bruijne, M., Loog, M., Lauze, F., Nielsen, M.: A family of principal component analyses for dealing with outliers. In: Ayache, N., Ourselin, S., Maeder, A. (eds.) MICCAI 2007, Part II. LNCS, vol. 4792, pp. 178–185. Springer, Heidelberg (2007)
14. Larsen, R., Eiriksson, H.: Robust and resistant 2d shape alignment. Technical report, Informatics and Mathematical Modelling Technical University of Denmark (2001)
15. Siegel, A.F., Benson, R.H.: A robust comparison of biological shapes. Biometrics 38, 341–350 (1982)
16. Larsen, R.: L1 generalized procrustes 2d shape alignment. Journal of Mathematical Imaging and Vision 32, 189–194 (2008)
17. Larsen, R.: Functional 2D procrustes shape analysis. In: Kalviainen, H., Parkkinen, J., Kaarna, A. (eds.) SCIA 2005. LNCS, vol. 3540, pp. 205–213. Springer, Heidelberg (2005)
18. Benameur, S., Mignotte, M., Parent, S., Labelle, H., Skalli, W., de Guise, J.: 3d/2d registration and segmentation of scoliotic vertebrae using statistical models. Computerized Medical Imaging and Graphics 27(5), 321–337 (2003)
19. Buxton, B.F., Dias, M.B.: Implicit, view invariant, linear flexible shape modelling. Pattern Recognition Letters 26, 433–447 (2005)
20. Bishop, C.M.: Pattern Recognition and Machine Learning (Information Science and Statistics). Springer, New York (2006)
21. Bagger, Y.Z., Tankó, L.B., Alexandersen, P., Hansen, H.B., Qin, G., Christiansen, C.: The long-term predictive value of bone mineral density measurements for fracture risk is independent of the site of measurement and the age at diagnosis: results from the prospective epidemiological risk factors study. Osteoporosis International 17, 1433–2965 (2006)
22. Wu, C.Y., Li, J., Jergas, M., Genant, H.K.: Comparison of semiquantitative and quantitative techniques for the assessment of prevalent and incident vertebral fractures. Osteoporosis International 5(5), 354–370 (2005)
23. Pedersen, J.H., Dirksen, A., Hansen, H., Bach, K.S., Tonnesen, P., Brodersen, J., Thorsen, H., Skov, B.G., Mortensen, J., Dossing, M.: The danish randomized lung cancer ct screening trial. results at baseline: A7-01. Thoracic Oncology 2, 329 (2007)
24. Chernoff, K., Nielsen, M.: Regularization based on local models. Submitted as technical report, Department of Computer Science, Copenhagen University (April 2009)

HARDI Denoising: Variational Regularization of the Spherical Apparent Diffusion Coefficient $sADC^\star$

Yunho Kim[1], Paul M. Thompson[2], Arthur W. Toga[2], Luminita Vese[1], and Liang Zhan[2]

[1] Mathematics Department, UCLA, Los Angeles, CA, USA
[2] LONI & Neurology Department, UCLA School of Medicine, Los Angeles, CA, USA

Abstract. We denoise HARDI (High Angular Resolution Diffusion Imaging) data arising in medical imaging. Diffusion imaging is a relatively new and powerful method to measure the 3D profile of water diffusion at each point. This can be used to reconstruct fiber directions and pathways in the living brain, providing detailed maps of fiber integrity and connectivity. HARDI is a powerful new extension of diffusion imaging, which goes beyond the diffusion tensor imaging (DTI) model: mathematically, intensity data is given at every voxel and at any direction on the sphere. However, HARDI data is usually highly contaminated with noise, depending on the b-value which is a tuning parameter preselected to collect the data. Larger b-values help to collect more accurate information in terms of measuring diffusivity, but more noise is generated by many factors as well. So large b-values are preferred, if we can satisfactorily reduce the noise without losing the data structure. We propose a variational method to denoise HARDI data by denoising the spherical Apparent Diffusion Coefficient (sADC), a field of radial functions derived from the data. We use vectorial total variation regularization, an L^1 data fidelity term and the logarithmic barrier function in the minimization. We present experiments of denoising synthetic and real HARDI data.

1 Introduction to the HARDI Data

Currently, HARDI data is used to map cerebral connectivity through fiber tractography in the brain. HARDI is a type of diffusion MRI, which was introduced in the mid-1980s by Le Bihan et al. [20,21,22] and Merboldt et al. [28]. It is based on the idea that the MR signal, which forms the basis of MRI, is attenuated when water diffuses out of a voxel, and the degree of attenuation can be used to measure the rate of water diffusion in any arbitrary 3D direction via the Stejskal-Tanner equation [33]. Water diffusion occurs preferentially in directions that are aligned with axonal fiber pathways, and is hindered in orthogonal directions by the myelin sheaths that coat the axons. Because of this diffusion anisotropy, initial approaches to assess fiber directions modeled the 3D diffusion

---

* Funded by the NIH Roadmap for Medical Research Grant U54 RR021813 (CCB).

J.L. Prince, D.L. Pham, and K.J. Myers (Eds.): IPMI 2009, LNCS 5636, pp. 515–527, 2009.
© Springer-Verlag Berlin Heidelberg 2009

profile at each point as a single tensor (Beaulieu et al. [4]), in which the principal eigenvector of the diffusion tensor can be used to recover the dominant fiber pathway at that voxel. The diffusion tensor model (Basser et al. [3]) describes the anisotropic nature of water diffusion in tissues (inside a typical 1-3mm sized voxel) by estimating, from a set of K diffusion-sensitized images, the 3x3 covariance matrix of a Gaussian distribution (Beaulieu et al. [4]). Each voxel's signal intensity in the k-th image is decreased, by water diffusion, according to the Stejskal-Tanner equation [33]: $S_k = S_0 \exp\left[-bg_k^T D g_k\right]$, where S_0 is the non-diffusion weighted signal intensity, D is the 3x3 diffusion tensor, g_k is the direction of the diffusion gradient and b is Le Bihan's factor with information on the pulse sequence, gradient strength, and physical constants.

Unfortunately, although it is widely used, the diffusion tensor model breaks down for voxels in which fiber pathways cross or mix together, and these are ubiquitous in the brain which is highly interconnected. More advanced image acquisition techniques, such as HARDI (Tuch et al. [39,40]), diffusion spectrum imaging [43], and q-ball imaging (Tuch et al. [41]), have been introduced in the past 5 years - these types of data recover the local microstructure of water diffusion more accurately than standard DTI data. HARDI, DTI and other similar modalities permit non-invasive quantification of the water diffusion in living tissues. The tissue structure will affect the Brownian motion of the water molecules which will lead to an anisotropic diffusion. By imaging diffusion in an arbitrary number of directions (often 100 or more), HARDI overcomes the limited accuracy of the tensor model in resolving the highly complex fiber structure of the brain, particularly in regions with fiber crossings.

HARDI data makes it possible to compute the orientation diffusion function over a sphere of possible directions. Tuch [38,40] developed the first HARDI acquisition and processing methods, and later Frank [15] used spherical harmonic expansions for processing HARDI data sets. A very active area of research has grown up in processing the HARDI signals, leading to methods for HARDI denoising, segmentation, and registration using metrics on spherical functions (Lenglet et al. [23]). Most of these signal processing methods still model the diffusion signal as a tensor, rather than exploiting the full information in the spherical harmonic expansion. For example, Khurd et al. [42] used isometric mapping and manifold learning (eigendecomposition of the distance matrix) to directly fit a manifold to the tensors, compute its dimensionality, and distinguish groups using Hotelling's T^2 statistics. Initial image processing on the full HARDI signal has focused on fitting a discrete mixture of k distinct tensors to the signal, and later on fitting a continuous mixture model for modeling the MR signal decay and multi-fiber reconstruction (Jian et al. [17], [18]), or fitting a continuous mixture of tensors using a unit-mass distribution on the symmetric positive definite tensor manifold (Leow et al. [24]).

Initial work on the nonlinear (fluid) matching of HARDI images has taken a more non-parametric approach, and has used the Kullback-Leibler divergence to measure the discrepancy between ODF fields (Chiang et al. [8,9]), using a 3D fluid transform to minimize the discrepancy between two fields of ODFs. As information theory can be used to measure the overlap between diffusion probability density functions, there is much promising work using metrics derived from information theory (e.g., the Fisher-Rao metric, von Mises-Fisher distribution, etc.; McGraw et al. [27]; Srivastava et al. [32]; Chiang et al. [9]). Other work has modeled the HARDI signal as high-order tensors (Barmpoutis et al. [2]) or as a stratification (mixture of manifolds with different dimensions; Haro et al. [16]).

The HARDI data is the MRI signal attenuation information after time $t > 0$ modeled by $S_t(x, \theta, \phi) = S_0(x) \exp(-b \cdot d_t(x, \theta, \phi))$, where Ω is a bounded open subset of $\mathbb{R}^3$, $x \in \Omega$, $\theta \in [0, 2\pi)$, $\phi \in [0, \pi)$. S_0 is the MRI signal that is obtained when no diffusion gradient vector is applied and this is considered to be a reference image, relative to which the diffusion-attenuated signal is measured. The function $d_t(x, \theta, \phi)$ is called the spherical Apparent Diffusion Coefficient (sADC), which measures how much the water molecules diffuse in the given direction $(\cos(\theta) \sin(\phi), \sin(\theta) \sin(\phi), \cos(\phi))$, and b is a parameter pre-selected to collect the data.

In reality, in experimental data, a higher b-value (e.g., 3000 s/mm^2) tends to lead to more noise in the obtained images [10]. Hence, we are led to consider the following simplified degradation model

$$S_t(x, \theta, \phi) = S_0(x) \exp(-b \cdot d_t(x, \theta, \phi)) + noise(x, \theta, \phi). \tag{1}$$

We may say that the baseline signal collected without any diffusion gradient applied, which is S_0, may also be contaminated by noise, but here we assume that this can be neglected, or we just consider the last noise term in (1) to encompass all types of noise. This is a reasonable approximation, because in practice, it is common to collect several non-diffusion weighted images $S_{0,i}$ whose average may be used as a reference signal S_0 (e.g. Zhan et al. [44]). If we let $\tilde{S}_t(x, \theta, \phi)$ be a denoised dataset, then we expect that for all x, ϕ, θ,

$$0 \leq \tilde{S}_t(x, \theta, \phi) \leq S_0(x). \tag{2}$$

As already mentioned, the data has to be first denoised before extracting the fibers, or before registration. Although HARDI is a relatively recent type of data acquisition, several HARDI processing methods have already been proposed: we mention a few more. In [26] and [7], curve evolution techniques are applied for the segmentation of HARDI data. Descoteaux, Deriche and collaborators, among others, have also proposed a segmentation of HARDI data [12], a regularized, fast and robust analytical solution for the Q-ball imaging reconstruction of the ODF [13], and for mapping of neuronal fiber crossings [14]. [11] deals with denoising and regularization of fields of ODFs (orientation distribution functions).

The prior work most relevant to ours is by Mc Graw et al. [25]: the noisy data $S_t(x, \theta, \phi)$ is regularized to remove noise in a functional minimization approach; a standard L^2 data fidelity term is used, combined with a weighted version of vectorial total variation regularization in space, and H^1 regularization of data at every voxel with respect to direction. The data is mapped into 2-dimensional space plane using spherical coordinates and discretized using finite elements. Denoising results for synthetic and real HARDI data are presented in [25]. In our proposed work, we also use vectorial total variation for the regularization. However, our proposed model differs from the one in [25], since we faithfully follow the signal degradation model (1) and we denoise $d_t(x, \theta, \phi)$ instead of $S_t(x, \theta, \phi)$. Results on synthetic data used in [25] will be shown for comparison.

2   Proposed Variational Denoising Model

We propose a variational denoising method that recovers a clean $d = d_t$. The HARDI data is a collection of intensity values at uniformly pre-selected directions on the sphere, to which the electromagnetic field is applied: at each position $x \in \Omega \subset \mathbb{R}^3$, we measure values at different directions. We note briefly that the actual set of directions is typically computed using an electrostatic repulsion PDE, to optimize the sampling of a spherical signal using a finite set of observations (see Tuch et al. [41] for a discussion of spherical sampling schemes).

In the continuous setting, we obtain a function defined on a manifold $\Omega \times S^2$; Ω is the spatial domain and the sphere S^2 is the space of gradient directions. It is not easy to work with the entire domain $\Omega \times S^2$ for computational purposes. Instead, we will use a discretized version of the sphere, given by n directions uniformly chosen. We drop the subscript t from S_t and thus the function that is given has the form $S = (S_1, \ldots, S_n)$ where each $S_i : \Omega \to \mathbb{R}$ corresponds to a given direction. The data S_0 has only spatial information and it is also given.

To impose the right amount of smoothness and discontinuity on the denoised data, we will use the vectorial total variation regularization, given by $|\nabla d|(\Omega) = \int_\Omega \sqrt{\sum_{i=1}^n |\nabla d_i(x)|^2} dx$ if $d \in W^{1,1}(\Omega; \mathbb{R}^n)$ (∇d is a $n \times 3$ matrix). For $d \in W^{1,1}(\Omega; \mathbb{R}^n)$, $\nabla d = (\frac{\partial d_i}{\partial x_k})_{i=1,\ldots,n, k=1,2,3}$ in the distributional sense and $|\nabla d|$ denotes the Frobenius norm of ∇d. The total variation has been successfully introduced and used in image denoising for gray-scale images by Rudin, Osher, Fatemi [31], being a convex edge-preserving regularization. The vectorial total variation for color images has been analyzed in Blomgren-Chan [6] and PhD manuscripts of Blomgren [5], Tschumperlé [34] (see also [35], [36]).

As we have mentioned, we wish to denoise the sADC (spherical Apparent Diffusion Coefficient) d_t in (1). We drop the subscript t and denote the sADC by d. We note that we can substitute $b \cdot d$ by d in (1), since b is a constant. From the HARDI data model (1), we see that knowing the true S is equivalent to knowing the true d. We directly impose the image formation model in our data-fidelity term and the constraint $d_i \geq 0$. Also, we use an L^1 noise term [1], instead of the more standard L^2 noise term, to penalize less the unknown. We minimize the energy $G(d) = G(d_1, \ldots, d_n)$.

We use the logarithmic barrier method [29] to realize the constraint: the energy should contain $-\mu \sum_{i=1}^n \log(d_i(x))$ (with a sequence of parameters $\mu > 0$ decreasing to zero), which realizes the constraint $d_i > 0$ for all i. Instead, we will use $-\mu \sum_{i=1}^n \left[H(S_i(x), S_0(x)) \cdot \frac{\log(d_i(x))}{d_i(x)} \right]$, with the function H depending only on the data S and S_0. One choice of the function H is: $H(a, b) = 0$ if $a \leq b$, $H(a, b) = 1$ if $a > b$. Using this weight H, we penalize the unknown only at those points $x \in \Omega$ with $S_i(x) - S_0(x) > 0$ which violate the second constraint in (2). Also, note that, if we would have used $-\mu \log(z)$ instead of $-\mu \log(z)/z$, with $z = d_i(x)$, then the energy would have no global minimizer since for any d such that $G(d) < \infty$, violating the constraint on a set of positive measure, then $\lim_{k \to \infty} G(k + d) = -\infty$. Another advantage of the function $-\mu \log(z)/z$ is that on one hand, unlike the logarithmic function $-\mu \log(z)$, it rather spreads uniform weights on $\{z > \epsilon\}$ for $\epsilon > 0$ when $\mu > 0$ is small. On the other hand, $-\mu \log(z)/z$ generates more repelling force from $z = 0$ than $-\mu \log(z)$. In this sense, $-\mu \log(z)/z$ realizes the constraints in (2) better than $-\mu \log(z)$.

Thus, our proposed minimization model for HARDI denoising is,

$$\inf_d G(d) = |\nabla d|(\Omega) + \lambda \int_\Omega \sum_{i=1}^n |S_i(x) - S_0(x)e^{-d_i(x)}|dx$$

$$- \mu \int_\Omega \sum_{i=1}^n \left[H(S_i(x), S_0(x)) \cdot \frac{\log(d_i(x))}{d_i(x)} \right] dx. \qquad (3)$$

In practice for computations, we use and discretize the Euler-Lagrange equations of model (3) in gradient descent form with respect to $d_i(t, x)$. For $i = 1, \ldots, n$, $t > 0$, these are

$$\frac{\partial d_i}{\partial t}(t, x) = \operatorname{div}\left(\frac{\nabla d_i(t, x)}{\sqrt{\sum_{j=1}^n |\nabla d_j(t, x)|^2}} \right) - \lambda \cdot S_0(x)e^{-d_i(t,x)} \qquad (4)$$

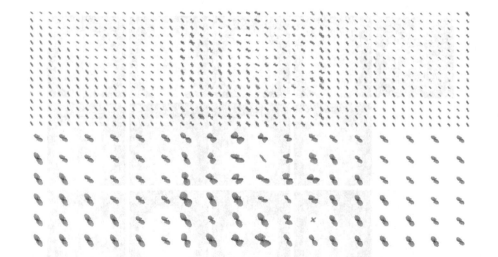

Fig. 1. ODFs. Left: noise-free synthetic data. Middle: noisy data, $M(original, noisy) = 4.2206$. Right: denoised data, $M(original, denoised) = 1.8243$. Ratio $\frac{M(original, noisy)}{M(original, denoised)} = \frac{4.2206}{1.8243} = 2.3135$, larger (better) than for the best result reported in McGraw et al. [25], $\frac{1.0409}{0.6576} = 1.5828$; $rmse(original, noisy) = 17.7079$, $rmse(original, denoised) = 7.7774$ (similar with $rmse(original, denoised) = 7.6367$ from [25]).

$$\cdot \ sign(S_i(x) - S_0(x)e^{-d_i(t,x)}) + \mu\frac{H(S_i(x), S_0(x))(1 - \log(d_i(t,x)))}{d_i(t,x)^2}$$

with boundary conditions. We use finite differences to discretize the above PDE's using an explicit scheme. The final C++ algorithm is computationally efficient.

3 Numerical Results

We recall that in practice we work with a decreasing sequence of values $\mu_k > 0$ and we find minimizers d_k^* for G, with μ substituted by μ_k. The minimizer d_k^* obtained for μ_k is the initial guess for the next minimization with $\mu_{k+1} < \mu_k$. We wish to mention that the visualization of noisy data and denoised results is done also through the ODFs (orientation distribution functions), which are obtained by a postprocessing from the HARDI signal (but the ODFs are not used in our denoising method). Note that calculating ODF of a noisy dataset means that we perform a process of smoothing the data. The ODF is typically calculated from the signal using the Fourier transform relationship between the signal and the diffusion propagator [37], [30]. Since the original noisy data usually violates the constraints we had in the model, if we want to visualize the ODF of the noisy data, then there has to be a pre-processing step to adjust those violating values.

We first show a denoising result of a synthetic 16×16 HARDI data, kindly provided by T. McGraw, for comparison with results from prior work of McGraw

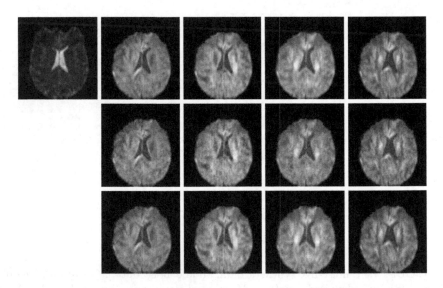

Fig. 2. Denoising experiment of real MRI data. Top: left, S_0; right, original clean slices. 2nd row: noisy slices (artificial Rician noise). 3rd row: denoised slices. $M(original, noisy) = 2.8350$, $M(original, denoised) = 1.1564$. $rmse(original, noisy) = 10.5448$, $rmse(original, denoised) = 4.7268$.

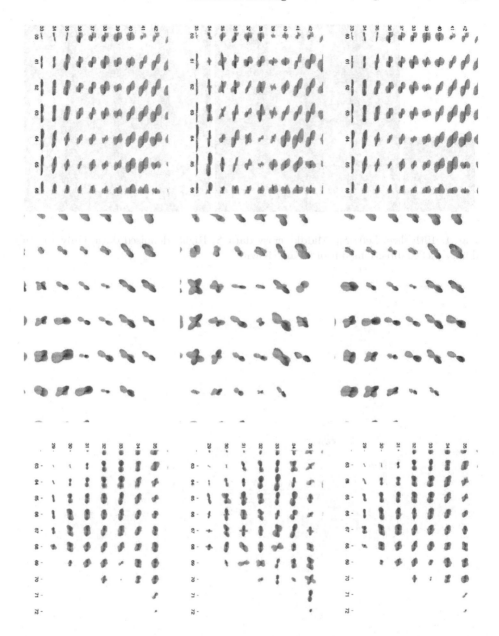

Fig. 3. ODFs of artificial denoising experiment of real MRI HARDI data from Fig. 2. Left: original clean ODFs. Middle: noisy ODFs (artificial Rician noise). Right: denoised ODFs.

et al. [25] (generated using the technique described in [30]). In Fig. 1 we show the ODF visualizations of synthetic, noise-free HARDI data and its noisy version, together with the denoised result.

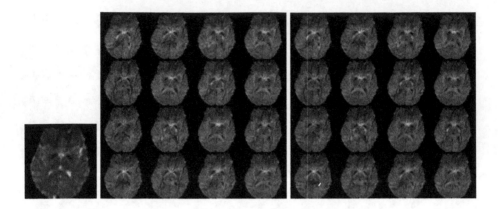

Fig. 4. 19th slice. Left: S_0. Middle: noisy data S. Right: denoised data. Only 16 randomly picked directions out of 94 are shown.

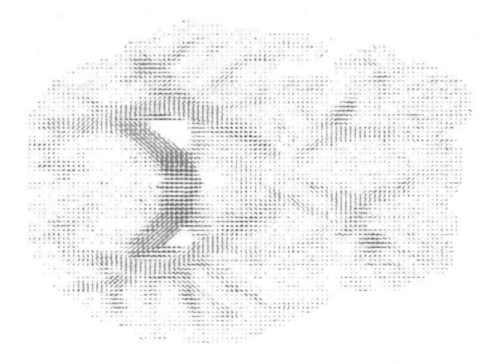

Fig. 5. ODFs: 19th slice of real clinical HARDI brain data

To assess the results'accuracy in the synthetic experiments (since we obtain the ODFs by postprocessing), we compute the mean M over all points of square root of symmetric Kullback-Leibler divergence between two probability densities $p(x), q(x)$ defined by $sKL(p, q) = \frac{1}{2} \int_\Omega \left\{ p(x) \log \left(\frac{p(x)}{q(x)} \right) + q(x) \log \left(\frac{q(x)}{p(x)} \right) \right\} dx$. We

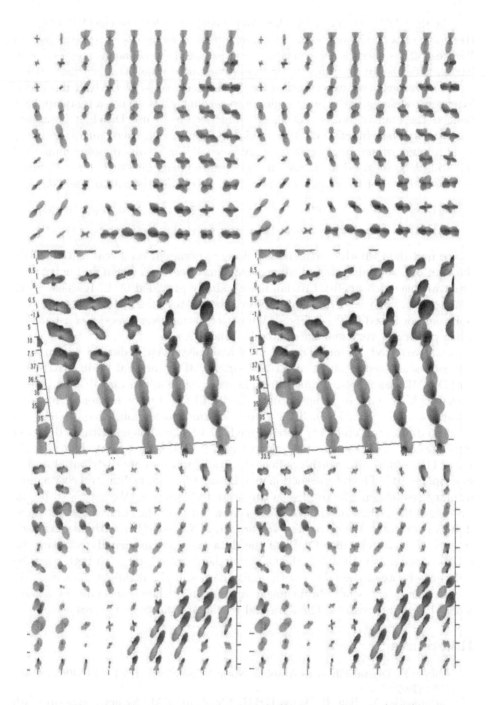

Fig. 6. ODFs of clinical noisy data (left), denoised result (right)

let q be the ODF of the noise free data and in each case, let p be the ODF of either the noisy data or the denoised data. The obtained mean distances are given in Figures 1-2. As another error measure, we also use the root mean square error in Fig. 2, which is obtained directly from our computed quantities, without ODFs.

We show next two experimental results on two real MRI HARDI data sets. We want to take only the brain region into account, thus we use a template that defined the brain region in the image. This led us to use Dirichlet boundary conditions. Since functional (3) is obviously nonconvex, there might be many local minima, which might cause visibly unsatisfying results or some numerical instability. So we need to choose an appropriate initial guess when $t = 0$. Since our minimizer d of (3) should satisfy $d_i \geq 0$, we choose the initial guess d_0 as

$$(d_0)_i(x) = \qquad\qquad 0.005 \qquad\qquad \text{on } \{x \in \Omega : \ H(S_i(x), S_0(x)) > 0\},$$
$$(d_0)_i(x) = \ -\log(S_i(x)/S_0(x)) + 0.1 \quad \text{on } \{x \in \Omega : \ H(S_i(x), S_0(x)) = 0\}.$$

We first show another artificial denoising experiment on a real MRI HARDI data set of $n = 30$ diffusion-sensitized gradient directions. Clean and noisy data are available (with artificial Rician noise), kindly provided by E. Iglesias. Slices of S_0, clean, noisy and restored data are shown in Fig. 2, with plots of clean, noisy and denoised ODFs in Fig. 3. We notice visually very good reconstruction while preserving very well the anatomic structure.

Next, we tested our model on a clinical real noisy HARDI dataset with $n = 94$ diffusion-sensitized gradient directions. Briefly, 3D structural brain MRI scans and DT-MRI scans were acquired from healthy young adults on a 4 Tesla Bruker Medspec MRI scanner using an optimized diffusion tensor sequence. Imaging parameters were: TE/TR 92.3/8250 ms, 55 x 2mm contiguous slices, FOV = 23 cm. 105 directional gradients were applied: 11 baseline images with no diffusion sensitization (i.e., T_2-weighted images) and 94 diffusion-weighted images (b-value 1159 s/mm^2) in which gradient directions were evenly distributed on the hemisphere [19]. The reconstruction matrix was 128x128, yielding a 1.8x1.8 mm^2 in-plane resolution. The total scan time was 14.5 minutes. We set S_0 to be the average of the 11 baseline images. Fig. 4 shows slices of the clinical dataset (non-diffusion weighted image S_0 and 16 directions S_i), together with the denoised results. Next we visualize ODFs of the data and we can visually compare the ODFs of the noisy data with the ODFs of the denoised data. To better see the difference between the ODFs of the noisy data and the denoised data, we take some parts of the whole brain image and magnify them especially in regions where fibers are crossing. The data and results are shown in Figures 5-6.

References

1. Alliney, S.: Digital Filters as Absolute Norm Regularizers. IEEE TSP 40(6), 1548–1562 (1992)
2. Barmpoutis, A., Jian, B., Vemuri, B.C., Shepherd, T.M.: Symmetric positive 4th order tensors & their estimation from diffusion weighted MRI. In: Karssemeijer, N., Lelieveldt, B. (eds.) IPMI 2007. LNCS, vol. 4584, pp. 308–319. Springer, Heidelberg (2007)

3. Basser, P.J., Pierpaoli, C.: Microstructural and physiological features of tissues elucidated by quantitative diffusion tensor MRI. JMR 111, 209–219 (1996)
4. Beaulieu, C., Allen, P.S.: Water diffusion in the giant axon of the squid: Implications for diffusion-weighted MRI of the nervous system. MRM 32(5), 579–583 (1994)
5. Blomgren, P.: Total Variation Methods for Restoration of Vector Valued Images (Ph.D. thesis), UCLA CAM Report 98-30 (1998)
6. Blomgren, P., Chan, T.F.: Color TV: Total variation methods for restoration of vector-valued images. IEEE TIP 7(3), 304–309 (1998)
7. Jonasson, L., Hagmann, P., Bresson, X., Thiran, J.-P., Wedeen, V.J.: Representing Diffusion MRI in 5D for Segmentation of White Matter Tracts with a Level Set Method. In: Christensen, G.E., Sonka, M. (eds.) IPMI 2005. LNCS, vol. 3565, pp. 311–320. Springer, Heidelberg (2005)
8. Chiang, M.C., Klunder, A.D., McMahon, K., de Zubicaray, G.I., Wright, M., Toga, A.W., Thompson, P.M.: Information-theoretic analysis of brain white matter fiber orientation distribution functions. In: Karssemeijer, N., Lelieveldt, B. (eds.) IPMI 2007. LNCS, vol. 4584, pp. 172–182. Springer, Heidelberg (2007)
9. Chiang, M.C., Leow, A.D., Dutton, R.A., Barysheva, M., Rose, S., McMahon, K.L., de Zubicaray, G.I., Toga, A.W., Thompson, P.M.: Fluid Registration of Diffusion Tensor Images Using Information Theory. IEEE TMI 2008 27(4), 442–456 (2008)
10. Cihangiroglu, M., Uluğ, A.M., Firat, Z., Bayram, A., Kovanlikaya, A., Kovanlikaya, İ.: High b-value diffusion-weighted MR imaging of normal brain at 3T. European Journal of Radiology 69(3), 454–458 (2009)
11. Deputte, S., Dierckx, H., Fieremans, E., D'Asseler, Y., Achten, R., Lemahieu, I.: Postprocessing of brain white matter fiber orientation distribution functions. In: Proc. IEEE ISBI: from Nano to Macro, pp. 784–787 (2007)
12. Descoteaux, M., Deriche, R.: High Angular Resolution Diffusion MRI Segmentation Using Region-Based Statistical Surface Evolution. JMIV 33(2), 239–252 (2009)
13. Descoteaux, M., Angelino, E., Fitzgibbons, S., Deriche, R.: Regularized, Fast and Robust Analytical Q-Ball Imaging. MRM 58(3), 497–510 (2007)
14. Descoteaux, M., Deriche, R.: Mapping neuronal fiber crossings in the human brain. SPIE Newsroom (August 2008)
15. Frank, L.R.: Characterization of anisotropy in high angular resolution diffusion-weighted MRI. MRM 47(6), 1083–1099 (2002)
16. Haro, G., Lenglet, C., Sapiro, G., Thompson, P.M.: On the Non-Uniform Complexity of Brain Connectivity. In: IEEE ISBI: from Nano to Macro, pp. 887–890 (2008)
17. Jian, B., Vemuri, B.C.: A Unified Computational Framework for Deconvolution to Reconstruct Multiple Fibers From Diffusion Weighted MRI. IEEE TMI 26(11), 1464–1471 (2007)
18. Jian, B., Vemuri, B.C., Özarslan, E., Carney, P.R., Mareci, T.H.: A novel tensor distribution model for the diffusion-weighted MR signal. NeuroImage 37(1), 164–176 (2007)
19. Jones, D.K., Horsfield, M.A., Simmons, A.: Optimal strategies for measuring diffusion in anisotropic systems by magnetic resonance imaging. MRM 42, 515–525 (1999)
20. Le Bihan, D., Breton, E.: Imagerie de diffusion in vivo par resonance magnétique nucléaire. CRAS 301, 1109–1112 (1985)
21. Le Bihan, D., Breton, E., Lallemand, D., Grenier, P., Cabanis, E., Laval-Jeantet, M.: MR imaging of intravoxel incoherent motions: Application to diffusion and perfusion in neurologic disorders. Radiology 161, 401–407 (1986)

22. Le Bihan, D., Poupon, C., Amadon, A., Lethimonnier, F.: Artifacts and Pitfalls in Diffusion MRI. JMRI 24, 478–488 (2006)
23. Lenglet, C., Campbell, J.S.W., Descoteaux, M., Haro, G., Savadjiev, P., Wassermann, D., Anwander, A., Deriche, R., Pike, G.B., Sapiro, G., Siddiqi, K., Thompson, P.M.: Mathematical Methods for Diffusion MRI Processing. NeuroImage. In: Thompson, P.M., Miller, M.I., Poldrack, R., Nichols, T. (eds.) Special Issue on Mathematics in Brain Imaging, November 13 (2008)
24. Leow, A.D., Zhu, S., Zhan, L., McMahon, K., de Zubicaray, G.I., Meredith, M., Wright, M.J., Toga, A.W., Thompson, P.M.: The Tensor Distribution Function. MRM 61(1), 205–214 (2008)
25. McGraw, T., Özarslan, E., Vemuri, B.C., Chen, Y., Mareci, T.: Denoising and visualization of HARDI data. REP-2005-360, CISE, Univ. of Florida (2005)
26. McGraw, T., Vemuri, B.C., Yezierski, B., Mareci, T.: Segmentation of High Angular Resolution Diffusion MRI Modeled as a Field of von Mises-Fisher Mixtures. In: Leonardis, A., Bischof, H., Pinz, A. (eds.) ECCV 2006. LNCS, vol. 3953, pp. 463–475. Springer, Heidelberg (2006)
27. McGraw, T., Vemuri, B.C., Yezierski, B., Mareci, T.: von Mises-Fisher Mixture model of the diffusion ODF. In: ISBI 2006: From Nano to Macro, pp. 65–68 (2006)
28. Merboldt, M., Hanicke, W., Frahm, J.: Self-diffusion NMR imaging using stimulated echoes. JMR 64, 479–486 (1985)
29. Nocedal, J., Wright, S.J.: Numerical Optimization. Springer Series in Operations Research. Springer, Heidelberg (1999)
30. Özarslan, E., Vemuri, B.C., Mareci, T.H.: Generalized scalar measures for diffusion MRI using trace, variance and entropy. MRM 53(4), 866–876 (2005)
31. Rudin, L.I., Osher, S., Fatemi, E.: Nonlinear total variation based noise removal algorithms. Physica D 60(1-4), 259–268 (1992)
32. Srivastava, A., Jermyn, I., Joshi, S.: Riemannian Analysis of Probability Density Functions with Application in Vision. In: IEEE CVPR, pp. 1–8 (2007)
33. Stejskal, E.O., Tanner, J.E.: Spin diffusion measurements: Spin echoes in the presence of a time-dependent field gradient. Journal of Chemical Physics 42, 288–292 (1965)
34. Tschumperlé, D.: PDE-Based Regularization of Multivalued Images and Applications. PhD Thesis Univ. of Nice-Sophia Antipolis, France (2002)
35. Tschumperlé, D., Deriche, R.: Anisotropic Diffusion Partial Differential Equations in Multi-Channel Image Processing: Framework and Applications. In: Book chapter in Advances in Imaging and Electron Physics (AIEP). Academic Press, London (2007)
36. Tschumperlé, D., Deriche, R.: Vector-Valued Image Regularization with PDE's: A Common Framework for Different Applications. IEEE TPAMI 27(4), 506–517 (2005)
37. Tuch, D.S.: Diffusion MRI of Complex Tissue Structure. Ph. D. Thesis, Harvard-MIT Division of Health Sciences and Technology (2002)
38. Tuch, D.S., Weisskoff, R.M., Belliveau, J.W., Wedeen, V.J.: High angular resolution diffusion imaging of the human brain. In: Proc. 7th Annual Meeting of ISMRM, Philadelphia, PA, p. 321 (1999)
39. Tuch, D.S., Reese, T.G., Wiegell, M.R., Makris, N., Belliveau, J.W., Wedeen, V.J.: High angular resolution diffusion imaging reveals intravoxel white matter fiber heterogeneity. MRM 48, 577–582 (2002)
40. Tuch, D.S., Reese, T.G., Wiegell, M.R., Wedeen, V.J.: Diffusion MRI of complex neural architecture. Neuron 40, 885–895 (2003)

41. Tuch, D.S.: Q-ball imaging. MRM 52, 1358–1372 (2004)
42. Verma, R., Khurd, P., Davatzikos, C.: On Analyzing Diffusion Tensor Images by Identifying Manifold Structure Using Isomaps. IEEE TMI 26(6), 772–778 (2007)
43. Wedeen, V.J., Hagmann, P., Tseng, W.Y., Reese, T.G., Weisskoff, R.M.: Mapping complex tissue architecture with diffusion spectrum magnetic resonance imaging. Magn. Reson. Med. 54(6), 1377–1386 (2005)
44. Zhan, L., Chiang, M.C., Barysheva, M., Toga, A.W., McMahon, K.L., de Zubicaray, G.I., Meredith, M., Wright, M.J., Thompson, P.M.: How Many Gradients are Sufficient in High-Angular Resolution Diffusion Imaging (HARDI)? In: MICCAI 2008, MICCAI DTI Workshop (2008)

Coronary Lumen Segmentation Using Graph Cuts and Robust Kernel Regression

Michiel Schaap[1,2], Lisan Neefjes[2,3], Coert Metz[1,2], Alina van der Giessen[4],
Annick Weustink[2,3], Nico Mollet[2,3], Jolanda Wentzel[4], Theo van Walsum[1,2],
and Wiro Niessen[1,2]

[1] Department of Medical Informatics
[2] Department of Radiology
[3] Department of Cardiology, Thoraxcenter
[4] Department of Biomedical Engineering
Erasmus MC - University Medical Center Rotterdam
michiel.schaap@erasmusmc.nl

Abstract. This paper presents a novel method for segmenting the coronary lumen in CTA data. The method is based on graph cuts, with edge-weights depending on the intensity of the centerline, and robust kernel regression. A quantitative evaluation in 28 coronary arteries from 12 patients is performed by comparing the semi-automatic segmentations to manual annotations. This evaluation showed that the method was able to segment the coronary arteries with high accuracy, compared to manually annotated segmentations, which is reflected in a Dice coefficient of 0.85 and average symmetric surface distance of 0.22 mm.

1 Introduction

Coronary artery disease (CAD) is one of the leading causes of death worldwide [1]. One of the imaging methods for diagnosing CAD is Computed Tomography Angiography (CTA) (see Figure 1(a) for a volume rendering of a CTA dataset), a non-invasive technique that allows the assessment of the coronary lumen and the evaluation of the presence, extent, and type (non-calcified or calcified) of coronary plaque [2]. Cardiac CTA therefore has large potential to improve risk stratification of CAD, requiring methods for objective and accurate quantification of coronary lumen and plaque parameters.

Since manual annotation of the lumen, calcium and soft plaque is very labor intensive, (semi-)automatic techniques are needed to efficiently quantify these parameters in cardiac CTA data. In this paper we focus on semi-automatic coronary lumen segmentation.

Coronary lumen segmentation is a challenging task owing to the small size of the coronary arteries (their size ranges from approximately 5 mm to less than 1 mm in diameter), the limited spatial resolution of CT (approximately 0.7 mm to 1.4 mm [3]), motion induced blurring, high intensity calcium close to the coronary lumen, and the presence of severe stenoses.

J.L. Prince, D.L. Pham, and K.J. Myers (Eds.): IPMI 2009, LNCS 5636, pp. 528–539, 2009.

Existing coronary segmentation methods can roughly be divided into two categories: methods that segment the coronaries in one pass and methods that first find the vessel centerline and then segment the vessel. The methods that segment the vessels in one pass can further be divided into methods that use region-growing or a combination of different morphology operators [4,5,6], methods that track the centerline and the radius of the vessel [7,8,9], and methods that evolve implicit surfaces [10,11].

The second group of methods first finds the centerline and then segments the vessel. A number of these methods uses the extracted centerline to segment the vessel with thresholding based on the image intensities on the centerline [12,13] or by finding multiple minimal cost paths along the vessel boundary in curved planes constructed with the centerline [14,15].

Most of the published coronary segmentation methods have been evaluated visually. Although a large body of centerline extraction methods have been quantitatively evaluated [16], to the best of our knowledge only Li et al. [8], Yang et al. [10], and Wesarg et al. [17,18] have evaluated their segmentation method quantitatively. The quantitative evaluation in these papers is done with the Dice coefficient [8], the average and maximum contour distance [10], and by assessing the performance of the method for calcium and stenosis detection [17,18].

In this paper we present a new semi-automatic coronary CTA lumen segmentation method. The method is based on graph cuts, with edge-weights depending on the intensity of the centerline, and robust kernel regression. A vessel centerline is used for initialization of the method. From recent work it has become clear that automatic coronary centerline extraction can be achieved with high precision and robustness [16].

A second major contribution of this paper is the quantitative evaluation of the method on 28 manually annotated coronary artery lumen boundaries from 12 patients. In this paper we quantitatively evaluate our method with the Dice coefficient and the average and maximum contour distance, the measures used by Li et al. [8] and Yang et al. [10].

2   Problem Formulation

Large CT intensity gradients can be observed on the boundary of the coronary lumen in CTA, while the CT intensity within the lumen varies smoothly. Therefore the problem of coronary lumen segmentation is similar to many image segmentation problems: find the strongest edge surrounding an area with relatively similar intensities. Formalizing such a problem quickly leads to balancing a gradient and an intensity term, while often the intensity term should only be used to prevent the segmentation of structures with very different intensities.

Because we segment the lumen given a centerline, we can tailor this approach to our task: find the strongest edge surrounding areas with intensities locally similar to the centerline intensity, while not segmenting areas with intensities dissimilar to the centerline intensity. The intensity information should only be used to steer the segmentation towards the regions with appropriate intensity values; the gradient information should be used to accurately detect the border.

An additional application specific constraint that we incorporate is that we aim to segment the vessel that contains the centerline; side branches of this vessel should not be segmented. This is specifically important for subsequent quantification of the degree of stenosis in a coronary artery. The surface should interpolate the boundary of the vessel of interest and not take into account the image information arising from the side-branch.

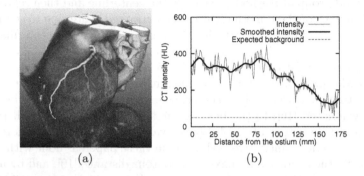

(a)   (b)

Fig. 1. (a) A 3D rendering of a cardiac CTA dataset with in yellow a manually annotated Left Anterior Descending (LAD) Coronary Artery. (b) A graph of the CT intensities I_x along the centerline of the LAD, a graph of the intensities after Gaussian kernel regression $\hat{I}_x$ and the expected background intensity I_{bg} (see section 3.1).

3   Method

In view of the above, we propose a two step approach for segmenting the coronary lumen given a centerline:

1. **Find an optimal labeling of lumen and background** using the strong edge and similar intensity prior. This is done by solving a Markov Random Field with image terms locally depending on the intensity of the centerline.
2. **Remove falsely segmented regions not belonging to the vessel of interest** using the fact that the segmented lumen should not contain any holes, the surface should be smooth, and side-branches should not be segmented. This is done by robust kernel regression on a cylindrical parameterization of the lumen boundary.

3.1   Step 1: Segmenting the Lumen with a Markov Random Field

In this first step we aim to find an optimal binary voxel labeling of the lumen and background. We do this by formalizing a binary Markov Random Field (MRF) which is solved using graph cuts [19,20,21].

A labeling $f = \{f_x | x \in \mathcal{X}\}$, with $f_x = \{0, 1\}$, is determined that has the maximum a posteriori likelihood given the CTA image $I = \{I_x | x \in \mathcal{X}\}$, with $\mathcal{X}$ being the set of voxels in the image. A labeling $f_x = 1$ corresponds to a voxel being lumen and $f_x = 0$ corresponds to a voxel being background. Each voxel x is associated with a set of neighborhood voxels $\mathcal{N} = \{\mathcal{N}_x | x \in \mathcal{X}\}$. The MRF is solved by factorizing the likelihood $Pr(f|I)$ as follows:

$$Pr(f|I) \propto \quad Pr(I|f)Pr(f)$$
$$Pr(f|I) \propto (\textstyle\prod_x Pr(I_x|f_x)) Pr(f) \tag{1}$$

with (see e.g. [20]):

$$Pr(f) = \exp\left(-\sum_x \sum_{y \in f_{\mathcal{N}_x}} \omega_{x,y}(1 - \delta(f_x - f_y))\right) \tag{2}$$

and rewriting it to the following energy functional that needs to be minimized:

$$E(f) = \sum_x -\log(Pr(I_x|f_x)) + \sum_x \sum_{y \in f_{\mathcal{N}_x}} \omega_{x,y}(1 - \delta(f_x - f_y)) \tag{3}$$

with $Pr(I_x|f_x = 1)$ and $\omega_{x,y}$ defined for our application below.

The minimization of the energy functional can be done with graph cuts. In this approach a graph is constructed where each node corresponds to a voxel x. Each voxel is connected (with *t-links*) to two additional nodes denoted respectively as 'source' and 'sink'. A weight of $\omega_s = -\log(1 - Pr(I_x|f_x = 1))$ is assigned to the source connection and a weight of $\omega_t = -\log(Pr(I_x|f_x = 1))$ is assigned to the sink connection.

Each voxel is also connected (with *n-links*) to 34 neighboring voxels $y \in \mathcal{N}_x$ and weights of $\omega_{x,y}$ are assigned to these connections (see section 3.3 for a description of the 34-connected neighborhood model $\mathcal{N}_x$). We subsequently find a cut in the graph with minimal summed weight that separates the source and the sink. This cut corresponds to the minimization of $E(f)$ [19,20,21]. Voxels still connected to the source are labeled as lumen.

Image Dependent Voxel Likelihood. We let the likelihood of a voxel being lumen $Pr(I_x|f_x = 1)$ depend on the difference between the voxel intensity and a local estimate of the lumen intensity, and a local estimate of the intensity difference between the lumen and the surrounding tissue. For notational purposes we ignore the dependency on these local estimates in $Pr(I_x|f_x = 1)$.

The local lumen intensity is estimated with a Nadaraya-Watson estimator [22]: image intensities $I_{x=c(s)}$ are sampled along the centerline, with $x = c(s)$ a position on the centerline and s the geodesic length from the start of the centerline c. This 1D function is smoothed with a Gaussian function with standard deviation σ_c to obtain a local estimate $\hat{I}_x$ of the lumen intensity.

Background tissue is modeled with a fixed intensity of I_{bg}, resulting in an estimated difference between the lumen and the background of $\hat{D}_{x'} = \hat{I}_{x'} - I_{bg}$ (see Figure 1(b)). Here x' denotes the position on the centerline closest to x, $D_x = |I_x - \hat{I}_{x'}|$ is the absolute difference between the intensity of a voxel I_x

and the local intensity estimate, and $\hat{D}_x = \hat{D}_{x'}$ describes the estimated local contrast in the image.

Using these local estimates we formalize the likelihood of a voxel given its intensity (and the intensities on the centerline) with a smooth step function (see also Figure 2(a)):

$$Pr(I_x|f_x = 1) = -0.5 \left(0.75 - 0.25 \mathrm{erf} \left(\frac{D_x - T_{\mathrm{in}}}{\sigma_i} \right) \right) \left(\mathrm{erf} \left(\frac{D_x - T_{\mathrm{out}}}{\sigma_i} \right) - 1 \right)$$

with

$$T_{\mathrm{out}} = \lambda \hat{D}_x \tag{4}$$

It can be appreciated that this function has two soft thresholds; differences D_x smaller than T_{in} correspond to a high lumen likelihood and differences higher than T_{out} correspond to a low lumen likelihood. The parameter T_{in} is user-defined and T_{out} depends locally on the contrast of the vessel with its background tissue.

By setting T_{in} relatively low and λ relatively high we make sure that the voxel term is only used to steer the segmentation towards the regions with appropriate intensity values; the edge term is used to accurately find the border in this region. In Figure 2 we show an example of $Pr(I_x|f_x = 1)$ applied to a randomly selected cross-sectional image.

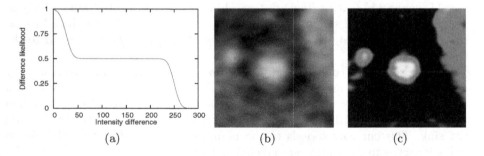

(a)   (b)   (c)

Fig. 2. (a) $Pr(I_x|f_x = 1)$ with $T_{\mathrm{in}} = 25$, $T_{\mathrm{out}} = 250$, and $\sigma_i = 15$. (b) A randomly selected cross-sectional image. (c) The application of $Pr(I_x|f_x = 1)$.

Edge Term. For the edge term we use a Gaussian function of the squared gradient magnitude on the boundary between voxel y and x $|\nabla I|(y, x)$. A high gradient magnitude corresponds to a high probability of a label switch between lumen and background:

$$Pr(f_x \neq f_y) \propto 1 - \exp \left(\frac{-|\nabla I|^2(x, y)}{2\sigma_g^2} \right). \tag{5}$$

Therefore we assign the following weight to a label switch between voxel x and y:

$$\omega_{x,y} = -\log \left(1 - \exp \left(\frac{-|\nabla I|^2(x, y)}{2\sigma_g^2} \right) \right). \tag{6}$$

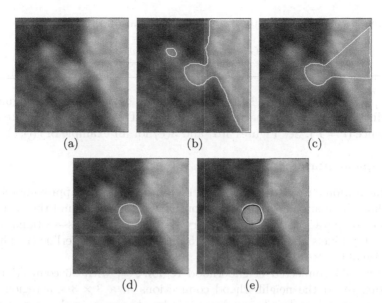

Fig. 3. A representative example (Dice=0.85, ASSD=0.18mm, AMCD=0.42mm, see section 4.3). (a) shows a cross-sectional slice of the input image, (b) shows the result after step 1, (c) shows the initialization of step 2, (d) shows the final segmentation, and (e) shows the automatic segmentation (white) together with the reference standard (black).

Segmentation after the First Step. In this first step of the algorithm a binary segmentation of the lumen is obtained. This segmentation is close to the optimal solution but it contains several false positives, corresponding to side-branches of the vessel of interest and other contrast-filled regions, voxels having a similar intensity as lumen while actually being blurred calcium, and some mis-segmentations caused by image artifacts. The result of step 1 can be seen in Figure 3(b).

3.2   Step 2: Removing Outliers from the Segmentation

In the second step of the algorithm we detect and remove regions not belonging to the vessel of interest with an iterative weighted kernel regression approach.

The segmented lumen is parameterized with cylindrical coordinates $r(\phi, s)$ by calculating the intersection of the boundary of the segmented lumen with a series of radial lines perpendicular to the centerline. We do this by extracting values from the masks obtained in step 1 with normalized Gaussian interpolation [23] and calculating the intersection point by linear interpolation (see Figure 3(c)).

Outliers are then removed from this parameterization by a simplified version of the reweighted kernel regression approach reviewed by Debruyne et al. in [24]. To each point $r(\phi, s)$ in the parameterization we iteratively assign a weight $w(\phi, s)$ describing the belief in this point. We use a Gaussian loss function, resulting in:

$$w(\phi, s)^t = exp\left(\frac{-(r(\phi, s)^t - r(\phi, s)^{t=0})^2}{2\sigma_r^2}\right) \qquad (7)$$

These weights are then used to improve the estimation of $r(.)$:

$$r(\phi,s)^{t+1} = \frac{\sum_{\phi',s'} G_{\sigma_\phi,\sigma_s}(\phi'-\phi,s'-s)w(\phi',s')^t r(\phi',s')^{t=0}}{\sum_{\phi',s'} G_{\sigma_\phi,\sigma_s}(\phi'-\phi,s'-s)w(\phi',s')^t} \tag{8}$$

with $G_{\sigma_\phi,\sigma_s}(.)$ a 2D Gaussian kernel with standard deviations in the angular and longitudinal direction of respectively σ_ϕ and σ_s. This process is repeated until convergence $(t = T)$. See Figures 3(d) and 3(e) for an example of $r(\phi,s)^T$.

3.3   Implementation

All segmentations are carried out in a region of 7.5 mm (approximately 50% larger than the maximum radius of a coronary arteries) around the centerlines to reduce computation time and memory requirements. Cross-sectional images of 128×128 pixels are created every 0.5 mm along the centerline (resulting in a voxelsize of $0.1 \times 0.1 \times 0.5$ mm^3).

We use a 34 connected neighborhood region $\mathcal{N}_x$, with 26 connections corresponding to all the neighborhood connections in a $3 \times 3 \times 3$ region and 8 connections corresponding to the 8 possible knight-moves in the cross-sectional plane. Using these knight-moves significantly improved the smoothness of the resulting segmentation (see also [25]).

3.4   Parameters

The parameters were empirically chosen by the authors; no extensive parameter-tuning was performed, with the exception of σ_ϕ and σ_s. These two parameters were tuned on one of the 28 vessels.

The following parameter settings were used for all the experiments in this paper: σ_c =2 mm, σ_i =15 HU, T_{in} = 25 HU, T_{bg} = 50 HU, $\lambda = 0.75$, σ_g =15 HU, σ_r =0.1 mm, $\sigma_\phi = 0.2$ rad, and $\sigma_s = 1$ mm.

4   Quantitative Evaluation

The method is quantitatively evaluated by comparing the segmentations with manually annotated lumen surfaces of 28 coronary arteries. The coronary arteries were segmented using manually annotated centerlines. These centerlines were also used to manually annotate the lumen boundary (see section 4.2).

4.1   Data

The cardiac CTA data of twelve patients was used for this study. Two main coronary arteries (RCA, LAD or LCX) were annotated in each dataset and an additional side-branch was annotated in four of the datasets. The observer annotated in total 8 RCAs, 8 LADs, 8 LCXs, and 4 side-branches.

The twelve CTA datasets were acquired in the Erasmus MC, University Medical Center Rotterdam, The Netherlands. The datasets were randomly selected from a series of patients who underwent a cardiac CTA examination between

June 2005 and June 2006. The datasets were acquired with a 64-slice CT scanner and a dual-source CT scanner (Sensation 64 and Somatom Definition, Siemens Medical Solutions, Forchheim, Germany). The datasets were reconstructed using a sharp (B46f) kernel or a medium-to-smooth (B30f) kernel.

4.2   Manual Annotation

One observer annotated the coronary arteries from the coronary ostium (i.e. the point where the coronary artery originates from the aorta), until the most distal point where the artery is still distinguishable from the background. On average the 28 coronary arteries were 147 mm long.

A tool was specifically designed for the manual annotation. The tool was developed in the free software package MeVisLab (http://www.mevislab.de) and has a workflow similar to the automatic approach used by Marquering et al. in [15]. After annotating a centerline the user annotates the lumen outlines longitudinally with B-splines in curved planar reformatted images created at three different angles. These curves are then intersected with planes perpendicular to the centerline spaced regularly with a distance of 1 mm. In the second annotation step the points resulting from the intersections are connected with closed B-splines to form initial contours in the cross-sectional planes. These contours can then be modified by the observer, resulting in the final annotation.

4.3   Evaluation Measures

The Dice measure, the average symmetric surface distance (ASSD), and the average maximum contour distance (AMCD) are used to quantify the difference between the manual annotations and the automatically extracted lumen surface (see [8] and [10] for the application of these measures on coronary artery segmentation evaluation).

The Dice measure represents the fraction of the volume of the overlap of the two segmentations and the average volume of the two segmentations:

$$\text{Dice} = \frac{2 \times \text{TP}}{2 \times \text{TP} + \text{FP} + \text{FN}} \tag{9}$$

The ASSD measure is determined by calculating for each point on both segmentations the distance to the closest point on the other segmentation and averaging these distances. The AMCD distance is calculated by averaging the maximum of all these distances per cross-sectional contour.

4.4   First 90 mm of the Vessel

Correctly segmenting the complete coronary shows the capability of the method to segment very small vessels, but segmenting the distal part of the vessel is not always needed in clinical practice, because disease occurs for more than 95% in the first 90 mm of the coronary arteries [26]. Therefore we also evaluate the capability of the method to segment the first 90 mm of the vessel.

536   M. Schaap et al.

5   Results

Table 1 shows the quantitative results. Figure 4 shows a series of cross-sectional
images with the manual annotation and an intersection of the automatic segmentation. Figure 5 shows two segmentations in 3D, color-coded with the distances
to the reference standard.

Table 1. An overview of the quantitative results. The Dice measure, average symmetric
surface distance (ASSD), and the average maximum contour distance (AMCD) are
reported for the complete vessel and for the first 90 mm of the vessel.

	Complete vessel			First 90 mm		
	Dice	ASSD	AMCD	Dice	ASSD	AMCD
LAD (8)	0.852	0.188	0.378	0.860	0.212	0.445
LCX (8)	0.831	0.250	0.514	0.862	0.229	0.495
RCA (8)	0.854	0.221	0.466	0.860	0.241	0.542
Side branch (8)	0.846	0.222	0.479	0.858	0.205	0.456
All (28)	0.846	0.220	0.456	0.859	0.226	0.491

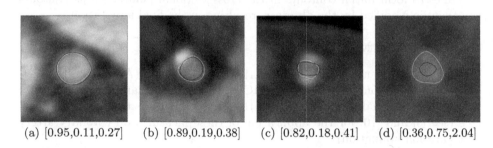

(a) [0.95,0.11,0.27]   (b) [0.89,0.19,0.38]   (c) [0.82,0.18,0.41]   (d) [0.36,0.75,2.04]

Fig. 4. Cross-sectional segmentation examples (15×15 mm^2) (in white) with corresponding reference standard (in black) and measures [Dice, ASSD in mm, AMCD in
mm]. The error in (d) was caused by the false segmentation of a stent.

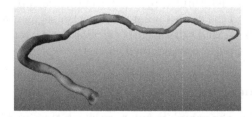

Fig. 5. 3D example of a coronary segmentation color-coded with the distance to the
reference standard. Red corresponds to the segmentation being locally 0.5 mm larger
than the reference standard, green corresponds to a perfect fit, and blue corresponds
to a 0.5 mm under-segmentation.

6   Discussion

We have presented a new CTA coronary lumen segmentation method, which uses a vessel centerline for initialization. The method accurately aligns the boundary of the segmentation with the strongest edge surrounding areas with intensities that are locally similar to the centerline intensity, while not segmenting intensities that are dissimilar to the centerline intensities. A successive robust regression step is used to remove outliers from the segmentation.

The method is quantitatively evaluated on 28 vessels in 12 cardiac CTA datasets. The average symmetric surface distance between the method and the manual reference is 0.22 mm, and the average maximum contour distance is 0.46 mm, with a mean voxel size of $0.32 \times 0.32 \times 0.40$ mm^3. Furthermore, the method obtains an average Dice coefficient of 0.85. As a rough reference one could compare these numbers to the quantitative results obtained by Li et al. and Yang et al. Li et al. obtain a Dice coefficient of 0.58 [8] and Yang et al. [10] obtain an ASSD of 0.37 mm and an AMCD of 1.36 mm. However, it should be noted that these two methods are evaluated in different patients and the datasets are most probably acquired with a different type of CT scanner. Furthermore, our method is initialized with a centerline in contrary to the methods of Li et al. and Yang et al. To objectively compare different coronary artery segmentation methods a standardized evaluation framework for coronary artery segmentation methods should be developed, e.g. using a similar approach as the coronary artery tracking evaluation framework [16].

A limitation of this study is that our algorithm uses the same centerlines as were used by the observers for annotating the coronary lumen, which may bias the results. In the future we will investigate the effect of perturbations of the centerline on the segmentation results.

Using the presented method for lumen segmentation can already reduce the amount of user-interaction with a factor of 10 (the manual annotation of a centerline takes approximately 5 minutes, while annotating the coronary lumen outline can take up to 50 minutes). A further reduction seems feasible, as results from the coronary artery tracking evaluation framework [16] show that semi-automated and fully automatic coronary artery centerline tracking methods that achieve high robustness and accuracy (comparable to inter-observer variability) are available. In the future we will also evaluate our method with (semi-)automatically extracted centerlines.

Another limitation is that at this moment we only have coronary lumen annotations of one observer. Manual annotations by multiple clinical experts are currently planned, and in future work we will therefore also relate the performance of the method to the inter-observer variability. Finally, we will investigate the possibility to quantify clinically relevant measures (such as the degree of stenosis) with the proposed method.

7   Conclusion

A high-precision coronary lumen segmentation method is presented. The method is based on graph cuts and robust kernel regression and segments the coronary lumen given a centerline. The method has been successfully applied for the segmentation of 28 coronary arteries. A quantitative evaluation showed that the method was able to segment the coronary arteries with high accuracy, compared to manually annotated segmentations.

References

1. Rosamond, W., et al.: Heart disease and stroke statistics–2008 update: a report from the American Heart Association Statistics Committee and Stroke Statistics Subcommittee. Circulation 117, e25–e146 (2008)
2. Leber, A.W., et al.: Accuracy of 64-slice computed tomography to classify and quantify plaque volumes in the proximal coronary system: a comparative study using intravascular ultrasound. Journal of the American College of Cardiology 47, 672–677 (2006)
3. Rollano-Hijarrubia, E., Stokking, R., van der Meer, F., Niessen, W.J.: Imaging of small high-density structures in CT; A phantom study. Academic Radiology 13, 893–908 (2006)
4. Boskamp, T., Rinck, D., Link, F., Kümmerlen, B., Stamm, G., Mildenberger, P.: New vessel analysis tool for morphometric quantification and visualization of vessels in CT and MR imaging data sets. Radiographics 24(1), 287–297 (2004)
5. Luengo-Oroz, M.A., Ledesma-Carbayo, M.J., Gómez-Diego, J.J., García-Fernández, M.A., Desco, M., Santos, A.: Extraction of the Coronary Artery Tree in Cardiac Computer Tomographic Images Using Morphological Operators. In: Sachse, F.B., Seemann, G. (eds.) FIMH 2007. LNCS, vol. 4466, pp. 424–432. Springer, Heidelberg (2007)
6. Bouraoui, B., Ronse, C., Baruthio, J., Passat, N., Germain, P.: Fully automatic 3D segmentation of coronary arteries based on mathematical morphology. In: Proceedings of ISBI 2008, pp. 1059–1062 (2008)
7. Lesage, D., Angelini, E., Bloch, I., Funka-Lea, G.: Medial-based Bayesian tracking for vascular segmentation: Application to coronary arteries in 3D CT angiography. In: Proceedings of ISBI 2008, pp. 268–271 (2008)
8. Li, H., Yezzi, A.: Vessels as 4-D Curves: Global Minimal 4-D Paths to Extract 3-D Tubular Surfaces and Centerlines. IEEE Transactions on Medical Imaging 26, 1213–1223 (2007)
9. Wesarg, S., Firle, E.: Segmentation of Vessels: The Corkscrew Algorithm. In: SPIE: Medical Imaging: Image Processing, vol. 9, p. 10 (2004)
10. Yang, Y., Tannenbaum, A., Giddens, D., Stillman, A.: Automatic segmentation of coronary arteries using bayesian driven implicit surfaces. In: Proceedings of ISBI 2007, pp. 189–192 (2007)
11. Nain, D., Yezzi, A., Turk, G.: Vessel Segmentation Using a Shape Driven Flow. In: Barillot, C., Haynor, D.R., Hellier, P. (eds.) MICCAI 2004. LNCS, vol. 3216, pp. 51–59. Springer, Heidelberg (2004)
12. Renard, F., Yang, Y.: Image analysis for detection of coronary artery soft plaques in MDCT images. In: Proceedings of ISBI 2008, pp. 25–28 (2008)
13. Lavi, G., Lessick, J., Johnson, P., Khullar, D.: Single-seeded coronary artery tracking in CT angiography. In: IEEE Nuclear Science Symposium Conference Record (2004)
14. Sonka, M., Winniford, M.D., Collins, S.M.: Robust simultaneous detection of coronary borders in complex images. IEEE Trans. Med. Imaging 14(1), 151–161 (1995)

15. Marquering, H.A., Dijkstra, J., de Koning, P.J.H., Stoel, B.C., Reiber, J.H.C.: Towards quantitative analysis of coronary CTA. Int. J. Cardiovasc. Imaging 21, 73–84 (2005)
16. Metz, C., Schaap, M., van Walsum, T., van der Giessen, A., Weustink, A., Mollet, N., Krestin, G., Niessen, W.: 3D segmentation in the clinic: A Grand Challenge II - Coronary Artery Tracking. In: IJ - 2008 MICCAI Workshop - Grand Challenge Coronary Artery Tracking (2008)
17. Wesarg, S., Khan, M.F., Firle, E.A.: Localizing calcifications in cardiac CT data sets using a new vessel segmentation approach. J. Digit. Imaging 19, 249–257 (2006)
18. Khan, M.F., Wesarg, S., Gurung, J., Dogan, S., Maataoui, A., Brehmer, B., Herzog, C., Ackermann, H., Assmus, B., Vogl, T.J.: Facilitating coronary artery evaluation in MDCT using a 3D automatic vessel segmentation tool. European Radiology 16, 1789–1795 (2006)
19. Boykov, Y., Funka-Lea, G.: Graph cuts and efficient n-d image segmentation. International Journal of Computer Vision 70, 109–131 (2006)
20. Boykov, Y., Veksler, O., Zabih, R.: Markov random fields with efficient approximations. In: IEEE Conference on Computer Vision and Pattern Recognition, pp. 648–655 (1998)
21. Kohli, P., Torr, P.H.S.: Dynamic graph cuts for efficient inference in markov random fields. IEEE Transactions on Pattern Analysis and Machine Intelligence 29(12), 2079–2088 (2007)
22. Nadaraya, E.A.: On estimating regression. Theory of Probability and its Applications 10, 186–190 (1964)
23. Knutsson, H., Westin, C.-F.: Normalized and differential convolution: Methods for interpolation and filtering of incomplete and uncertain data. In: Proceedings of Computer Vision and Pattern Recognition 1993, pp. 515–523 (1993)
24. Debruyne, M., Hubert, M., Suykens, J.: Model selection in kernel based regression using the influence function. Journal of Machine Learning Research 9, 2377–2400 (2008)
25. Boykov, Y., Kolmogorov, V.: Computing geodesics and minimal surfaces via graph cuts. In: ICCV (2003)
26. Hong, M.-K., et al.: The site of plaque rupture in native coronary arteries: a three-vessel intravascular ultrasound analysis. J. Am. Coll. Cardiol. 46, 261–265 (2005)

Dense Registration with Deformation Priors

Ben Glocker[1,2], Nikos Komodakis[3],
Nassir Navab[2], Georgios Tziritas[3], and Nikos Paragios[1,4]

[1] Laboratoire MAS, Ecole Centrale Paris, Chatenay-Malabry, France
[2] Computer Aided Medical Procedures (CAMP), Technische Universität München, Germany
[3] Computer Science Department, University of Crete, Greece
[4] Equipe GALEN, INRIA Saclay - Ile-de-France, Orsay, France
glocker@in.tum.de

Abstract. In this paper we propose a novel approach to define task-driven regularization constraints in deformable image registration using learned deformation priors. Our method consists of representing deformation through a set of control points and an interpolation strategy. Then, using a training set of images and the corresponding deformations we seek for a weakly connected graph on the control points where edges define the prior knowledge on the deformation. This graph is obtained using a clustering technique which models the co-dependencies between the displacements of the control points. The resulting classification is used to encode regularization constraints through connections between cluster centers and cluster elements. Additionally, the global structure of the deformation is encoded through a fully connected graph on the cluster centers. Then, registration of a new pair of images consists of displacing the set of control points where on top of conventional image correspondence costs, we introduce costs that are based on the relative deformation of two control points with respect to the learned deformation. The resulting paradigm is implemented using a discrete Markov Random Field which is optimized using efficient linear programming. Promising experimental results on synthetic and real data demonstrate the potential of our approach.

1 Introduction

Image deformation estimation consists of recovering a transformation which aligns two images. Optical flow estimation [1] or fusion of medical images [2] are prominent applications in the fields of computer vision and medical image analysis. Starting from the pioneering formulation of the visual preservation constraint [3], it has been an active problem for almost two decades. The spatial transformation to be recovered establishes correspondences between the two images according to some similarity measure. The task of registration often involves three aspects, the transformation model, the similarity measure, and the optimization strategy used to estimate the transformation parameters.

Variational techniques [4], statistical methods [5] and more recently discrete optimization approaches [6] were considered to address this task. The main challenge to be addressed is related with the ill-posedness definition of the problem. In the most general case, one has to determine a vector of variables from a single constraint, while at the same time signals can be non-linearly related with an unknown spatial transformation (registration). The use of regularization techniques [7] is often used as a soft

J.L. Prince, D.L. Pham, and K.J. Myers (Eds.): IPMI 2009, LNCS 5636, pp. 540–551, 2009.
© Springer-Verlag Berlin Heidelberg 2009

prior to deal with the above limitation which often deteriorates estimation along region boundaries.

In medical imaging, if one neglects the global component of the transformation, and since observed signals measure information on anatomical structures, the notion of repetitive behavior is present, for example the deformation of the heart during the cardiac cycle. The use of prior models can be an excellent choice to address the ill-posedness of the registration task, in particular when considering intra-modal registration of challenging, emerging imaging modalities (functional MRI, diffusion tensor imaging, ultrasound, ...), or in case of inter-modal registration for pairs of images where the similarity metric is ill-defined. A lot of work has been done in modeling variations in shape in a more global sense using principal component analysis (PCA). Active shape models (ASMs) [8] have been successfully and widely used in automatic segmentation and shape matching. However, despite enormous investment on model-free deformable registration, one can observe limited work on registration with deformation priors.

The main challenge of dense registration with deformation priors is with regard to the dimensionality of the problem. Opposite to conventional learning problems, in the most general case, learning the deformations corresponding to the entire image domain requires a huge number of training examples. One can overcome this limitation through a rough dimensionality reduction of the deformation fields [9], but then the performance of the model is compromised in terms of ability to capture local deformations. An alternative to such an approach is to consider a rather dense sampling and determine dependencies between deformations. If such a task can be addressed, then one can model prior knowledge on the deformation through decomposition into several local parts where each exhibits similar behavior. This will introduce two novel priors, one that encodes local dependencies and one that accounts for the global structure of the deformation.

In this paper, we propose a novel approach to deformable image registration with priors on the deformation. The deformation field is represented using a set of control points and an interpolation strategy. Using a training set, we perform clustering on the determined deformations according to the displacements of the control points. The aim is to determine pairs with statistical correlation in terms of deformation behavior. Recent advances from linear programming are used to address the clustering task. The outcome of the process is integrated within a discrete Markov Random Field (MRF) [10] approach for dense image registration. Conventional regularization constraints – e.g. penalizing the gradients of the displacement field – are replaced in order to encode co-dependencies between the cluster centers and the corresponding cluster elements. The global structure of the learned deformation is modeled through a fully connected graph on the cluster centers. The resulting graph structure involves a very small number of connections and can be learned from a rather small training set. Experimental results using these two novel deformation priors demonstrate the potential of our approach.

The remainder of this paper is organized as follows: in Section 2 we present the construction of the deformation priors, while in Section 3 the registration paradigm is presented. Experimental results and validation are part of Section 4, while the last Section concludes the paper.

2   Learning and Construction of Deformation Priors

Let us consider a set of N training examples (pairs of images). The corresponding deformation fields $\{D_1, D_2, \ldots, D_N\}$ are assumed to be known (e.g. obtained through dense registration). Considering a transformation model such as Free Form Deformations (FFD) [11], a deformation field D can be efficiently represented through a set of M control points $P = \{\mathbf{p}_1, \mathbf{p}_2, \ldots, \mathbf{p}_M\}$ defined on a regular grid where each control point $\mathbf{p}_i$ is associated with a displacement vector $\mathbf{d}_i$. Then, the displacement $D(\mathbf{x})$ of any pixel $\mathbf{x}$ in the image domain can be determined through interpolation between control point displacements, or

$$D(\mathbf{x}) = \sum_{i=1}^{M} \eta(\mathbf{x}) \mathbf{d}_i \ , \tag{1}$$

with $\eta(\cdot)$ being the interpolation function (often based on B-spline basis functions [12]).

Modeling prior knowledge based on observed deformations aims at determining a probability density function (pdf) $\psi(D)$. Such a pdf could then be incorporated into the registration procedure and hopefully would improve the estimation of the deformation. In order to construct a compact representation of such a prior, we assume that correlations exist between the behavior of control points. We further assume that we can separate the control points into two groups – the masters and the slaves. The master control points are the ones that encode the most important information, while the slaves are the ones which can be determined to some extent from the master ones. This can be viewed as a clustering problem where cluster centers will correspond to master control points and cluster elements to the slave ones. Each of the slaves will be attributed to a single cluster according to their statistical dependency, while one should reduce the number of retained clusters to a minimum. Such a clustering task involves the following unknown variables: (i) number of clusters K, (ii) identity of the cluster centers $C = \{\mathbf{c}_1, \mathbf{c}_2, \ldots, \mathbf{c}_K\}$, and (iii) assignment of elements to clusters $A = \{a_1, a_2, \ldots, a_M\}$ with $a_i \in [1, K]$. Additionally, let κ be a multivariate probability distribution determined from the N observed displacement vectors of a control point $\mathbf{p}$. Then, the statistical dependency between two control points $\mathbf{p}_i$ and $\mathbf{p}_j$ can be obtained by a distance function $\xi(\kappa_i, \kappa_j)$. From a mathematical perspective, we try to minimize the following function

$$\min_{K,C,A} \sum_{i=1}^{M} \xi(\kappa_{\mathbf{p}_i}, \kappa_{\mathbf{c}_{a_i}}) + \sum_{k=1}^{K} f(\mathbf{c}_k) \ , \tag{2}$$

where $f(\cdot)$ is a cluster penalty term which avoids the trivial solution of choosing all elements as cluster centers.

A common drawback of many popular clustering techniques (such as the K-means algorithm) is that they need to be given the number of clusters K beforehand (which simplifies Eq. (2)). This is, however, problematic as this number is very often not known in advance. Another very bad symptom of many clustering techniques is that they are particularly sensitive to initialization. To address these issues, we make use of a recently proposed clustering method based on linear programming [13] which automatically estimates the optimal number of clusters and works independent from the initialization. Due to the limited space we refer the reader to the given reference which also discusses the right choice of the cluster penalty term. However, other clustering approaches might be considered as well.

Still, a crucial part is the choice of an appropriate distance function $\xi(\cdot,\cdot)$. It can be for instance the Kullback-Leibler divergence [14] or the Bhattacharyya divergence [15] which is considered in this paper. The Bhattacharyya measure is defined as

$$B(\kappa_i,\kappa_j) = \int_{-\infty}^{\infty} \sqrt{\kappa_i(\mathbf{x})\kappa_j(\mathbf{x})}d\mathbf{x} \ , \tag{3}$$

which satisfies the properties $0 \leq B(\kappa_i,\kappa_j) \leq 1$, $B(\kappa_i,\kappa_j) = B(\kappa_j,\kappa_i)$ and $B(\kappa_i,\kappa_j) = 1$ if and only if $\kappa_i = \kappa_j$. The corresponding Bhattacharyya divergence is defined as $\xi_B(\kappa_i,\kappa_j) = -\log B(\kappa_i,\kappa_j)$. For Gaussian distributions the Bhattacharyya divergence has a closed form expression, while for more complex distributions such as Gaussian mixture models (GMMs) closed form expressions do not exist and sampling strategies [16] have to be used.

2.1 Deformation Prior

The outcome of the clustering consists of a set of cluster centers $C \subseteq P$ and disjunct clusters of control points $\{P_1, P_2, \ldots, P_K\}$ with $\bigcup_{k=1}^{K} P_k = P$. Then, in order to capture the local dependencies within a cluster, we consider the pairwise probability distributions on the relative deformation between cluster elements $\mathbf{p} \in P_k$ and the corresponding cluster center $\mathbf{c}_k \in P_k, C$, or

$$\psi_k^{\text{local}}(D) = \prod_{\mathbf{p},\mathbf{c}_k \in P_k, \mathbf{c}_k \in C, \mathbf{p} \neq \mathbf{c}_k} \kappa_{\mathbf{p}\mathbf{c}_k}(\|\mathbf{d}_\mathbf{p} - \mathbf{d}_{\mathbf{c}_k}\|) \ . \tag{4}$$

Additionally, in order to capture the global structure of the learned deformation, we consider the distributions between cluster centers

$$\psi^{\text{global}}(D) = \prod_{\mathbf{c}_i,\mathbf{c}_j \in C, i \neq j} \kappa_{\mathbf{c}_i\mathbf{c}_j}(\|\mathbf{d}_{\mathbf{c}_i} - \mathbf{d}_{\mathbf{c}_j}\|) \ . \tag{5}$$

The pairwise distributions for the relative deformation of two control points are estimated from the training data, once the clustering is computed.

We can now approximate the overall pdf $\psi(\mathcal{D})$ by combining the above terms into a prior on the deformation, or

$$\psi(D) = \psi^{\text{global}}(D) \prod_{k=1}^{K} \psi_k^{\text{local}}(D) \tag{6}$$

One should note that such a representation is invariant to global translation. Implementing this prior into a registration framework constraints the space of feasible deformations. This could be of great benefit in cases where the similarity measure deteriorates due to noise or data corruption. Also, conventional soft priors – e.g. penalizing the gradients of the displacement field – might result in oversmoothed displacement fields which could also be overcome by incorporating the above priors.

Throughout this paper, we represent the probability density functions by GMMs. Other representations can be considered, however the main advantage of GMMs is their compact representation for complex distributions while being efficient in terms of evaluation and implementation. The density estimation from the training data is performed through the EM algorithm [17] while the optimal number of Gaussians is determined in a brute force manner. To this end, we evaluate the minimum description length (MDL) for 1 to 5 Gaussians and keep the GMM with the lowest MDL.

3 MRF Registration with Deformation Priors

In order to prove the concept of using the proposed deformation priors for image registration, we implemented the proposed paradigm in a dense registration framework based on discrete MRFs [18]. In our case, the main advantage of such a framework is that MRFs naturally allow for encoding dependencies between pairs of variables (here, the FFD control points). We show that simple changes in the MRF topology and the replacement of conventional regularization costs are sufficient to enhance the registration algorithm with the learned deformation priors.

3.1 Dense Registration through MRF Labeling

We will briefly recall the principles of the intensity-based registration framework described in [18]. Considering the common approach of energy minimization for the registration of two images I and J, or

$$D^* = \arg\min_D \int_\Omega \phi(I(\mathbf{x}), J(\mathbf{x} + D(\mathbf{x}))) \, d\mathbf{x} \tag{7}$$

one seeks for recovering the optimal deformation D^* w.r.t. a similarity measure ϕ. Considering the FFD transformation model defined Eq. (1), we can define the objective function based on the control points as

$$E_{\text{data}}(D) = \sum_{\mathbf{p} \in P} \int_\Omega \hat{\eta}(\mathbf{x}) \cdot \phi(I(\mathbf{x}), J(\mathbf{x} + D(\mathbf{x}))) \, d\mathbf{x}. \tag{8}$$

where $\hat{\eta}(\cdot)$ is a weighting function determining the influence of a pixel $\mathbf{x}$ to the local similarity at control point $\mathbf{p}$. Different approaches for the weighting function can be considered (cp. [18]), depending on the nature of the similarity measure.

The key idea in this approach is now to reformulate the registration problem as a *discrete labeling problem*. Based on the previous assumptions, the control points P of the deformation grid are considered as a set of discrete variables. Additionally, a discrete set of labels $L = \{l_1, ..., l_i\}$ corresponding to a quantized version of the deformation space $\Theta = \{\mathbf{d}_1, ..., \mathbf{d}_i\}$ is introduced. A label assignment $l_\mathbf{p}$ to a grid node $\mathbf{p}$ is associated with displacing the node by the corresponding vector $\mathbf{d}_{l_\mathbf{p}}$. Once a label is assigned to every node we obtain a discrete labeling **l**. A popular and efficient model for representing such discrete labeling problems are second-order MRFs [19]:

$$E_{\mathrm{mrf}}(\mathbf{l}) = \sum_{\mathbf{p} \in P} V_{\mathbf{p}}(l_{\mathbf{p}}) + \lambda \sum_{(\mathbf{p},\mathbf{q}) \in S} V_{\mathbf{pq}}(l_{\mathbf{p}}, l_{\mathbf{q}}) \; , \qquad (9)$$

where $V_{\mathbf{p}}(\cdot)$ are the unary potentials representing the data term, $V_{\mathbf{pq}}(\cdot,\cdot)$ are the pairwise potentials representing dependencies between neighboring nodes, and S defines the neighborhood system through a set of edges. Additionally, λ acts as a weighting factor controlling the influence of the pairwise term. We define the unary potentials (in iteration t) according to our data term as

$$V_{\mathbf{p}}(l_{\mathbf{p}}) = \int_{\Omega} \hat{\eta}(\mathbf{x}) \cdot \phi \left(I(\mathbf{x}), J(\mathbf{x} + D^{t-1}(\mathbf{x}) + \mathbf{d}_{l_{\mathbf{p}}}) \right) d\mathbf{x} \; . \qquad (10)$$

The pairwise potentials can encode penalty costs for assigning different labels to connected nodes. The FFD transformation model already inherits implicit smoothness. Additionally, one can consider explicit regularization constraints on the grid domain. A common, but rather heuristic, approach is to consider regularization on the squared differences of displacement vectors – i.e. an approximation of penalizing the gradients of the deformation field. This can be defined as

$$V_{\mathbf{pq}}(l_{\mathbf{p}}, l_{\mathbf{q}}) = \left((\mathbf{d}_{\mathbf{p}}^{t-1} + \mathbf{d}_{l_{\mathbf{p}}}) - (\mathbf{d}_{\mathbf{q}}^{t-1} + \mathbf{d}_{l_{\mathbf{q}}}) \right)^2 \; , \qquad (11)$$

where $\mathbf{d}_{\mathbf{p}}^{t-1}$ and $\mathbf{d}_{\mathbf{q}}^{t-1}$ are the accumulated displacements for the control points **p** and **q** in iteration t.

Many optimization algorithms exist for efficiently solving discrete labeling problems in form of an MRF. We use a recently proposed method called FastPD [20] which is also used in [6,18]. Due to the limited space, we refer the reader to the given references for more details about the algorithm.

3.2 Local and Global Prior Costs

Conventional regularization techniques as introduced in Eq. (11) can be seen as soft priors which are used to deal with the ill-posedness of the registration problem. Still, these approaches may deteriorate the estimation along region boundaries or result in oversmoothed displacement fields, since there is no relationship between the penalty function based on the grid topology and the actual local dependencies of object deformations. To overcome this limitation, we propose a novel regularization term based on the results of the control point clustering. One can claim that variations on the deformation of nodes belonging to one cluster should be penalized w.r.t. to the relative deformation learned from the training data while discontinuities between nodes of different clusters should be explicitly allowed (even desired). We propose to remove the conventional regularization term which simply imposes smoothness for neighboring nodes. Instead, we define an intra-cluster regularization that accounts for the local dependencies of control points. For each cluster k, we connect its elements $\mathbf{p} \in P_k$ with the cluster center $\mathbf{c}_k$ and define edge penalty costs derived from Eq. (4) as:

$$V_{\mathbf{pc}_k}(l_{\mathbf{p}}, l_{\mathbf{c}_k}) = -\log \left(\kappa_{\mathbf{pc}_k}(\| (\mathbf{d}_{\mathbf{p}}^{t-1} + \mathbf{d}_{l_{\mathbf{p}}}) - (\mathbf{d}_{\mathbf{c}_k}^{t-1} + \mathbf{d}_{l_{\mathbf{c}_k}}) \|) \right) \; . \qquad (12)$$

The advantage of this cluster-based regularization is on one hand its direct relation to the learned local dependencies on the level of control points, and on the other hand, it allows for discontinuities between neighboring control points belonging to different clusters. Additional to the cluster-based regularization, we propose a second prior term that accounts for the global structure of the deformation. Using the concept of pairwise densities defined in Eq. (5), we can impose a global prior cost on the desired deformations by introducing connections between all cluster centers (fully connected graph), or

$$V_{\mathbf{c}_i \mathbf{c}_j}(l_{\mathbf{c}_i}, l_{\mathbf{c}_j}) = -\log \left(\kappa_{\mathbf{c}_i \mathbf{c}_j}(\|(\mathbf{d}_{\mathbf{c}_i}^{t-1} + \mathbf{d}_{l_{\mathbf{c}_i}}) - (\mathbf{d}_{\mathbf{c}_j}^{t-1} + \mathbf{d}_{l_{\mathbf{c}_j}})\|) \right) . \qquad (13)$$

The overall pdf derived in Eq. (6) can then be encoded by combining the two terms which leads to the proposed registration approach using learned deformation priors. The new energy function of the MRF registration is then defined as

$$E_{\mathrm{mrf}}(\mathbf{l}) = \underbrace{\sum_{\mathbf{p} \in P} V_{\mathbf{p}}(l_{\mathbf{p}})}_{\text{Data Costs}} + \lambda \underbrace{\left(\sum_{\mathbf{c}_i, \mathbf{c}_j \in C} V_{\mathbf{c}_i \mathbf{c}_j}(l_{\mathbf{c}_i}, l_{\mathbf{c}_j}) + \sum_{k=1}^{K} \sum_{\mathbf{p}, \mathbf{c}_k \in P_k} V_{\mathbf{p}\mathbf{c}_k}(l_{\mathbf{p}}, l_{\mathbf{c}_k}) \right)}_{\text{Deformation Prior Costs}} . \qquad (14)$$

4 Experimental Validation

In our first experiment, we investigate the performance of the proposed approach in a synthetic scenario. On the one hand, this experiment should illustrate the single steps of our method from the training phase to the final application of image registration. On the other hand, we will compare its performance to conventional regularization techniques – i.e. penalizing the vector difference between neighboring control points [18]. The second experiment is on real data where the idea is to learn the deformation on images of good quality which are suitable for conventional registration. After the learning, the registration with deformation priors is used to register images of bad quality showing the same anatomy as in the training data.

4.1 Experiments on Synthetic Deformations

In the absence of a gold standard, evaluation in deformable registration settings is a challenging task. One option is to consider synthetic deformations where everything is known by construction. To this end, we generate a 2D image with a resolution of 128×96 showing a bone like structure and define a deformation grid of size 17×13 (see Fig. 1(e)). We separate the control points into nine clusters from which eight clusters are used to generate random deformations and the ninth cluster is without deformation. Random displacements of elements belonging to the same cluster are following a similar Gaussian distribution. In total we generate 500 deformations. Examples are shown in Fig. 1(a)-(d) where the dense displacement field is overlaid. We use 400 deformations for the training and the prior construction. A Gaussian density with zero mean and standard deviation one is assumed for the control points of the ninth cluster without deformation. All other densities are estimated from the training data. Based on the clustering result (see Fig. 1(f)) we define the new MRF topology using intra-cluster

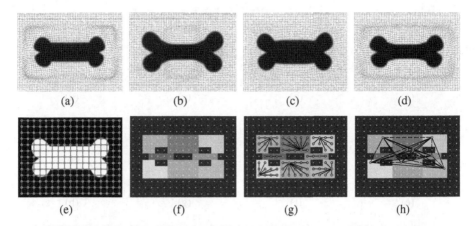

(a)   (b)   (c)   (d)

(e)   (f)   (g)   (h)

Fig. 1. Synthetic experiment: the upper row shows exemplary deformations and overlaid the corresponding dense displacement fields. The lower row illustrates the clustering (f) and the resulting MRF topology consisting of intra-cluster edges (g) and the fully connected graph on the cluster centers (h).

edges for the local prior as shown in Fig. 1(g) and for the global prior we define a fully connected graph on the cluster centers as shown in Fig. 1(h). For better visibility all connections within and to the ninth cluster are discarded from the drawings.

We compare the performance of the proposed method to conventional regularization as defined in Eq. (11) and used for instance in [18]. To this end, the source image (see Fig. 1(e)) is registered to different target images where either varying amount of Gaussian noise is added or the image data is heavily corrupted. We use the sum of squared differences (SSD) as the similarity measure. The SSD is very sensitive to noise and allows us to investigate the important role of regularization. The weighting factors λ are individually determined empirically for the conventional and the approach using learned priors such that smooth and reasonable deformations are obtained. In particular, the conventional method is sensitive to λ such that too less regularization leads the SSD measure to smear the source image while too much regularization constraints the deformation to rigid translations. Once a good compromise is found on exemplary images, the values are fixed throughout the experiments for both methods.

Target	Conventional	Learned Priors
Noise σ=0.1	0.42 ($\pm$ 0.11)	0.16 ($\pm$ 0.06)
Noise σ=1.0	0.73 ($\pm$ 0.18)	0.42 ($\pm$ 0.15)
Noise σ=5.0	1.17 ($\pm$ 0.26)	0.79 ($\pm$ 0.25)
Corrupted	1.52 ($\pm$ 0.49)	0.69 ($\pm$ 0.12)

Fig. 2. Synthetic experiment: on the left, the average boundary distance (ABD) after registration using the conventional regularization and the approach using learned priors. Before registration the overall ABD is 2.16 ($\pm$0.46) pixels. On the right, the initial alignment of source (in green) and an exemplary target image (in blue) also used in Fig. 3. For this example, the ABD is 1.77 pixels.

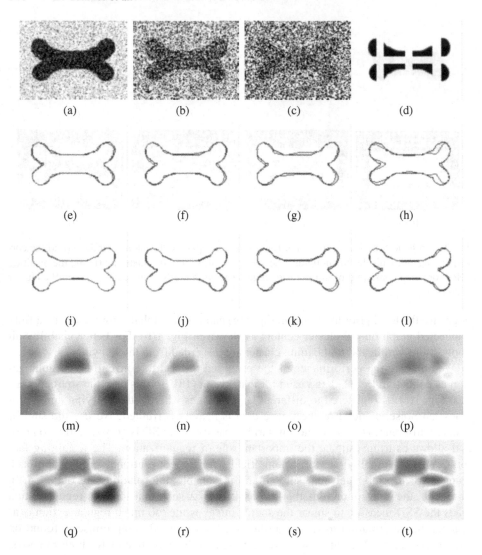

Fig. 3. Synthetic experiment: the first row illustrates exemplary target images with varying amounts of noise and corruption. The second row shows the registration results for the conventional registration while the third row shows the results for using learned priors. The target shape boundary is drawn in blue, the shape boundary of the deformed source image is drawn in red. The initial alignment before registration is illustrated in Fig. 2. The fourth and fifth row show the color encoded displacement fields for both methods. The color represents the angle, the intensity the magnitude of the displacement vectors. Note, how well the clustering topology is reflected in all fields for registration with deformation priors (compare Fig. 1(f)).

Exemplary target images are shown in Fig. 3(a)-(d). After registration, we compare the original shape boundary of the target image with the warped boundary of the deformed source image and compute the symmetric average boundary distance (ABD). Visually, we observe that conventional regularization tends to result in oversmoothed displacement fields (see Fig. 3(m)) while the registration with deformation priors reflects the single clusters in the recovered deformations (see Fig. 3(q)). Visual registration results and the color encoded displacement fields are illustrated in Fig. 3(e)-(t). Quantitative

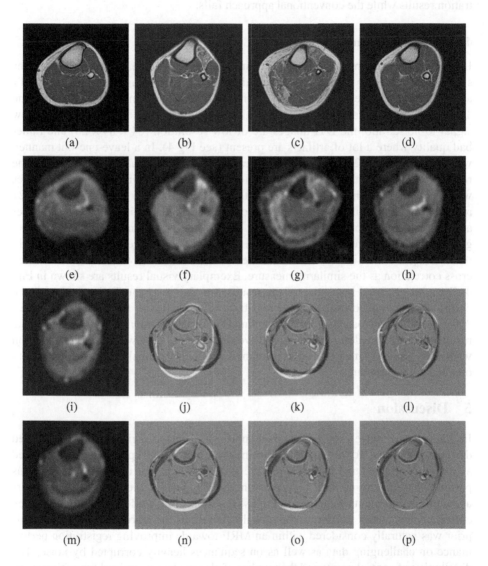

Fig. 4. Real data experiment: Upper row shows exemplary T1 images from the training set. Middle row shows the corresponding B0 DTI images. The two last rows show from left to right the target image, the difference image for the initial alignment, the alignment after conventional registration, and the result for the registration with deformation priors when using (e) as the source image. Note, for better visual inspection of the registration results, the difference images (j)-(l) are computed from the warped T1 images using the deformations obtained from the DTI registrations.

measurements of the ABD after registration are summarized in Fig. 2. The overall ABD before registration is $2.16\,(\pm0.46)$ pixels. The approach using learned priors clearly outperforms the conventional regularization. In particular under extreme conditions of noise and corruption, the priors on the deformation help to achieve meaningful registration results while the conventional approach fails.

4.2   Experiments on Real Data

In our second experiment, we consider clinical data of a myopathy study. MRI scans showing the lower leg muscles are acquired from 23 subjects. Each scan consists of T1 and DTI images. Note, that from the DTI images only the B0 image is used. While the T1 images have a very good contrast, a high resolution ($256 \times 256 \times 20$), and a low signal-to-noise ratio, the DTI images are of low resolution ($64 \times 64 \times 20$) and rather bad quality where a lot of artifacts are present (see Fig 4). In a leave-one-out manner, we randomly select 22 subjects for the training where one subject is chosen as the reference. We perform a series of conventional registrations using only the T1 images where the reference is aligned with all other training images. The results of the 21 registrations are then used for the learning of the deformation priors. Since we consider a multi-resolution approach, we separately learn the deformation prior for each control grid level. For evaluation, we register the DTI image of the reference with the DTI of the subject which is not included in the training set. Here, we use the normalized cross correlation as the similarity measure. Exemplary visual results are shown in Fig. 4. For a better visual inspection of the results, we also warp the T1 images using the deformations obtained from the DTI registration, and visualize the difference images. A perfect alignment based on the challenging DTI images is not achieved. However, the results show that the deformation prior drives the registration towards the right solution where the similarity measure alone combined with conventional regularization fails to obtain a good alignment.

5   Discussion

In this paper we have proposed a novel approach to image registration using learned deformation priors. To this end, the deformation of the control points were considered as random variables and clustering on the statistical behavior of these variables was performed to determine their co-dependencies. Connections between cluster centers and attributed elements were used to impose regularization, while connections between cluster centers aimed to capture the global structure of the learned deformation. This prior was naturally considered within an MRF towards improving registration performance on challenging data as well as on sequences heavily corrupted by noise. The distribution of control points and the number of clusters being retained are critical components of our process as well as the distance between variables. Non-uniform transformation models (such as NURBS) might be a more appropriate selection for the graph construction. Further investigation on the above mentioned components of the method could improve the performance. The use of this concept to address registration within modalities that do exhibit low signal to noise ratio is a natural extension of our approach. Ultrasound images, diffusion tensor imaging, or functional MRI are examples where conventional registration techniques might often fail to provide meaningful results. Therefore, we believe that our approach has great potential in such applications.

References

1. Fleet, D., Weiss, Y.: Optical Flow Estimation. In: Handbook of Mathematical Models in Computer Vision, pp. 239–256. Springer, Heidelberg (2006)
2. Hajnal, J., Hill, D.L.G., Hawkes, D.J. (eds.): Medical Image Registration. CRC Press, Boca Raton (2001)
3. Horn, B., Schunck, B.: Determining optical flow. Artificial Intelligence 17, 185–204 (1981)
4. Bruhn, A., Weickert, J., Schnörr, C.: Lucas/kanade meets horn/schunck: Combining local and global optic flow methods. International Journal of Computer Vision (IJCV) 61(3) (2005)
5. Viola, P., Wells, W.M.: Alignment by maximization of mutual information. International Journal of Computer Vision (IJCV) 24(2), 137–154 (1997)
6. Glocker, B., Komodakis, N., Paragios, N., Tziritas, G., Navab, N.: Inter and intra-modal deformable registration: Continuous deformations meet efficient optimal linear programming. In: Karssemeijer, N., Lelieveldt, B. (eds.) IPMI 2007. LNCS, vol. 4584, pp. 408–420. Springer, Heidelberg (2007)
7. Tikhonov, A.: Ill-posed problems in natural sciences, Coronet (1992)
8. Cootes, T.F., Taylor, C.J., Cooper, D.H., Graham, J.: Active shape models — their training and application. Computer Vision and Image Understanding (CVIU) 61(1), 38–59 (1995)
9. Black, M.J., Anandan, P.: The robust estimation of multiple motions: parametric and piecewise-smooth flow fields. Computer Vision and Image Understanding (CVIU) 63(1), 75–104 (1996)
10. Geman, S., Geman, D.: Stochastic relaxation, gibbs distributions, and the bayesian restoration of images. IEEE Transactions on Pattern Recognition and Machine Learning (PAMI) 6 (1984)
11. Sederberg, T.W., Parry, S.R.: Free-form deformation of solid geometric models. In: SIGGRAPH. ACM Press, New York (1986)
12. Rueckert, D., Sonoda, L., Hayes, C., Hill, D., Leach, M., Hawkes, D.: Nonrigid registration using free-form deformations: application to breast MR images. IEEE Transactions on Medical Imaging (TMI) 18(8), 712–721 (1999)
13. Komodakis, N., Paragios, N., Tziritas, G.: Clustering via lp-based stabilities. In: Neural Information Processing Systems (NIPS) (2008)
14. Kullback, S.: Information Theory and Statistics. Dover Publications Inc., New York (1968)
15. Bhattacharyya, A.: On a measure of divergence between two statistical populations defined by probability distributions. Bull. Calcutta Math. Soc. 35, 99–109 (1943)
16. Olsen, P., Hershey, J.: Bhattacharyya error and divergence using variational importance sampling. In: Interspeech, Antwerp, Belgium (August 2007)
17. Bishop, C.M.: Pattern Recognition and Machine Learning. Springer, Heidelberg (2006)
18. Glocker, B., Komodakis, N., Tziritas, G., Navab, N., Paragios, N.: Dense image registration through mrfs and efficient linear programming. Medical Image Analysis 12(6) (2008)
19. Li, S.Z.: Markov random field modeling in image analysis. Springer, Heidelberg (2001)
20. Komodakis, N., Tziritas, G., Paragios, N.: Fast, approximately optimal solutions for single and dynamic mrfs. In: Computer Vision and Pattern Recognition (CVPR) (2007)

Multivariate High-Dimensional Cortical Folding Analysis, Combining Complexity and Shape, in Neonates with Congenital Heart Disease

Suyash P. Awate[1], Paul Yushkevich[1], Zhuang Song[1], Daniel Licht[2], and James C. Gee[1]

[1] Penn Image Computing and Science Lab (PICSL), University of Pennsylvania
awate@mail.med.upenn.edu
[2] Children's Hospital of Philadelphia, USA*

Abstract. The paper presents a novel statistical framework for cortical folding pattern analysis that relies on a rich *multivariate descriptor* of folding patterns in a region of interest (ROI). The ROI-based approach avoids problems faced by spatial-normalization-based approaches stemming from the severe deficiency of homologous features between typical human cerebral cortices. Unlike typical ROI-based methods that summarize folding complexity or shape by a single number, the proposed descriptor unifies *complexity* and *shape* of the surface in a *high-dimensional* space. In this way, the proposed framework couples the reliability of ROI-based analysis with the richness of the novel cortical folding pattern descriptor. Furthermore, the descriptor can easily incorporate additional variables, e.g. cortical thickness. The paper proposes a novel application of a nonparametric permutation-based approach for statistical hypothesis testing for any multivariate high-dimensional descriptor. While the proposed framework has a rigorous theoretical underpinning, it is straightforward to implement. The framework is validated via simulated and clinical data. The paper is the first to quantitatively evaluate cortical folding in neonates with complex congenital heart disease.

1 Introduction

Cerebral cortical folding forms an underpinning for the cognitive skills and behavioral traits in humans. It is one of the major maturational processes of the human brain that occurs rapidly throughout fetal and early postnatal life. For the last few decades, the use of magnetic resonance (MR) imaging has enabled in vivo studies of human cortical folding patterns. Several studies relate abnormalities in the *complexity* of folding patterns to neurodevelopmental disorders [1,2].

* The authors gratefully acknowledge the support of this work via NIH grants HD042974, HD046159, NS045839, EB06266, DA14129, DA22807, UL1RR024234, K23 NS052380, NS061111, K25 AG027785, the Dana Foundation, the June and Steve Wolfson Family Foundation, and the Institute for Translational Medicine and Therapeutics' (ITMAT) Transdisciplinary Awards Program in Translational Medicine and Therapeutics at the University of Pennsylvania.

J.L. Prince, D.L. Pham, and K.J. Myers (Eds.): IPMI 2009, LNCS 5636, pp. 552–563, 2009.

While several pioneering studies track the progress of normal cortical folding in foetuses and neonates [3,4,5], others study cortical-folding abnormalities in neonates [6,7] based on subjective clinical protocols.

This paper studies cortical folding in the operculum in neonates with complex congenital heart disease (CHD). The operculum includes language areas and the sensory motor cortex for the mouth, tongue, and throat. There is growing evidence of immature features or frankly delayed maturation of the brains of full-term infants with complex CHD [8,9]. This immaturity likely gives rise to unexpected vulnerability to a white matter injury termed periventricular leukomalacia (PVL), an injury previously seen only in premature infants. Abnormally low fetal blood oxygenation and blood flow and the brain are likely the cause of this maturational delay. While direct evidence is lacking, there are differences in the circulatory patterns in fetuses with different forms of complex CHD. This paper quantitatively evaluates cortical folding in the operculum in two key subtypes of CHD, namely hypoplastic left heart syndrome (HLHS) and transposition of the great arteries (TGA). The paper reports differences in *not* only the complexity of opercular folding patterns, but also their *shape*.

One class of approaches to folding analysis rely on spatial normalization, either volumetric [10,4] or surface-based [2], and subsequently perform statistical hypothesis testing at every voxel or surface-element in the normalized space. Such methods can employ folding descriptors that are curvature-based [10], wavelet-based, etc. In typical cortical studies, however, "dramatic individual differences in the specific pattern of convolutions" [11] make it extremely difficult to find sufficiently-many homologous features [12] that could guarantee a consistent parameterization between cortical surfaces [12,13,11] (see [11] for brain images). Essen and Dierker [11] observe that "no registration that respects the topology of the cortical sheet can successfully match every major and minor fold". While lack of homologies are indeed observed for minor folds, they may occur for some major folds as well [13,11]. The reliability of normalization, because of this natural variability, may directly affect the reliability of findings in the clinical study. Furthermore, because the phenomenon of cortical folding has an inherent large-scale or non-local character, the rationale for point-by-point analysis of folding differences seems unclear.

A second class of approaches propose region-based folding descriptors to quantify folding complexity [14,15,3,5]. Such approaches avoid the problems associated with normalization by reducing spatial sensitivity from a voxel to a region of interest (ROI). ROIs considered in such folding studies can indeed be reliably defined in each individual based on observed homologous features. Such ROIs can be specific structures (e.g. hippocampus), regions around sulci/gyri that are always observable (e.g. operculum), lobes (e.g. frontal), etc.

Most studies in literature based on both aforementioned classes of approaches measure only the complexity of folding patterns, *ignoring* information related to shape, orientation, etc. Although some very recent ROI-based approaches propose descriptors incorporating shape information [16], they fail to integrate all the information on shape and complexity in a single descriptor. Furthermore, typical

ROI-based approaches produce scalar or low-dimensional summary statistics for the entire ROI, risking serious information loss.

This paper makes several contributions. First, the paper presents a novel ROI-based statistical framework for folding pattern analysis relying on a rich multivariate non-local descriptor that captures the spectrum of complexity and shape. Specifically, the descriptor is a joint probability density function (PDF) of two variables, one capturing surface complexity and the other capturing surface shape. Second, the paper proposes a novel application of a nonparametric permutation-based approach for statistical hypothesis testing for the proposed descriptor. In these ways, the proposed framework couples the reliability of ROI-based analysis with the richness of the proposed descriptor. This paper shows that the proposed framework has a rigorous theoretical underpinning and it is straightforward to implement. Third, the proposed hypothesis-testing approach can be easily applied to any multivariate descriptor, e.g. one that augments the proposed cortical-folding descriptor to include cortical-thickness information. Fourth, to the best of our knowledge, this paper is the first to report the affects of HLHS and TGA on opercular folding.

2   Background

2.1   Univariate Low-Dimensional Complexity Descriptors

It is generally important to design folding descriptors that (i) are invariant to *translation* and *rotation* of the cortical surface representation (changes in the location or orientation of the slice planes during MR imaging), and (ii) capture all aspects of folding including *complexity* as well as *shape*.

Some of the earliest folding descriptors were intended to capture *only* the complexity of the cortical surface. Fractal dimension [17,14] captures the increases in surface area over multiscale representations of the surface. Gyrification index [18] is the ratio of the length of a planar curve to the length of the curve's envelope. Convexity ratio [3] is the ratio of the area of the surface to the area of the convex hull/envelope of the surface. Isoperimetric ratio [3] is the ratio of the surface area to the two-third power of the volume enclosed by the surface. Average curvedness (AC) [16] measure the deviation of the surface from a plane. [5] proposes the 2D centroid of the histogram of a curvature.

Some folding descriptors were designed to inform about specific aspects (*not* all) of surface shape. Intrinsic curvature index (ICI) [15] sums up degrees of hemisphericity of all surface patches, but ignores cylindrical or saddle-shaped patches. Mean curvature norm (MCN) [3] sums up degrees of hemisphericity and cylindricity of all surface patches, but ignores saddle-shaped patches. Gaussian curvature norm (GCN) [3] sums up degrees of hemisphericity and saddle-likeness of all surface patches, but ignores cylindrical patches.

While some aforementioned descriptors ignore the *shape* of surface patches, all aforementioned descriptors ignore the *orientation* of surface patches. For instance, they fail to distinguish pimples from dimples or ridges from valleys; these might be compared to cortical gyri and sulci, respectively. Indeed, for every surface patch, ICI, MCN, GCN, and AC project the space of principal curvatures, having two degrees of freedom, to derive a single scalar descriptor. [5] condense the histogram of a curvature measure to 2 numbers.

2.2   Univariate Low-Dimensional Shape Descriptors

Recent works incorporate information regarding local surface-patch orientation and shape for cortical surface analysis [10,16]. These approaches rely on Koenderink and van Doorn's orthogonal reparameterization of the 2D space of principal curvatures into *shape index* and *curvedness* [19]. Consider a surface $\mathcal{M}$. Let $d\mathcal{M}$ represent the area measure of a small surface patch at point $m \in \mathcal{M}$. At point m, the minimum and maximum principal curvatures of a local patch are denoted by $K_{\min}(m)$ and $K_{\max}(m)$, respectively. Shape index $S : \mathcal{M} \to [-1, 1]$ for a patch at point m is $S(m) = [2/\pi] \arctan\{[K_{\max}(m) + K_{\min}(m)]/[K_{\max}(m) - K_{\min}(m)]\}$. Shape index values for some standard shapes are: $-1 \equiv$ hemispherical concave, $-0.5 \equiv$ hemicylindrical valley, $0 \equiv$ saddle, $0.5 \equiv$ hemicylindrical ridge, and $1 \equiv$ hemispherical convex. Curvedness $C : \mathcal{M} \to [0, \infty)$ for a patch at point m is $C(m) = \{0.5[K_{\max}^2(m) + K_{\min}^2(m)]\}^{0.5}$.

Tosun et al. [10] employ the shape index in a voxel-based cortical morphometry scheme. For ROI-based analyses, Awate et al. [16] propose an average shape index, $\text{AS}(\mathcal{M}) = \int_{m \in \mathcal{M}} S(m)\, d\mathcal{M}$, that averages shape indices of all patches in the ROI. In computer vision, a descriptor corresponding to values of the shape-index histogram at 9 predetermined locations, was proposed recently [20].

All aforementioned approaches in this section ignore cortical complexity in the description of folding patterns. Furthermore, they reduce the information in the shape-index histogram to at most a few numbers (low dimensional).

3   New Multivariate High-Dimensional Folding Descriptor

This section presents a high-dimensional multivariate surface descriptor that captures the spectrum of complexity and shape.

At every point m of a cortical surface $\mathcal{M}$, the principal curvatures *completely* describe the geometry of the local surface patch. The orthogonal parameterization of principal curvatures $< K_{\min}, K_{\max} >$ is, however, unintuitive. This probably motivated reparameterizing $< K_{\min}, K_{\max} >$ into $< C, S >$ [19] to cleanly separate notions of bending and shape, while retaining the orthogonality. Figure 1 shows values of C and S at all points on a typical cortical surface.

We propose the following generative statistical model of cortical surfaces. Let us consider $C : \mathcal{M} \to [0, \infty]$ and $S : \mathcal{M} \to [-1, 1]$ as random fields [21]. Let us also consider the joint PDF that captures the dependencies between $C(m)$ and $S(m)$ for a specific class of surfaces. Consider a finite collection $\mathcal{O} = \{d\mathcal{M}^1, \ldots, d\mathcal{M}^T\}$ of T surface patches, located at points $\{m^1, \ldots, m^T\} \in \mathcal{M}$ *uniformly* distributed over the surface $\mathcal{M}$, which form a cover for $\mathcal{M}$. Then, the set $\{(C(m^1), S(m^1)), \ldots, (C(m^T), S(m^T))\}$ is an instantiation of the field of random vectors at locations $\{m^1, \ldots, m^T\}$. We assume that the random

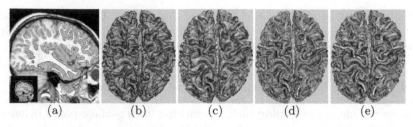

| (a) | (b) | (c) | (d) | (e) |

Fig. 1. (a) MR image overlapped with the extracted cortical gray-white interface parcellated by lobe. (b)-(c) Curvedness $C(m) \geq 0$ values (red→blue ≡ low→high curvature) at each point m on the extracted surface $\mathcal{M}$ and its smoothed version $\mathcal{M}^{\text{smooth}}$, respectively. Note that $\mathcal{M}$ has many more high-curvedness regions than $\mathcal{M}^{\text{smooth}}$. (d)-(e) Shape-index $S(m) \in [-1, 1]$ values painted on $\mathcal{M}$ and $\mathcal{M}^{\text{smooth}}$, respectively. Unlike C, S exhibits little change between $\mathcal{M}$ and $\mathcal{M}^{\text{smooth}}$.

field is *stationary* [21], i.e. each observation $(C(m^t), S(m^t))$, is randomly drawn from a single PDF $P_{\mathcal{M}}(C, S)$. The tremendous complexity and inter-individual variability in cortical folding suggests that dependencies between random variables $(C(m^t), S(m^t))$ and $(C(m^s), S(m^s))$ decrease at a fast rate with increasing geodesic distance between the locations m^t and m^s. Thus, we assume that the random field is *mixing* [21].

We propose the joint PDF $P_{\mathcal{M}}(C, S)$ as the multivariate high-dimensional descriptor of cerebral cortical folding patterns for surface $\mathcal{M}$. It is clear that many of the aforementioned univariate descriptors (e.g. ICI, MCN, GCN, AC, AS, histogram centroid, and [20]) are subsumed by the proposed descriptor.

For a given surface $\mathcal{M}$, we propose to estimate $P_{\mathcal{M}}(C, S)$ as follows. Using the sample $\{(C(m^1), S(m^1)), \ldots, (C(m^T), S(m^T))\}$ drawn from a stationary mixing random field, a consistent [22] nonparametric kernel density estimate for the folding descriptor is $P_{\mathcal{M}}(C, S) \approx \frac{1}{T} \sum_{t=1}^{T} G((C(m^t), S(m^t)), \Sigma_t)$, where $G((\mu_1, \mu_s), \Sigma)$ is a 2D Gaussian kernel with mean (μ_1, μ_2) and covariance Σ. Consistency requires an optimal choice of Σ_t, dependent on the sample size T, and we employ a cross-validation-based penalized maximum likelihood scheme to estimate Σ_t [23]; the literature provides a variety of schemes.

It is crucial that the sample $\{m^1, \ldots, m^T\}$ is uniformly distributed over the surface $\mathcal{M}$, eliminating any bias in over/undersampling specific surface features. Nonuniform sampling can undesirably bias $P_{\mathcal{M}}(C, S)$. For instance, adaptively refined meshes will generate more surface patches in areas with larger C and artificially boost the PDF for larger C. Thus, we propose to obtain uniformly-distributed points/patches by representing the surface as a level set of a distance transform on a Cartesian grid [24] sampled at a resolution much higher than the highest C values (see next paragraph). Figure 1 shows a level-set surface colored by the values of C and S, respectively.

This paper represents the level set in a grid of isotropic voxels of size v^3 mm^3 with $v = 0.4$ mm (Figures 1). To reduce effects of noise, level-set fitting incorporates smoothing. Empirically, we find that values $C(m)$ virtually never exceed $c_{\max} = (15v)^{-1}$ mm^{-1} equivalent to a minimum radius of curvature of

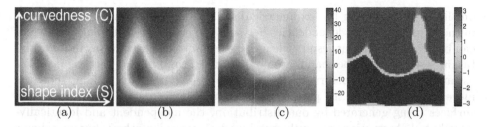

Fig. 2. Validation : a cross sectional study between the group of gray-white interfaces of 20 BrainWeb [26] images and a second group of smoothed versions of the same surfaces. For all plots in this paper, horizontal axis $\equiv S$, vertical axis $\equiv C$, coordinates for the bottom left corner : $(C, S) = (c_{min}, -1)$; bottom right corner : $(C, S) = (c_{min}, 1)$; top left corner : $(C, S) = (c_{max}, -1)$. **(a)-(b)** Mean of the multivariate surface descriptors $P_{\mathcal{M}^n}(C, S)$ for the $n = 1, \ldots, 20$ original and smoothed surfaces, respectively, as proposed in Section 3; red$\equiv$high and blue$\equiv$low values. **(c)** The t-statistic map for the original and smoothed surfaces; $t > 0 \Rightarrow P_{\text{original}} > P_{\text{smoothed}}$. **(d)** The significant locations ($p < 0.05$) produced via SnPM [25]. For all plots in this paper, p values for significant locations/clusters are indicated by coloring them by the associated z score [21], e.g. $z(p = 0.05) = 1.65$, $z(p = 0.005) = 2.58$.

$15v = 6$ mm. Figures 1 suggests that this degree of smoothing continues to capture essential folding pattern information in typical pediatric cortical surfaces. The lower limit of 6 mm is more conservative than the limit of 3 mm in [5]. Imaging limitations on voxel sizes and signal-to-noise ratios risk less fidelity in capturing sharper surface features.

Figure 2(a) shows a typical $P_{\mathcal{M}}(C, S)$, which is multimodal and far from standard parametric PDFs, thus justifying nonparametric PDF estimation for reliability. In practice, typical ROIs yield sample sizes T in the range of thousands or tens of thousands, producing (i) very small kernel bandwidth estimates such that $P_{\mathcal{M}}(c < 0, s \notin [-1, 1])$ is desirably close to zero and (ii) robust estimations. Moreover, the PDF mass very close to the $c = 0$ axis (shape index is undefined for a plane) is also negligible: $P_{\mathcal{M}}(c < c_{min}, s \in [-1, 1]) < \delta$ for sufficiently small c_{min}, δ. This paper sets $c_{min} = 0.001$.

4   New Approach to Multivariate Histogram Testing

Having estimated the folding pattern descriptors for a group of N surfaces in a clinical study, namely $P_{\mathcal{M}^1}(C, S), \ldots, P_{\mathcal{M}^N}(C, S)$, this section proposes a novel application of a known nonparametric permutation-based approach for statistical hypothesis testing for multivariate histograms.

Typical hypothesis tests (cross-sectional, longitudinal, regression) are subsumed in the framework of general linear models (GLM). The GLM framework has been applied extensively for *voxel-based* neuroimaging studies of brain function and structure, which entail running parametric GLM tests at each voxel in the image followed by corrections for multiple comparisons via, for instance, random field theory. However, this parametric approach makes strong assumptions on the data concerning the parametric distributions of the values at each point in the domain and the dependencies between the neighborhoods. Such strategies can be prone to spurious results when these assumptions become invalid. Permutation tests, on the other hand, are nonparametric and rely on the *less inclusive* assumption that the observations are *exchangeable*, thereby making the tests more stringent. Under the permutation-test null hypothesis, i.e. both groups of surfaces being generated by one distribution, the independent and identically-distributed observations are exchangeable. A rigorous hypothesis testing scheme based on nonparametric permutation testing for *voxel-based* studies is statistical nonparametric mapping (SnPM) [25].

We propose a novel application of SnPM for multivariate high-dimensional histogram analysis. This scheme differs from (i) conventional use of SnPM for studies in the image domain [25] or surface domain [27] domain, and (ii) typical parametric tests (e.g. Hotelling T^2) for histogram analysis which fail to inform the location, in the histogram domain, for a significant difference/effect. The algorithm is as follows:

1. Empirically select thresholds $c_{\min} > 0$ and $c_{\max}$ for curvedness values and a very small ϵ such that, $\forall n = 1, \ldots, N$; $P_{\mathcal{M}^n}(c \notin [c_{\min}, c_{\max}], s \notin [-1, 1]) < \epsilon$.
2. For the domain $[c_{\min}, c_{\max}] \times [-1, 1]$, construct a regular rectangular tessellation of the desired resolution. Denote the resulting IJ rectangular bins by $\{b_{ij} :: i = 1, \ldots, I; j = 1, \ldots, J\}$. This paper sets $I = J = 64$; finer resolutions increase computation time.
3. For all surfaces $n = 1, \ldots, N$ and all bins $\{b_{ij}\}$, compute the probabilities $P_{\mathcal{M}^n}((c, s) \in b_{ij})$ denoted in short by $P_n(i, j)$. Note that $0 \leq P_n(i, j) \leq 1$ justifying a nonparametric testing approach for accuracy and reliability.
4. Use the N 2D images of probability values, $P_1, \ldots, P_N$, as input for SnPM [25]. SnPM will produce (i) a set of *locations* ij and (ii) a set of *clusters* exhibiting statistical significance for the underlying GLM experiment. Figure 2 shows an example study which is explained in detail later in Section 5.2.

5   Validation and Results

5.1   Cortical Folding Pattern Analysis Pipeline

The clinical study in this paper employed the following processing sequence: (i) brain extraction, ROI parcellation [28], denoising, inhomogeneity correction, and contrast enhancement via adaptive histogram equalization (ii) automatic intensity-based probabilistic tissue segmentation [29]; (iii) resample the segmentation to an isotropic voxel size of 0.4 mm^3; (iv) define $\mathcal{M}$ to be the cortical gray-white interface corresponding to a cortical-white-matter membership of 0.5 (gray-white interface estimated much more reliably than gray-fluid interface, especially in neonatal/pediatric populations); (v) represent cortical surface $\mathcal{M}$ in the ROI, to subvoxel accuracy, as a level set [24] (vi) compute curvedness $C(m)$ and shape-index $S(m)$ values at every voxel m on the level set $\mathcal{M}$, (vii) estimate the proposed multivariate folding pattern descriptor $P_{\mathcal{M}}(C, S)$ in the operculum as described in

Section 3, (viii) perform multivariate statistical hypothesis testing as described in Section 4. The implementation and visualization in this paper relied on the Insight Toolkit (ITK), Matlab, ITK-SNAP, and the Visualization Toolkit (VTK).

5.2   Validation via Clinical and Simulated Adult Data

Cortical Shape Asymmetry in Normal Adults: The first validation experiment used 50 MR images of normal adults and measured the average fraction of cortical surface area embedded in sulci. The left halves, i.e. $S < 0$, of the plots concern concave patches (associated with sulci), while the right halves, i.e. $S > 0$, concerns convex patches (associated with gyri). The mass in the left half of the mean PDF of all images, i.e. $P_{mean}(S < 0; C \geq 0)$ is a robust estimate of the fraction of the surface area of the cortical surface buried in sulci. We estimated this fraction to be 0.58 for the frontal, parietal, and temporal lobes in adults, which comes very close to the published value of 0.61 for gray-white interfaces of entire brains [18,15]. For the occipital lobes, however, our estimate of this fraction was lower, equal to 0.54. Figure 3 shows this phenomenon clearly, i.e. the PDF in Figure 3(d) has more mass (red) on the right (convex gyral regions) relative to the PDFs in Figure 3(a)-(c). These experiments demonstrate that the proposed descriptor is sensitive to changes in cortical *shape*.

Simulated Complexity Differences using BrainWeb Data: We validated the proposed framework for folding pattern analysis using 20 simulated images from the BrainWeb [26] repository having ground-truth segmentations. We conducted a cross sectional study between (i) the group of gray-white surfaces in the BrainWeb images and (ii) another group of surfaces obtained after slightly smoothing the surfaces in the first group (mean curvature flow, time step 0.24, iterations 4). Figure 1(d)-(g) show values of C and S painted on a cortical surface and its smoothed version. Figure 2(a) and (b) show the means of the surface descriptors $P_{\mathcal{M}^n}(C, S)$ in the two groups. As expected, the smoothed surfaces have a mean PDF (Figure 2(b)) shifted slightly downwards, i.e. regions of low curvature, relative to Figure 2(a). The t-statistic map (Figure 2(c)) clearly reveals the

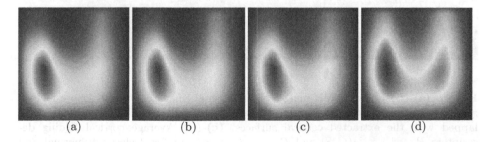

(a)   (b)   (c)   (d)

Fig. 3. Validation : measuring the fraction of surface area of the cortical gray-white surface embedded in sulci (concave surface patches) in 50 normal adults. **(a)-(d)** Proposed surface descriptors for the frontal, parietal, temporal, and occipital lobes, respectively.

difference between the two groups. The blue (or red) significant locations (Figure 2(d)), at level of significance $\alpha = 0.05$, correspond to those locations whose t statistics were less than (or greater than) the lowest (or greatest) 100α-th percentile of the permutation distribution of the smallest (or largest) t statistic over the $< C, S >$ domain. Similarly, significant clusters (in all figures in this paper) are shown in blue (or red) when the sizes of the clusters formed by thresholding the negative (or positive) t statistics are larger than the 100α-th percentile of the permutation distribution of the maximum cluster size obtained after thresholding the negative (or positive) t statistics. Figure 2(d) shows that the proposed framework correctly indicates that the differences between the groups are in cortical complexity alone, *not* in cortical shape.

5.3   Neonatal CHD Cohort, Imaging, and Image Analysis

The clinical cohort comprised 42 neonates with complex CHD (29 with HLHS, 13 with TGA) between $1-2$ weeks of age, *before* undergoing corrective heart surgery. MR images were acquired on a 3T scanner (Siemens Trio) with voxel sizes around $0.88\text{x}0.88\text{x}1.5$ mm^3 using T1-weighted, T2-weighted, and FLAIR schemes. The HLHS and TGA groups were well matched by age *and brain volume*. The left and right opercula in every image were parcellated semi-automatically with expert supervision. Brain tissue segmentation was performed via [29].

5.4   Folding Differences between Normal and Abnormal Opercula

Before studying opercular differences in HLHS and TGA, we first study the differences between normal and abnormal opercular folding complexity and shape. Figure 4 shows the differences in the surface descriptors of two neonates selected by a pediatric neurologist from the clinical cohort, one with the closest-to-normal operculum (mature, "closed", folded) and another with the farthest-from-normal

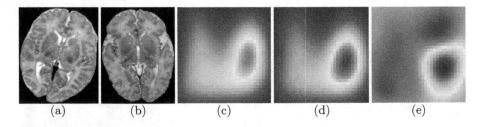

(a)   (b)   (c)   (d)   (e)

Fig. 4. **(a)-(b)** Example MR images of the normal (mature, "closed", more folded) and farthest-from-normal (immature, "open", less folded) opercula, respectively, overlapped with the extracted cortical surfaces. **(c)-(d)** Average cortical folding descriptors $P_{\text{average normal}}(C, S)$ and $P_{\text{average abnormal}}(C, S)$ for 2 closest-to-normal and 4 significantly-abnormal opercula, respectively, chosen by a medical expert based on a subjective clinical scoring protocol [9]. **(e)** $P_{\text{average normal}}(C, S) - P_{\text{average abnormal}}(C, S)$; blue $\equiv$ negative and red $\equiv$ positive values.

operculum (immature, "open", less folded). Figure 4(e) indicates that normal opercula have (i) a larger fraction of surface patches that have higher curvature (implying more complex folding) and (ii) a larger fraction of surface patches that are concave (implying more "closed" shape). We compared these findings to qualitative studies of immature opercula in neonates [6,7] that provide drawings of immature opercular cortical surfaces. The analysis in this paper shows that, relative to normal opercula, abnormal opercula in CHD may exhibit lesser folding complexity and may be more "open". This also indicates that brain maturation concerns *not* only cortical complexity, but cortical shape as well.

5.5   Folding Differences between HLHS and TGA Opercula

Figure 5 shows the differences in folding complexity and shape between HLHS and TGA. Establishing analogies between Figure 5 and Figure 4, we find that while TGA neonates have a larger fraction of high-curvature patches, HLHS neonates have a large fraction of concave low-curvature surface patches. Since it is known via subjective clinical-scoring-based studies that the opercula are immature in both HLHS and TGA [9], the analysis in this paper suggests that HLHS and TGA might affect opercular development in different ways, i.e. while HLHS might cause greater reductions in opercular folding complexity, TGA might cause more "open" opercula. A cross-sectional study between CHD neonates and normal neonates would be very interesting and probably yield much more significant differences, but such data has been elusive so far. Nevertheless, this is an important aspect of future work.

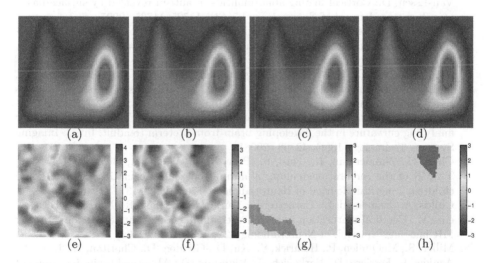

Fig. 5. **(a)-(b)** Average of cortical folding descriptors $P(C, S)$ in right and left opercula, respectively, for 29 neonates with HLHS. **(c)-(d)** Average of the descriptors in right and left opercula, respectively, for 12 neonates with TGA. **(e)-(f)** t-statistic maps; $t > 0 \Rightarrow P_{\text{HLHS}} > P_{\text{TGA}}$. for right and left opercula, respectively. **(g)-(h)** Significant clusters found via SnPM [25] for right and left opercula, respectively.

6   Conclusion

The paper proposes a novel multivariate statistical descriptor of folding patterns in a high-dimensional space. PDF-based shape descriptors in the literature that come closest to the proposed method analyze histograms of either shape-indices or curvatures (*not* both) and produce low-dimensional descriptors: [5] and [20] propose 2-valued and 9-valued descriptors, respectively. On the other hand, the proposed descriptor is a continuous function informing about both surface shape and complexity. Unlike [20] which shows concern about the dimensionality of their descriptor, the proposed framework effectively deals with dimensionality by a novel application of a rigorous hypothesis-testing framework. The experiments establish a link between the proposed descriptor and published qualitative studies of normal/abnormal opercular folding [6,7] to demonstrate how the proposed descriptor can be interpreted for opercular studies. The proposed framework can be easily extended to (i) include other cortical information, e.g. thickness, and (ii) study other specific anatomical structures or ROIs. The rigorous theoretical underpinning coupled with the ease of implementation can facilitate sophisticated studies of surfaces with relatively less effort.

References

1. Thompson, P., Lee, A., Dutton, R., Geaga, J., Hayashi, K., Eckert, M., Bellugi, U., Galaburda, A., Korenberg, J., Mills, D., Toga, A., Reiss, A.: Abnormal cortical complexity and thickness profiles mapped in Williams syndrome. J. Neuroscience 25(16), 4146–4158 (2005)
2. Nordahl, C., Dierker, D., Mostafavi, I., Schumann, C., Rivera, S., Amaral, D., Van-Essen, D.: Cortical folding abnormalities in autism revealed by surface-based morphometry. Journal of Neuroscience 27(43), 11725–11735 (2007)
3. Batchelor, P., Castellano-Smith, A., Hill, D., Hawkes, D., Cox, T., Dean, A.: Measures of folding applied to the development of the human fetal brain. IEEE Trans. Med. Imaging 21(8), 953–965 (2002)
4. Yu, P., Grant, P.E., Qi, Y., Han, X., Segonne, F., Pienaar, R., Busa, E., Pacheco, J., Makris, N., Buckner, R.L., Golland, P., Fischl, B.: Cortical surface shape analysis based on spherical wavelets. IEEE Trans. Med. Imaging 26(4), 582–597 (2007)
5. Pienaar, R., Fischl, B., Caviness, V., Makris, N., Grant, P.E.: A methodology for analyzing curvature in the developing brain from preterm to adult. Int. J. Imaging Systems Technology 18(1), 42–68 (2008)
6. Chen, C., Zimmerman, R., Faro, S., Parrish, B., Wang, Z., Bilaniuk, L., Chou, T.: MR of the cerebral operculum: abnormal opercular formation in infants and children. American Journal of Neuroradiology 17(7), 1303–1311 (1996)
7. Childs, A., Ramenghi, L., Cornette, L., Tanner, S., Arthur, R., Martinez, D., Levene, M.: Cerebral maturation in premature infants: Quantitative assessment using MR imaging. Amer. J. of Neuroradiology 22, 1577–1582 (2001)
8. Miller, S., McQuillen, P., Hamrick, S., Xu, D., Glidden, D., Charlton, N., Karl, T., Azakie, A., Ferriero, D., Barkovich, J., Vigneron, D.: Abnormal brain development in newborns with congenital heart disease. New Eng. J. Med. 357, 1928–1938 (2007)
9. Licht, D., Shera, D., Clancy, R., Wernovsky, G., Montenegro, L., Nicolson, S., Zimmerman, R., Spray, T., Gaynor, W., Vossough, A.: Brain maturation is delayed in infants with complex congenital heart defects. J. Thorac. Cardiovasc. Surg. 137, 529–537 (2009)

10. Tosun, D., Duchesne, S., Rolland, Y., Toga, A., Verin, M., Barillot, C.: 3D analysis of cortical morphometry in differential diagnosis of Parkinson's Plus Syndromes. In: Ayache, N., Ourselin, S., Maeder, A. (eds.) MICCAI 2007, Part II. LNCS, vol. 4792, pp. 891–899. Springer, Heidelberg (2007)
11. Van-Essen, D., Dierker, D.: Surface-based and probabilistic atlases of primate cerebral cortex. Neuron 56, 209–225 (2007)
12. Mangin, J., Riviere, D., Cachia, A., Duchesnay, E., Cointepas, Y., Papadopoulos-Orfanos, D., Scifo, P., Ochiai, T., Brunelle, F., Regis, J.: A framework to study the cortical folding patterns. NeuroImage 23(1), S129–S138 (2004)
13. Lyttelton, O., Boucher, M., Robbins, S., Evans, A.: An unbiased iterative group registration template for cortical surface analysis. NeuroImage 34, 1535–1544 (2007)
14. Thompson, P., Schwartz, C., Lin, R., Khan, A., Toga, A.: Three-dimensional statistical analysis of sulcal variability in the human brain. J. Neurosci. 16(13), 4261–4274 (1996)
15. Van-Essen, D., Drury, H.: Structural and functional analyses of human cerebral cortex using a surface-based atlas. J. Neuroscience 17(18), 7079–7102 (1997)
16. Awate, S.P., Win, L., Yushkevich, P., Schultz, R.T., Gee, J.C.: 3D cerebral cortical morphometry in autism: Increased folding in children and adolescents in frontal, parietal, and temporal lobes. In: Proc. Int. Conf. Med. Image Comput. Comp. Assist. Interv., vol. 1, pp. 559–567 (2008)
17. Griffin, L.: The intrinsic geometry of the cerebral cortex. J. Theor. Biol. 166(3), 261–273 (1994)
18. Zilles, K., Armstrong, E., Schleicher, A., Kretschmann, H.: The human pattern of gyrification in the cerebral cortex. Anat. Embryol. 179, 173–179 (1988)
19. Koenderink, J., van Doorn, A.: Surface shape and curvature scales. Image and Vision Computing 10(8), 557–565 (1992)
20. Akgul, C., Sankur, B., Schmitt, F., Yemez, Y.: Multivariate density-based 3D shape descriptors. In: Int. Conf. Shape Modeling and Appl., pp. 3–12 (2007)
21. Papoulis, A., Pillai, S.U.: Probability, Random Variables, and Stochastic Processes, 4th edn. McGraw-Hill, New York (2001)
22. Lu, Z., Chen, X.: Spatial kernel regression estimation: weak consistency. Stat. and Prob. Letters 68(2), 125–136 (2004)
23. Chow, Y., Geman, S., Wu, L.: Consistant cross-validated density estimation. Annals of Statistics 11(1), 25–38 (1983)
24. Osher, S., Paragios, N.: Geometric Level Set Methods in Imaging, Vision, and Graphics. Springer, Heidelberg (2003)
25. Nichols, T., Holmes, A.: Nonparametric permutation tests for functional neuroimaging: a primer with examples. Human Brain Mapping 15(1), 1–25 (2002)
26. Aubert-Broche, B., Collins, D., Evans, A.: Twenty new digital brain phantoms for creation of validation image data bases. IEEE Trans. Med. Imag. 25(11), 1410–1416 (2006)
27. Styner, M., Gerig, G.: Correction scheme for multiple correlated statistical tests in local shape analysis. In: SPIE Medical Imaging, pp. 233–240 (2003)
28. Avants, B., Gee, J.: Geodesic estimation for large deformation anatomical shape averaging and interpolation. Neuroimage 23(1), 139–150 (2004)
29. Song, Z., Awate, S.P., Licht, D., Gee, J.: Clinical neonatal brain MRI segmentation using adaptive nonparametric data models and intensity-based Markov priors. In: Proc. Med. Image Comput. Comp. Assist. Interv., vol. 1, pp. 883–890 (2007)

The 3D Moore-Rayleigh Test for the Quantitative Groupwise Comparison of MR Brain Images

Alize E.H. Scheenstra[1], Michael Muskulus[2], Marius Staring[1],
Arn M.J.V. van den Maagdenberg[3,4], Sjoerd Verduyn Lunel[2],
J. Hans C. Reiber[1], Louise van der Weerd[3], and Jouke Dijkstra[1]

[1] Department of Radiology, Division of Image processing
[2] Department of Neurology
[3] Department of Anatomy and Embryology,
Leiden University Medical Center, Leiden, the Netherlands
[4] Leiden University, Mathematical Institute, Postbus 9600, 2300 RC Leiden, The Netherlands

Abstract. Non-rigid registration of MR images to a common reference image results in deformation fields, from which anatomical differences can be statistically assessed, within and between populations. Without further assumptions, nonparametric tests are required and currently the analysis of deformation fields is performed by permutation tests. For deformation fields, often the vector magnitude is chosen as test statistic, resulting in a loss of information. In this paper, we consider the three dimensional Moore-Rayleigh test as an alternative for permutation tests. This nonparametric test offers two novel features: first, it incorporates both the directions and magnitude of the deformation vectors. Second, as its distribution function is available in closed form, this test statistic can be used in a clinical setting. Using synthetic data that represents variations as commonly encountered in clinical data, we show that the Moore-Rayleigh test outperforms the classical permutation test.

1 Introduction

Mice have been used in genetic research as models for a variety of diseases occurring in the human population. They allow researchers to study the development of genetic diseases, to improve early diagnoses and subsequent treatment. Non-invasive imaging techniques, e.g. MRI, allow localized investigation of 3D anatomical structures of interest [1]. This provides a useful tool for *in vivo* structural and functional phenotyping, especially in the brain [2]. Since the introduction of non-rigid registration of brain images, a variety of new applications for brain research have emerged. Non-rigid registration is used in clinical practice to register MR images taken from different biological populations to a common average. The resulting deformation fields indicate and localize differences between pairs of images. Their second order statistics are stored in atlases to characterize variability within a population (intra-group variability) [3,4].

J.L. Prince, D.L. Pham, and K.J. Myers (Eds.): IPMI 2009, LNCS 5636, pp. 564–575, 2009.
© Springer-Verlag Berlin Heidelberg 2009

A major challenge in this area of research is not only to highlight the intra-group variability but to also assess inter-group variability, especially with regard to structural anatomical differences and their possible causes. For instance, in genetic research with transgenic mice, mutants are compared with their wild-types, where the group difference is determined by only one gene. To test and localize possible anatomical differences, statistical testing is required. In human brain research, similar problems have been addressed in functional brain images. BOLD signals are compared between and within groups to characterize differences in brain activation. A logical first choice for the statistical analysis of such data are permutation tests with their minimal assumptions [5,6].

In contrast to the statistical analysis of fMRI signals, the statistical analysis of deformation fields requires handling vector data instead of scalars. Furthermore, in genetic research, usually transgenic mouse with the same genetic background (apart from the gene of interest) are compared, resulting in populations with low intra-variability[3], but often also very subtle inter-group differences, thus requiring a highly sensitive test. Chen et al. presented a test statistic using the standard deviation of the lengths of deformation vectors, for which different mouse strains (129S1, SvImJ, C57/B16 and CD1) were subjected to permutation tests [7]. However, since they were analyzing the complete brain, they had to limit their tests to 500 permutations because of time considerations. In mouse strains for which there result large inter-group differences, this might be sufficient. The minimal p-value that can be resolved with 500 permutations is $\frac{1}{500+1}$, without correcting for multiple comparisons. Obviously, a larger number of permutations is required to resolve smaller significance probabilities. Furthermore, by using only the lengths of the deformation vectors, valuable information, in particular that encoded in the directionality, is lost. A first step to improve on this situation is the use of Hotelling's t^2-test with voxelwise estimated covariances of the vector field. This test statistic can also be used in the setting of a permutation test as in [6]. Unfortunately permutation tests are highly computationally expensive, even taking into account algorithmic improvements [8], so alternatives for the permutation tests have been considered: among others, the Brunner - Munzel test[9].

The goal of this work is to show the applicability of the 3D Moore-Rayleigh test for the quantitative groupwise comparison of images, and to propose the Moore-Rayleigh test as an alternative to permutation testing. The 2D case of this test was first introduced by Moore [10] who numerically obtained critical values. We generalized his idea to k dimensions and determined the closed form of the density and the distribution function for three dimensional vector data. Because its test statistic is available in closed form, the test does not require much computational effort. We evaluate it empirically with simulated clinical data of known ground-truth and compare it to the performance of a permutation test and a variant of the Mann-Whitney test. Furthermore, we show that the Moore-Rayleigh test outperforms permutation testing on account of sensitivity. For the compactness of this paper, in Section 2 we introduce the Moore-Rayleigh test only for the three-dimensional case and describe how this method is applied in the two-sample problem. In Section 3 experimental results on simulated data are given and the method is compared to currently popular methods. Finally, we conclude the paper with a summary and discussion in Section 4.

2   3D Moore-Rayleigh Test

We consider a finite sample of N real-valued vectors $X = (X_1, ..., X_N)$. For the application to deformation fields we only consider vectors in $\mathbb{R}^3$, such that $X_n = (X_{n,1}, X_{n,2}, X_{n,3})$. For the general Moore-Rayleigh test in k dimensions, we refer to our publication [?].

If we assume that the X_n are independently drawn from a common continuous distribution, the null-hypothesis is that the probability density $f : \mathbb{R}^3 \to [0, \infty)$ is spherically symmetric. This implies that the density f factors into the product of a radial probability density $p_r : [0, \infty) \to [0, \infty)$ and the uniform distribution on each hypersphere $r\,S^2 = \{x \in \mathbb{R}^3 \mid \|x\| = r\}$, such that $f(x) = p_r(\|x\|)/\mathrm{vol}(rS^2)$. The random sum $\sum_{n=1}^N X_n$ represents a random flight with N steps whose lengths are distributed according to p_r. In the one dimensional case (not discussed here), this sum corresponds to a random walk.

To render the test nonparametric, the vectors are scaled by the rank of their lengths:

$$S_N = \sum_{n=1}^N \frac{n X_{(n)}}{\|X_{(n)}\|}, \tag{1}$$

where $X_{(n)}$ is the nth largest vector in the sample. The distribution of S_N is now independent of the actual p_r. Note that $\sum_{n=1}^N \frac{X_{(n)}}{\|X_{(n)}\|}$ is a Rayleigh random flight [11], and our S_N is a Rayleigh random flight with increasing steps. The addition of the vectors incorporates the directionality information and by weighting the vectors by their ranks, also the vector magnitude influences the test statistic.

The test statistic of interest R_N^* is then obtained by scaling S_N by $N\sqrt{N}$ for asymptotic simplicity:

$$R_N^* = \frac{S_N}{N^{3/2}} \tag{2}$$

Let $\alpha_N = N^{3/2}$. The distribution function of $R_N = \alpha_N R_N^*$ in 3 dimensions is given by:

$$\mathrm{pr}(R_N = r) = \frac{2r}{\pi} \int_0^\infty t \frac{\sin rt/\alpha_N}{r} \prod_{n=1}^N \frac{\sin nt}{nt} \, dt \tag{3}$$

This function can be derived by way of characteristic functions [11].

Asymptotically the distribution of R_N^* approaches a χ_3^2 distribution. Of course, for small values of N, the exact form of $\mathrm{pr}(R_N = r)$ should be used whenever possible. As shown in [?] the oscillating integral in eq. (3) can be evaluated in the form of a finite series.

2.1   The Two-Sample Problem

In the two sample problem, we are given two vector-valued random variables $X = (X_1, ..., X_N)$ and $Y = (Y_1, ..., Y_N)$. Under the null hypothesis that X_i and Y_j are identically and independently distributed according to a common probability density $f : \mathbb{R}^3 \rightarrow [0, \infty)$, the differences $X_i - Y_j$ are distributed according to the symmetrizing convolution $f * (-f)$, whose density is given by

$$\mathrm{pr}(X - Y = x) = \int \mathrm{pr}(X = u)\mathrm{pr}(Y = u + x)\,\mathrm{d}u \qquad (4)$$

Under the null hypothesis that f is spherically symmetric around its mean, significance probabilities can be calculated from eq.(3). If it is assumed that X is distributed according to a multivariate normal distribution, the use of the Moore-Rayleigh test is justified. However the distribution of $g = f * (-f)$ is in general only symmetric, i.e. $g(x) = g(-x)$ for all $x \in \mathbb{R}^3$ and therefore the Moore-Rayleigh test is only approximately valid.

Of course, one would prefer to test conservatively for mere symmetry, but the available tests are either only asymptotically nonparametric or require further randomization of the underlying distribution [12,13,14,15,16,17].

Therefore, we suggest to use the Moore-Rayleigh test, but to bootstrap the empirical distributions of the two samples X and Y by random sampling without replacement (to avoid degeneracy issues when two or more vector differences are equal) and to compare the mean of R_N^* obtained under M such samples with eq. (3). In theory, the bootstrapping reduces the error made when the assumptions of the Moore-Rayleigh test are only approximately fulfilled by a factor of almost $1/\sqrt{M}$, although these considerations are beyond the scope of this paper. Here, the properties of the test so obtained are evaluated by computer experiments.

2.2   Clinical Interpretation

Consider two sets of 3D MR images taken from different populations of equal size. The first step in the analysis is the affine registration to an atlas A. This normalization step brings all images to the same coordinate system and removes all non-specific anatomical differences, like global orientation and the scale parameters. From now on, we consider only the normalized sets of images $I = (I_1, ..., I_N)$ and $J = (J_1, ..., J_N)$.

A non-rigid registration defines the relation between the average and an image I, which is found by the minimum of a similarity measure ρ:

$$\mathcal{T}_I = \min \rho(I, A) \qquad (5)$$

Assuming that the similarity measure returns the best approximation of the unknown relation between I and A, $\mathcal{T}_I$ indicates the local anatomical differences between I and A, which are coded by vectors in $\mathbb{R}^3$.

Non-rigidly registering I and J to the atlas results in two sets of deformation fields $\mathcal{T}_I = (\mathcal{T}_{I1}, ..., \mathcal{T}_{IN})$ and $\mathcal{T}_J = (\mathcal{T}_{J1}, ..., \mathcal{T}_{JN})$. Each anatomically homologous point h in T_I and T_J can then be subjected to the two sample Moore-Rayleigh test, as described in Section 2.1.

The resulting p-value in a point h indicates the probability that an observed difference between groups I and J occurs by chance. A small p-value is an indication that there is a difference between I and J. It can occur that both groups I and J are significantly different from A, but as long as the difference of I with A is similar to the difference of J with A, the Moore-Rayleigh test will not return a significant difference between I and J.

3   Validation

3.1   Image Formation

For the validation of the Moore-Rayleigh test an average MR volume of the C57Bl6/Jico mouse brain was used, which was cropped to a volume of 50 x 50 x 80 voxels due to considerations of running time. This subvolume included the ventricles, thalamus, and several fiber tracts, as illustrated in Figure 1(a).

Individual subjects ($n = 30$) were simulated by the introduction of artificial, spherically shaped deformations. Each such local deformation is completely characterized by a center point c and a radius r. The length of each deformation vector in the sphere takes a maximum of $\frac{1}{2}r$ at the center and drops radially and linearly until the edge of the sphere, where the deformation is zero to ensure continuity (in fact, smoothness) with the surrounding field. By varying the parameters c and r two groups (G_1 and G_2) were generated with 15 individuals each.

The goal of this numerical experiment was to test whether and under which conditions the Moore-Rayleigh test picks up group differences (the inter-group variation) only or whether also inter-group variation is detected. For this reason two spherical deformations were used in each subject, which are referred to as *sphere 1* (S_1) and *sphere 2* (S_2) and which are shown in Figure 1(b). The average radius and center of S_1 was taken to be identical for both groups, but in S_2 a systematic difference of 5 voxels in the average radius ($\Delta r = 5$) between G_1 and G_2 was introduced, the average center was kept constant. Intra-group variation was simulated in both groups by randomly adding small variations in the center point and uniform radius of the spheres ($r \pm 5$ and $c \pm 2.5$) from an uniform distribution. The values for the inter-group and intra-group variability, are corresponding to the ones described in the literature[3,7].

After the creation of the individual subjects, Gaussian noise ($\mu=0$, sd=300) was superimposed on each image. The result is shown in Figure 1(c) for one subject. A spherical mask was created (Figure 1(d)) that indicates the average locations of the spherical deformations S_1 and S_2, and which is later used for validation purposes. Figure 1(d) shows the average locations of S_1 (lower sphere) and S_2 (upper sphere), where in S_2 also the differences between the two groups (G_1 and G_2) is shown.

The non-rigid registration of the 30 subjects to the average was performed using the symmetric demons algorithm [18], as implemented in ITK [19]. This

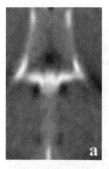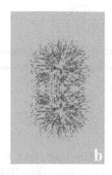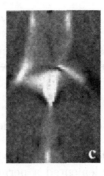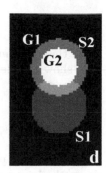

Fig. 1. The various stages during the creation of one of the synthetic images: The midsection of the average image (a), which is deformed by two spheres (b), and the final image after adding gaussian noise (c). For each dataset a sphere mask is created (d) which indicates the average locations of the spherical deformations S_1 and S_2 for G_1 (outer sphere) and G_2 (inner sphere).

registration algorithm uses the mean squared difference with a smoothing factor of 1.0 and was performed with 60 iterations. The output of the non-rigid registration is a deformation field, i.e. vectors in $\mathbb{R}^3$ that represent the geometric translations of voxels to their corresponding points in the atlas image.

3.2   Validation Method

The output of the two-sample Moore-Rayleigh test is a probability image with a p-value per voxel that indicates how likely it is that the null hypothesis holds at that particular point, thus indicating how likely it is that an observed difference between groups I and J occurs by chance in that voxel. Thresholding the probability image with a critical value α results in a binary image that shows the regions where a significant group difference has been detected. For the synthetically generated data the locations are known where there exists a simulated structural difference between the two groups; these are all the voxels lying in S_2 (Figure 1(d)) and this knowledge is taken as ground-truth for the assessment of the statistical tests. We use this information to quantify the performance of the Moore-Rayleigh test by calculating the following:

True positives (TP). Amount of voxels found significant inside S_2
False positives (FP). Amount of voxels found significant outside S_2
false negatives (FN). Amount of voxels found not significant inside S_2
true negatives (TN). Amount of voxels found not significant outside S_2

For the various tests, we report the sensitivity and specificity for $\alpha=0.05$. The sensitivity is the ratio of significant voxels which are detected correctly and specificity is the ratio of not significant voxels which are detected correctly.

$$\text{sensitivity} = \frac{\text{TP}}{\text{TP} + \text{FN}} \qquad (6)$$

$$\text{specificity} = \frac{TN}{TN + FP} \tag{7}$$

From these two measures we also calculated Receiver Operator Curves (ROCs) that show the dependence of sensitivity and specificity on the critical values $0.0 \le \alpha \le 1.0$.

3.3 Comparison of Test Statistic

To compare the performance of the Moore-Rayleigh test to other nonparametric methods, we implemented a permutation test (m=10.000 labellings) with Hotelling's t^2 as test statistic as in [6]. Furthermore, we also implemented the Mann–Whitney test [20], which is the nonparametric equivalent of the t-test, on a rank one approximation (see Appendix A for details).

A visualization of the significant voxels for the three test statistics are given in Figure 2. By visual inspection, better classification results were obtained using the Moore-Rayleigh test. The performance of the three test statistics are given in Figure 3. The sensitivity and the specificity of the cut-off value of $\alpha = 0.05$ is given for the three test statistics in Table 1. The relatively low sensitivity of the permutation tests, might be increased if more permutations were used. Furthermore, the sensitivity of the Mann-Whitney test is comparable with the Moore-Rayleigh test, where the Moore-Rayleigh test outperforms the Mann-Whitney on specificity. Furthermore, the presented p-values are not corrected for multi testing[22]. If multitest correction would have been applied, the Mann-Whitney test would have shown no significance, since the Mann-Whitney test classified voxels significantly different with a probability between 0.01 and 0.05, whereas the Moore-Rayleigh test indicates significance with a probability of between 10^{-2} and 10^{-10}.

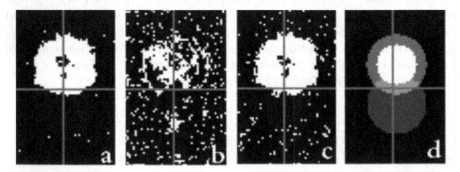

Fig. 2. The classification result with cut-off value $\alpha = 0.05$ for the Moore-Rayleigh test (a), the permutation test (b), and the Mann-Whitney test (c) as compared to the ground truth(d)

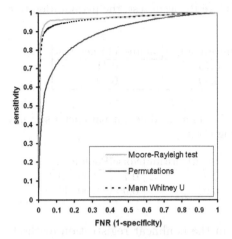

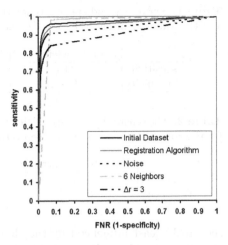

Fig. 3. The ROC of the different non-parametric test statistics for the quantitative analysis of deformation fields

Fig. 4. The ROC of the different parameter settings for the robustness testing of the Moore-Rayleigh test

3.4 Robustness Testing

Several parameters have been varied to investigate the robustness of the Moore-Rayleigh test under various conditions. The dataset as described in 3.1 was used as input and for each experiment only one parameter was changed to measure its effect. The several tests are described below:

Registration Algorithm. Instead of using the Demons non-rigid registration method, a B-Spline transform[23] was applied, as implemented in elastix[24]. Since the Moore-Rayleigh test is a voxel based test, the gridspacing was set at 2.5 voxels with a 3-level pyramid registration. Furthermore, the mutual information metric was used.

Noise. Noise is known for having a major influence on the quality of the images and their postprocessing. The influence of noise on the hypothesis testing is quantified by increasing the standard deviation from 300 (used in Section 3.1) to a value of 700.

6 Neighbors. With the hope of increasing the sensitivity of the test and decreasing the influence of noise, the deformation vectors of the six closest neighbors (two in each coordinate dimension) for each voxel z are pooled.

Δr. In this test, 15 subjects of one group are generated with a systematic difference in radius of 3 voxels between G_1 and G_2 (for S_2), instead of 5 voxels as in Section 3.1. The intra-group variation is kept constant at ± 5 voxels as before.

The ROCs of the Moore-Rayleigh test for these various settings are shown in Figure 4. The sensitivity and the specificity for the cut-off value $\alpha = 0.05$ are additionally given in Table 2. The performance of the Moore-Rayleigh test is

Table 1. Sensitivity and specificity for the Moore-Rayleigh test, the permutation test and the Mann-Whitney test ($\alpha = 0.05$ each)

	Moore-Rayleigh test	Permutation test	Mann-Whitney test
sensitivity	0.91	0.73	0.41
specificity	0.97	0.89	0.99

Table 2. The sensitivity and specificity ($\alpha = 0.05$) for the different parameter settings for the robustness testing of the Moore-Rayleigh test

	Moore-Rayleigh test	Registration Algorithm	Noise	Pooling	Δr
sensitivity	0.91	0.88	0.77	0.99	0.70
specificity	0.97	0.97	0.99	0.90	0.98

seen to be least influenced by the change in the nonlinear registration method. However, the Moore-Rayleigh test is quite sensitive on the influence of noise, loosing sensitivity when the noise level is increased. Pooling neighboring voxels, however, increases the sensitivity, with an accompanying loss in specificity due to the smoothing effect this introduces. As can also be seen in Figure 4, a decrease in inter-group variation (scenario Δr) decreases the sensitivity. This is well explained, as the intra-group variation was kept constant, while the inter-group variation was decreased to only 3 voxels.

4   Discussion

In this paper we presented a novel nonparametric statistical method to detect and quantify anatomical differences between groups of MR images. Our method is based on (a generalization of)the nonparametrical Moore-Rayleigh test, which tests for spherical symmetry in vector data. This method uses as input the deformation fields which are obtained by the non-rigid registration of all subjects to a common reference image. Under the assumption that no registration errors were made in the creation of the deformation fields, significant anatomical differences between the two groups can be assessed.

Permutation tests are not routinely applicable in a clinical setting because of the large number of permutations required. In clinical practice the number of labellings is often reduced to speed up the analysis, which reduces the power of the permutation test severely and makes it almost impossible to correct for multiple comparisons. The method presented here, on the other hand, is computationally fast and offers an interesting alternative to permutation tests. Although the null hypothesis of mere symmetry is not tested, i.e. the Moore-Rayleigh test is only approximately valid, the results are quite convincing, as shown in Section 3.3.

A further advantage of the Moore-Rayleigh test is that it is completely nonparametric and needs no assumptions on the underlying dataset. As the test statistic is continuous, the significance probabilities can be very low (up to 10^{-18} or less is numerically possible), so the Moore-Rayleigh test also results in significant voxels under correction for multiple comparisons (not shown). It was also found to be relatively unaffected by the (non-rigid) registration method used. The sensitivity was most influenced by the decrease of the inter-variation to 3 voxels, but considering that the intra-variation was 5 voxels and that still more than 70 percent of all voxels assessed as significant were true positives, it can be concluded that the Moore-Rayleigh test is able to detect small differences between groups. Furthermore, it was expected and indeed observed that noise, which affects the registration algorithm, results in an increase of false positives. As the results in Section 3.4 indicate, this problem could be addressed by pooling the deformation vectors from neighboring voxels. Although this would result in a loss of specificity, it is plausible that the Moore-Rayleigh test would then be more robust to the effect of noise.

One important topic of our future work concerns the evaluation of this algorithm on real clinical data. For now, we have only assessed the Moore-Rayleigh test on simulated images, with spherically deformations. Although, it can be argued that these deformations are representative for structural deformations, as brain atrophy. Furthermore, the main goal of this paper is to show the performance of the Moore-Rayleigh test on the quantification of inter-group variability. This performance can only be validated on a dataset with known inter-group and intra-group variability. Therefore, to stay close to real data, the variabilities from the synthetic dataset are simulated according to the descriptions of variations of real mouse brain MRI data[3,7].

Finally, we would like to encourage the reader to apply this method on their own data. Therefore, the code is made publicly available and can be obtained by sending an e-mail to the corresponding author.

Acknowledgments. This work was supported in part by funds from CYT-TRON within the BSIK program (Besluit subsidies investeringen kennisinfrastructuur). Furthermore, the authors would like to than Boudewijn Lelieveldt and Luca Ferrarini for their useful comments on the manuscript and method development.

References

1. Driehuys, B., Nouls, J., Badea, A., Bucholz, E., Ghaghada, K., Petiet, A., Hedlund, L.W.: Small animal imaging with magnetic resonance microscopy. ILAR Journal 49, 35–53 (2008)
2. Benveniste, H., Blackband, S.: MR microscopy and high resolution small animal MRI: applications in neuroscience research. Progress in Neurobiology 67, 393–420 (2002)
3. Kovacević, N., Henderson, J.T., Chan, E., Lifshitz, N., Bishop, J., Evans, A.C., Henkelman, R.M., Chen, X.J.: A Three-dimensional MRI Atlas of the Mouse Brain with Estimates of the Average and Variability. Cerebral Cortex 15, 639–645 (2005)
4. Pohl, K.M., Fisher, J., Bouix, S., Shenton, M., McCarley, R.W., Grimson, W.E.L., Ron Kikinis, R., Wells, W.M.: Using the logarithm of odds to define a vector space on probabilistic atlases. Medical Image Analysis 11, 465–477 (2007)

5. Nichols, T.E., Holmes, A.P.: Nonparametric Permutation Tests For Functional Neuroimaging: A Primer with Examples. Human Brain Mapping 15, 1–25 (2001)
6. Ferrarini, L., Palm, W.M., Olofson, H., van Buchem, M.A., Reiber, J.H.C., Admiraal-Behloul, F.: Shape differences of the brain ventricles in Alzheimer's disease. NeuroImage 32, 1060–1069 (2006)
7. Chen, X.J., Kovacevic, N., Lobaugh, N.J., Sled, J.G., Henkelman, R.M., Henderson, J.T.: Neuroanatomical differences between mouse strains as shown by high-resolution 3D MRI. Neuroimage 29, 99–105 (2005)
8. Heckel, D., Arndt, S., Cizadlo, T., Andreasen, N.C.: An efficient procedure for permutation tests in imaging research. Computers and Biomedical Research 31, 164–171 (1998)
9. Rorden, C., Bonilha, L., Nichols, T.E.: Rank-Order versus mean based statistics for neuroimaging. NeuroImage 35, 1531–1537 (2007)
10. Moore, B.R.: A modification of the Rayleigh test for vector data. Biometrika 67, 175–180 (1980)
11. Dutka, J.: On the problem of random flights. Archive for History of Exact Sciences 32, 351–375 (1985)
12. Aki, S.: On nonparametric tests for symmetry in $\mathcal{R}^m$. Annals of the Institute of Statistical Mathematics 45, 787–800 (1993)
13. Ngatchou-Wandji, J.: Testing for symmetry in multivariate distributions. Statistical Methodology (in press)
14. Henze, N., Klar, B., Meintanis, S.G.: Invariant tests for symmetry about an unspecified point based on the empirical characteristic function. Journal of Multivariate Analysis 87, 275–297 (2003)
15. Fernández, V.A., Gamero, M.D.J., García, J.M.: A test for the two-sample problem based on empirical characteristic functions. Computational Statistics & Data Analysis 52, 3730–3748 (2008)
16. Diks, C., Tong, H.: A test for symmetries of multivariate probability distributions. Biometrika 86, 605–614 (1999)
17. Jupp, P.E.: A nonparametric correlation coefficient and a two-sample test for random vectors or directions. Biometrika 74, 887–890 (1987)
18. Thirion, J.P.: Image matching as a diffusion process: an analogy with Maxwell's demons. Medical Image Analysis 2, 243–260 (1998)
19. Yoo, T.S., Ackerman, M.J., Lorensen, W.E., Schroeder, W., Chalana, V., Aylward, S., Metaxes, D., Whitaker, R.: Engineering and Algorithm Design for an Image Processing API: A Technical Report on ITK - The Insight Toolkit. In: Proc. of Medicine Meets Virtual Reality, pp. 586–592 (2002)
20. Mann, H.B., Whitney, D.R.: On a test of whether one of 2 random variables is stochastically larger than the other. The Annals of Mathematical Statistics 18, 50–60 (1947)
21. Siegel, S., Castellan, N.J.: Nonparametric Statistics for the Behavioural Sciences, 2nd edn. McGraw-Hill, New York (1988)
22. Shaffer, J.P.: Multiple Hypothesis Testing. Annual Review of Psychology 46, 561–584 (1995)
23. Rueckert, D., Sonoda, L.I., Hayes, C., Hill, D.L.G., Leach, M.O., Hawkes, D.J.: Non-rigid registration using free-form deformations: Application to breast MR images. IEEE Transactions on Medical Imaging 18, 712–721 (1999)
24. Staring, M.: Intrasubject Registration for Change Analysis in Medical Imaging. PhD thesis, Utrecht University, The Netherlands (2008), http://elastix.isi.uu.nl ISBN 978-90-8891-063-0

A   Mann-Whitney Test

The Mann Whitney test is the nonparametric equivalent to the t–test. It makes the following assumptions:

1. The two samples are randomly and independently drawn from the same underlying distribution.
2. The dependent variable is continuous.
3. The values of the dependent variable are at least ordinal.

As item 3 is stating, the vectors for a point need to be ordered, based on a measure of a continuous scale (item 2). To order vectors in R^3, a rank–1 approximation has been performed: for each point of the average image, a covariance matrix Σ is calculated based on all subjects in the two groups under consideration. Using the singular value decomposition of this covariance matrix (principal component analysis), the eigenvectors V and eigenvalues Λ are obtained and represent the principal modes of variation. $\Sigma = U\Lambda V$,

The first mode of variation V_1, corresponding to the largest eigenvalue $\Lambda_{1,1}$, represents the direction of largest variance between the vectors considered for that particular point in the average. Projecting the vectors on this direction results in vectors all pointing in the same direction, and their lengths are then used in the usual Mann-Whitney test. A disadvantage of this test is that only the first principal mode of the covariance matrix is used, and therefore only partial information on the orientation of the vectors is used, decreasing the power of the test.

A Framework for Brain Registration via Simultaneous Surface and Volume Flow

Anand Joshi[1], Richard Leahy[2], Arthur W. Toga[1], and David Shattuck[1,*]

[1] Laboratory of Neuro Imaging,
UCLA school of Medicine, Los Angeles, CA 90095, USA
anand.joshi@loni.ucla.edu, toga@loni.ucla.edu, shattuck@loni.ucla.edu
[2] Signal and Image Processing Institute,
University of Southern California, Los Angeles 90089, USA
leahy@sipi.usc.edu

Abstract. Volumetric registration of brain MR images presents a challenging problem due to the wide variety of sulcal folding patterns. We present a novel volumetric registration method based on an intermediate parameter space in which the shape differences are normalized. First, we generate a 3D harmonic map of each brain volume to unit ball which is used as an intermediate space. Cortical surface features and volumetric intensity are then used to find a simultaneous surface and volume registration. We present a finite element method for the registration by using a tetrahedral volumetric mesh for registering the interior volumetric information and the corresponding triangulated mesh at the surface points. This framework aligns the convoluted sulcal folding patterns as well as the subcortical structures by allowing simultaneous flow of surface and volumes for registration. We describe the methodology and FEM implementation and then evaluate the method in terms of the overlap between segmented structures in coregistered brains.

1 Introduction

Inter-subject studies for detecting systematic patterns of brain structure and function in human populations require that the data first be transformed to a common coordinate system in which anatomical structures are aligned [1, 2]. Similarly, inter-subject longitudinal studies or group analyses of functional data also require that the images first be anatomically aligned. Such an alignment is commonly performed either with respect to the entire volumetric space or is restricted to the cortical surface [3–7]. While volumetric approaches [8–10] perform well at aligning the interior of the brain e.g. subcortical structures, they often fail to align the folding patterns of the sulcal anatomy [11]. On the other hand, surface based registration techniques align the sulcal folds, but they do not define a volumetric correspondence between points in the interior. In order to overcome the shortcomings of these two types of methods, approaches have

---

* This work is supported under grants U54 RR021813 and P41 RR013642.

J.L. Prince, D.L. Pham, and K.J. Myers (Eds.): IPMI 2009, LNCS 5636, pp. 576–588, 2009.

been developed recently to combine surface and volume registration [12, 13]. In these methods surface registration is performed first and then used to constrain the full volumetric registration. In contrast to these methods, we present a novel framework in which both surface and volume registrations are performed simultaneously. This is achieved by using an intermediate unit ball parameter space in which the shape differences in the two brain volumes are normalized.

The motivation for using an intermediate parameter space for volumetric registration is derived from surface registration approaches in which the challenging problem of normalizing large folding pattern differences is solved by mapping the surface to a flat space such as a sphere [5, 14, 15] or a square [3]. We extend this idea to volume registration where we first generate a harmonic map of the two volumes to a unit ball and thus generate an initial diffeomorphism between between two volumes exhibiting very different folding patterns on their surfaces. The point correspondence defined by this initial mapping is further refined by using additional information in the form of intensity values and surface curvature information. This approach presents a unified framework in which surface and volume data can be combined together for their joint registration.

2   Methods

2.1   Problem Statement and Formulation

Given two 3D manifolds Ω_1 and Ω_2 representing subject and target brain volumes, with boundaries $\partial\Omega_1$ and $\partial\Omega_2$ representing corresponding cortical surfaces, we want to find a map from Ω_1 to Ω_2 such that $\partial\Omega_1$, the surface of Ω_1, maps to Ω_2, the surface of Ω_2, and the intensities of the images in the interior of Ω_1 and Ω_2 are matched. The boundaries, $\partial\Omega_1$ and $\partial\Omega_2$, representing the cortical surfaces of the two brain volumes are assumed to have a spherical topology. We perform this registration in the following steps:

- The two surfaces $\partial\Omega_1$ and $\partial\Omega_2$ are flattened and are mapped to spheres.
- The interior volumes of the two brains Ω_1 and Ω_2 are mapped to the interior of unit balls by 3D harmonic maps.
- The induced mapping from subject brain Ω_1 to Ω_2 is refined by minimizing a cost function with intensity matching and surface curvatures matching terms.

Parameterization-based methods are commonly used for surface registrations especially for registration of the cortical sheet because the intermediate flat space, either a square or a sphere, provides a convenient common space in which structural and functional surface data can be used for performing the alignment. The large-scale differences are normalized in this representation and so the registration problem is simplified to some extent. The disadvantage of this approach is that the metric distortion that takes place during the flat mapping can affect the registration results in locations where the Jacobian of the map is not close to unity. However this can be accounted for by weighting the cost function by the determinant of the Jacobian for the transformation from subject brain to the target brain.

2.2   Surface-Volume Parameter Space

In this section we describe the unit ball parameter space [16–18] used for simultaneous surface and volume registration. As a first step, the cortical surfaces
of subject and target denoted by $\partial\Omega_1$ and $\partial\Omega_2$ are mapped to unit balls [19].
We choose the unit ball as a parameter space because the harmonic maps from
brain to the ball are known to be diffeomorphic [18]. To compute mappings of
the brain manifolds to the unit ball, we first compute a mapping of the brain
surface to the unit sphere. To map the interior of the manifold to the interior of
the unit ball $B(0,1)$, the mapping energy

$$E(v) = \int_{\Omega_i} \|\nabla v\|^2 dV, i = 1, 2 \tag{1}$$

is minimized to get v with the constraint that the surface ∂N maps to the unit
sphere, the boundary of $B(0,1)$. Here ∇ is the usual gradient operator in 3D
Euclidean space and dV denotes the volume integral. This mapping is performed
for both the brains Ω_1 and Ω_2. The minimization is performed by using numerical integration over the voxel lattice and finite differences to approximate the
gradients. The resulting discretized cost function is minimized by conjugate gradient. The result of this minimization is a harmonic map to the unit ball. This
map is known to be diffeomorphic [18]. The one-to-one point correspondence between the brain volume and the unit ball is then used to map the intensity data
to the interior of the unit ball and the curvature data to the spherical boundary
of the ball (see Fig. 2). In this manner we generate harmonic maps v_1 and v_2
from subject and target brains to the unit ball.

2.3   Generation of the Tetrahedral Mesh

We applied TetGen [20] to create a standard unit ball using using $2,663,731$
tetrahedrons and $81,920$ triangles (see Fig. 1) on its surface. The mapped intensity volumes and curvature maps for the two brains were resampled to the nodes
of the tetrahedral mesh, representing the common parameter space, by using
linear interpolation. The resampled image intensities and curvatures as shown
in figure 2 are used in the subsequent sections for the registration. We denote
the resampled intensities are denoted by I_1 and I_2 and curvatures by I_1^c and I_2^c.

2.4   Cost Function

In order to register the surface and volume data of the brain, a dissimilarity
cost function is minimized. We develop a cost function for registration with four
terms designed to control different requirements of the registration warp:

- We want the intensity across the two brain volumes to match
- We want the curvature on the surface of the brains to match
- The deformation from one brain to the other should be smooth
- The Jacobian of the transformation should be non-negative

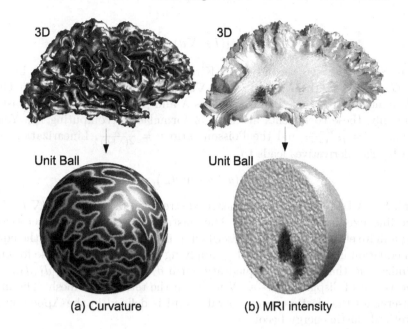

Fig. 1. Mapping of (a) the surface curvature to the unit sphere and (b) MRI intensities to the interior of the unit ball

Let $x = (x_1, x_2, x_3)$ denote 3D coordinates of the subject, $y = (y_1, y_2, y_3)$ denote 3D coordinates of the target and $z = (z_1, z_2, z_3)$ denotes the 3D coordinates of the unit ball.

Intensity and Curvature Mismatch. The intensity mismatch term is computed with respect to the target coordinates. Let U denotes the unit ball. Therefore we define a intensity mismatch cost:

$$C_1(u) = \int_U \left(I_1(x + d(x)) - I_2(x)\right)^2 dV \tag{2}$$

where the integration is over the whole brain volume V. The mapping from subject to target u is $u(x) = x + d(x)$. Similarly, for curvature,

$$C_2(u) = \int_{\partial U} \left(I_1^c(x + d(x)) - I_2^c(x)\right)^2 dS \tag{3}$$

where the integration is over the whole brain surface $\partial \Omega_1$.

Smoothness of the Deformation. We want the displacement vector field from the subject brain to the target be smooth. This is done by penalizing the displacement by an elastic energy, i.e., $C_3(d)$ corresponding to deformation d [13, 21]:

$$C_3(d) = f = -\text{div}\left[(I + \nabla d)\,\hat{S}\right] \quad \hat{S} : \Omega \to \mathbb{R}^3, \tag{4}$$

where $\hat{S}$ denotes the second Piola-Kirchoff stress tensor defined by $\hat{S} = \lambda\,\text{Tr}\,(\hat{G})I + 2\mu\hat{G}$ with $\hat{G} = \frac{1}{2}\left(\nabla d^T + \nabla d + \nabla d^T \nabla d\right)$ representing the Green-St. Venant strain tensor. The coefficients λ and μ are Lamés elastic constants. Commonly, these coefficients are used in formulae for computing the Young's modulus $Y = \mu\frac{3\lambda+2\mu}{\lambda+\mu}$ and the Poisson ratio $\nu = \frac{\lambda}{2(\lambda+\mu)}$. Linearization of (4) using Fréchet derivatives leads to

$$C_3(d) = -\text{div}(S), \tag{5}$$

where, $S = \lambda\,\text{Tr}(G) + 2\mu G$ is the linearized stress tensor and $G = \frac{1}{2}\left(\nabla d + \nabla d^T\right)$ is the linearized strain tensor [13]. The elasticity operator C_3 is discretized by using a finite element method as described in the Appendix. In brief, the equilibrium equation in (5) is formulated by applying a variational principle for energy minimization, that leads to a quadratic form $d^T K d$, where $d = [d_1, d_2..., d_N]^T$ is the vector of displacements at N nodes in the tetrahedral mesh. The matrix K discretizes the elastic energy operator and is defined in the Appendix. The discretized elastic energy becomes:

$$C_3(d) = d^T K d. \tag{6}$$

Non-positive Jacobian. We want the transformation to be non-singular and hence we would like to have a large penalty on negative and small Jacobian. We use the chain rule to compute the Jacobian

$$D(u)|_x = D(v^{-1} \circ \tilde{u})|_x = D(v_2^{-1})|_{v_1(x)} \circ D(\tilde{v_1})|_x \tag{7}$$

where D denotes the derivative operator. Therefore, its determinant is calculated as

$$|D(u)|_x| = \left|D(v_2^{-1})|_{v_1(x)}\right| |D(v_2)|_x| \tag{8}$$

$$= \left|D(v_2)|_{v_1(x)}\right|^{-1} |D(v_2)|_x| \tag{9}$$

the associated cost function can be calculated

$$C_4(u) = \int (1 - \text{sgm}(|D(u)|_x|))^2 dV \tag{10}$$

where $\text{sgm}(x) = \frac{1}{1+e^{-t}}$. This cost function penalizes small and negative Jacobians and thus reduces the probability of folding in the registration maps.

3   Volume Image Displacement Vector Field

The key to the function minimization is computing derivatives of the intensity difference cost function (eq. 2) on the tetrahedral mesh inside of the unit ball, and curvature difference cost function (eq. 3) on the triangulated mesh of the sphere.

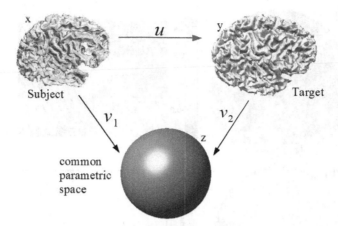

Fig. 2. Schematic of our method. The intermediate unit ball is used as a common space for volumetric registration.

Here we show the discretization of the intensity image for the tetrahedral mesh using finite elements. Discretization of the curvature image on the triangulated mesh is performed similarly, except that in case of surface, the vector field on the sphere is constrained to be tangential to the sphere.

3.1 Tetrahedral Mesh Image Similarity Cost Function

The intensity dissimilarity cost function (eq. 2) for a tetrahedral mesh is given by:

$$C(d_1, d_2, d_3) = \int \int \int [I_1(z_1 + d_1(z), z_2 \\ + d_2(z), z_3 + d_3(z)) - I_2(z_1, z_2, z_3)]^2 dz_1 dz_2 dz_3$$

Let $I_1(z_1 + d_1(z), z_2 + d_2(z), z_3 + z_3(z)) = \sum_{j \in V} \hat{I}_1^j \phi_j(z_1, z_2, z_3)$ where V is the set of vertices and $\phi_j(z_1, z_2, z_3)$ denotes piecewise linear interpolating basis functions [22], $\hat{I}_1^j$ is the warped subject image $I_1(z_1 + d_1, z_2 + d_2, z_3 + d_3)$ interpolated at the set of vertices and $I_2(z_1, z_2, z_3) = \sum_{j \in V} I_2^j \psi_j(z_1, z_2, z_3)$ where I_2^j is $I_2(z_1, z_2, z_3)$ interpolated at the vertex points. Also let $d_1(z_1, z_2, z_3) = \sum_{j \in V} z_1^j \psi_j(z_1, z_2, z_3)$, $d_2(z_1, z_2, z_3) = \sum_{j \in V} d_2^j \psi_j(z_1, z_2, z_3)$ and $d_3(z_1, z_2, z_3) = \sum_{j \in V} d_3^j \psi_j(z_1, z_2, z_3)$.
Therefore the intensity dissimilarity cost function becomes

$$C(d_1, d_2, d_3) = \int \int \int \left(\sum_{j \in V} (\hat{I}_1^j - I_2^j) \psi_j(z_1, z_2, z_3) \right)^2 dz_1 dz_2 dz_3$$

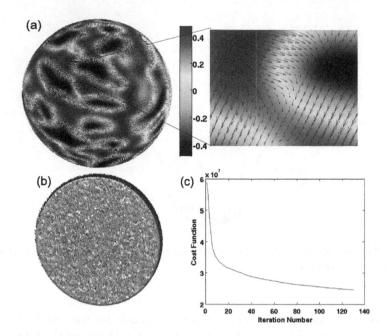

Fig. 3. (a) Displacement field on the surface overlaid on the curvature map, (b) volumetric displacement field (c) cost function as a function of iteration number

We minimize the intensity difference cost function by using gradient descent. Therefore the gradient of the cost function needs to be calculated. The derivative with respect to one coordinate is given by:

$$\frac{\partial C}{\partial d_1^k} = \int\int\int \sum_{j \in V} 2(\hat{I}_1^j - I_2^j)\psi_j(z_1, z_2, z_3)\frac{\partial I_1(z_1 + d_1(z), z_2 + z_2(z), z_3 + d_3(z))}{\partial(z_1 + d_1^k)}\frac{\partial(z_1 + d_1(z))}{\partial(d_1^k)}dz_1dz_2dz_3$$

$$= \int\int\int \sum_{j \in V} 2(\hat{I}_1^j - I_2^j)\psi_j(z)\frac{\partial I_1(z_1 + d_1(z), z_2 + d_2(z), z_3 + d_3(z))}{\partial(z_1 + d_1^k)}\psi_k(z)dz_1dz_2dz_3$$

$$= 2\sum_{j \in V}\left(\int_z \psi_j(z)\psi_k(z)dz_1dz_2dz_3\right)W^j,$$

where W^j indicate the rest of terms. Derivatives with respect to coordinates u_2^j are found similarly. The terms in the integral have a closed form for the tetrahedral mesh and are given by:

$$\int_{z_1, z_2, z_3} \psi_j(z_1, z_2, z_3)\psi_k(z_1, z_2, z_3)dxdydz = \begin{cases} 20\sum_{t \in T_{jk}} V_t & j = k \\ 10\sum_{t \in T_{jk}} V_t & j \neq k \end{cases}$$

where T_{jk} denotes a set tetrahedrons with vertices j and k [22]. The cost function $C(d) = C_1(d) + C_2(d) + C_3(d) + C_4(d)$ is minimized by using steepest descent. The point correspondence between the two brains induced in their unit-ball representations is then applied to the 3D volumes to find a displacement field in 3D using linear interpolation.

4   Implementation and Results

Assuming T1 weighted MR images of the subject and the target brains, the method assumes extracted cortical surface and pial surface, as well as, the brain masks corresponding to the subject and target brains. Here we used a combination of BrainSuite [23] and FreeSurfer [5] for surface extraction, spherical mapping and computation of the curvature. This spherical representation was then used as described in Sec. 2.3 for generating a volumetric harmonic map. This sequence of operations is performed for both target and subject brains to generate a unit ball representation of the two brains. The registration of the two unit ball representations of the brains is then performed and the mapping induced by this intermediate unit ball space is applied to the 3D volumes. The registration results are shown in Fig. 4. For validating our method we used manually labeled brain data from IBSR database at the Center for Morphometric Analysis at Massachusetts General Hospital. These data include volumetric MR data and hand segmented and labeled structures. We then applied the HAMMER software and our method. HAMMER is an automated method for volume registration which is able to achieve improved alignment of geometric features by basing the alignment on an attribute vector that includes a set of geometric moment invariants rather than simply the voxel intensities. To evaluate accuracy, we computed the Dice coefficients [24] for each subcortical structure, where the structure names and boundaries were taken from the IBSR database. The method was implemented in Matlab and in a current non-optimized implementation takes 8 hours to perform a total of 100 iterations of gradient descent on a Pentium IV 3.2GHz desktop workstation. We performed 100 iterations of gradient descent. Reduction of the cost function with iteration number is shown in Fig. 3(c). Dice coefficients averaged over all structures show a small improvement

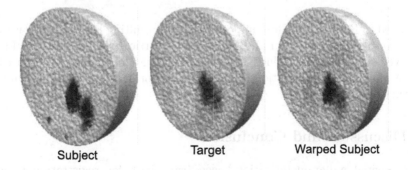

Subject   Target   Warped Subject

Fig. 4. MR intensity images in the tetrahedral mesh of the unit ball space for subject, target and warped subject

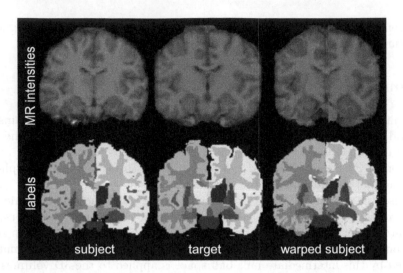

Fig. 5. MR intensity images as well as subcortical labels for subject, target MR and warped subject

Table 1. Comparison of Dice coefficients

Subcortical Structure	HAMMER	Our Method
Left Thalamus	0.7365	0.8463
Left Caudate	0.5820	0.6912
Left Putamen	0.5186	0.7700
Left Hippocampus	0.6837	0.8918
Right Thalamus	0.8719	0.8291
Right Caudate	0.8107	0.6474
Right Putamen	0.6759	0.7862
Right Hippocampus	0.5974	0.8188
Average dice coeffs	0.7658	0.7920

compared to HAMMER. More importantly, the resulting registration has one to one correspondence between all points on the cortical surface and should have improved sulcal alignment due to the curvature matching term in our cost function. A more detailed validation will quantify performance in terms of volumetric and surface alignment.

5   Discussion and Conclusion

We presented a parameterization-based framework for registration in which surface-based and volumetric features can be combined together for registration. We used MR intensity as a volumetric features and curvature as surface-based feature. For multimodality images, additional volumetric features can be used if available. By mapping the two brains to the unit ball and performed the registration in the parameter space, instead of the 3D space, the sulcal folding pattern differences between the two brains are normalized. This framework also allows for the surfaces to flow while internal MR intensity values register. Note that our method is limited to brain representations with a genus zero surface which might not be the case for abnormal anatomy, e.g. when legions are present. In such cases, a mask could be used for the brains with abormalities, with cost function modified appropriately to exclude the differences in the masked region. The method presented aligns cortical surface as well as subcortical structures accurately in the volumetric space by performing their simultaneous alignment.

Acknowledgment

The authors would like to thank the Center for Morphometric Analysis at Massachusetts General Hospital for providing the MR brain data sets and their manual segmentations. The MR and segmentation data sets are available at http://www.cma.mgh.harvard.edu/ibsr/. HAMMER was made available for download by Dr. Shen.

References

1. Changeux, J.P.: Drug use and abuse. In: Edelman, G.M., Changeux, J. (eds.) The Brain. Transaction Publishers (2001)
2. Nahas, G.G., Burks, T.F. (eds.): Drug Abuse in the Decade of the Brain. IOS Press, Amsterdam (1997)
3. Joshi, A.A., Shattuck, D.W., Thompson, P.M., Leahy, R.M.: A finite element method for elastic parameterization and alignment of cortical surfaces using sulcal constraints. In: Proc. of ISBI (2007)
4. Tosun, D., Rettmann, M.E., Prince, J.L.: Mapping techniques for aligning sulci across multiple brains. Medical Image Analysis 8(3), 295–309 (2005)
5. Fischl, B., Sereno, M.I., Tootell, R.B.H., Dale, A.M.: High-resolution inter-subject averaging and a coordinate system for the cortical surface. Human Brain Mapping 8, 272–284 (1998)
6. Ray, N., Levy, B.: Hierarchical least squares conformal map. In: PG 2003: Proceedings of the 11th Pacific Conference on Computer Graphics and Applications, Washington, DC, USA, p. 263. IEEE Computer Society, Los Alamitos (2003)
7. Yeo, B.T.T., Sabuncu, M.R., Vercauteren, T., Ayache, N., Fischl, B., Golland, P.: Spherical demons: Fast surface registration. In: Metaxas, D., Axel, L., Fichtinger, G., Székely, G. (eds.) MICCAI 2008, Part I. LNCS, vol. 5241, pp. 745–753. Springer, Heidelberg (2008)
8. Shen, D., Davatzikos, C.: HAMMER: hierarchical attribute matching mechanism for elastic registration. IEEE Transactions on Medical Imaging 21(11), 1421–1439 (2002)
9. Lester, H., Arridge, S.: A survey of hierarchical non-linear medical image registration. Pattern Recognition 32(1), 129–149 (1999)
10. Christensen, G., et al.: Consistent Linear-Elastic Transformations for Image Matching. LNCS, pp. 224–237. Springer, Heidelberg (1999)

11. Zitová, B., Flusser, J.: Image registration methods: a survey. Image and Vision Computing 21(11), 977–1000 (2003)
12. Joshi, A.A., Shattuck, D.W., Thompson, P.M., Leahy, R.M.: Surface-constrained volumetric brain registration using harmonic mappings. IEEE Trans. Med. Imaging 26(12), 1657–1669 (2007)
13. Postelnicu, G., Zollei, L., Fischl, B.: Combined volumetric and surface registration. IEEE Transactions on Medical Imaging (2008) (to apprear)
14. Thompson, P.M., Mega, M.S., Toga, A.W.: Disease-specific probabilistic brain atlases. In: Procedings of IEEE International Conference on Computer Vision and Pattern Recognition, pp. 227–234 (2000)
15. Joshi, A.A., Leahy, R.M., Thompson, P.M., Shattuck, D.W.: Cortical surface parameterization by p-harmonic energy minimization. In: ISBI, pp. 428–431 (2004)
16. Li, X., Guo, X., Wang, H., He, Y., Gu, X., Qin, H.: Harmonic volumetric mapping for solid modeling applications. In: Proceedings of the 2007 ACM symposium on Solid and physical modeling, pp. 109–120. ACM Press, New York (2007)
17. Joshi, A., Shattuck, D., Thompson, P., Leahy, R.: Brain Image Registration Using Cortically Constrained Harmonic Mappings. In: Karssemeijer, N., Lelieveldt, B. (eds.) IPMI 2007. LNCS, vol. 4584, pp. 359–371. Springer, Heidelberg (2007)
18. Wang, Y., Gu, X., Yau, S.: Volumetric harmonic map. Communications in Information and Systems 3(3), 191–202 (2004)
19. Van Essen, D., Drury, H., Dickson, J., Harwell, J., Hanlon, D., Anderson, C.: An Integrated Software Suite for Surface-based Analyses of Cerebral Cortex (2001)
20. Si, H., Gaertner, K.: Meshing Piecewise Linear Complexes by Constrained Delaunay Tetrahedralizations. In: Proceedings of the 14th International Meshing Roundtable, pp. 147–163. Springer, Heidelberg (2005)
21. Holden, M.: A review of geometric transformations for nonrigid body registration. IEEE Transactions on Medical Imaging 27(1), 111–128 (2008)
22. Hughes, T.: The finite element method. Prentice-Hall, Englewood Cliffs (1987)
23. Shattuck, D.W., Leahy, R.M.: Brainsuite: An automated cortical surface identification tool. Medical Image Analysis 8(2), 129–142 (2002)
24. Kondrak, G., Marcu, D., Knight, K.: Cognates can improve statistical translation models. In: Proceedings of HLT-NAACL, pp. 44–48 (2003)

Appendix

The solution to the elastic energy minimization problem in section 2.4 is obtained by finite element method. We use tetrahedral elements in order to perform the volumetric discretization of the elastic energy. The objective is to get the displacement field at every point in the unit ball. The 3D unit ball is divided into tetrahedral elements such that every point in the space lies inside exactly one tetrahedron. We denote the 3 spatial coordinates by x, y, z for simplicity. We assume that the displacement field $d(x, y, z)$ is piecewise linear. i.e., if the point is inside tetrahedron, then

$$d(x, y, z) = a_0^i + a_1^i x + a_2^i y + a_3^i z, \tag{11}$$

for some coefficients $a_0^i, a_1^i, a_2^i, a_3^i$. Therefore, for the tetrahedron i with nodes $(x_1^i, y_1^i, z_1^i), (x_2^i, y_2^i, z_2^i), (x_3^i, y_3^i, z_3^i)$ and (x_4^i, y_4^i, z_4^i), we can write expressions for u in matrix form as:

$$\begin{bmatrix} d(x_1^i, y_1^i, z_1^i) \\ d(x_2^i, y_2^i, z_2^i) \\ d(x_3^i, y_3^i, z_3^i) \\ d(x_4^i, y_4^i, z_4^i) \end{bmatrix} = \underbrace{\begin{bmatrix} 1 & x_1^i & y_1^i & z_1^i \\ 1 & x_2^i & y_2^i & z_2^i \\ 1 & x_3^i & y_3^i & z_3^i \\ 1 & x_4^i & y_4^i & z_4^i \end{bmatrix}}_{M} \begin{bmatrix} a_0^i \\ a_1^i \\ a_2^i \\ a_3^i \end{bmatrix}. \tag{12}$$

Therefore, the derivative operators for a tetrahedral element el are given by

$$D_x^{el} = \frac{1}{|M|} \begin{bmatrix} z_3 y_4 - y_3 z_4 + y_2 z_4 - y_4 z_2 - y_2 z_3 + y_3 z_2 \\ y_3 z_4 - z_3 y_4 - y_1 z_4 + y_4 z_1 + y_1 z_3 - y_3 z_1 \\ z_2 y_4 - y_2 z_4 + y_1 z_4 - y_4 z_1 - y_1 z_2 + y_2 z_1 \\ y_2 z_3 - z_2 y_3 - z_3 y_1 + z_1 y_3 + y_1 z_2 - z_1 y_2 \end{bmatrix}^T, \tag{13}$$

$$D_y^{el} = -\frac{1}{|M|} \begin{bmatrix} z_3 x_4 - x_3 z_4 + x_2 z_4 - x_4 z_2 - x_2 z_3 + x_3 z_2 \\ x_3 z_4 - z_3 x_4 - x_1 z_4 + x_4 z_1 + x_1 z_3 - x_3 z_1 \\ z_2 x_4 - x_2 z_4 + x_1 z_4 - x_4 z_1 - x_1 z_2 + x_2 z_1 \\ x_2 z_3 - z_2 x_3 - z_3 x_1 + z_1 x_3 + x_1 z_2 - z_1 x_2 \end{bmatrix}^T, \tag{14}$$

$$D_z^{el} = \frac{1}{|M|} \begin{bmatrix} y_3 x_4 - x_3 y_4 + x_2 y_4 - x_2 y_4 - x_2 y_3 + x_3 y_2 \\ x_3 y_4 - y_3 x_4 - x_1 y_4 + x_4 y_1 + x_1 y_3 - x_3 y_1 \\ y_2 x_4 - x_2 y_4 + x_1 y_4 - x_4 y_1 - x_1 y_2 + x_2 y_1 \\ x_2 y_3 - y_2 x_3 - y_3 x_1 + y_1 x_3 + x_1 y_2 - y_1 x_2 \end{bmatrix}^T, \tag{15}$$

and,

$$D_x = \sum_{el} r(D_x^{el}), D_y = \sum_{el} r(D_y^{el}), D_z = \sum_{el} r(D_z^{el}), \tag{16}$$

where r is a resizing function that keeps track of indices of the individual nodes in the whole mesh. This kind of re-indexing is commonly done in FEM techniques [22]. Let the matrices L, L^W and K be defined as

$$L = \begin{bmatrix} D_x & 0 & 0 \\ 0 & D_y & 0 \\ 0 & 0 & D_z \\ D_y & D_x & 0 \\ 0 & D_z & D_y \\ D_z & 0 & D_x \end{bmatrix},$$ (17)

$$L^W = \begin{bmatrix} (1-\nu)D_x & \nu D_y & \nu D_z \\ \nu D_x & (1-\nu)D_y & \nu D_z \\ \nu D_x & \nu D_y & (1-\nu)D_z \\ \frac{1-2\nu}{2}D_y & \frac{1-2\nu}{2}D_x & 0 \\ 0 & \frac{1-2\nu}{2}D_z & \frac{1-2\nu}{2}D_y \\ \frac{1-2\nu}{2}D_z & 0 & \frac{1-2\nu}{2}D_x \end{bmatrix},$$ (18)

$$K = \frac{Y}{(1+\nu)(1-2\nu)} L^T L^W.$$ (19)

Let the x, y, z components of the displacement (U_x, U_y, U_z) at nodal points is arranged in a column $U = [U_x, U_y, U_z]^T$. Then the elastic energy, without any external forces, is given by

$$E_{elastic}(U) = U^T K U.$$ (20)

Level Set Image Segmentation with a Statistical Overlap Constraint

Ismail Ben Ayed[1], Shuo Li[1], and Ian Ross[2]

[1] GE Healthcare, London, ON, Canada
[2] London Health Sciences Centre, London, ON, Canada

Abstract. This study investigates active curve image segmentation with a *statistical overlap constraint*, which biases the overlap between the non-parametric (kernel-based) distributions of image data within the segmentation regions–a foreground and a background–to a statistical description learned *a priori*. We model the overlap, measured via the Bhattacharyya coefficient, with a Gaussian prior whose parameters are estimated from a set of relevant training images. This can be viewed as a generalization of current intensity-driven constraints for difficult situations where a significant overlap exists between the distributions of the segmentation regions. We propose to minimize a functional containing the overlap constraint and classic regularization terms, compute the corresponding Euler-Lagrange curve evolution equation, and give a simple interpretation of how the statistical overlap constraint influences such evolution. A representative number of statistical, quantitative, and comparative experiments with Magnetic Resonance (MR) cardiac images and Computed Tomography (CT) liver images demonstrate the desirable properties of the statistical overlap constraint. First, it outperforms significantly the likelihood prior commonly used in level set segmentation. Second, it is *easy-to-learn*; we demonstrate experimentally that the Gaussian assumption is sufficient for cardiac images. Third, it can relax the need of both complex geometric training and accurate learning of the background distribution, thereby allowing more flexibility in clinical use.

1 Introduction

Image segmentation is a fundamental task in medical image analysis [2]–[9], [23]–[25]. It consists of partitioning an image into two regions: a target object (foreground), for instance a specific organ, and a background. Level set functional minimization, which uses an active curve to delineate the target object, has resulted in the most effective and flexible segmentation algorithms [10]–[20], mainly because it allows introducing a wide range of photometric and geometric constraints on the solution. It has become very popular in medical image analysis [2]–[9], [23]–[25] because there are several applications where anatomical entities can be enclosed within a closed contour. Furthermore, the level set representation of curve evolution extends readily to higher dimensions, and allows to compute easily the geometric characteristics of objects.

J.L. Prince, D.L. Pham, and K.J. Myers (Eds.): IPMI 2009, LNCS 5636, pp. 589–601, 2009.

Level set segmentation consists of evolving a curve to delineate the target object. The curve evolution equation is obtained by optimizing a functional which, generally, contains a data term measuring the conformity of photometric image data (e.g. intensity) within each region to a given statistical description. Chan and Vese [1] pioneered a data term, which measures the conformity of image data within each region to the piecewise constant model. Albeit applicable only to segmentation regions where image data is approximately constant, the Chan-Vese model has established the potential of region-based active contours, and has been widely used in medical image analysis [2]–[5], [7]. More generally, most of segmentation algorithms are stated as a Bayesian inference problem [8]–[14], [21]–[22], [26] where optimization of the data term amounts to maximizing the *likelihood* of the image. This corresponds to maximizing the conditional probability of pixel data given the assumed model distributions within the object and background. The way of estimating model distributions divides segmentation methods into two categories: unsupervised methods, where model distributions are estimated from the current image along with the segmentation process, and methods using *likelihood priors*, where model distributions are learned *a priori*[1] from a set of segmented training images [8], [9], or interactively from user-specified pixels [21]–[22]. Embedding likelihood priors in image segmentation has significantly improved the performances of unsupervised methods [10]. It has led to promising results in medical image segmentation [8], [9], [21]. Unfortunately, likelihood priors require both object and background models. This can be a limitation in medical image analysis because, within a class of images depicting the same object, the background distribution generally undergoes high variations and, therefore, is difficult to learn. More importantly, they can not incorporate information about the *overlap* between the distributions of image data within the object and background–they measure only pixelwise information and, as such, are not sufficient to segment images where a significant overlap (or similarity) exists between the actual distributions within the foreground and background (cf. the typical example in Fig. 1). Recent studies have shown the advantages and effectiveness of using *distributions measures* in object tracking [18]–[20] and image segmentation [15]–[17]. In the context of image segmentation, curve evolution is derived so that, at convergence, the final curve minimizes the overlap (or similarity) between the photometric distributions of the foreground and background regions [15]–[17].

Whether based the likelihood principle or distribution measures, existing segmentation methods assume, implicitly or explicitly, that the overlap between the distributions of image data within the object and its background has to be minimal. The assumption of minimal overlap may not be valid in many applications in medical image analysis where segmentation is often complicated by the similarity in photometric properties between the segmentation regions (cf. the

---

[1] For instance, segmenting a class of images depicting the same organ and having similar photometric patterns is common in medical image analysis [8]. In this case, learning model distributions from segmented training images is very useful.

typical example in Fig. 1). In this case, adding complex training-based geometric[2] constraints to existing photometric constraints was inevitable to prevent curve spilling and obtain satisfying results [5], [7], [8].

This study investigates image segmentation with a *statistical overlap constraint*, which biases the overlap between the distributions of photometric data within the segmentation regions to a statistical description learned *a priori*. We model the overlap, measured via the Bhattacharyya coefficient, with a Gaussian prior whose parameters are estimated from a set of relevant training images. The overlap constraint can be viewed as a *generalization* of current intensity-driven constraints for difficult situations where a significant overlap exists between the intensity distributions of the foreground and background regions (cf. the typical example in Fig. 1). Used in conjunction with classic regularization terms, the statistical overlap constraint is minimized by curve evolution via the Euler-Lagrange equation. A quantitative and comparative performance evaluation over a representative number of experiments with Magnetic Resonance (MR) cardiac images and Computed Tomography (CT) liver images demonstrate that the proposed constraint outperforms significantly the likelihood prior commonly used in image segmentation. Furthermore, it is *easy-to-learn*; we demonstrate experimentally that the overlap between the intensity distributions within the heart myocardium and the background in cardiac images can be modeled accurately with the Gaussian distribution (cf. Fig. 2 a and b). The proposed method can relax, on one hand, the need of complex geometric constraints and, on the other hand, accurate learning of the background distribution, thereby leading to more flexibility in clinical use.

2   The Proposed Statistical Overlap Constraint

Let $I_{\mathbf{x}} - I(\mathbf{x}) : \Omega \subset \mathbb{R}^2 \to \mathcal{Z} \subset \mathbb{R}$ be an image function from the domain Ω to the space $\mathcal{Z}$ of photometric variables. Let $\Gamma(s) : [0, 1] \to \Omega$ be a closed planar parametric curve. The purpose of this study is to evolve Γ in order to divide Ω into two regions: $\mathbf{R}_{in} = \mathbf{R}_\Gamma$, corresponding to the interior of Γ (foreground), and $\mathbf{R}_{out} = \mathbf{R}_{in}^c = \mathbf{R}_\Gamma^c$, corresponding to the exterior of Γ (background). The evolution equation of Γ is sought by optimizing a statistical overlap constraint. To introduce such constraint, we first consider the following definitions:

* $\mathbf{P}_{out}$ is the nonparametric (kernel-based) estimate of the distribution of image data outside Γ

$$\forall z \in \mathcal{Z} \quad \mathbf{P}_{out}(z) = \frac{\int_{\mathbf{R}_{out}} K(z - I_{\mathbf{x}}) d\mathbf{x}}{\mathbf{A}_{out}}, \tag{1}$$

where $\mathbf{A}_{out}$ is the area of region $\mathbf{R}_{out}$: $\mathbf{A}_{out} = \int_{\mathbf{R}_{out}} d\mathbf{x}$. Typical choices of K are the Dirac function and the Gaussian kernel [16]: $K(y) = \frac{1}{\sqrt{2\pi h^2}} exp^{-\frac{y^2}{2h^2}}$, where h is the kernel width.

---

[2] Geometric properties include object shape, spatial position, and inter-object spatial relations.

• $\mathcal{B}(f/g)$ is the Bhattacharyya coefficient measuring the amount of overlap between two statistical samples f and g

$$\mathcal{B}(f/g) = \sum_{z \in \mathcal{Z}} \sqrt{f(z)g(z)} \qquad (2)$$

Note that the values of $\mathcal{B}$ are always in $[0, 1]$, where 0 indicates that there is no overlap, and 1 indicates a perfect match.

We assume that the foreground region, i.e., the target object to be segmented, is characterized by a model distribution, $\mathcal{M}_{in}$, which can be learned over a set of training images and segmentation examples. Consider the following measure of *overlap* between the sample distribution outside the curve (background) and the model distribution of the object (foreground)

$$\mathcal{O}(\Gamma, \mathcal{M}_{in}) = \mathcal{B}(\mathbf{P}_{out}/\mathcal{M}_{in}) = \sum_{z \in \mathcal{Z}} \sqrt{\mathbf{P}_{out}(z)\mathcal{M}_{in}(z)} \qquad (3)$$

In order to incorporate prior statistical information about the photometric similarities between the object and the background, we assume that $\mathcal{O}(\Gamma, \mathcal{M}_{in})$ is a random variable following a Gaussian distribution

$$\mathcal{N}\left(\mathcal{O}(\Gamma, \mathcal{M}_{in}), \mu, \sigma\right) = \frac{1}{\sqrt{2\pi\sigma^2}} exp^{-\frac{(\mathcal{O}(\Gamma, \mathcal{M}_{in}) - \mu)^2}{2\sigma^2}} \qquad (4)$$

Parameters μ and σ are learned beforehand over a set of relevant segmented training images different from the test images (images of interest). Parametric distributions other than the Gaussian distribution can be employed to model the overlap prior. This would change the final curve evolution equation, but would not change the method *conceptually*. We will show in the experiments that the Gaussian assumption is sufficient in many practical cases in medical image analysis. For instance, the overlap between the intensity distributions within the heart myocardium and the background in Magnetic Resonance Images (MRI) can be modeled accurately with the Gaussian distribution (refer to Fig. 2 b).

We propose to minimize with respect to Γ a *statistical overlap term* which measures the conformity of $\mathcal{O}(\Gamma, \mathcal{M}_{in})$ to a Gaussian model described by μ and σ

$$\mathcal{F}\left(\mathcal{O}(\Gamma, \mathcal{M}_{in}), \mu, \sigma\right) = \sqrt{-\log \mathcal{N}\left(\mathcal{O}(\Gamma, \mathcal{M}_{in}), \mu, \sigma\right)} \qquad (5)$$

The *statistical overlap* term can be viewed as a *generalization* of the *distribution-based* terms proposed recently for image segmentation [15], [16], [17], and object tracking [18], [19], [20]. The particular case corresponding to $\mu = 0$ is an *explicit* form of assuming that the overlap between the intensity distributions of the object and background is *minimal*. Such assumption is *implicit* in existing level set segmentation methods. The proposed overlap term is more *versatile* than existing data terms. It addresses cases in which a significant overlap (cf. the typical example in Fig. 1) exists between the intensity distributions within the object and background and, as such, the ensuing algorithm is more widely applicable than existing level set segmentation algorithms.

We propose to minimize an active curve segmentation functional containing the proposed statistical overlap term and classic regularization terms [1], namely, the length of curve Γ and the area of the region within Γ

$$\mathcal{E}_{\mathbf{O}} = \lambda \mathcal{F}\left(\mathcal{O}(\Gamma, \mathcal{M}_{in}), \mu, \sigma\right) + \alpha \oint_{\Gamma} ds + \nu \int_{\mathbf{R}_{in}} d\mathbf{x}, \qquad (6)$$

where λ, α, and ν are positive constants to weigh the contribution of each constraint.

3   Minimization Equation via Curve Evolution

The curve evolution equation is obtained by minimizing $\mathcal{E}_{\mathbf{O}}$ with respect to Γ. To this end, we derive the *Euler-Lagrange* gradient descent equation by embedding curve Γ in a one-parameter family of curves: $\Gamma(s, t) : [0, 1] \times \mathbb{R}_{+} \to \Omega$, and solving the partial differential equation:

$$\frac{\partial \Gamma}{\partial t} = -\frac{\partial \mathcal{E}_{\mathbf{O}}}{\partial \Gamma} = -\lambda \frac{\partial \mathcal{F}\left(\mathcal{O}(\Gamma, \mathcal{M}_{in}), \mu, \sigma\right)}{\partial \Gamma} - \alpha \frac{\partial \oint_{\Gamma} ds}{\partial \Gamma} - \nu \frac{\partial \int_{\mathbf{R}_{in}} d\mathbf{x}}{\partial \Gamma}, \qquad (7)$$

where t is an artificial time parameterizing the descent direction, and $\frac{\partial \mathcal{E}_{\mathbf{O}}}{\partial \Gamma}$ denotes the functional derivative of $\mathcal{E}_{\mathbf{O}}$ with respect to Γ.

To derive the final curve evolution equation, we need to compute the functional derivative of the statistical overlap term with respect to Γ. We have

$$\frac{\partial \mathcal{F}\left(\mathcal{O}(\Gamma, \mathcal{M}_{in}), \mu, \sigma\right)}{\partial \Gamma} = \frac{(\mathcal{O}(\Gamma, \mathcal{M}_{in}) - \mu)}{2\sigma^2 \, \mathcal{F}\left(\mathcal{O}(\Gamma, \mathcal{M}_{in}), \mu, \sigma\right)} \frac{\partial \mathcal{O}(\Gamma, \mathcal{M}_{in})}{\partial \Gamma} \qquad (8)$$

Now we need to compute $\frac{\partial \mathcal{O}(\Gamma, \mathcal{M}_{in})}{\partial \Gamma}$ in (8). We have

$$\frac{\partial \mathcal{O}(\Gamma, \mathcal{M}_{in})}{\partial \Gamma} - \frac{1}{2} \int_{z \in \mathcal{Z}} \sqrt{\frac{\mathcal{M}_{in}(z)}{\mathbf{P}_{out}(z)}} \frac{\partial \mathbf{P}_{out}(z)}{\partial \Gamma} \qquad (9)$$

To derive the final expression of $\frac{\partial \mathcal{O}(\Gamma, \mathcal{M}_{in})}{\partial \Gamma}$, we need to compute $\frac{\partial \mathbf{P}_{out}(z)}{\partial \Gamma}$. To this end, we use the result in [26], which shows that for a scalar function g and a curve Γ, the functional derivative with respect to Γ of the integral of g over the region outside Γ, i.e., $\mathbf{R}_{\Gamma}^c = \mathbf{R}_{out}$, is given by $\frac{\partial \int_{\mathbf{R}_{out}} g(\mathbf{x}) d\mathbf{x}}{\partial \Gamma(s,t)} = -g\left(\Gamma(s,t)\right) \mathbf{n}(s, t)$, where $\mathbf{n}(s, t)$ is the outward unit normal to Γ at (s, t). Applying this proposition to $\mathbf{A}_{out}$ and $\int_{\mathbf{R}_{out}} K(z - I_{\mathbf{x}}) d\mathbf{x}$ in $\frac{\partial \mathbf{P}_{out}(z)}{\partial \Gamma}$ yields, after some algebraic manipulations

$$\frac{\partial \mathbf{P}_{out}(z)}{\partial \Gamma(s,t)} = \frac{1}{\mathbf{A}_{out}} \left(\mathbf{P}_{out}(I_{\Gamma(s,t)}) - K(z - I_{\Gamma(s,t)})\right) \mathbf{n}(s, t) \qquad (10)$$

Embedding (10) into (9), and after some algebraic manipulations, we obtain:

$$\frac{\partial \mathcal{O}(\Gamma, \mathcal{M}_{in})}{\partial \Gamma(s,t)} = \frac{1}{2\mathbf{A}_{out}} \left(\mathcal{O}(\Gamma, \mathcal{M}_{in}) - \int_{z \in \mathcal{Z}} K(z - I_{\Gamma(s,t)}) \sqrt{\frac{\mathcal{M}_{in}(z)}{\mathbf{P}_{out}(z)}} dz\right) \mathbf{n}(s, t)$$

$$\qquad (11)$$

Using (11) and the classic derivative of the regularization terms [1] in (8) gives
the final curve evolution equation:

$$\frac{\partial \boldsymbol{\Gamma}(s,t)}{\partial t} = \{ \underbrace{\frac{(\mathcal{O}(\boldsymbol{\Gamma}, \mathcal{M}_{in}) - \mu)}{2\sigma^2 \mathcal{F}(\mathcal{O}(\boldsymbol{\Gamma}, \mathcal{M}_{in}), \mu, \sigma)}}_{Overlap\ constraint\ influence}$$

$$\underbrace{\frac{\lambda}{2\mathbf{A}_{out}} \left(\int_{z \in \mathcal{Z}} K(z - I_{\boldsymbol{\Gamma}(s,t)}) \sqrt{\frac{\mathcal{M}_{in}(z)}{\mathbf{P}_{out}(z)}} dz - \mathcal{O}(\boldsymbol{\Gamma}, \mathcal{M}_{in}) \right)}_{Flow\ optimizing\ the\ overlap\ measure\ \mathcal{O}(\boldsymbol{\Gamma}, \mathcal{M}_{in})}$$

$$+ \alpha\kappa(s,t) - \nu\}\boldsymbol{n}(s,t), \tag{12}$$

where $\kappa(s,t)$ is the mean curvature function of $\boldsymbol{\Gamma}$. Note that $\mathcal{O}(\boldsymbol{\Gamma}, \mathcal{M}_{in})$, $\mathbf{P}_{out}$, and $\mathbf{A}_{out}$ depend on the curve and, consequently, *need to be updated along with the evolution process*. The level-set framework [27] is used to implement the evolution equation in (12). Level sets have well-known advantages over explicit curve discretization and can be effected by stable numerical schemes [27].

Interpretation: Let us give an interpretation of how the overlap constraint guides the curve. The learned mean μ influences the sign of the multiplicative coefficient (*overlap constraint influence*) affected to the flow optimizing the overlap measure $\mathcal{O}(\boldsymbol{\Gamma}, \mathcal{M}_{in})$, i.e., $\frac{\partial \mathcal{O}(\boldsymbol{\Gamma}, \mathcal{M}_{in})}{\partial \boldsymbol{\Gamma}}$. This coefficient is *negative* when the overlap $\mathcal{O}(\boldsymbol{\Gamma}, \mathcal{M}_{in})$ is *superior* to its most likely value μ. In this case, the overlap constraint results in a curve evolution which *decreases* $\mathcal{O}(\boldsymbol{\Gamma}, \mathcal{M}_{in})$. By contrast, when $\mathcal{O}(\boldsymbol{\Gamma}, \mathcal{M}_{in})$ is *inferior* to μ, the coefficient becomes *positive* and the curve evolution *increases* $\mathcal{O}(\boldsymbol{\Gamma}, \mathcal{M}_{in})$. The overlap constraint leads to a curve evolution which keeps $\mathcal{O}(\boldsymbol{\Gamma}, \mathcal{M}_{in})$ close to its most likely value. The learned variance σ affects the weight of the overlap constraint. The smaller σ, the higher such weight. This is intuitive because a small variance σ indicates that μ is a reliable estimation of the overlap and, as such, it gives more importance to the overlap constraint flow. On the contrary, a high variance gives more importance to the other functional terms.

3.1   Experiments

To demonstrates clearly the advantage of using overlap constraint over commonly used likelihood priors [8], [9], [21], [22], we first give a typical example. Then we describe a *quantitative* and *comparative* performance evaluation over a representative number of experiments on cardiac images. Evaluation of the segmentation method we propose, referred to as Overlap Constraint Method (**OCM**), is supported by extensive comparisons with a Likelihood Prior Method (**LPM**). *The same training images, curve initializations, and parameters were used for both methods.* We also demonstrate experimentally that the overlap prior is *easy-to-learn* in an important application, namely segmentation of the Left Ventricle (LV) in cardiac Magnetic Resonance Images (MRI), where the overlap between the intensity distributions within the heart myocardium and the background can be modeled accurately with a Gaussian distribution. Finally, we show a representative sample of the tests with Computed Tomography (CT) images and cardiac MRI, which illustrates the effectiveness of the proposed method.

Overlap constraint vs. likelihood prior: We first show a typical example of our extensive testing with cardiac MRI. Fig. 1 (a) depicts the expected (manual) segmentations of the LV cavity (region inside the green curve) and the myocardium (ring between the green and blue curves). Fig. 1 (b) illustrates the significant overlap between the intensity distributions of the myocardium, considered as a foreground (or object), and the background. Our purpose is to use

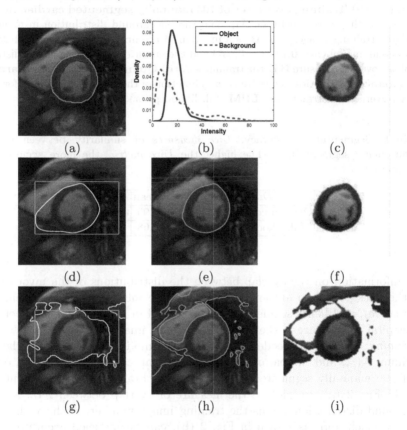

Fig. 1. A typical example of the Left Ventricle (LV) segmentation. First line: (a) expected (manual) delineations of the LV (region inside the green curve) and the myocardium (ring between the green and blue curves); (b) overlap between the intensity distributions of the myocardium and the background (region outside the green curve); (c) manual LV segmentation. Segmentation *with the overlap constraint*, i.e., with **OCM** (second line): (d) initial (green) and intermediate (yellow) curves; (e) curve obtained at convergence; (f) LV segmentation with **OCM**. Segmentation *with the likelihood prior*, i.e., with **LPM** (third line): (g) initial (green) and intermediate (yellow) curves; (h) curve obtained at convergence; (i) LV segmentation with **LPM**. $\mu = 0.72$, $\sigma = 0.037$, $\lambda = 10^3$, $\alpha = 10$, $\nu = 0.1$. *The overlap constraint prevents the curve from spilling.*

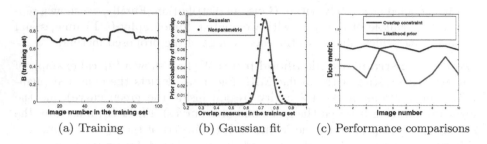

(a) Training   (b) Gaussian fit   (c) Performance comparisons

Fig. 2. (a)–(b) Training over a set of 100 manually segmented cardiac images (**B** measures the overlap between $\mathcal{M}_{in}$ and the background distribution in manually segmented training images): (a) **B** as a function of the image number; (b) fit between the Gaussian model ($\mu = \mathbf{0.72}$, $\sigma = \mathbf{0.037}$) and the empirical (nonparametric) distribution of the overlap measure **B** in the training set. **(c) Quantitative and comparative performance evaluation**: *Dice Metric* as a function of the test image number for both **OCM** (Overlap constraint) and **LPM** (Likelihood prior). $\lambda = 10^3$, $\alpha = 10$, $\nu = 0.1$.

Table 1. Segmentation accuracy: *Dice measures* of similarity between manual and automatic segmentations. The higher the *Dice metric*, the more accurate the segmentation.

Dice metrics	Mean	Std
Overlap constraint (**OCM**)	0.95	0.026
Likelihood prior (**LPM**)	0.68	0.15

prior information on the overlap between the distributions of the myocardium and the background to automatically detect the interface between them (the green curve), and hence segment the LV depicted in Fig. 1 (c). The latter task is of capital importance in the analysis of cardiac images.

Training: We first proceeded to learning the model distribution of the myocardium, $\mathcal{M}_{in}$, and the parameters of the overlap constraint, μ and σ, over a set of **100** manually segmented training images obtained from **5** different subjects. In Fig. 2 (a), we plotted the measure of overlap between $\mathcal{M}_{in}$ and the background distribution versus the training image number. Such overlap does not vary much and, as shown in Fig. 2 (b), can be modeled accurately with a Gaussian distribution. Our training yielded an overlap mean $\mu = \mathbf{0.72}$ and standard deviation $\sigma = \mathbf{0.037}$. These overlap parameters were used for all our tests on cardiac images. Note that the training images are different from the test images.

Likelihood Prior: The likelihood prior has been commonly used in image segmentation as a data term, such as in [8], [9], [21], [22], and many others. We proceeded to a comparison between the proposed method (**OCM**) and a Likelihood Prior Method (**LPM**) that corresponds to minimizing the following active curve functional:

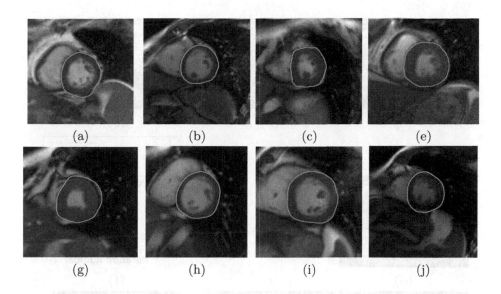

$$
\begin{array}{cccc}
\text{(a)} & \text{(b)} & \text{(c)} & \text{(e)}
\end{array}
$$

$$
\begin{array}{cccc}
\text{(g)} & \text{(h)} & \text{(i)} & \text{(j)}
\end{array}
$$

Fig. 3. A representative sample of the tests: height examples of the left ventricle segmentation. $\lambda = 10^3$, $\alpha = 10$, $\nu = 0.1$. The proposed overlap constraint prevents the curves from spilling into the background, which yielded accurate segmentation results, although no additional training-based geometric constraints were used.

$$
\mathcal{E}_{\mathbf{L}} = \underbrace{-\lambda \left(\int_{\mathbf{R}_{in}} \log \mathcal{M}_{in}(I_{\mathbf{x}}) d\mathbf{x} + \int_{\mathbf{R}_{out}} \log \mathcal{M}_{out}(I_{\mathbf{x}}) d\mathbf{x} \right)}_{Likelihood\ prior} + \alpha \oint_{\Gamma} ds + \nu \int_{\mathbf{R}_{in}} d\mathbf{x},
$$

(13)

i.e., we replaced our overlap constraint in (6) by a commonly used likelihood prior. The latter minimizes minus the image log-likelihood, i.e., maximizes the conditional probability of pixel intensity given the assumed model distributions, $\mathcal{M}_{in}$ and $\mathcal{M}_{out}$, within, respectively, the foreground and background. The same training images, segmentation examples, curve initializations, and weighting parameters were used for both methods (**OCM** and **LPM**). Note that, different from our method, **LPM** needs a prior estimation of the background model distribution $\mathcal{M}_{out}$. For the tests we run with **LPM** for comparisons, we used the actual background distribution, i.e., the correct distribution estimated from a manual segmentation of the current test image. Note that this is advantageous to **LPM** and would not bias our comparative appraisal of the proposed method.

Weighting parameters: The parameters weighting the relative contribution of the intensity terms and the regularization terms were fixed for all the experiments: $\lambda = 10^3$, $\alpha = 10$, $\nu = 0.1$.

Quantitative and comparative evaluation: The typical example in Fig. 1 demonstrates clearly the advantage of using an overlap constraint over a likelihood prior. The third line in Fig. 1 depicts segmentation results with the **LPM**.

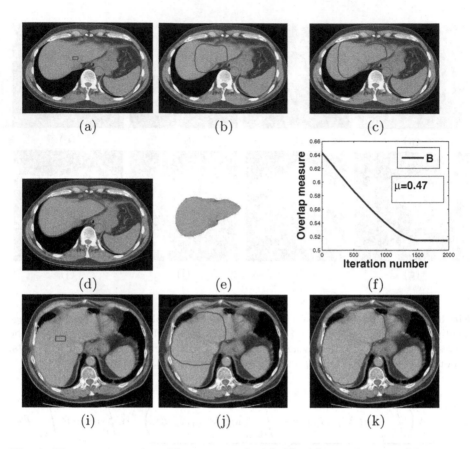

Fig. 4. Liver segmentation. **First example** (a)–(f): (a) initial curve; (b) iteration 400 (intermediate); (c) iteration 800 (intermediate); (d) iteration 1600 (final curve); (e) obtained liver segmentation; (f) evolution of the overlap measure during curve evolution: $\mathbf{B} = \mathcal{O}(\boldsymbol{\Gamma}, \mathcal{M}_{in})$ as a function of the iteration number. Overlap measure obtained at convergence: $\mathbf{B} = 0.51$. **Second example** (i)–(k): (i) initial curve; (j) intermediate curve; (k) final curve. Overlap measure obtained at convergence: $\mathbf{B} = \mathcal{O}(\boldsymbol{\Gamma}, \mathcal{M}_{in}) = 0.50$. Parameters for both examples: $\mu = 0.47$, $\sigma = 0.03$ (μ and σ were learned from 6 images). $\lambda = 10^3$, $\alpha = 10$, $\nu = 0.1$.

Fig. 1 (g) shows initial (green) and intermediate (yellow) curves. The final curve at convergence with the **LPM** is displayed in Fig. 1 (h), and the corresponding left ventricle segmentation in (i). As expected, parts of the background, which have intensity profiles similar to the myocardium, were included inside the final curve. The result with the **LPM** is affected by the significant overlap between the distributions of the myocardium and the background (Fig. 1 (b)). By contrast, the proposed method delineated accurately the left ventricle (Fig. 1 e) and yielded a result (Fig. 1 (f)) which is very similar to the manual segmentation (Fig. 1 (c)). The proposed overlap constraint prevents the curve from spilling into the background, thereby relaxing the need of complex geometric training. Initial (green) and intermediate (yellow) curves are depicted in (d).

To demonstrate that the overlap constraint is an effective alternative to the likelihood prior, we proceeded to a *quantitative* and *comparative* performance evaluation over a representative number of experiments. We run tests with both **OCM** and **LPM** on 10 cardiac MR images obtained from 10 different subjects. Performance analysis was carried out by assessing the similarities between automatic segmentations, obtained with both **OCM** and **LPM**, and independent manual segmentations approved by a radiologist. We used the *Dice Metric (DM)* to measure the *similarity* between manual and automatic segmentations. Let $\mathbf{A}_a$, $\mathbf{A}_m$ and $\mathbf{A}_{am}$ be the areas of, respectively, the automatically detected region, the corresponding hand-labeled region and the intersection between them. *DM* is given by $\frac{2\mathbf{A}_{am}}{\mathbf{A}_a+\mathbf{A}_m}$. Area measurements are expressed as the number of pixels within the region. Note that *DM* is always in $[0, 1]$, where *DM* equal to 1 indicates a perfect match between manual and automatic segmentation. Our method yielded a *DM* equal to 0.95 ± 0.026, whereas **LPM** gave a *DM* equal to 0.68 ± 0.15 (refer to table 1). *DM* is expressed as mean $\pm$ standard deviation. Fig. 2 (c) plots the obtained *DM* as a function of the test image number for both **LPM** and **OCM**. The higher *DM*, the more accurate the segmentation result. *Using the same training images, curve initializations, and weighting parameters for both methods, the proposed method (**OCM**) outperforms significantly **LPM**.*

A representative sample of the tests: Here following a representative sample of the results obtained with the proposed method in two challenging segmentation tasks: left ventricle segmentation in MRI and liver segmentation in Computed Tomography (CT) images.

Left ventricle segmentation in MRI: In Fig. 3, we give a representative sample of the tests we run with cardiac images for visual inspection. The green curve represents Γ at convergence. The proposed overlap constraint prevents the active curves from spilling into the background, which yielded accurate left ventricle segmentation results, although no additional training-based geometric constraints were used.

Liver segmentation in CT images: Liver segmentation is challenging and has recently attracted research attention [25]. We applied our method to liver segmentation in CT images. The overlap constraint parameters were learned from six training images independent from the test images: $\mu = 0.47$ and $\sigma = 0.03$. Fig. 4 depicts two typical examples. For the first example, initial curve, two intermediate steps, and the curve obtained at convergence are shown, respectively, in Figs. 4 (a), (b), (c), and (d). The obtained liver is depicted in (e). In Fig. 4 (f), we plotted the optimized overlap measure, $\mathbf{B} = \mathcal{O}(\Gamma, \mathcal{M}_{in})$, as a function of the iteration number. At convergence, the obtained overlap measure is equal to 0.51, and is close to the learned overlap mean μ. Although parts of the background have intensity profiles similar to the liver, the proposed method yielded an accurate segmentation. The second example of our tests on liver images is depicted in Figs. 4 (i)–(k). Initial curve, one intermediate step, and the curve obtained at convergence are shown, respectively, in Fig. 4 (i), (j), and (k).

The proposed method delineated accurately the liver as visual inspection can show. The overlap measure obtained at convergence is equal to **0**.50, and is also close to μ. These results demonstrate the effectiveness of the proposed method in various challenging image segmentation tasks.

4   Conclusion

We investigated a statistical overlap constraint for active curve segmentation. This led to an algorithm that relaxes the assumption of minimal overlap and, as such, is more widely applicable than existing level set algorithms. A representative number of statistical, quantitative, and comparative experiments demonstrated the desirable effects of the statistical overlap constraint.

References

1. Chan, T.F., Vese, L.A.: Active Contours without Edges. IEEE Transactions on Image Processing 10(2), 266–277 (2001)
2. Li, C., Huang, R., Ding, Z., Gatenby, C., Metaxas, D.N., Gore, J.C.: A Variational Level Set Approach to Segmentation and Bias Correction of Images with Intensity Inhomogeneity. In: Metaxas, D., Axel, L., Fichtinger, G., Székely, G. (eds.) MICCAI 2008, Part II. LNCS, vol. 5242, pp. 1083–1091. Springer, Heidelberg (2008)
3. Wang, L., Li, C., Sun, Q., Xia, D., Kao, C.-Y.: Brain MR Image Segmentation Using Local and Global Intensity Fitting Active Contours/Surfaces. In: Metaxas, D., Axel, L., Fichtinger, G., Székely, G. (eds.) MICCAI 2008, Part I. LNCS, vol. 5241, pp. 384–392. Springer, Heidelberg (2008)
4. Sun, W., Çetin, M., Chan, R., Reddy, V., Holmvang, G., Chandar, V., Willsky, A.: Segmenting and Tracking the Left Ventricle by Learning the Dynamics in Cardiac Images. In: Christensen, G.E., Sonka, M. (eds.) IPMI 2005. LNCS, vol. 3565, pp. 553–565. Springer, Heidelberg (2005)
5. Kohlberger, T., Cremers, D., Rousson, M., Ramaraj, R., Funka-Lea, G.: 4D Shape Priors for a Level Set Segmentation of the Left Myocardium in SPECT Sequences. In: Larsen, R., Nielsen, M., Sporring, J. (eds.) MICCAI 2006. LNCS, vol. 4190, pp. 92–100. Springer, Heidelberg (2006)
6. Pohl, K.M., Kikinis, R., Wells, W.M.: Active mean fields: Solving the mean field approximation in the level set framework. In: Karssemeijer, N., Lelieveldt, B. (eds.) IPMI 2007. LNCS, vol. 4584, pp. 26–37. Springer, Heidelberg (2007)
7. Tsai, A., Yezzi, A., Wells, W., Tempany, C., Tucker, D., Fan, A., Grimson, W.E., Willsky, A.: A shape-based approach to the segmentation of medical imagery using level sets. IEEE Transactions on Medical Imaging 22(2), 137–154 (2003)
8. Rousson, M., Cremers, D.: Efficient Kernel Density Estimation of Shape and Intensity Priors for Level Set Segmentation. In: Duncan, J.S., Gerig, G. (eds.) MICCAI 2005, Part I. LNCS, vol. 3749, pp. 757–764. Springer, Heidelberg (2005)
9. Paragios, N.: A Variational Approach for the Segmentation of the Left Ventricle in Cardiac Image Analysis. International Journal of Computer Vision 50(3), 345–362 (2002)
10. Cremers, D., Rousson, M., Deriche, R.: A Review of Statistical Approaches to Level Set Segmentation: Integrating Color, Texture, Motion and Shape. International Journal of Computer Vision 62, 249–265 (2007)

11. Ben Ayed, I., Mitiche, A., Belhadj, Z.: Multiregion Level Set Partitioning on Synthetic Aperture Radar Images. IEEE Transactions on Pattern Analysis and Machine Intelligence 27(5), 793–800 (2005)
12. Ben Ayed, I., Mitiche, A., Belhadj, Z.: Polarimetric Image Segmentation via Maximum Likelihood Approximation and Efficient Multiphase Level Sets. IEEE Transactions on Pattern Analysis and Machine Intelligence 28(9), 1493–1500 (2006)
13. Ben Ayed, I., Hennane, N., Mitiche, A.: Unsupervised Variational Image Segmentation/Classification using a Weibull Observation Model. IEEE Transactions on Image Processing 15, 3431–3439 (2006)
14. Rousson, M., Paragios, N.: Prior Knowledge, Level Set Representations and Visual Grouping. International Journal of Computer Vision 76(3), 231–243 (2008)
15. Michailovich, O.V., Rathi, Y., Tannenbaum, A.: Image Segmentation Using Active Contours Driven by the Bhattacharyya Gradient Flow. IEEE Transactions on Image Processing 16(11), 2787–2801 (2007)
16. Georgiou, T., Michailovich, O., Rathi, Y., Malcolm, J., Tannenbaum, A.: Distribution Metrics and Image Segmentation. Linear Algebra and its Applications 425, 663–672 (2007)
17. Kim, J., Fisher III, J.W., Yezzi, A., Cetin, M., Willsky, A.S.: A nonparametric statistical method for image segmentation using information theory and curve evolution. IEEE Transactions on Image processing 14(10), 1486–1502 (2005)
18. Zhang, T., Freedman, D.: Improving performance of distribution tracking through background mismatch. IEEE Transactions on Pattern Analysis and Machine Intelligence 27(2), 282–287 (2005)
19. Ben Ayed, I., Li, S., Ross, I.: Tracking Distributions with an Overlap Prior. In: CVPR, Anchorage, AK (2008)
20. Freedman, D., Zhang, T.: Active contours for tracking distributions. IEEE Transactions on Image Processing 13(4), 518–526 (2004)
21. Boykov, Y., Funka-Lea, G.: Graph Cuts and Efficient N-D Image Segmentation. International Journal of Computer Vision 70(2), 109–131 (2006)
22. Rother, C., Kolmogorov, V., Blake, A.: Grabcut-interactive foreground extraction using iterated graph cuts. In: SIGGRAPH 2004 (2004)
23. Ben Ayed, I., Lu, Y., Li, S., Ross, I.: Left Ventricle Tracking Using Overlap Priors. In: Metaxas, D., Axel, L., Fichtinger, G., Székely, G. (eds.) MICCAI 2008, Part I. LNCS, vol. 5241, pp. 1025–1033. Springer, Heidelberg (2008)
24. Lynch, M., Ghita, O., Whelan, P.F.: Segmentation of the Left Ventricle of the Heart in 3-D+t MRI Data Using an Optimized Nonrigid Temporal Model. IEEE Transactions on Medical Imaging 27(2), 195–203 (2008)
25. Ling, H., Kevin Zhou, S., Zheng, Y., Georgescu, B., Suehling, M., Comaniciu, D.: Hierarchical, Learning-based Automatic Liver Segmentation. In: CVPR, Anchorage, AK (2008)
26. Zhu, S.C., Yuille, A.L.: Region Competition: Unifying Snake/balloon, Region Growing and Bayes/MDL/Energy for multi-band Image Segmentation. IEEE Transactions on Pattern Analysis and Machine Intelligence 18(9), 884–900 (1996)
27. Sethian, J.: Level Set Methods and Fast Marching Methods. Cambridge University Press, Cambridge (1999)

Estimating the Confidence of Statistical Model Based Shape Prediction

Rémi Blanc[*], Ekaterina Syrkina, and Gábor Székely

Computer Vision Laboratory, ETHZ, Sternwartstrasse 7,
8092 Zürich, Switzerland
{blanc,syrkina,szekely}@vision.ee.ethz.ch

Abstract. We propose a method for estimating confidence regions around shapes predicted from partial observations, given a statistical shape model. Our method relies on the estimation of the distribution of the prediction error, obtained non-parametrically through a bootstrap resampling of a training set. It can thus be easily adapted to different shape prediction algorithms. Individual confidence regions for each landmark are then derived, assuming a Gaussian distribution. Merging those individual confidence regions, we establish the probability that, on average, a given proportion of the predicted landmarks actually lie in their estimated regions. We also propose a method for validating the accuracy of these regions using a test set.

Keywords: Statistical shape model, shape prediction, confidence regions.

1 Introduction

Statistical shape models are widely employed in medical image analysis [1]. They allow making use of prior anatomical knowledge for compensating low contrast or noise in the data. Statistical shape models are also used for regularizing elastic registration algorithms [2], so that the estimated shape is both anatomically plausible and matches the image information.

During the past years, the possibility to rely on statistical shapes models for predicting shapes from a partial observation has been extensively studied. Applications range from 3D face estimation from a partial 2D view [3], supervised segmentation for which a registration algorithm is initialized from manually positioned points on the object's surface [4,5], reconstruction of a 3D bone from sparse observations [6,7] or even from the shape of another one [8], to hierarchical segmentation of brain structures starting from the most visible structures [9]. In some cases, one can only rely on the available model without any image information about the shape to be predicted.

Different shape prediction methods have been proposed so far. A scheme proposed by [3] relies on a regularized least square estimation of the model parameters for optimally matching the predictors and preserving plausible shape parameters. Regression based approaches have also been employed, such as Canonical Correlation Analysis

---

[*] Corresponding author.

J.L. Prince, D.L. Pham, and K.J. Myers (Eds.): IPMI 2009, LNCS 5636, pp. 602–613, 2009.
© Springer-Verlag Berlin Heidelberg 2009

(CCA) in [10], or Partial Least Squares (PLS) in [9,8]. The basic idea behind these methods is to find projection directions for both the predictors and the variables to be predicted, so as to optimize a given criterion (correlation for CCA, and covariance for PLS). Those can thus be categorized as subspace methods, for which one has to choose or estimate the optimal number of modes to use, while the remaining dimensions orthogonal to this basis is considered to correspond to noise. No extensive testing has been done yet for comparing the quality of the results provided by the different methods. According to our experience, none of these methods seems to be outstandingly superior to the others, though they all require appropriate parameter tuning.

Whichever prediction method is chosen, the accuracy of such predictions can be vital in many surgical applications. For example, neurosurgical interventions such as implantation of electrodes for deep brain stimulation require an accurate localization of specific nuclei, while these are not directly visible with current imaging techniques. It is therefore highly desirable to estimate confidence regions for the provided prediction, so that appropriate safety margins can be designed when planning the intervention. Indeed, it is relatively clear that the related uncertainty is highly dependent on the available model, determined by the number of training samples, the quality of the parameterization and of the correspondences between those shapes, as well as on the degree of correlation between the observed part and the part to predict. Unfortunately, to our knowledge, no method has been published so far allowing to estimate the confidence of statistical model based shape prediction and to estimate error margins around a predicted shape.

In this paper, we propose an approach for estimating confidence regions for the predicted shape, based on an already available shape model generated from training samples, which are already aligned and parameterized in correspondence. Section 2 introduces the notations and recalls some basics about statistical shape models. Section 3 briefly presents the least square fitting algorithm proposed by [3], and develops a method to estimate the regularization parameter. Our contribution in establishing confidence regions for the shape prediction is presented in Section 4, together with a method for validating these estimations on set of test shapes. The feasibility of the approach is then demonstrated by an application example in section 5. Conclusions and perspective for future work are given in Section 6.

2   Notations and Problem Specification

Statistical shape models aim at describing the natural variability of a shape, e.g. the morphological manifestations of an organ over different individuals or through time. Such models usually rely on a specific parameterization of a set of training shapes, which consists in identifying p landmarks in correspondence in the various shapes [11]. Through this parameterization, a continuous k-dimensional shape, $k \in \{2;3\}$, is represented as a single point in a d – dimensional space, $d = kp$. A collection of different instances of a shape, e.g. the same organ observed for different individuals, then corresponds to a point cloud in the parameterized space, which contains the information about the shape's variability observed from the available samples, and which can be analyzed using multivariate statistics techniques such as PCA [12,13].

More precisely, we denote the available training shapes in their parameter space as n column vectors $\mathbf{z}_i, i \in \{1,...,n\}$, each containing d elements corresponding to the landmark coordinates. The mean shape $\mathbf{m}$ and the covariance matrix $\mathbf{S}$ representing the shapes' variability can be calculated using the classical unbiased estimators. Without loss of generality, we also re-order the elements of $\mathbf{z}$ so that the actual observations – or *predictors* - $\mathbf{x}$ are the first d_x variables, and the remaining $d_y = d - d_x$ coordinates correspond to the *dependent variables* $\mathbf{y}$ we want to predict:

$$\mathbf{m} = \frac{1}{n}\sum_{i=1}^{n}\mathbf{z}_i = \frac{1}{n}\sum_{i=1}^{n}\begin{bmatrix}\mathbf{x}_i \\ \mathbf{y}_i\end{bmatrix} = \begin{bmatrix}\mathbf{m}_x \\ \mathbf{m}_y\end{bmatrix}$$
$$\mathbf{S} = \frac{1}{n-1}\sum_{i=1}^{n}(\mathbf{z}_i - \mathbf{m})(\mathbf{z}_i - \mathbf{m})^T = \begin{bmatrix}\mathbf{S}_{xx} & \mathbf{S}_{xy} \\ \mathbf{S}_{yx} & \mathbf{S}_{yy}\end{bmatrix}$$

(1)

Since we will often have to rely on centered variables, we introduce a notation convention where a dot on top of a variable means that it is centered: $\dot{\mathbf{x}} = \mathbf{x} - \mathbf{m}_x$, etc.

The usual representation of a statistical shape model is based on the mean shape $\mathbf{m}$ and a set of orthogonal modes of variation $\mathbf{U}$, which are the eigenvectors of $\mathbf{S}$. As $\mathbf{S}$ is a $d \times d$ matrix, it can easily become extremely large for complex 3-D shapes, where more than 10^5 landmarks may be needed for achieving a reasonably detailed characterization. In such cases, even the storage of $\mathbf{S}$ can become problematic. Fortunately, the Singular Value Decomposition (SVD) of $\dot{\mathbf{Z}} = [\dot{\mathbf{z}}_1 \ \dot{\mathbf{z}}_2 \ ... \ \dot{\mathbf{z}}_n] = \mathbf{U}\mathbf{D}\mathbf{V}^T$ provides the sought eigenvectors $\mathbf{U}$, while the singular values $\mathbf{D}$ are directly related to the eigenvalues $\mathbf{\Lambda} = \mathbf{D}\mathbf{D}^T / (n-1)$ of $\mathbf{S}$. Moreover, as only at most $n-1$ eigenvalues are non-zero, the size of the model can remain acceptable. The dimensionality of the model is usually even further reduced by keeping only the first r modes representing e.g. 95% of the total variance.

The retained modes of deformation $\mathbf{U}$ allow to define a linear model space, where any shape $\mathbf{z}$ can be approximately represented by a set of parameters $\mathbf{b} = \mathbf{U}^T\dot{\mathbf{z}}$. The residual representation error $\mathbf{\eta} = \dot{\mathbf{z}} - \mathbf{U}\mathbf{b}$ indicates how well the shape can be be described by the selected model. This error is minimized for the shapes in the training set. The domain covered by the eigenvectors and the distribution of the PCA parameters observed on the training shapes represent the available knowledge about shape variability. When assuming Gaussian distribution, the classical rule of thumb is that a shape is plausible if each of its parameters $\mathbf{b}_i$ lies in the $[-3\sigma_i; +3\sigma_i]$ interval, σ_i^2 being the ith eigenvalue of the model.

3 Shape Prediction by Fitting Model Parameters

In the following, we present a shape prediction method similar to the one proposed in [3], using the notations introduced above. Given a potentially noisy, partial observation $\mathbf{x}$, a sensible approach is to find optimal parameters $\mathbf{b}^*$ for the statistical shape model so that the predicted shape fits the observed points as closely as possible. If we decompose $\mathbf{U} = [\mathbf{U}_x; \mathbf{U}_y]$, according to the predictors and independent variables, the sought parameters can be obtained by the following minimization:

$$\mathbf{b}_\lambda^* = \underset{\mathbf{b}}{Argmin} \left(\|\mathbf{U}_x \mathbf{b} - \dot{\mathbf{x}}\| + \lambda \mathbf{b}^T \Lambda^{-1} \mathbf{b} \right) = \left(\mathbf{U}_x^T \mathbf{U}_x + \lambda \Lambda^{-1} \right)^{-1} \mathbf{U}_x^T \dot{\mathbf{x}} \qquad (2)$$

where λ is an additional regularization hyper-parameter introduced to avoid problems of potentially ill-conditioned matrix inversion, and the over-fitting of the predictors. The matrix Λ of the retained non-zero eigenvalues of $\mathbf{S}$ is employed so as to give equivalent weights to the different PCA parameters. The resulting predicted shape $\hat{\mathbf{z}}_\lambda$ is the one which both best fits the observation and which is still plausible given the shape model.

$$\hat{\mathbf{z}}_\lambda = \mathbf{U}\mathbf{b}_\lambda^* + \mathbf{m} \qquad (3)$$

The iterative LSQR algorithm [14] can also be used, but the algorithm needs to be stopped before convergence to avoid over-fitting, which allow only a coarse control over the regularization and cannot generally achieve shape optimality.

A practical approach for tuning a hyper-parameter is cross-validation, i.e. to generate numerous models based on different subsets of the original collection of training shapes. For every such replicate, shapes that were not included in the model generation can be used for prediction, and thus provide samples allowing to estimate the prediction error $\varepsilon_\lambda = \hat{\mathbf{z}}_\lambda - \mathbf{z}$. Different strategies can be employed here, such as bootstrap, jackknife or leaving multiple samples out for each replicate [15].

The optimal regularization parameter λ^* is then estimated by minimizing the average norm of the prediction error, i.e.:

$$\lambda^* = \underset{\lambda}{Argmin} \left(\|\varepsilon_\lambda\| \right) \qquad (4)$$

4 Confidence Regions

In many applications, e.g. related to navigated surgery, it is essential to provide not only the predicted shape, but also information about the uncertainty of the prediction. Obviously, the corresponding confidence region should be as small as possible but most importantly provide correct information about the probability that it effectively contains the true shape. The first problem is addressed by selecting the optimal regularization hyper-parameter of the prediction. Indeed, a sub-optimal selection would lead to a larger prediction error on average, and thus to enlarged uncertainty margins.

In general, a confidence region with significance level α defines a region in space which has a *nominal probability* $1 - \alpha$ to cover the true shape. In practice, those confidence regions can only be estimated, and several factors may affect the quality of this estimate. Among those factors are the relevance of the chosen model, the number of samples used to create it, the prediction method selected and the quality of the predictors. As a consequence, the *effective probability* $1 - \hat{\alpha}$ that the estimated region actually contains the true shape may be different from the nominal probability $1 - \alpha$ introduced above. In the ideal case $\alpha = \hat{\alpha}$, the confidence regions are said to be *nominal*. If

$1 - \hat{\alpha} > 1 - \alpha$, then the confidence region is broader than necessary, and the estimate will be called *under-confident*. As long as the uncertainty is not becoming excessively large, this case may not be critical from the clinical point of view. On the other hand, $1 - \hat{\alpha} < 1 - \alpha$ implies that the generated confidence region is too small, i.e. *over-confident*, and what we would consider as being a safe localization may prove to be an erroneous guess. Such a situation should be avoided by all means, or at least properly detected, as it can seriously threaten treatment success. Unfortunately, this effective probability $1 - \hat{\alpha}$ also has to be determined, requiring further independent test samples.

4.1 Confidence Regions around Individual Landmarks

Following the non-parametric resampling presented in section 3, we extract a collection of samples for estimating the prediction error ε_{λ^*} when using the optimal regularization parameter λ^*. Assuming a multivariate Gaussian distribution for ε_{λ^*} with $\mathbf{0}$ mean and $d \times d$ covariance matrix $\mathbf{E}$, the confidence region $C_\alpha(\hat{\mathbf{z}})$ around the optimal predicted shape $\hat{\mathbf{z}}_{\lambda^*} = \hat{\mathbf{z}}$, with significance level α, is the interior of a d-dimensional ellipsoid centered around $\hat{\mathbf{z}}$, with axes defined by the eigenvalue decomposition of $\mathbf{E}$, and satisfying:

$$P\left[\mathbf{z} \in C_\alpha(\hat{\mathbf{z}})\right] = 1 - \alpha \tag{5}$$

Decreasing α values result in growing homothetic ellipsoids. When taking a random sample from the Gaussian distribution of mean $\hat{\mathbf{z}}$ and covariance $\mathbf{E}$, the probability $1 - \alpha$ that it falls within $C_\alpha(\hat{\mathbf{z}})$ is equal to the integral of the probability density function over the interior of this ellipsoid. The boundary of this ellipsoid is defined by the set of d-dimensional points $\boldsymbol{\rho}$ which have a constant Mahalanobis distance D_α to the mean $\hat{\mathbf{z}}$:

$$D_\alpha = \sqrt{(\boldsymbol{\rho} - \hat{\mathbf{z}})^T \mathbf{E}^{-1} (\boldsymbol{\rho} - \hat{\mathbf{z}})} \tag{6}$$

Therefore, the sought integral can be calculated from the cumulative χ^2 distribution function with d degrees of freedom [13, p.86], noted $K\left(D_\alpha^2, d\right)$:

$$1 - \alpha = K\left(D_\alpha^2, d\right) = \frac{\gamma\left(D_\alpha^2/2, d/2\right)}{\Gamma(d/2)} \tag{7}$$

where Γ is the gamma function, γ is the lower incomplete gamma function.

Conversely, for a given significance level α, the confidence region $C_\alpha(\hat{\mathbf{z}})$ is defined as the interior of the ellipsoid centered on $\hat{\mathbf{z}}$, with axes defined by $\mathbf{E}$, and with Mahalanobis 'radius' D_α:

$$D_\alpha^2 = K^{-1}(1 - \alpha, d) \tag{8}$$

Unfortunately, the confidence region estimation procedure described above requires the ability to estimate the large $d \times d$ covariance matrix $\mathbf{E}$. Considering that, under realistic conditions where the number of samples n will be much smaller than the number of variables d, estimates will certainly be rank-deficient, the problem of its inversion becomes even more problematic. Completely non-parametric confidence regions could, in theory, be produced e.g. by calculating a kernel density for ε_{λ^*} with an optimized multivariate bandwidth [16]. However, to our knowledge, no algorithm is available, which can be used for such high dimensional distributions.

Nonetheless, even for very high number of parameters, we can always calculate the $k \times k$ marginal covariance matrices $\{\mathbf{E}_i ; i = 1..p\}$ about each predicted landmark $\hat{\ell}_i$. These can be used to estimate individual confidence regions $C_\alpha^{(i)}(\hat{\ell}_i)$ for the true landmarks ℓ_i of the shape, using the same methodology as presented above.

4.2 Overall Confidence for Shape Prediction

The stochastic event $\ell_i \in C_\alpha^{(i)}(\hat{\ell}_i)$ will be denoted by $A_\alpha^{(i)}$. $1(A_\alpha^{(i)})$ is its indicative function, which takes value 1 when the event is true, and 0 otherwise. $1(A_\alpha^{(i)})$ follows a Bernoulli distribution with parameter $P[1(A_\alpha^{(i)}) = 1] = 1 - \alpha$, so its expected value is also $E[1(A_\alpha^{(i)})] = 1 - \alpha$. For any given shape, the portion of its landmarks which are effectively within their own α − confidence region is denoted $\pi_\alpha = \sum_{i=1}^{p} 1(A_\alpha^{(i)}) / p$.

A proper way to define a global confidence for the full shape $\mathbf{z}$ is then to calculate the probability β that at least a portion τ of its landmarks ℓ_i are actually within $C_\alpha^{(i)}(\hat{\ell}_i)$, that is:

$$P[\pi_\alpha \geq \tau] = \beta \qquad (9)$$

Unfortunately, examining the full distribution of π_α and estimating β requires knowledge of the full joint distribution of the events $A_\alpha^{(i)}$. We can nonetheless state that, on average, for any significance level α, a portion $1 - \alpha$ of the true landmarks shall be within their estimated confidence region:

$$E[\pi_\alpha] = E\left[\frac{1}{p} \sum_{i=1}^{p} 1(A_\alpha^{(i)})\right] = 1 - \alpha \qquad (10)$$

The average portion $E[\pi_\alpha] = 1 - \alpha$ of correctly estimated landmarks, at significance level α, will be considered as the nominal level of the overall confidence region for the predicted shape, which is defined by the collection of the individual regions $C_\alpha^{(i)}(\hat{\ell}_i)$.

4.3 Validation of the Confidence Regions

As discussed in the beginning of section 4, the confidence regions calculated above are only estimates, and thus may not correspond exactly to their *nominal* significance level. Thus, it is necessary to validate the resulting uncertainty margins by estimating their *effective* significance level, and compare it to the nominal value. This validation has to be done on a *test set*, for which the number of shapes is noted n_{test}.

For each test shape $\mathbf{z}_j$, we can compute the α − confidence regions $C_\alpha^{(i)}(\hat{\ell}_{i,j})$ for each of its landmarks as described above. The probability that the true landmark $\ell_{i,j}$

is within its estimated region can be estimated as the effective frequency $1 - \hat{\alpha}^{(i)}$ with which this happens for the n_{test} test shapes:

$$1 - \hat{\alpha}^{(i)} = \frac{1}{n_{test}} \sum_{j=1}^{n_{test}} 1\left(\ell_{i,j} \in C_{\alpha}^{(i)}\left(\hat{\ell}_{i,j}\right)\right) \xrightarrow[n_{test} \to \infty]{} P\left[\ell_i \in C_{\alpha}^{(i)}\left(\hat{\ell}_i\right)\right] \tag{11}$$

Similarly, we can observe for each test shape z_j the effective portion of its landmarks $\hat{\pi}_{\alpha}^{(j)} = \sum_{i=1}^{p} 1(\ell_{i,j} \in C_{\alpha}^{(i)}(\hat{\ell}_{i,j}))/p$ which actually fall within their estimated region. The sample mean $\hat{\pi}_{\alpha}$ over all test shapes will estimate the effective average portion of landmarks which are correctly estimated:

$$\hat{\pi}_{\alpha} = \frac{1}{n_{test}} \sum_{j=1}^{n_{test}} \hat{\pi}_{\alpha}^{(j)} \xrightarrow[n_{test} \to \infty]{} E\left[\frac{1}{p} \sum_{i=1}^{p} 1(A_{\alpha}^{(i)})\right] \tag{12}$$

The quality of the estimated confidence regions can then be validated through the comparison between the *effective* values $1 - \hat{\alpha}^{(i)}$, and $\hat{\pi}_{\alpha}$ and their *nominal* value $1 - \alpha$. For the practical applicability on the method, it is perhaps even more important to validate the quality of the confidence regions for each individual test shape, through the *effective* portions $\hat{\pi}_{\alpha}^{(j)}$, which are stochastic variable that can clearly deviate from their expected value $(1 - \alpha)$. If for some test shapes, the corresponding proportion $\hat{\pi}_{\alpha}^{(j)}$ takes values significantly lower than the expected $1 - \alpha$, then the estimated confidence regions would be misleading and potentially dangerous to use.

However, even in such a case, it could still be possible to detect when the confidence region may be erroneous. Indeed, up to now, we treated the predictors x and the originally unseen variables y equally. Observing how the model is able to represent the predictors should provide information about the overall quality of the prediction. It is indeed likely that if the model cannot find a shape that matches closely the predictors, the rest of the shape may also be difficult to predict accurately. It is thus sensible to analyze the correlation between the error $\|x_j - \hat{x}_j\|$ and the deviation $\hat{\pi}_{\alpha}^{(j)} - (1 - \alpha)$. If one finds a large negative correlation between those values, then it should still be possible to detect individual cases for which the estimated regions could be misleading.

5   Results

In this section, we illustrate our concepts on a statistical shape model consisting of a total of 71 samples of corpus callosum outlines, obtained from manual delineations on 2-D mid-sagittal MR images, parameterized with $p = 258$ landmarks in correspondence, leading to $d = 516$ variables [5]. Two of these landmarks correspond to the Anterior (AC) and Posterior (PC) Commissures and are used for aligning the shapes in translation and rotation. As the original images are of similar resolution, no scaling has been applied. We retained $n = 50$ shapes for training the statistical shape model, and kept the $n_{test} = 21$ remaining shapes for validation.

The estimation of the model parameters $\mathbf{U}$ and Λ where done using SVD as described in section 2. The importance of the regularization parameter λ is demonstrated on Fig. 1, where Fig. 1(a) illustrates over-fitting if no regularization is used ($\lambda = 0$), and Fig. 1(b) shows the shape predicted using the optimal parameter λ^*. The resampling procedure chosen for estimating the distribution of the prediction error was a classical bootstrapping approach. We generated 500 bootstrap replicate sets, each composed of $n = 50$ shapes drawn with replacement from the original set of training shapes. A replicate set contained about 32 different shapes on average. For each replicate, we obtained samples for the prediction error by investigating the shapes excluded. The total number of predicted samples obtained from this procedure was around 9000 on average.

Having defined the bootstrap replicate sets, the value λ^* was estimated simply by varying λ, and choosing the value which minimizes the average norm of the prediction error $\|\boldsymbol{\varepsilon}_\lambda\| = \|\hat{\mathbf{z}}_\lambda - \mathbf{z}\|$, with $\hat{\mathbf{z}}_\lambda$ defined by (3), averaged over the available prediction samples. As can be seen in Fig. 1(c), the norm of the prediction error $\|\boldsymbol{\varepsilon}_\lambda\|$ is varying rather smoothly, so this simple selection method should lead to a value very close to optimal. Fig. 1(c) also shows that the prediction is not very sensitive to the removal of a few modes with low eigenvalues. We nonetheless kept all the available modes in the following experiments.

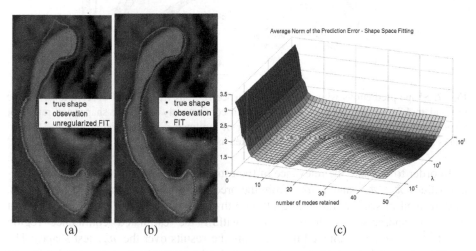

(a)   (b)   (c)

Fig. 1. (a) Illustration of over-fitting using $\lambda = 0$, (b) regularized estimation using λ^*. (c) Average norm of the prediction error as a function of the number of modes retained and λ.

From the results obtained using the optimal λ^*, we could then estimate the marginal covariance matrices $\{\mathbf{E}_i ; i = 1..p\}$, and the $\alpha-$ confidence regions around each landmark, as described in section 4.1. Fig. 2 presents the union of such confidence regions, estimated for three different choices of the predictors and dependent variables. As expected, the confidence regions are much wider around the independent variables than around the predictors.

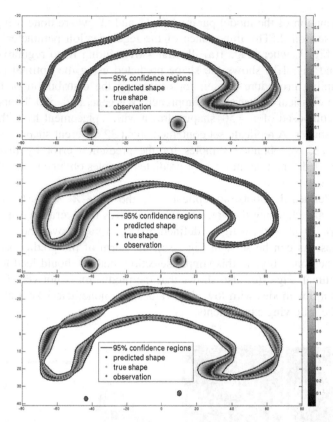

Fig. 2. Shape predictions with union of confidence regions from partial observations. On the top and middle figures, the predictors are taken continuously along the shape, and represent respectively 80% and 60% of the total number of landmarks. On the bottom figure, 15 landmarks scattered around the shape have been taken as predictors.

In order to validate the relevance of the estimated regions, we computed the *effective* values $\hat{\pi}_\alpha$, $\hat{\pi}_\alpha^{(j)}$ and $1-\hat{\alpha}^{(i)}$ from the prediction results on the set of test shapes, as described in section 4.3. We recall here that $1-\hat{\alpha}^{(i)}$ indicates the probability that the true landmark i effectively lies within the estimated confidence region $\ell_i \in C_\alpha^{(i)}(\hat{\ell}_i)$, and is computed by averaging the results over the n_{test} test shapes. The quantity $\hat{\pi}_\alpha^{(j)}$ indicates, for a given shape j, the percentage of its true landmarks which are correctly estimated. Finally, $\hat{\pi}_\alpha$ corresponds to the average result over both the individual landmarks and the test shapes. The comparisons between these values and the *nominal* level $1-\alpha$ are displayed on Fig. 3. As can be seen on Fig. 3, the estimated regions appear to have a tendency for under-confidence ($\hat{\pi}_\alpha \geq \alpha$), i.e. they are slightly larger than necessary. Nevertheless, for most test shapes, the proportion $\hat{\pi}_\alpha^{(j)}$ of landmarks correctly predicted is almost always larger or equal than expected, even at the highest probability levels, which is probably the most important for defining proper security margins in surgery. Consequently, such results indicate that the estimated confidence regions are clinically useful.

Nonetheless, without questioning the validity of the estimated confidence regions, the detailed results from Fig. 3 need to be commented further, especially concerning $\hat{\pi}_\alpha^{(j)}$ and $1 - \hat{\alpha}^{(i)}$. As shapes are usually relatively smooth, neighboring landmarks are likely to be highly correlated. It is therefore probable that if the confidence region for one given landmark diverges from its nominal level, the same will happen for its neighbors. Consequently, the fact that we neglected the inter-landmark correlations significantly increases the variance of the $\hat{\pi}_\alpha^{(j)}$.

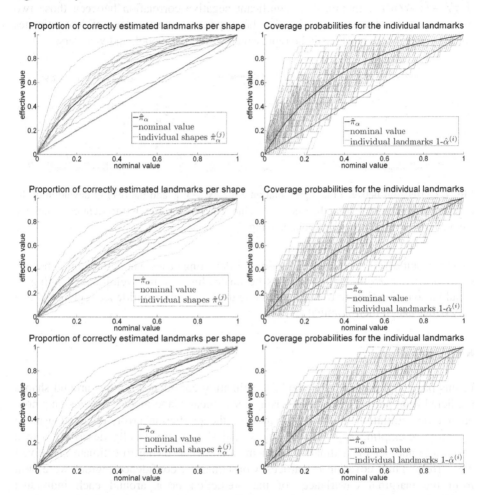

Fig. 3. The left column indicates the values $\hat{\pi}_\alpha^{(j)}$, and on the right are displayed the $1 - \hat{\alpha}^{(i)}$. The average, $\hat{\pi}_\alpha$, is displayed on both. On every image, the diagonal represents the nominal value $1 - \alpha$. The plots from top to bottom correspond to the same choices of predictors as in Fig. 2.

Concerning the individual $1 - \hat{\alpha}^{(i)}$, besides the fact that they are estimated only a finite set of n_{test} test shapes, an important reason why they can diverge from their nominal values is that the individual confidence regions $C_\alpha^{(i)}\left(\hat{\ell}_i\right)$ are derived from the estimated distribution of the prediction error, which bases on an insufficiently representative training set. As more samples are used, the model should better represent the true shape distribution, and these regions should converge towards their nominal level. Nonetheless, the right column of Fig. 3 shows that the confidence regions tend to be larger than necessary for most landmarks, and they are too narrow for only a small minority of them (curves which go below the diagonal).

As proposed in section 4.3, we also investigated, for the test shapes, the correlation between $\|\mathbf{x}_j - \hat{\mathbf{x}}_j\|$ and a global measure of the deviation of $\hat{\pi}_\alpha^{(j)}$ from $1 - \alpha$, namely $\int_0^1 \hat{\pi}_\alpha^{(j)} - (1 - \alpha) d\alpha$. In Fig. 4, a significant negative correlation between those two measures can be observed, meaning that the shapes with most underconfident estimates are those which can most easily be represented within the model, and vice versa.

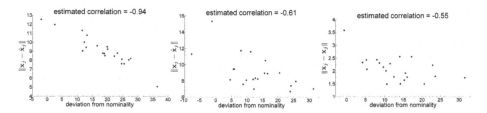

Fig. 4. Correlation between the representation error $\|\mathbf{x}_j - \hat{\mathbf{x}}_j\|$ and the overall deviation of the confidence regions $\hat{\pi}_\alpha^{(j)}$ from their nominal value. The images from left to right correspond to the predictor settings from top to bottom in Fig. 2.

This result offers an interesting option for detecting cases where the confidence regions are too narrow, and could thus be misleading for interventional planning. It should also be possible to use this for tuning the size of the confidence regions, so that they better match their nominal level.

6 Conclusion

In this paper, we propose a method for estimating confidence regions around shapes predicted from partial observations using a statistical shape model. It relies on a non-parametric estimation of the distribution of the prediction error, obtained using a bootstrap resampling approach. As individual shapes are usually described with a very large number of landmarks, problems arise when trying to estimate and invert the corresponding covariance matrices. Consequently, confidence regions were built from the marginal covariances of the prediction error around each individual landmark, assuming a Gaussian distribution. By combining these individual regions, we derived the probability that a given portion of landmarks would be correctly estimated, i.e. truly lying within their own confidence region. Validation on a test set showed that the obtained confidence regions are generally slightly larger than necessary. However, this can be considered as a safeguard when establishing security margins in surgery, at least as long as the regions are not excessively large. Moreover, significant negative correlation has been found between the ability of the shape model to represent the observed part of the shape to predict and the quality of the predicted confidence regions, indicating that the shapes which can be most accurately represented by the model are also those for which the predictions are the most underconfident.

Paths for future work include the refinement of the estimated confidence regions, in particular by taking into account the ability of the model to represent a given partial shape observation. Considering correlations between landmarks should also help in more accurately estimating the confidence regions. Another direction should be the incorporation of assumed uncertainties about the predictors and of possible errors in establishing the correspondences between the individual shapes. Uncertainties related to the estimation of the rigid registration parameters, i.e. translation, rotation and possibly scaling should also be evaluated.

References

1. Cootes, T.F., Edwards, G.J., Taylor, C.J.: Active Appearance models. In: Burkhardt, H., Neumann, B. (eds.) ECCV 1998. LNCS, vol. 1407, pp. 484–498. Springer, Heidelberg (1998)
2. Kelemen, A., Székely, G., Gerig, G.: Elastic model-based segmentation of 3-D neuroradiological data sets. IEEE Trans. on Medical Imaging 18(10), 828–839 (1999)
3. Blanz, V., Vetter, T.: Reconstructing the Complete 3D Shape of Faces from Partial Information. Informationstechnik und Technische Informatik 44(6), 295–302 (2002)
4. Bailleul, J., Ruan, S., Constans, J.-M.: Statistical shape model-based segmentation of brain MRI images. In: Proc. IEEE 29th EMBS, pp. 5255–5258 (2007)
5. Hug, J., Brechbühler, C., Szekely, G.: Model-Based Initialisation for Segmentation. In: Vernon, D. (ed.) ECCV 2000. LNCS, vol. 1843, pp. 290–306. Springer, Heidelberg (2000)
6. Zheng, G.: A robust and accurate approach for reconstruction of patient-specific 3D bone models from sparse point sets. In: Proc. SPIE, vol. 6509 (2007)
7. Rajamani, K.T., Hug, J., Nolte, L.-P., Styner, M.: Bone Morphing with statistical shape models for enhanced visualization. In: Proc. SPIE, vol. 5367, pp. 122–130 (2004)
8. Yang, Y.M., Rueckert, D., Bull, A.M.J.: Predicting the shapes of bones at a joint: application to the shoulder. Computer Methods in Biomechanics and Biomedical Engineering 11(1), 19–30 (2008)
9. Rao, A., Aljabar, P., Rueckert, D.: Hierarchical statistical shape analysis and prediction of sub-cortical brain structures. Medical Image Analysis 12, 55–68 (2008)
10. Liu, T., Shen, D., Davatzikos, C.: Predictive Modeling of Anatomic Structures using Canonical Correlation Analysis. In: Proc. ISBI, pp. 1279–1282 (2004)
11. Styner, M., Rajamani, K.T., Nolte, L.-P., Zsemlye, G., Székely, G., Taylor, C.J., Davies, R.H.: Evaluation of 3D Correspondence Methods for Model Building. In: Taylor, C.J., Noble, J.A. (eds.) IPMI 2003. LNCS, vol. 2732, pp. 63–75. Springer, Heidelberg (2003)
12. Cooley, W.W., Lohnes, P.R.: Multivariate Data Analysis. J. Wiley & Sons, NY (1971)
13. Rencher, A.C.: Methods of Multivariate Analysis, 2nd edn. Wiley Series in Probability and Statistics. J. Wiley & Sons, Chichester (2003)
14. Paige, C., Saunders, M.: LSQR: An Algorithm for Sparse Linear Equations and Sparse Least Squares. ACM Trans. Math. Softw. 8(1), 43–71 (1982)
15. Efron, B.: Nonparametric estimates of standard error: The jackknife, the bootstrap and other methods. Biometrika 68, 589–599 (1981)
16. Zhang, X., King, M.L., Hyndman, R.J.: Bandwidth Selection for Multivariate Kernel Density using MCMC. Econometric Society, Australasian Meetings 120 (2004)

Oriented Morphometry of Folds on Surfaces

Maxime Boucher[1,*], Alan Evans[2], and Kaleem Siddiqi[1]

[1] School of Computer Science, McGill University, Canada
boucher@bic.mni.mcgill.ca
[2] McConnell Brain Imaging Center, Montreal Neurological Institute, McGill
University, Canada

Abstract. The exterior surface of the brain is characterized by a juxtaposition of crests and troughs that together form a folding pattern.
The majority of the deformations that occur in the normal course of
adult human development result in folds changing their length or width.
Current statistical shape analysis methods cannot easily discriminate
between these two cases. Using discrete exterior calculus and Tikhonov
regularization, we develop a method to estimate a dense orientation field
in the tangent space of a surface described by a triangulated mesh, in the
direction of its folds. We then use this orientation field to distinguish between shape differences in the direction parallel to folds and those in the
direction across them. We test the method quantitatively on synthetic
data and qualitatively on a database consisting of segmented cortical
surfaces of 92 healthy subjects and 97 subjects with Alzheimer's disease.
The method estimates the correct fold directions and also indicates that
the healthy and diseased subjects are distinguished by shape differences
that are in the direction perpendicular to the underlying hippocampi,
a finding which is consistent with the neuroscientific literature. These
results demonstrate the importance of direction specific computational
methods for shape analysis.

1 Introduction

The exterior surface of the human brain has a characteristic shape formed by a
collection of folds. A fold can be described in loose terms as an oriented structure
where the surface curvature has a greater magnitude in the direction perpendicular to its orientation than in the direction parallel to it. The study of the shape
of folds on surfaces is particularly relevant in medical imaging. For example, it
has been hypothesized by [1] that folds on the exterior surface of the brain are
the result of the underlying mechanical tensions that force the surface to sink
at certain locations. Thus, numerous mechanical models have been developed to
analyze the shape of folding patterns and to find correlations among particular
folds as a function of disease or other factors, such as age [2–5].

---

* Corresponding author.

J.L. Prince, D.L. Pham, and K.J. Myers (Eds.): IPMI 2009, LNCS 5636, pp. 614–625, 2009.
© Springer-Verlag Berlin Heidelberg 2009

If one wishes to mathematically characterize the variability of surface shape in a population, a statistical shape model must be used and two ingredients are necessary. The first is a notion of the average shape and the second is an appropriate metric to provide a distance measure between two exemplars. In the case of brain imaging, the cortical surface is often represented as a single surface and continuous deformation models are built using diffeomorphic maps to match the fold on each exemplar surface with those on a population average. Several metrics has been proposed to describe how two surfaces are locally dissimilar (see e.g. [3, 6, 7]). These metrics however lack specificity when it comes to differentiating between a deformation that occurs in the direction parallel to a fold and one in the direction perpendicular to it. Certain shape differences, such as a relative depth difference between two folds, can only occur when the spacing between two consecutive crests is altered. Thus, in the context of medical image analysis, the interpretation of the results can strongly depend on the orientation of the shape deformation.

To address the above problem, we develop a method to estimate a dense orientation field on a surface, such that it is optimally oriented along the direction of its folds[1]. A fold on a surface is comprised by locations where the principal curvature is high in the direction perpendicular to it, and is low in the direction along it. We thus use this description of a fold to estimate an orientation field using Tikhonov regularization. The approach we develop is motivated by the literature on smoothing direction fields in images, such as the techniques in [8–10]. These methods cannot be directly applied to our problem. For example, in the method in [8] the underlying vector field is embedded in Euclidean space whereas we need to embed the orientation field into the tangent space of the surface. For this purpose, we use the discrete exterior calculus framework of [11] to develop a simple computational method for a discrete triangulated mesh. The triangles provide an estimate of the tangent space and the orientation field is embedded within each triangle. The mesh surface is then unfolded locally to solve the variational problem. Once the orientation field is found, we provide a statistical measure of shape difference to determine if two folds differ in length or in width.

We validate our approach quantitatively on synthetic surfaces, where the underlying ground truth fold orientation is known, and qualitatively on a database comprised of a combination of cortical surfaces of healthy subjects and those of patients with Alzheimer's disease. We find that on a surface with known ground-truth, the estimated orientation fields follow the expected orientation. We then provide a metric for oriented shape differences and test this metric on the population affected by Alzheimer's disease. We find that the hippocampi are atrophied ($p < 0.001$) in the direction perpendicular to an associated fold, which is consistent with the neuroscientific literature. Our results thus imply that increased specificity is achieved by orienting the analysis of shape difference.

---

[1] In this paper, a direction field is a vector field where all vectors are constrained to have unit length. An orientation field is a direction field where opposing vectors are considered equivalent.

2   Finding the Orientation of Folds

We begin by developing an energy functional which when minimized results in a smooth orientation field on a surface, which follows the direction of a folding pattern. To get an intuitive sense of our goals, consider Fig. 1 which illustrates a portion of a cortical surface. A crest (or ridge) is shown in red, with a nearby parallel trough (or valley) in yellow. A fold is characterized by a juxtaposition of crests and troughs with the same orientation. In the case of the human brain this is an approximation that is correct for the most part, except at pattern singularities. The dense orientation field estimated by our method corresponds to the local orientation of crests and troughs. In Section 2.2 we describe how our solution can be discretized and solved numerically on a triangulated mesh. Then, in Section 2.3, we present a statistical shape model which uses the estimated orientation field to differentiate between shape differences which occur in the direction of a fold and those which occur across it.

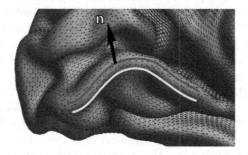

Fig. 1. A dense orientation field that follows crests and troughs

2.1   A Minimum Principal Curvature Orientation Field

We first develop a mathematical model of a fold on a surface. Consider a Riemannian manifold $(\mathcal{S}, g)$, where g is a Riemannian metric. Let the unit normal vector to the surface be $\mathbf{n}$. Let $\mathbf{v}$ be a vector field tangent to the surface $\mathcal{S}$ and let ∇ be the torsion-free affine connection on $\mathcal{S}$. Using this notation, the associated covariant derivative along $\mathbf{v}$ is $\nabla_{\mathbf{v}}$ and the shape operator $S(\mathbf{v})$ is given by $\nabla_{\mathbf{v}}\mathbf{n}$. Covariant derivation being a linear operation, with a slight abuse in notation the action of the shape operator S on the vector field can be expressed as

$$S(\mathbf{v}) = S\mathbf{v}. \tag{1}$$

Because the affine connection ∇ is torsion free, the second fundamental form is symmetric, i.e., $S = S^t$.

We first define an orientation field on a surface and provide a differentiable metric on orientation fields, which will later be used to set up an appropriate variation problem. Let a unit-norm vector field within the tangent space of the surface $\mathcal{S}$ be defined such that the norm of any vector is equal to 1:

$$\mathbf{v} : \mathcal{S} \mapsto \mathcal{T}_{\mathbf{p}}\mathcal{S}, \|\mathbf{v}(\mathbf{p})\| = 1 . \tag{2}$$

We define an orientation field as a unit-norm vector field which is invariant under rotations of π radians. For example, the structure tensor, defined as

$$M(\mathbf{v}) = \mathbf{v} \otimes \mathbf{v}, \tag{3}$$

is invariant under rotations of π radians $(M(\mathbf{v}) = M(-\mathbf{v}))$. It is often more convenient to parametrize the space of possible orientations using angles θ. A unit length vector $\mathbf{v}$ is then expressed as $\mathbf{v}_\theta = (cos(\theta), sin(\theta))$. The θ parameterization allows us to define a natural Riemannian metric between two orientations $\mathbf{v}_{\theta_1}$ and $\mathbf{v}_{\theta_2}$ as

$$d_{Riemann}(\mathbf{v}_{\theta_1}, \mathbf{v}_{\theta_2})^2 = min_n(\theta_1 - \theta_2 + n\pi)^2, n \in \mathbb{Z}. \tag{4}$$

However, this metric lacks differentiability at the point $\theta_1 - \theta_2 + n\pi = \pi/2$. In practice, the lack of differentiability makes it difficult to find a global minimum of a variational problem using a gradient descent approach. For this reason, we follow the approach described in [8, 9] which is to approximate the Riemannian metric by a differentiable metric which is locally equivalent to Equation 4 if the orientation field is continuous. Let the structure tensor be given as

$$M(\mathbf{v}_\theta) = \begin{pmatrix} cos^2(\theta) & sin(\theta)cos(\theta) \\ sin(\theta)cos(\theta) & sin^2(\theta) \end{pmatrix}. \tag{5}$$

Let $M_\theta = M(\mathbf{v}_\theta)$, and let a basis vector of the tangent space of M_θ be given as

$$T_\theta = \frac{\partial M_\theta}{\partial \theta} = \begin{pmatrix} -sin(2\theta) & cos(2\theta) \\ cos(2\theta) & sin(2\theta) \end{pmatrix}. \tag{6}$$

Let the contraction : be defined between two matrices A and B as $A : B = trace$ $(A^t B)$ and the associated Frobenius norm defined as $\|A\|_F^2 = A : A$. We define the Euclidean orthonormal projection of M_{θ_2} onto the tangent space of M_{θ_1} as

$$\Pi_{M_{\theta_1}}(M_{\theta_2}) = M_{\theta_2} - T_{\theta_1} \frac{T_{\theta_1} : M_{\theta_2}}{\|T_{\theta_1}\|_F^2}. \tag{7}$$

We then define a differentiable metric between M_1 and M_2 as

$$d(M_{\theta_1}, M_{\theta_2}) = \frac{1}{2}\|\Pi_{M_{\theta_1}}(M_{\theta_2})\|_F. \tag{8}$$

The following theorem shows $d(M_{\theta_1}, M_{\theta_2})$ and $d_{Riemann}(\mathbf{v}_{\theta_1}, \mathbf{v}_{\theta_2})$ are locally equivalent if the orientation field is continuous.

Theorem 21
$$lim_{\theta_2 \to \theta_1} \frac{d(M_{\theta_1}, M_{\theta_2})}{d_{Riemann}(\mathbf{v}_{\theta_1}, \mathbf{v}_{\theta_2})} = 1$$

Proof. Choose $\theta_2' = \theta_2 + n\pi, n \in \mathbb{Z}$ such that $(\theta_1 - \theta_2' + n\pi)^2$ is minimum for $n = 0$ and perform a Taylor series expansion of $d(M_{\theta_1}, M_{\theta_2'})$ around M_{θ_1} to obtain that

$$d(M_{\theta_1}, M_{\theta_2}) = d_{Riemann}(\mathbf{v}_{\theta_1}, \mathbf{v}_{\theta_2}) \left(1 + \mathcal{O}\left(d_{Riemann}(\mathbf{v}_{\theta_1}, \mathbf{v}_{\theta_2})^2\right)\right).$$

Thus, in the limit, the two metrics are equivalent.   □

We now use this differentiable structure to set up a variational problem whose solution will provide a direction field oriented along the crest lines and trough lines of a surface. A crest on a surface is given by a curve $\gamma \subset \mathcal{S}$ such that the curvature of $\mathcal{S}$ in the direction perpendicular to γ is positive, and reaches a maximum in magnitude. A trough has the same property, except that the sign of the curvature in the direction perpendicular to γ is now negative. Hence, to estimate the presence of a fold in a given orientation we define the following surface curvature energy function

$$E_{curvature}(\mathbf{v}_\theta) = \int_\mathcal{S} \|S\mathbf{v}_\theta\|^2 d\mathcal{S}. \tag{9}$$

If $\lambda_1^2 < \lambda_2^2$ are the eigenvalues of S^tS with associated eigenvectors $\mathbf{v}_1, \mathbf{v}_2$, then the minimum value of $E_{curvature}$ is achieved for $\mathbf{v} = \mathbf{v}_1$.

A fold is characterized by a juxtaposition of crests and troughs with the same orientation (see Fig. 1). To capture this idea, we define a second energy functional which measures the local smoothness of the orientation field

$$E_{smoothness}(M_\theta) = \int_\mathcal{S} \|\nabla M_\theta\|^2 d\mathcal{S}. \tag{10}$$

We will deem a crest γ_1 and a trough γ_2 to have roughly the same orientation if there is an orientation field $\mathbf{v}$ on $\mathcal{S}$ such that $\mathbf{v}$ is tangent to both γ_1 and γ_2 and such that the energy functional $E_{smoothness}(M_\theta)$ is small. Our goal is not to explicitly locate the crests and troughs but rather to *directly* find an orientation field that minimizes both Equations 9 and 10. This leads to the following estimate for a fold orientation, based on a regularization functional:

$$M_\theta = argmin_{M_\theta^*} \left(\alpha E_{smoothness}(M_\theta^*) + E_{curvature}(M_\theta^*)\right). \tag{11}$$

Here $E_{smoothness}$ is the smoothness term, $E_{curvature}$ is the data attachment term and α is a constant to balance to the two.

We can then find the first variation of Equation 11 to find a minimum via the gradient descent equation

$$\frac{\partial M_\theta}{\partial t} = \Pi_{M_\theta} \left(\alpha \Delta_\mathcal{S} M_\theta - S^tS\right). \tag{12}$$

2.2 Discrete Heat Diffusion of the Orientation Field on a Triangulated Mesh

To solve Equation 11 on a discrete triangulated mesh, we need to be able to smooth an orientation field on a surface. The initial orientation field is given by the eigendirection with lowest absolute eigenvalue of the shape operator. We thus first describe an expression for the shape operator S and then provide a numerical scheme to diffuse the orientation field on each triangle. We assume that the orientation field is constant over each triangle and use finite volume methods. Since the normal vector of a triangle is constant on it, the tangent space of a triangle is uniquely defined. More importantly, we can use parallel transport to transport the orientation field between any two neighboring triangles in a unique fashion.

The shape operator simply describes the rate of change of the unit normal between two neighboring triangles, as explained in [12]. On an orientable triangulated mesh, the unit normal vector is uniquely defined for every triangle, by choosing one of the two possible directions. Let the set of all triangles be denoted $\{\triangle_i, i = 1, \ldots, N\}$ and let $\mathbf{p}_{i,j}, j = 1, 2, 3$, be the three vertices of triangle $\triangle_i$. We denote the oriented edges of the triangle as $\mathbf{l}_{i,1} = \mathbf{p}_{i,2} - \mathbf{p}_{i,1}, \mathbf{l}_{i,2} = \mathbf{p}_{i,3} - \mathbf{p}_{i,2}, \mathbf{l}_{i,3} = \mathbf{p}_{i,1} - \mathbf{p}_{i,3}$ and by $\mathbf{e}_{i,j}$ the unit normal vector that points in the same direction as $\mathbf{l}_{i,j}$. We denote by $\mathbf{n}_i$ the unit normal of the triangle and by $\mathbf{n}_{i,j}, j = 1, 2, 3$ the unit normals of the neighboring triangles (those with which an edge is shared). Finally, let A_i be the area of the triangle and $\mathbf{e}_{i,j}^{\perp}$ the unit outward pointing vector that is perpendicular to both $\mathbf{e}_{i,j}$ and $\mathbf{n}_i$. The shape operator S_i then measures the difference in the orientation of the normal vectors $\mathbf{n}_i$ with the one of its neighboring triangles $\mathbf{n}_{i,j}$ weighted by length of the adjacent edges [12]:

$$S_i = \frac{1}{A_i} \sum_{j \in \{1,2,3\}} \|\mathbf{l}_{i,j}\| M(\mathbf{e}_{i,j}^{\perp}) < \mathbf{e}_{i,j}^{\perp}, \mathbf{n}_{i,j} - \mathbf{n}_i > . \tag{13}$$

We now need to diffuse the orientation field on a discrete triangulated surface so that it is restricted to the tangent space of a surface. The solution we propose to this problem is to locally unfold the surface around a triangle to place the neighboring triangles within the same Euclidean plane. Once the solution is computed, it can be mapped back onto the original surface. We write the orientation vector M_θ as a general Euclidean tensor in $\mathbb{R}^3 \times \mathbb{R}^3$. Suppose that $M_{\theta,i}$ is our current estimate at $\triangle_i$ and $M_{\theta,i,j}, j = 1, 2, 3$ is the estimate at the neighboring triangles. To locally unfold the surface, we need to rotate the estimate at the neighboring triangles $M_{\theta,i,j}$ such that they lie in the same plane as $M_{\theta,i}$. To do this, we need to pick a rotation matrix such that $\mathbf{n}_{i,j}$ is mapped onto $\mathbf{n}_i$. Also, we already know that an edge $\mathbf{e}_{i,j}$ that separates two triangles is already in the tangent space of both triangles and hence should remain fixed. These two constraints uniquely define the orientation matrix that maps the tangent space of neighboring triangles:

$$R_{i,j} = \mathbf{e}_{i,j} \otimes \mathbf{e}_{i,j} + \mathbf{n}_i \otimes \mathbf{n}_{i,j} + (\mathbf{e}_{i,j} \times \mathbf{n}_i) \otimes (\mathbf{e}_{i,j} \times \mathbf{n}_{i,j}). \tag{14}$$

Obviously, since the orientation field is always perpendicular to the normal vector to the triangle, it is not necessary to rotate the entire space, but only the plane that contains the triangle. On $\triangle_i$, we use local coordinates $\mathbf{u}_{i,k}, k = 1, 2$ such that $\mathbf{u}_{i,1} \times \mathbf{u}_{i,2} = \mathbf{n}_i$, as a basis to describe the orientation field. We express the orientation field using the $\mathbf{u}_{i,j}$ coordinates for each triangle. Let $\mathbf{u}_{i,j,k}$ be the coordinate frame of the triangle $\triangle_{i,j}$. Then the rotation matrix between the tangent space of $\triangle_i$ and $\triangle_{i,j}$ is given as

$$R_{i,j} = [\mathbf{u}_{i,1}, \mathbf{u}_{i,2}] \big(\mathbf{e}_{i,j} \otimes \mathbf{e}_{i,j} + (\mathbf{e}_{i,j} \times \mathbf{n}_i) \otimes (\mathbf{e}_{i,j} \times \mathbf{n}_{i,j}) \big) [\mathbf{u}_{i,j,1}, \mathbf{u}_{i,j,2}]^t \tag{15}$$

To perform diffusion on a triangulated mesh, we also need a discrete Laplace-Beltrami operator. In the case of a scalar density field over a triangle, an expression for the discrete Laplace-Beltrami operator in terms of differences between the value of the density field at $\triangle_i$ and its neighboring triangles is given in [12]. Let $A_{i,j}$ be the area of triangle $\triangle_{i,j}$ and let F be a scalar function on the mesh such that $F(\triangle_i) = F_i$. We denote by $\beta_{i,j}$ and $\gamma_{i,j}$ the opposite angles of triangles $\triangle_i$ and $\triangle_{i,j}$. Then, the discrete Laplace-Beltrami operator is

$$(\Delta_S F)_i = \frac{1}{A_i} \sum_{j=1}^{3} \frac{1}{cot(\beta_{i,j}) + cot(\gamma_{i,j})} (F_i - F_{i,j}). \qquad (16)$$

If we write $\mathbf{F} = (F_1, \ldots, F_N)^t$ as a vector, over a discrete triangular mesh Δ_S can be written as a product of two matrices $\Delta_S = A^{-1}L$, where A is a diagonal matrix whose diagonal entries are given by A_i and L is a sparse positive semi-definite symmetric matrix whose entries are given by Equation 16.

We can now express the Laplace-Beltrami operator for an orientation field using the rotation matrices given by Equation 15:

$$(\Delta_S M_\theta)_i = \frac{1}{A_i} \sum_{j=1}^{3} \frac{1}{cot(\beta_{i,j}) + cot(\gamma_{i,j})} \left(M_{\theta,i} - R_{i,j} M_{\theta,i,j} R_{i,j}^t\right). \qquad (17)$$

Now let $M_{\theta,i}$ be expressed as a vector of coordinates $a_1 \mathbf{u}_{i,1} \otimes \mathbf{u}_{i,1} + b_i(\mathbf{u}_{i,1} \otimes \mathbf{u}_{i,2} + \mathbf{u}_{i,2} \otimes \mathbf{u}_{i,1}) + c_i \mathbf{u}_{i,2} \otimes \mathbf{u}_{i,2}$. Then, if we write $\mathbf{M}_\theta = [a_1, b_1, c_1, \ldots, a_N, b_N, c_N]$, Δ_S can be written as $\Delta_S = A^{-1}L$ with L a sparse symmetric positive semi-definite matrix with entries given by Equation 17. This provides us with an efficient numerical scheme to find a minimum of the variational problem given in Equation 11.

2.3   An Oriented Shape Deformation Model

Once a dense orientation field $\mathbf{v}$ in the direction of folds has been found it is possible to develop a shape deformation model that is specific to deformations that occur either along the orientation of a fold or in the direction parallel to it. Assume that we have a set of surfaces $S_l, l = 1, \ldots, n$ with a set of diffeomorphisms that map these surfaces onto a template average $\bar{S}$:

$$\phi_l : S_l \to \bar{S}. \qquad (18)$$

Examples of algorithms to find diffeomorphisms that match the shape of the surfaces based on the folding patterns can be found in [4, 13]. Suppose that $\bar{\triangle}_i$ is a triangle on $\bar{S}$ and ϕ_l^{-1} is its mapping on S_l. We note by $D\bar{S}$ the differential in the triangle's coordinate, given as

$$D_i \bar{S} = [\bar{\mathbf{l}}_{i,1}, \bar{\mathbf{l}}_{i,2}]. \qquad (19)$$

The *grad* operator, given by the dual of the differential is

$$\nabla_i \bar{S} = (D_i \bar{S}^t D_i \bar{S})^{-1} D_i \bar{S}^t. \qquad (20)$$

The dilation of the triangle $\bar{\triangle}_i$ by the diffeomorphism ϕ_l is then given by

$$D_{i,l} = (D_i \mathcal{S}_l \nabla_i \bar{\mathcal{S}})^t (D_i \mathcal{S}_l \nabla_i \bar{\mathcal{S}}). \tag{21}$$

The directional dilatation is then given as

$$D_{i,l,\mathbf{v}} = \mathbf{v}_{i,euc}^t D_{i,l} \mathbf{v}_{i,euc}, \tag{22}$$

where $\mathbf{v}_{i,euc}$ is the projection of the tangent vector onto the corresponding 3×1 vector in Euclidean space $\mathbb{R}^3$. From Equation 21, we see that $D_{i,l,\mathbf{v}}$ is always positive. This means that the dilation can be modeled using a log-normal distribution as

$$log(D_{i,l,\mathbf{v}}) \sim \widetilde{log(D_{i,\mathbf{v}})} + \epsilon_{i,l}, \tag{23}$$

where $\widetilde{log(D_{i,\mathbf{v}})}$ is the average dilation over all surfaces $\mathcal{S}_l$ and $\epsilon_{i,l}$ is a random variable which is normally distributed and has finite variance. The likelihood of such a model can be determined using a standard Student t-test while correcting for multiple comparisons, using the method described in [14].

3   Results

In this section we validate our method on synthetic data, for which the ground truth (desired) orientation field is known. We then present experimental results on a population of surfaces extracted from MRI scans of elderly humans.

3.1   Quantitative Validation

We created a circle relief on a flat background as our first test surface (see Fig. 2(a)). On this surface, we expect that the detected fold orientation will be tangential to the radial direction. To generate the figure, we used a simple grayscale image of the desired circle relief and randomly placed points on the resulting height function. These points were then triangulated using the approach of [15]. A second "T" relief surface, shown in Fig. 2(b), was also used. On this surface, we expect that the detected fold orientation will be tangential to the edges of the "T" . Equation 12 was solved on both of these surfaces. We stopped the simulation whenever the following ratio fell below a chosen threshold:

$$\frac{sup\left(\|\Pi_{M_\theta}\left(\alpha \triangle_\mathcal{S} M_\theta - S^t S\right)\|\right)}{sup\left(\|\Pi_{M_\theta}\left(\alpha \triangle_\mathcal{S} M_\theta\right)\| + \|\Pi_{M_\theta}\left(S^t S\right)\|\right)} < \epsilon . \tag{24}$$

For the circle relief, we initialized our algorithm using random orientations. We picked a constant of $\alpha = 10$ for the smoothness term and an ϵ of $1e - 4$ in Equation 24. Visual results for the circle relief are shown in Fig. 2(c). The colormap shows the difference between the estimated orientation of the fold and the expected orientation. The recovered orientation field is accurate everywhere, with the exception of the center of the relief, where the notion of a fold orientation is not evident. On Fig. 2(a), we see there are two singularities in opposition to

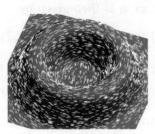 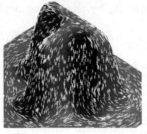 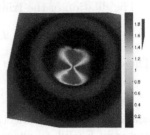

(a) Recovered Fold Orienta- (b) Recovered Fold Orienta- (c) Accuracy of Fold Orien-
tion for the Circle Relief   tion for the T Relief   tation for the Circle Relief
                                                               (in radians)

Fig. 2. Validation on synthetic surfaces

one another, which gives an arbitrary orientation. However, on cortical surfaces, most orientation singularities would arise from junctions of prominent crests and troughs. For the second synthetic surface, the results are shown in Fig. 2(b). The method recovers the expected orientations, as well as a singularity at the junction of the three segments of the "T".

3.2 Results on Cortical Surfaces

We used the OASIS database, which consists of 97 healthy subjects and 92 subjects (aged 60 and above) affected with mild and very-mild dementia [16]. We used the same surface extraction pipeline as in [13, 17, 18], which produces one mid-surface representation of the gray-matter cortical sheet, and obtained mappings ϕ_l for each surface onto a common template average. As with every surface analysis algorithm, mesh resolution can be a concern. Validations of the mesh generation and registration technique can be found in [13, 17, 18]. Once this mapping was found, we computed the average surface of the entire population and used this average surface to compute orientation fields.

To compute the fold orientation, we solved Equation 11 using both $\alpha = 1$ and $\alpha = 100$. A close up result for the left hemisphere is shown in Figure 3, while a result for the right hemisphere is shown in Figure 1. As can be visually assessed on Figure 3, the estimated orientations accurately follow the folds of the surface. For $\alpha = 1$, the recovered orientation field is less smooth and closely follows every ridge on the surface. For $\alpha = 100$, however, the orientation field is smoothed out and folds that are separated by a small ridge are connected. This allows us to obtain a global picture of the folding pattern of the surface, which is used for oriented shape analysis in the following section.

3.3 Oriented Deformation Morphometry

The direction of the fold on a surface allows us to test if its shape is influenced by an exterior factor, such as a particular disease. For example, in the neuroscience

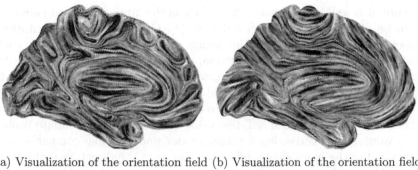

(a) Visualization of the orientation field (b) Visualization of the orientation field
for $\alpha = 1$ for $\alpha = 100$

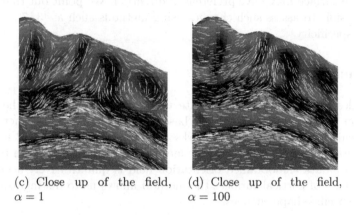

(c) Close up of the field,   (d) Close up of the field,
    $\alpha = 1$ $\alpha = 100$

Fig. 3. Estimated Fold Orientation in a saggital cut of the left hemisphere. The orientation field is smoother for $\alpha = 100$. Visualization of the orientation field produced by integrating a random image along the orientation field (see [19]).

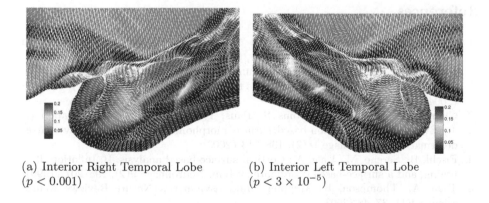

(a) Interior Right Temporal Lobe   (b) Interior Left Temporal Lobe
$(p < 0.001)$ $(p < 3 \times 10^{-5})$

Fig. 4. Shape difference perpendicular to fold orientation due to Alzheimer's disease. The perpendicular orientation field is shown with its p value as a colorbar.

literature, it is well known that regions such as the hippocampus are among the first to be affected by Alzheimer's disease [2]. Our estimate of orientation on surfaces allows us to determine the nature of the deformation on the cortical surface. As explained in the introduction, a shorter fold corresponds to a deformation parallel to the fold orientation, whereas a shallower one corresponds to a deformation perpendicular to the fold. We used Equation 22 to produce two deformation maps, one that is parallel to the folds, and one that is perpendicular to them. We then performed a T-test using Equation 23 to compute probability (p) values, after correcting for age, gender and multiple comparisons [14]. We found that the main shape differences occur in the direction perpendicular to the folds, as illustrated in Figure 4. These results indicate that atrophy on the cortical surface may have preferential direction. We point out that it would not be possible to assess such changes using methods such as [3, 7], which lack direction specificity.

4   Conclusion

We have described a method to estimate a dense orientation field in the direction of folds on a surface. The method is based on a regularization functional and a numerical implementation that works directly on a triangulated mesh. The experimental results indicate that this method has great promise. In particular, for synthetic data the obtained orientation field is quantitatively accurate and for a database of cortical surfaces the method allows us to distinguish between direction specific shape changes.

Acknowledgments

This work was supported by funds from NSERC, FQRNT and CIHR.

References

1. Van Essen, D.: A tension-based theory of morphogenesis and compact wiring in the central nervous system. Nature 385, 313–318 (1997)
2. Buckner, R.: Memory and Executive Function in Aging and AD Multiple Factors that Cause Decline and Reserve Factors that Compensate. Neuron 44(1), 195–208 (2004)
3. Chung, M., Worsley, K., Robbins, S., Paus, T., Taylor, J., Giedd, J., Rapoport, J., Evans, A.: Deformation-based surface morphometry applied to gray matter deformation. NeuroImage 18(2), 198–213 (2003)
4. Fischl, B., Sereno, M., Dale, A.: Cortical surface-based analysis. II: Inflation, flattening, and a surface-based coordinate system. Neuroimage 9(2), 195–207 (1999)
5. Toga, A., Thompson, P.: Mapping brain asymmetry. Nature Reviews Neuroscience 4(1), 37–48 (2003)
6. Fillard, P., Arsigny, V., Ayache, N., Pennec, X.: A Riemannian Framework for the Processing of Tensor-Valued Images. In: Fogh Olsen, O., Florack, L.M.J., Kuijper, A. (eds.) DSSCV 2005. LNCS, vol. 3753, pp. 112–123. Springer, Heidelberg (2005)

7. Lepore, N., Brun, C., Chou, Y., Chiang, M., Dutton, R., Hayashi, K., Luders, E., Lopez, O., Aizenstein, H., Toga, A., et al.: Generalized Tensor-Based Morphometry of HIV/AIDS Using Multivariate Statistics on Deformation Tensors. IEEE Transactions on Medical Imaging 27(1), 129–141 (2008)

8. Tang, B., Sapiro, G., Caselles, V.: Diffusion of General Data on Non-Flat Manifolds via Harmonic Maps Theory: The Direction Diffusion Case. International Journal of Computer Vision 36(2), 149–161 (2000)

9. Perona, P.: Orientation diffusions. IEEE Image Processing 7, 457–467 (1998)

10. Kimmel, R., Sochen, N.: Orientation Diffusion or How to Comb a Porcupine. Visual Com. and Image Representation 13(1-2), 238–248 (2002)

11. Hirani, A.: Discrete exterior calculus. PhD thesis, California Institute of Technology (2003)

12. Grinspun, E., Gingold, Y., Reisman, J., Zorin, D.: Computing discrete shape operators on general meshes. In: Computer Graphics Forum, vol. 25, pp. 547–556. Blackwell Synergy, Malden (2006)

13. Lyttelton, O., Boucher, M., Robbins, S., Evans, A.: An unbiased iterative group registration template for cortical surface analysis. Neuroimage 34(4), 1535–1544 (2007)

14. Worsley, K., Andermann, M., Koulis, T., MacDonald, D., Evans, A.: Detecting changes in nonisotropic images. Human Brain Mapping 8(2-3), 98–101 (1999)

15. Fisher, M., Springborn, B., Schröder, P., Bobenko, A.: An algorithm for the construction of intrinsic delaunay triangulations with applications to digital geometry processing. Computing 81(2), 199–213 (2007)

16. Marcus, D., Wang, T., Parker, J., Csernansky, J., Morris, J., Buckner, R.: Open Access Series of Imaging Studies (OASIS): Cross-sectional MRI Data in Young, Middle Aged, Nondemented, and Demented Older Adults. Journal of Cognitive Neuroscience 19(9), 1498–1507 (2007)

17. Boucher, M., Whitesides, S., Evans, A.: Depth potential function for folding pattern representation, registration and analysis. Medical Image Analysis (2008)

18. Kim, J., Singh, V., Lee, J., Lerch, J., Ad-Dabbagh, Y., MacDonald, D., Lee, J., Kim, S., Evans, A.: Automated 3-D extraction and evaluation of the inner and outer cortical surfaces using a Laplacian map and partial volume effect classification. Neuroimage 27, 210–221 (2005)

19. Cabral, B., Leedom, L.: Imaging vector fields using line integral convolution. In: Proceedings of the 20th annual conference on Computer graphics and interactive techniques, pp. 263–270. ACM, New York (1993)

Diffusion MRI Registration Using Orientation Distribution Functions

Xiujuan Geng[1], Thomas J. Ross[1], Wang Zhan[2], Hong Gu[1], Yi-Ping Chao[3], Ching-Po Lin[4], Gary E. Christensen[5], Norbert Schuff[2], and Yihong Yang[1]

[1] National Institute on Drug Abuse, NIH
gengx@mail.nih.gov
[2] Department of Radiology, University of California, San Francisco
[3] Department of Electrical Engineering, National Taiwan University, Taiwan
[4] Institute of Neuroscience, National Yang-Ming University, Taiwan
[5] Department of Electrical and Computer Engineering, University of Iowa

Abstract. We propose a linear-elastic registration method to register diffusion-weighted MRI (DW-MRI) data sets by mapping their diffusion orientation distribution functions (ODFs). The ODFs were reconstructed using a q-ball imaging (QBI) technique to resolve intravoxel fiber crossing. The registration method is based on mapping the ODF maps represented by spherical harmonics which yield analytic solutions and reduce the computational complexity. ODF reorientation is required to maintain the consistency with transformed local fiber directions. The reorientation matrices are extracted from the local Jacobian and directly applied to the coefficients of spherical harmonics. The similarity cost of the registration is defined by the ODF shape distance calculated from the spherical harmonic coefficients. The transformation fields are regularized by linear elastic constraints. The proposed method was validated using both synthetic and real data sets. Experimental results show that the elastic registration improved the affine alignment by further reducing the ODF shape difference; reorientation during the registration produced registered ODF maps with more consistent principle directions compared to registrations without reorientation or simultaneous reorientation.

1 Introduction

Diffusion-weighted magnetic resonance imaging (DW-MRI) is an emerging technique and plays an important role in studying white matter structure and anatomical connectivity. Non-rigid registration of DW-MRI images is crucial for building a white matter and fiber tract atlas and group analysis. With the assumption of a Gaussian diffusion profile, the second order diffusion tensor MRI (DTI) [1] provides a relatively simple approach for quantifying diffusion anisotropy as well as extracting local fiber directions. DTI Registration [2,3,4] has been studied and utilized in brain MRI analyses and produces additional information compared to conventional imaging modalities. However, a major drawback of DTI is that it fails to accurately characterize the diffusion in complex white matter, where fiber tracts with different orientations intersect within

J.L. Prince, D.L. Pham, and K.J. Myers (Eds.): IPMI 2009, LNCS 5636, pp. 626–637, 2009.

a voxel. Extension of DTI to higher orders [5] and multi-tensor models of the diffusivity profiles were recently introduced to solve this limitation. Another approach is q-space imaging (QSI) [6] which measures the diffusion function directly by employing the Fourier relation between the diffusion signal and the diffusion function. Due to the sampling burden and large pulse gradient requirements, q-ball imaging (QBI) techniques [7] haven been proposed, which sample the diffusion signals on a spherical shell and apply the Funk-Radon transform to reconstruct the model-free diffusion orientation distribution function (ODF) based on radial basis functions or spherical harmonics [8]. Spherical harmonics lead to an analytic solution for the ODF reconstruction and are widely utilized in various applications, such as shape modeling in molecular sciences and real-time lighting in computer graphics.

In this work we present a novel registration method for ODF maps represented by spherical harmonics. The potential of the ODF-based registration techniques is to align structures accordingly in locations where other image modalities are unable to characterize, for example, fiber crossings. However, the proposed technique is not restricted to ODF registration, it can also be applied to align the apparent diffusion profiles represented by spherical harmonics.

The registration is based on optimizing a cost function including the ODF shape similarity cost defined with a L^2 norm and an elastic regularization constraint. During the optimization, a rotation matrix is extracted at each voxel from the local Jacobian and converted to a general spherical harmonic rotation matrix to reorient the ODFs. The reorientation is directly applied to the coefficients without detecting principle directions ODFs which may have multiple directions and involve significant computation. We demonstrated the reorientation using both synthetic and real data sets. Experimental results show that the proposed registration method provides better performance in terms of smaller ODF shape difference and more consistent principle directions of the registered images, compared to registration without or with reorientation after registration.

2   Method

2.1   Diffusion ODFs Represented as Spherical Harmonics

The ODF characterizes the relative likelihood of water diffusion along any given angular direction $\mathbf{u}$ with $\mathbf{u}(\theta, \phi) = [\sin\theta\cos\phi \ \sin\theta\sin\phi \ \cos\theta]$ where θ and ϕ are the polar and azimuthal angles. Our registration method is applied to the reconstructed ODF maps from the QBI technique proposed by Hess et al. [8]. The ODF is approximated by a great circle integration on the sphere, i.e., $F(\mathbf{u}) = \oint_{\mathbf{q} \perp \mathbf{u}} E(\mathbf{q})d\mathbf{q}$. $E(\mathbf{q})$ represents an underlying diffusion-attenuated signal at a finite set of points on a sphere and $\mathbf{q}$ is the wavevector which describes diffusion encoding in a pulsed-gradient spin-echo experiment. The software "Camino" [9] is used to calculate and visualize ODFs.

As a single-valued spherical function, the function $F(\mathbf{u}) : S^2 \rightarrow R^+$, can be represented as a linear combination of a set of spherical harmonic basis $Y_l^m(\mathbf{u})$

with order l and phase factor m: $F(\mathbf{u}) = \sum_{l=0}^{L} \sum_{m=-l}^{l} y_l^m Y_l^m(\mathbf{u})$, where y_l^m denotes the harmonic series coefficient, and L is the maximum harmonic order. Since F is real, it is sufficient to utilize a real basis function set Y_{lm}, expanded as linear combinations of the complex harmonics:

$$Y_{lm}(\mathbf{u}) = \begin{cases} Y_l^0(\mathbf{u}) & , \text{ if } m = 0, \\ \frac{1}{\sqrt{2}}(Y_l^m(\mathbf{u}) + (-1)^m Y_l^{-m}(\mathbf{u})) & , \text{ if } m > 0, \\ \frac{i}{\sqrt{2}}((-1)^m Y_l^m(\mathbf{u}) - Y_l^{-m}(\mathbf{u})) & , \text{ if } m < 0. \end{cases} \tag{1}$$

F is also assumed to be antipodal symmetric, such that the order l only takes even numbers and the function can be expressed as

$$F(\mathbf{u}) = \sum_{l=0,\text{ even}}^{L} \sum_{m=-l}^{l} c_m^l Y_{lm}(\mathbf{u}), \tag{2}$$

where c_m^l represents the real harmonic series coefficient. In general, ODFs form an open subset of the space of complex-valued L^2 spherical functions with the induced L^2 norm $||F|| = \sqrt{<F,F>}$ [10]. In this work, we define the ODF shape difference with the L^2 norm. Other metrics, such as the Kullback-Leibler Divergence introduced by Chiang et al. [11], can also be applied to define the shape similarity. Given that the ODFs are represented with a complete set of orthonormal basis functions, they thus form a vector space analogue to unit basis vectors. The invariant shape norm and the distance between two functions can be defined as

$$||F|| = \sqrt{<F,F>} = \sqrt{\sum_{l=0,\text{even}}^{L} \sum_{m=-l}^{l} ||c_m^l||^2} \quad \text{and} \tag{3}$$

$$D(F_1, F_2) = ||F_1 - F_2|| = \sqrt{\sum_{l=0,\text{even}}^{L} \sum_{m=-l}^{l} ||c_{1m}^l - c_{2m}^l||^2}. \tag{4}$$

2.2   Rotation of Real Spherical Harmonics

A $3D$ rotation can be decomposed to three Euler angles using the zyz convention with three subsequent rotations around the z, y and z axes by angles α_1, α_2 and α_3, respectively: $\mathbf{R} = \mathbf{R}_Z(\alpha_3)\mathbf{R}_Y(\alpha_2)\mathbf{R}_Z(\alpha_1)$.

The coefficients of real spherical harmonics can be rotated in the same way as vectors with so-called Wigner matrices [12]. The coefficients λ_m^l for the rotated function $\mathbf{R}(F(\mathbf{u})) = \sum_l \sum_m \lambda_m^l Y_{lm}(\mathbf{u})$ can be represented as a linear transformation of the original coefficients:

$$\lambda_m^l(\alpha_1, \alpha_2, \alpha_3) = \sum_{m'=-l}^{l} R_{mm'}^l(\alpha_1, \alpha_2, \alpha_3) c_{m'}^l. \tag{5}$$

The Wigner matrix $\mathbf{R}$ can be represented as a sparse block matrix:

$$R = \begin{bmatrix} 1 & 0 & 0 & \cdots \\ 0 & R^1 & 0 & \cdots \\ 0 & 0 & R^2 & \cdots \\ \vdots & \vdots & \vdots & \ddots \end{bmatrix} \qquad (6)$$

where R^l corresponds to the l-order. For complex spherical harmonics, a rotation operator expressed in terms of the Euler angle parametrization can be represented with a Wigner matrix with the matrix elements given by

$$D^l_{m'm}(\alpha_1, \alpha_2, \alpha_3) = e^{-im'\alpha_1} d^l_{m'm}(\alpha_2) e^{-im\alpha_3}, \quad \text{where} \qquad (7)$$

$$d^l_{m'm}(\alpha_2) = \left[\frac{(l+m')!(l-m')!}{(l+m)!(l-m)!}\right]^{1/2}$$
$$\times \sum_{k=\max(0,m-m')}^{\min(l-m',l+m)} [(-1)^{k+m'-m} \binom{l+m}{k} \times \binom{l-m}{l-m'-k} \qquad (8)$$
$$\times (\cos \alpha_2/2)^{2l+m-m'-2k} (\sin \alpha_2/2)^{2k+m'-m}]$$

Re-define the linear combination in Eq.(1) as $y_{lm}(\mathbf{u}) = \sum_{m'} A^l_{mm'} Y^l_{m'}(\mathbf{u})$, then the rotation matrix for real spherical harmonics is given by

$$R^l = A^l D^l A^{l\dagger}, \qquad (9)$$

where $\dagger$ is the complex conjugate transpose. The z-axis rotation of spherical harmonics is straightforward and can be calculated as follows, without constructing R_Z:

$$\lambda^l_m = c^l_{-m} \sin(-m\alpha) + c^l_m \cos(m\alpha). \qquad (10)$$

To implement R_Y, we followed Eq.(20) in [13]. A fast spherical harmonic rotation approximation using a truncated Taylor expansion of R_Z [14] can be used to speed up the calculation, however the accuracy is compromised.

2.3   Reorientation of Diffusion ODFs

Image registration searches for transformations to map structures in the source to corresponding ones in the reference. By assumption, the water diffusion orientation distributions reflect the underlying fiber structures; therefore, ODF reorientation along the transformation is required. The Jacobian of the spatial transformations is the first order linear approximation to the differentiable functions at a given spatial location. Therefore, a natural thought is to apply the Jacobian to the ODF at each location to reorient it. Using this strategy, the shape and size of the ODFs are subject to change. To keep the shape invariant, we apply the rotation matrix extracted from the Jacobian to reorient the ODFs, which is similar to the "finite strain" tensor reorientation technique proposed by Alexander et al. [2]. Since a diffusion ODF may have multiple local maxima indicating multiple crossing fibers, which are computationally expensive to detect, direct implementation of the "preservation of principal directions

(PPD)" method [2] may not work efficiently. A convenience of formulating ODFs with spherical harmonics is that the shape rotation can be achieved by apply a rotation matrix directly to the coefficients (see Sec.2.2) without changing of the basis functions and without reconstruction of the ODFs after reorientation during each registration step. The invariance of the basis functions simplifies the calculation of the shape difference which can be always preformed using the corresponding coefficients as described in Eq.(4).

Chiang *et al.* [11] proposed a reorientation method that first detected the principle direction of the diffusivity functions by shape-based PCA, and then applied PPD to reorient the diffusivity function. A major difference of our approach is that, instead of computing the diffusion attenuation signal at each reoriented direction, we apply the rotation matrices directly to the coefficients to get the reoriented ODF. As QBI techniques normally acquire several hundred sampling directions, performing operations on much fewer coefficients reduces the computation cost significantly. Barmpoutis *et al.* [5] noted limitations of the re-orientation of diffusivity functions, and provided a full affine "re-transform" of diffusion functions instead of reorientation under a 4th order tensor model.

2.4   Registration of ODFs

The ODF-based registration can be stated as an optimization problem of finding spatial transformation h_{12} that minimizes the following cost function:

$$
\begin{aligned}
C &= C_{SIM} + C_{REG} \\
&= \sigma \int_{\Omega} ||D(\mathbf{R}_{12}(F_1(h_{12}(x))), F_2(x))||^2 dx + \rho \int_{\Omega} ||\mathcal{L}(u_{12}(x))||^2 dx \\
&= \sigma \int_{\Omega} \sum_{l=0,even}^{L} \sum_{m=-l}^{l} ||\lambda_{1m}^l(h_{12}(x)) - c_{2m}^l(x)||^2 dx \\
&\quad + \rho \int_{\Omega} ||\nabla^2(u_{12}(x))||^2 dx
\end{aligned}
\tag{11}
$$

where Ω represents the ODF map space, σ and ρ are weighting parameters for the similarity and regularization costs, respectively, $\mathbf{R}_{12}$ is the associated reorientation matrix of the ODF F_1 at $h_{12}(x)$, λ_m^l is the rotated coefficient defined in Eq.(5), and $u_{12}(x)$ is the displacements satisfying $h_{12}(x) = x + u_{12}(x)$. The similarity term was defined using the shape difference metric in Eq.4. $\mathcal{L}$ is a linear differential operator and was defined to be the Laplacian operator in this work, i.e., $\mathcal{L} = \nabla^2 = \left[\frac{\partial^2}{\partial x_1^2} + \frac{\partial^2}{\partial x_2^2} + \frac{\partial^2}{\partial x_3^2} \right]$. The transformations were initialized as identities, and updated by gradient descent iteratively. At each iteration, linear interpolation of the reoriented coefficients λ_m^l was used to generate the deformed ODF maps.

The transformation fields are defined in Eulerian space, therefore the reorientation matrix operating on the deforming ODF should be extracted from the inverse of $J(h_{12})$ with the following equation

$$
\mathbf{R}_{12} = ((J(h_{12}) \cdot J(h_{12})^T)^{-\frac{1}{2}} J(h_{12}))^T.
\tag{12}
$$

To apply the rotation to the spherical harmonic coefficients, $\mathbf{R}_{12}$ is decomposed into three Euler angles using the zyz convention. Let c_1 denote $cos(\alpha_1)$, s_1 denote $sin(\alpha_1)$, and define c_2, s_2, c_3 and s_3 accordingly. Then $\mathbf{R}(\alpha_1\alpha_2\alpha_3)$ is expressed as:

$$\begin{bmatrix} c_1c_2c_3 - s_1s_3 & -c_2c_3s_1 - c_1s_3 & c_3s_2 \\ c_3s_1 + c_1c_2s_3 & c_1c_3 - c_2s_1s_3 & s_2s_3 \\ -c_1s_2 & s_1s_2 & c_2 \end{bmatrix} \tag{13}$$

Therefore, the three Euler angles can be obtained as:

$$\alpha_1 = -\arctan(R_{32}, R_{31}), \quad \alpha_2 = \arccos(R_{33}), \quad \text{and} \quad \alpha_3 = \arctan(R_{23}, R_{13}), \quad (14)$$

with the constraints of $\alpha_1 \in [-\pi\ \pi]$, $\alpha_2 \in [-\frac{\pi}{2}\ \frac{\pi}{2}]$, and $\alpha_3 \in [-\pi\ \pi]$. R_{ij} represents the element of $\mathbf{R}$ in the ith row and jth column, and (R_{ij}, R_{kl}) represents the angle vector coordinate in the plane. Note that $\arctan(a, b)$ is almost equivalent to $\arctan(a/b)$ except that we also take into account the quadrant in which the point (a,b) is located.

3   Experiments and Results

3.1   Synthetic Experiments of Reorientation

Diffusion tensors with three mixtured zero-mean Gaussians under low intravoxel water exchange model were simulated with SNR of 100 using "Camino". The largest eigenvalues of the three tensors were set to be $3 \times 10^{-9}m^2/s$, $2 \times 10^{-9}m^2/s$ and $1.5 \times 10^{-9}m^2/s$ along the x, y and z axes, respectively. The other two eigenvalues had a value of $0.6 \times 10^{-9}m^2/s$ along the y and z axes, the x and z axes, and the x and y axes. 162 encoding directions were used for the QBI acquisition with $b = 3000\ s/mm^2$. Fig. 1 (a) shows the reconstructed ODF projected on the xy and the xz planes. 30° rotations along the z-axis and along y-axis were applied separately on the spherical harmonic coefficients according to Eq.(9), (7), (8) and (10). The reconstructed ODF are shown in Fig. 1 (b) and (c). Fig. 1 (d) plots the coefficients of the original and rotated ODFs. Fig.2 demonstrates a spatial rotation of 25° of a real DW-MRI data set without and with ODF reorientation. A rotation transformation without ODF reorientation resulted in an inconsistency between the principle directions of the ODFs and the underlying fiber directions. With ODF reorientation of the coefficients, the principle directions were rotated to follow the transformed fiber structures.

3.2   Registration Experiments with Real Data

Human brain QBI data from five healthy subjects were acquired on a 3T TrioTim Siemens MRI scanner. Isotropic axial diffusion-weighted images were obtained using a single shot diffusion spin-echo echo-planar imaging (EPI) sequence with TR/TE = 9,500/116 ms, FOV= 192 mm, matrix size = 96×96, yielding a 2mm image resolution. 162 diffusion encoding directions (using an electrostatic repulsion model) with a b value of 3000 s/mm² and one reference image with $b = 0$

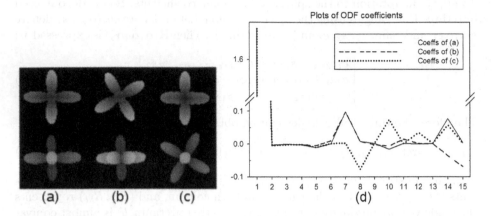

Fig. 1. Illustration of the ODF reorientation with simulated 3-tensor data sets. (a) the original ODF projected on the xy plane on the top and the xz plane at the bottom; (b) the ODF rotated 30° along the z-axis; (c) the ODF rotated 30° along the y-axis; and (d) the plots of corresponding ODF coefficients stored in a $1d$ array $[c_0^0, c_{-2}^2, c_{-1}^2 \cdots, c_3^4, c_4^4]$.

were acquired. 60 slices with slice thickness of 2mm were obtained to cover the whole brain. The total scan time was 25.65 minutes.

ODF maps of each data set were reconstructed with real spherical harmonics following the technique in [8]. The maximum harmonic order was set to 4 in this preliminary study resulting in $(4 + 1) \times (4 + 2)/2 = 15$ coefficients to represent the diffusion functions. The proposed method is general to any order of spherical harmonics. One data set was selected as the reference and the other four were registered to it. The mean shape of the ODF at each voxel location was calculated following Eq.(4) and used to perform the scalar-based affine registration. The affine matrices were then decomposed to Euler rotation angles using Eq.(12) and Eq.(14) and applied to transform the coefficients to reorient the ODFs. The affine aligned images were regarded as inputs to register to the reference using the elastic registration described in Sec.2.4. The parameters were set to: the similarity weight $\sigma = 1$, the regularization weight $\rho = 0.4$, and the number of iterations $= 100$. A Gaussian filter with $FWHM = 1.77mm$ was applied to smooth the deformation fields at each iteration. The similarity error converged after around 50 iterations for all registrations.

To demonstrate the contribution of the ODF reorientation, the experiments were designed to compare the proposed method with reorientation at each iteration to registration methods without reorientation, and with reorientation after registration. All three methods used the same registration parameters.

Two metrics were computed for evaluation and comparison: the average of ODF shape difference defined in Eq.(4) and the average directional consistency of the largest principle direction of the registered ODF maps. The average directional consistency is defined as $adc = \frac{1}{N} \sum_i |\mathbf{u}_1(i) \cdot \mathbf{u}_2(i))|$, where $\mathbf{u}_1$ is the

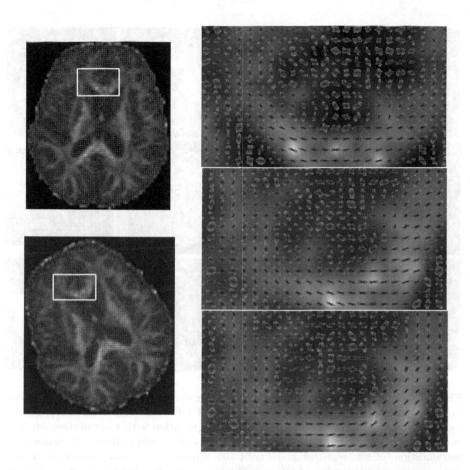

Fig. 2. Illustration of ODF reorientation using real qball imaging (QBI) data with a $25°$ rotation along the z-axis. The underlays are the fractional anisotropy (FA) maps calculated by a single tensor model. The overlays are reconstructed ODFs using QBI. The enlarged figures on the right from top to bottom are: original ODFs on the original FA image; ODFs without reorientation on the rotated FA image; and ODFs with reorientation on the rotated FA image.

largest principle direction of the deformed ODF map at voxel i, $\mathbf{u}_2$ is the largest principle direction of the reference ODF map at voxel i and N is the number of voxels where both deformed and reference maps have nonzero values. The closer to 1 that the measure is, the more consistent the largest principle directions between the deformed and the reference map are. The reason for taking the absolute value of the dot product is due to the assumption of antipodal symmetry of the ODFs. The peak direction was calculated by searching the local maximum within a fixed search radius of 0.4 and randomly rotating a unit icosahedron 8672 times using "Camino".

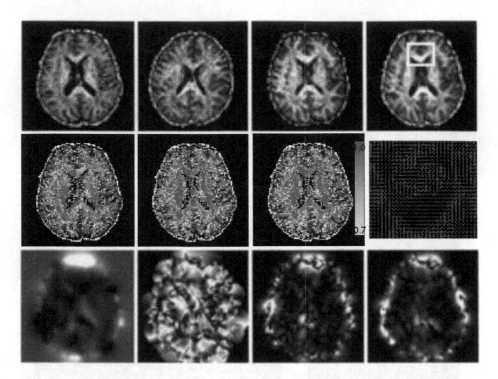

Fig. 3. Typical ODF registration results with various registration methods. The top row from left to right: the mean shape of the ODF maps of the reference, source, source after affine alignment and after elastic registration with reorientation; the second row from left to right: directional consistency maps after affine registration with reorientation, elastic registration without reorientation and elastic registration with reorientation, and the enlarged ODFs of the boxed region in the above figure; the bottom row from left to right: the norm of the transformation fields, the rotation angle α_1 along z-axis, α_2 along y-axis and the sum of the first rotation angle α_1 and second angle α_3 along z-axis.

The mean shape of the ODF maps of the reference, original source, source after affine alignment and after elastic registration are shown in the top row of Fig.3. The alignment of brain structures is improved from affine to elastic registration around several regions such as the corpus callosum and the ventricles. Fig.3 also shows the enlarged ODFs after elastic registration with reorientation of the selected box region. We found that the ODF maps are smooth and follow the structural directions. The directional consistency maps after affine registration with reorientation, elastic registration without reorientation and elastic registration with reorientation are shown in the second row of Fig.3. The values are color-coded from 0.707 (corresponding to 45° angular difference) to 1. Larger values from affine to elastic registration are observed which indicate greater consistency of the direction peaks between the deformed and reference maps. The

Table 1. Registration results for the four subjects measured by average shape difference and directional consistency metrics. Affine without reorientation (ro) and with ro, elastic without ro, with ro after registration (roa) and with ro during registration methods were compared.

method	ave shape difference				ave directional consistency			
	1	2	3	4	1	2	3	4
affine wo/ro	4.905	3.332	3.333	4.239	0.475	0.479	0.472	0.468
affine w/ro	4.900	3.320	3.331	4.220	0.481	0.483	0.504	0.480
elastic wo/ro	2.011	1.589	1.617	1.987	0.595	0.598	0.580	0.566
elastic w/roa	1.987	1.580	1.612	1.976	0.599	0.601	0.590	0.572
elastic w/ro	1.976	1.576	1.604	1.962	0.609	0.608	0.598	0.585

difference is subtle to be seen between with and without reorientation using elastic registration. Slightly greater values in the genu and splenium of the corpus callosum can be observed. The norm of the transformation fields, the rotation angle α_1 along z-axis, α_2 along y-axis and the sum of the first and second rotation angles α_1 and α_3 along z-axis are displayed in the bottom row of Fig.3. The composition of α_1 and α_3 play the major role in the rotation along the z-axis, given that the rotation angles along y-axis are small (which is the case in this experiment). Therefore the unsmooth α_1 map does not imply the unsmooth rotation fields along the z-axis, but the sum of α_1 and α_2 gives an indication of the degree of smoothness of rotation fields along the z-axis. This can be seen by the fact that a first large rotation along the z-axis can be canceled out by a second large but negative direction rotation along z-axis. There are some places around the boundary that the rotation angle fields are not very smooth. A regularization term on the rotation fields may help to produce a smoother rotation.

Tab.1 shows the affine and elastic registration results with and without reorientation measured by the average shape difference and directional consistency metrics. In general, the elastic registration methods significantly reduced the ODF shape difference and improved directional consistency compared to the affine methods. The reorientation after affine alignment slightly improved the shape similarity and directional consistency. All elastic methods used the affine aligned ODF maps as inputs. Based on the four sets of registration results, reorientation after registration produced slightly better results compared to registration without reorientation, which demonstrates the need of reorienting ODFs to keep them consistent with the deformed local structures. Simultaneous reorientation further improved the performance in terms of smaller average shape difference and larger directional consistency, which shows that it has the potential to help the registration process to get out of local minima.

The small improvements of shape similarity caused by ODF reorientation may be due to the relatively insensitive shape metric under rotation. The shape difference metric used here includes the 0-order spherical harmonics which are invariant under rotation and take a large portion in the distance calculation (see Fig.3 (d)). Metrics more sensitive to rotation, such as computing the difference using all but the 0 order coefficients would potentially magnify the improvement. One reason of the small amount of improvement measured by the directional consistency metric is because it was averaged over the whole brain instead of in specific regions. Due to the relatively low SNR (around 10) in QBI data, in many gray matter regions, the ODF peaks may not truly reflect the underlying structures. The peaks in those regions between source and reference have large differences to begin with and are hard to match even with ODF reorientation. The calculation of the differential of the ODF reorientation is ignored in this work, and taking into account it may improve the registration performance [15].

4   Conclusions and Discussion

We presented a novel DW-MRI registration algorithm based on reconstructed ODFs represented by spherical harmonics. The ODF reorientation was performed during the elastic registration procedure. The reorientation matrices were obtained by extracting the rotation part from the local Jacobian and directly applied to the spherical harmonic coefficients to rotate the ODF. Computation of the principal directions and reconstruction of the ODFs during each registration iteration are avoided. The similarity cost was computed based on a shape difference metric defined using the L^2 norm. A linear elastic regularization term was added to constrain the transformation fields. ODF reorientation was tested using synthetic q-ball data and real q-ball data with known rotation angles. The registration method was evaluated and compared with affine registration and elastic registration without reorientation or with reorientation after registration. Average shape difference and directional consistency were measured and compared with various registration techniques. Results show that the elastic registration model significantly reduced ODF shape difference and improved directional consistency; simultaneous reorientation further improved the registration performance.

A limitation of the proposed ODF-based registration is that it fully depends on the quality of the reconstructed ODF maps. Metrics derived from other models (such as fractional anisotropy from DTI) or directly from diffusion attenuation signals (i.e., mean shape of the acquired signals instead of the reconstructed ones) may help to validate the registration performance and analyze how much the reconstructed ODF would affect the registration results. Other possible areas to improve the method include to apply the motion correction of the EPI data sets to get more accurate ODFs and therefore better registration; to use a multi-resolution registration scheme to avoid local minima; and to include the differential of ODF reorientation in the registration optimization procedure.

Acknowledgments

This work was supported by the Intramural Research Program of the National Institute on Drug Abuse (NIDA), National Institute of Health (NIH).

References

1. Basser, P.J., Pierpaoli, C.: Microstructural and physiological features of tissues elucidated by quantitative-diffusion-tensor MRI. Journal of Magnetic Resonance, Series B 111, 209–219 (1996)
2. Alexander, D., Pierpaoli, C., Basser, P., Gee, J.: Spatial transformations of diffusion tensor magnetic resonance images. IEEE Trans. Med. Imaging 20(11) (2001)
3. Verma, R., Khurd, P., Davatzikos, C.: On analyzing diffusion tensor images by identifying manifold structure using isomaps. IEEE Trans. Med. Imaging 26(6), 772–778 (2007)
4. Zhang, H., Avants, B.B., Yushkevich, P.A., Woo, J.H., Wang, S., McCluskey, L.F., Elman, L.B., Melhem, E.R., Gee, J.C.: High-dimensional spatial normalization of diffusion tensor images improves the detection of white matter differences: An example study using amyotrophic lateral sclerosis. IEEE Trans. Med. Imaging 26(11) (2007)
5. Barmpoutis, A., Jian, B., Vemuri, B.C., Shepherd, T.M.: Symmetric positive 4th order tensors & their estimation from diffusion weighted MRI. In: Karssemeijer, N., Lelieveldt, B. (eds.) IPMI 2007. LNCS, vol. 4584, pp. 308–319. Springer, Heidelberg (2007)
6. Gilbert, R., Magnusson, L., Napadow, V., Benner, T., Wang, R., Wedeen, V.: Mapping complex myoarchitecture in the bovine tongue with diffusion- spectrum-magnetic resonance imaging. Biophys. 91, 1014–1022 (2006)
7. Tuch, D.S.: Q-ball imaging. Magnetic Resonance in Medicine 56, 1358–1372 (2004)
8. Hess, C., Mukherjee, P., Han, E., Xu, D., Vigneron, D.: Q-ball reconstruction of multimodal fiber orientations using the spherical harmonic basis. Magnetic Resonance in Medicine 56, 104–117 (2006)
9. Cook, P.A., Bai, Y., Nedjati-Gilani, S., Seunarine, K.K., Hall, M.G., Parker, G.J., Alexander, D.C.: Camino: Open-source diffusion-mri reconstruction and processing. In: 14th Scientific Meeting of the International Society for Magnetic Resonance in Medicine (2006)
10. Zhang, H., Yushkevich, P.A., Gee, J.C.: Registration of diffusion tensor images. In: 2004 Conference on Computer Vision and Pattern Recognition (CVPR 2004), pp. 842–847. IEEE Computer Society, Los Alamitos (2004)
11. Chiang, M., Klunder, A., McMahon, K., de Zubicaray, G., Wright, M., Toga, A., Thompson, P.: Information-theoretic analysis of brain white matter fiber orientation distribution functions. In: Karssemeijer, N., Lelieveldt, B. (eds.) IPMI 2007. LNCS, vol. 4584, pp. 172–182. Springer, Heidelberg (2007)
12. Edmonds, A.: Angular Momentum in Quantum Mechanic. Princeton University Press, Princeton (1996)
13. Ritchie, D.W., Kemp, G.J.L.: Fast computation, rotation, and comparison of low resolution spherical harmonic molecular surfaces. Journal of Computational Chemistry 20(4), 383–395 (1999)
14. Krivanek, J., Konttinen, J., Pattanaik, S., Bouatouch, K., Zara, J.: Fast approximation to spherical harmonic rotation. In: International Conference on Computer Graphics and Interactive Techniques (2006)
15. Yeo, B.T.T., Vercauteren, T., Fillard, P., Pennec, X., Golland, P., Ayache, N., Clatz, O.: Dti registration with exact finite-strain differential. In: Proceedings of the International Symposium on Biomedical Imaging (2008)

Robust Joint Entropy Regularization of Limited View Transmission Tomography Using Gaussian Approximations to the Joint Histogram

Dominique Van de Sompel and Sir Michael Brady

University of Oxford, Oxford, United Kingdom
dominique@robots.ox.ac.uk

Abstract. Information theoretic measures to incorporate anatomical priors have been explored in the field of emission tomography, but not in transmission tomography. In this work, we apply the joint entropy prior to the case of limited angle transmission tomography. Due to the data insufficiency problem, the joint entropy prior is found to be very sensitive to local optima. Two methods for robust joint entropy minimization are proposed. The first approximates the joint probability density function by a single 2D Gaussian, and is found to be appropriate for reconstructions where the ground truth joint histogram is dominated by two clusters, or multiple clusters that are roughly aligned. The second method is an extension to the case of multiple Gaussians. The intended application for the single Gaussian approximation is digital breast tomosynthesis, where reconstructed volumes are approximately bimodal, consisting mainly of fatty and fibroglandular tissues.

1 Introduction

Limited view transmission tomography is a branch of computed tomography that is of increasing practical importance. It is widely used in industrial as well as clinical applications, where it is commonly motivated by geometric design constraints on the imaging machinery, limitations on time for image acquisition, and/or efforts to reduce patient radiation dose. Common clinical applications include intra-operative imaging for reference with a pre-operative planning CT, angiography, chest tomosynthesis, dental tomosynthesis, cardiac CT, and orthopaedic imaging [7].

Recently, a new limited angle application known as digital breast tomosynthesis (DBT) has attracted much attention in the tomography literature as well as in the medical imaging industry, and its outstanding challenges have provided much of the inspiration for this work. DBT has been proposed as a way to overcome some of the limitations of standard two-view X-ray mammography. While cost effective, the projective nature of mammography results in the superposition of tissue structures, which can lead either to the occlusion of cancers, or falsely suspicious appearances. To overcome mammography's loss of depth information, digital breast tomosynthesis typically involves taking 10-20 low-dose X-ray images of the breast over a limited angular range. The set of images

J.L. Prince, D.L. Pham, and K.J. Myers (Eds.): IPMI 2009, LNCS 5636, pp. 638–650, 2009.

is then processed digitally to produce a three-dimensional reconstruction of the breast, enabling radiologists to 'page through' reconstructions slice by slice. This is expected to increase sensitivity and specificity, at substantially reduced breast compressions.

However, digital breast tomosynthesis faces many issues that have yet to be resolved satisfactorily. First, DBT's low radiation dose requirements challenge even the most advanced x-ray detectors. Second, because of the limited number of views, DBT reconstructions are underdefined. As a result, standard reconstruction algorithms as developed for full angular range CT and emission tomography do not perform satisfactorily. In practice, this leads to blurry reconstructions which often contain streak artifacts along the projection directions.

This paper addresses the data insufficiency problem of DBT. The long term goal of our work is to develop an algorithm that uses follow-up breast MR scans to retrospectively regularize DBT reconstructions. This work will involve both a reconstruction and non-rigid registration component. The current paper is part of the first stage of this work, where it has been assumed that the reconstruction and the anatomical prior are aligned *a priori*.

The remainder of this paper is structured as follows. Section 1.1 situates the current contribution in the reconstruction literature, and explains how anatomical priors can be used to attack the data insufficiency problem of DBT. Section 2 explains the regularizers explored in this paper, and Section 3 presents results on a number of 2D mathematical phantoms as well as 2D clinical data. Finally, Section 4 draws conclusions on the applicability of the regularizers proposed.

1.1 Tomographic Reconstruction Algorithms

The literature on computed tomography is vast, and an exhaustive overview is beyond the scope of this paper. It is however possible to identify three broad reconstruction paradigms, namely those based on Fourier analysis, and those based on algebraic and penalized maximum likelihood principles. More extensive overviews are given in [8] and [4]. Of interest here are penalized maximum likelihood (PML) algorithms, which enable the incorporation of various image priors. In this work we use PML methods to incorporate anatomical prior information, and thereby to attack the problem of missing information faced by limited view tomography, which is explained next.

Null Space Problem. The data insufficiency problem of limited view tomography (aka the 'null space' problem) can be understood in terms of the Fourier Slice Theorem [8]. This theorem states that the Fourier transform of a parallel projection of an image f gives a slice through its Fourier domain F perpendicular to the direction of the projection. Hence, as illustrated in Fig. 1, the incomplete angular sampling of limited view tomography leaves large swathes of the Fourier space unmeasured. In theory, the unsampled regions could be occupied by any Fourier coefficients that exhibit Hermitian symmetry, i.e. an infinity of solutions is possible, but of course some solutions will be more likely than others (Fig. 1, right). It is possible to introduce plausible constraints by, for example,

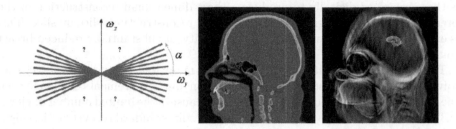

Fig. 1. Left: Insufficient angular sampling leaves regions of the Fourier domain unmeasured. Right: illustration of the null space problem for a 384x370 head CT image. Both images satisfy the same projection data (15 noiseless projections distributed uniformly over $\pm 30°$), but the reconstruction on the right is undesirable.

Gerchberg-Papoulis extrapolation [13,12], but the extrapolation of Fourier coefficients remains problematic because of the global and oscillatory nature of the Fourier transform [3]. In this work, we estimate the unsampled information by incorporating an anatomical prior into the reconstruction process.

Anatomical Priors. Previous studies have considered the use of anatomical priors in both emission and transmission tomography. The work done so far in limited view transmission tomography, however, has focused mainly on direct intensity-based distance regularizers, for example between planning CT's and intraoperative tomosynthesis views [1]. Some work in emission tomography has also considered the simulation of template PET volumes from CT or MRI volumes followed by the use of an intensity-based distance measure [9]. Only a small number of recent studies have looked at the use of information theoretic similarity measures such as mutual information [14] and joint entropy [11,15], and this only in the field of emission tomography. Due to its succes in image registration, mutual information was considered first, but it was later demonstrated by Nuyts [11] that joint entropy introduces less bias into the reconstruction and is therefore more appropriate. In this work, we build on Nuyts' results and apply joint entropy (JE) regularization to limited view transmisson tomography. To the best of our knowledge, this is the first study to do so. As a further contribution, we identify JE's vulnerability to local optima and propose methods to increase robustness against them which have not yet been proposed in emission tomography.

2   Methods

2.1   Penalized Maximum Likelihood (PML) Reconstruction

Penalized maximum likelihood (aka maximum a posteriori, or MAP) algorithms incorporate prior information about the reconstruction by means of Bayes' rule:

$$P(x|r) = \frac{P(r|x)P(x)}{P(r)} \tag{1}$$

where x and r represent the attenuation map and the observed projection data, respectively. The prior distribution $P(r)$ is commonly assumed to be uniform, and Eqn. 1 is log transformed to convert any multiplications into summations. This yields an objective function in x of the form $\psi(x) = L(x) - \beta R(x)$, where $L(x)$ is the data log-likelihood term, β is a tuning hyperparameter, and $R(x)$ is the regularizing penalty term. The data likelihood term can be written as a sum of concave functions $h_i(l_i)$, yielding an expression of the form $L(x) = \sum_{i=1}^{M} h_i(l_i)$, where M is the number of projection rays or observations made. For transmission tomography, the functions $h_i(l_i)$ are given by $h_i(l_i) = - \left(r_{0,i} e^{-l_i} + b_i \right) + r_i \log \left(r_{0,i} e^{-l_i} + b_i \right)$, where $l_i = \sum_{j=1}^{N} a_{ij} x_j$. In this notation, N is the number of pixels in the discretized attenuation map, a_{ij} is the length of traversal of the ith ray through the jth pixel, r_i is the photon count observed by the ith detector, $r_{0,i}$ is the number of photons leaving the source for the ith ray, and b_i accounts for scatter events. Here we minorize the data term $L(x)$ by fitting quadratic surrogate functions of optimal curvature to the cost function at the current image estimate $x = x^n$, as described in [5]. This gives

$$L(x) = \sum_{i=1}^{M} h_i(l_i) \geq Q(x; x^n) = \sum_{i=1}^{M} q_i(l_i; l_i^n) \tag{2}$$

In the following sections, we discuss the regularizers $R(x)$ explored in this paper.

2.2   Joint Entropy

The superiority of joint entropy over mutual information, first suggested by Nuyts [11], was confirmed in our own experiments (not reported here). We then set out to improve some of joint entropy's shortcomings. The joint entropy penalty term is given by

$$R(x) = H(A, B) = - \sum_a \sum_b p_{A,B}(a, b) \log p_{A,B}(a, b) \tag{3}$$

where $p_{A,B}(a, b)$ denotes the joint probability density function between images A and B. To ensure differentiability with respect to the image intensities A_j, we estimated $p_{A,B}(a, b)$ using symmetric Gaussian kernels as Parzen windows:

$$p_{A,B}(a, b) = \frac{1}{N} \sum_{j=1}^{N} w_{\sigma,j} = \frac{1}{N} \sum_{j=1}^{N} \alpha^2 e^{-\beta\left((A_j-a)^2+(B_j-b)^2\right)} \tag{4}$$

where $\alpha = \frac{1}{\sqrt{2\pi}\sigma}$ and $\beta = \frac{1}{2\sigma^2}$. The variables a and b represent the (discrete) coordinates of the joint histogram bin centers[1].

We can optimize the surrogate objective function $\psi(x) = Q(x; x^n) - \beta R(x)$ using a general steepest ascent algorithm. The intensities A_j are denoted as x_j

---

[1] Note that it is also possible to consider continuous intensity coordinates a and b, in which case the summations in Eqn. 3 turn into integrals. However, the derivatives with respect to A_j and B_j would not have a closed form.

in the remainder of the paper to align the notation with that used in Section 2.1. The direction of steepest ascent is given by the gradient vector with components $\frac{\partial \psi}{\partial x_j} = \frac{\partial Q(x)}{\partial x_j} - \beta \frac{\partial R(x)}{\partial x_j} = x'_j$, where

$$\frac{\partial Q(x)}{\partial x_j} = \sum_{i=1}^{M} \dot{h}_i(l_i)a_{ij} \tag{5}$$

and

$$\frac{\partial R(x)}{\partial x_j} = \frac{-2\beta}{N} \sum_a \sum_b w_{\sigma,j}(x_j - a) \left[\log\left(\frac{1}{N}\sum_{j=1}^{N} w_{\sigma,j} \right) + 1 \right] \tag{6}$$

To compute the steepest ascent update step, we parametrize the cost function in terms of a single variable λ, which yields $\psi(\lambda; x^n) = Q(\lambda; x^n) - \beta R(\lambda; x^n)$. This is done by writing the image x as $x = x^n + \lambda x'$, where x^n is the image estimate at the beginning of the nth iteration. The terms of the parametrized cost function are given by

$$Q(\lambda; x^n) = \sum_{i=1}^{M} h_i(l_i^n) + \lambda \dot{h}_i(l_i^n)\left(\sum_{j=1}^{N} a_{ij}x'_j \right) + \lambda^2 \frac{1}{2}c_i \left(\sum_{j=1}^{N} a_{ij}x'_j \right)^2 \tag{7}$$

where constant terms have been dropped, and

$$R(\lambda; x^n) = \sum_a \sum_b \left(\frac{1}{N}\sum_{j=1}^{N} G_j(\lambda) \right) \log\left(\frac{1}{N}\sum_{j=1}^{N} G_j(\lambda) \right) \tag{8}$$

where $G_j(\lambda) = \alpha^2 e^{-\beta\left((x_j^n - a)^2 + 2\lambda(x_j^n - a)x'_j + \lambda^2 x'^2_j + (B_j - b)^2 \right)}$. The Newton-Raphson update step is now given by

$$\lambda^{n+1} = -\frac{\frac{d}{d\lambda}\left[Q(\lambda; x^n) - \beta R(\lambda; x^n) \right]|_{\lambda=0}}{\frac{d^2}{d\lambda^2}\left[Q(\lambda; x^n) - \beta R(\lambda; x^n) \right]|_{\lambda=0}} \tag{9}$$

The derivatives of Eqn. 7 with respect to λ are trivial. The derivatives of Eqn. 8 are more involved but can be computed efficiently by convolving standard binning joint histograms with either Gaussian kernels or their first or second derivatives in x_j (not described here due to space limitations). Reconstruction results using the joint entropy regularizer are presented in Section 3.

2.3   Single Gaussian (SG) Approximation

As demonstrated in the results section, the joint entropy regularizer is sensitive to local optima in limited angle transmission tomography. To eliminate this problem, we propose to approximate the joint pdf using a single 2D Gaussian approximation, and then to optimize the joint entropy of this distribution. The sum of N multivariate Gaussians can be approximated by a single multivariate Gaussian of the same first and second moments by using the expressions

$$\mu^* = \frac{1}{N} \sum_{j=1}^{N} \mu_j, \qquad \text{and} \qquad \Sigma^* = \frac{1}{N} \sum_{j=1}^{N} \left(\Sigma_j + \mu_j \mu_j^T \right) - \mu^* \mu^{*T} \qquad (10)$$

where $\mu_j = \begin{bmatrix} x_j \\ B_j \end{bmatrix}$, and $\Sigma_j = \begin{bmatrix} \sigma^2 & 0 \\ 0 & \sigma^2 \end{bmatrix}$. The entropy of the fitted single Gaussian is then given by

$$H = \frac{1}{2} \ln \left((2\pi e)^2 |\Sigma^*| \right) \qquad (11)$$

From Eqn. 11 we can see that the penalty function $R(x) = H$ can be minimized simply by minimizing the variance $|\Sigma^*|$ of the Gaussian used to approximate the joint histogram. This yields a quadratic cost function, which enables relatively cheap update steps and fast convergence rates, and guarantees convergence to a global optimum. Considering the intensities B_j to be constant, the variance $|\Sigma^*|$ reduces to

$$R(x) = \frac{C}{N} \left[\sum_{j=1}^{N} x_j^2 - \frac{1}{N} \left(\sum_{j=1}^{N} x_j \right)^2 \right] - \left(\frac{1}{N} \sum_{j=1}^{N} x_j B_j - \frac{c}{N} \sum_{j=1}^{N} x_j \right)^2 \qquad (12)$$

after dropping constant terms, and where the constants c and C are given by $c = \frac{1}{N} \sum_{j=1}^{N} B_j$ and $C = \sigma^2 + \frac{1}{N} \sum_{j=1}^{N} B_j^2 - c^2$.

The overall cost function $\psi(x) = Q(x) - \beta R(x)$ can again be parametrized using $x_j = x_j^n + \lambda x_j'$, and the Newton-Raphson update step, which guarantees monotonic convergence for quadratic objective functions, found using the expression given in Eqn. 9.

2.4 Multiple Gaussian (MG) Approximation

Our experiments have shown that the single Gaussian (SG) approximation works well for object-prior combinations whose joint histograms are roughly bimodal (have two clusters in the joint histogram)[2], or contain multiple clusters that are more or less aligned. More generally however, joint histograms may show multiple clusters that appear anywhere in the joint histogram at any orientation, often overlapping. Hence we propose an extension that models the joint histogram as a sum of a limited number of 2D Gaussians. The MG method retains the advantage over the JE prior that the number of local optima can be suppressed by declaring only a limited number of Gaussian clusters.

Using Bayes' rule, we can construct the following cost function

$$P(x, p, \theta | r, B) = \frac{1}{Z} P(r|x) P(B|x, p, \theta) P(x) P(p) P(\theta), \qquad (13)$$

---

[2] This makes it a potential candidate for DBT regularization, as discussed later.

where B is the anatomical prior image, p is the hidden measure field proposed by Marroquin [10], and θ is the set of parameters that describe each Gaussian cluster. The p field is essentially a vector field giving the probability of each pixel x_j belonging to the cluster k.

The data match term $P(r|x)$ is the standard Poisson likelihood term, which was given in Section 2.1. The term $P(B|x, p, \theta)$ relates to the joint segmentation of the ongoing reconstruction, and can be decomposed as:

$$P(B|x,p,\theta) = \prod_{j=1}^{N} P(B_j|x,p,\theta) = \prod_{j=1}^{N} \sum_{k=1}^{K} P(B_j|f_j = k, x_j, \theta_k)p_{j,k} \quad (14)$$

where the class labels f have been marginalized out as described in Marroquin [10]. We define

$$v_{j,k} = P(B_j|f_j = k, x_j, \theta_k) = \frac{1}{2\pi|\Sigma_k|^{1/2}} \exp\left(-\frac{1}{2}(X_j - M_k)^T \Sigma_k^{-1}(X_j - M_k)\right) \quad (15)$$

where $X_j = \begin{bmatrix} x_j \\ B_j \end{bmatrix}$, $M_k = \begin{bmatrix} \mu_{x,k} \\ \mu_{B,k} \end{bmatrix}$ and Σ_k is the variance of the kth Gaussian cluster in the joint histogram. The means $\mu_{x,k}$ and $\mu_{B,k}$ give the coordinates of the kth Gaussian cluster in the joint histogram. Note that we have chosen a Gaussian probability density function to illustrate the method, but that other variational models could be specified as well.

Next, we assume a uniform prior for x, and the prior $P(p)$ is given by

$$P(p) = \frac{1}{Z_p} \exp\left[-\sum_C V_C(p) - \sum_{j=1}^{N} H(p_j)\right] \quad (16)$$

where Z_p is a normalizing constant, C denotes the cliques, V_C is an appropriate smoothness penalty function, and $H(p_j)$ denotes the Shannon entropy of the probability vector p_j. The entropy term of the prior encourages peaked distributions, and hence minimizes the number of Gaussians needed to model the joint histogram. This allows us to overdeclare the number of Gaussians, and thereby increases robustness to cases where additional, anomalous clusters appear in the joint histogram. Finally, we assume a uniform (non-informative) distribution for $P(\theta)$. Of course, in real clinical applications there is a prior expectation on the clusters seen in the joint histogram, but a formulation of such priors is postponed to future work. Taking the logarithm of Eqn. 13 to turn multiplication into summation, we obtain

$$\psi(x,p,\theta) = \sum_{i=1}^{M} h_i(l_i) + \beta \sum_{j=1}^{N} \log\left(\sum_{k=1}^{K} v_{j,k}p_{j,k}\right) - \gamma \sum_C V_C(p) - \omega \sum_{j=1}^{N} H(p_j) \quad (17)$$

after dropping constant terms and adding hyperparameters to control the strength of each term. Note that in the case $K = 1$, Eqn. 17 yields a cost function that is similar but not identical to the one used for the single Gaussian approximation. Since the cluster parameters would still need to be optimized for, it is more efficient to use the previously proposed SG approximation, where the cluster parameters are defined explicitly.

The above generalization of the Gaussian approximation framework has been successful in preliminary experiments on phantom-prior combinations with multiple out-of-line clusters. The simpler SG approximation is however expected to be already sufficiently powerful for the intended application of DBT (see later). Hence, to remain within space limitations, we restrict this discussion to a short summary of the methodology and focus on the single Gaussian case in the remainder of the paper. It is our intention to report more extensively on the multiple Gaussian case in a future journal or conference submission.

3   Results and Discussion

3.1   Limitations of the Joint Entropy Prior

The main weakness of the joint entropy prior in limited angle tomography is demonstrated in Fig. 2. As illustrated, the JE prior is very sensitive to local optima (even though stable on the correct answer). When viewed in the space of the joint histogram, trapping in local optima amounts to a breaking up of the initial joint histogram into many small clusters, after which the algorithm converges. This behaviour was confirmed for multiple phantoms using various initial guesses, namely the zero image, unfiltered backprojections (UBP), filtered backprojections (FBP) and initial guesses obtained by unregularized steepest ascent reconstructions.

Nutys [11] suggested in the context of emission tomography that the sensitivity to local optima could be reduced by gradually increasing the weight of the joint entropy prior, rather than applying it at full strength from the beginning. However, this strategy was not successful in our experiments with limited angle tomography. The failure of this approach is presumably due to the null space problem: once the projection data are satisfied, the data term becomes uninformative (i.e. the data cost function becomes flat), and hence possesses no power to drive the joint entropy towards a superior optimum.

3.2   Improved Performance by Single Gaussian pdf Estimation

To counter the problem of fragmentation into many clusters, we proposed a single Gaussian (SG) approximation to the joint histogram, whose joint entropy was then optimized jointly with the data match term. As mentioned above, however, the SG prior turned out to be powerful only for bimodal or roughly in-line clusters. Fortunately, since the 1D histogram of breast tissue is approximately bimodal in both CT [2] and MR scans (the two modes corresponding to fatty and fibroglandular tissue), it is plausible that the joint histogram of correctly aligned breast MR's and breast CT's will also show two clusters. Hence the single

Gaussian approximation may be a useful regularizer for DBT. We are looking to confirm this assumption on clinical data in a future conference submission.

The following results evaluate the performance of SG on cases with bimodal and roughly in-line clusters. As seen in Fig. 2, the single Gaussian approximation outperforms the JE prior by a significant margin. Fig. 2 (third row from bottom) shows that, even though the SG prior was formulated to minimize the joint entropy of an approximation to the joint histogram, it in effect minimizes the joint entropy of the actual joint histogram much more efficiently than the original JE prior. In addition, it was found that the SG prior yields a much higher convergence rate ($\sim$ 30 vs. $\sim$ 300 iterations to convergence), and is computationally lighter (0.045 vs. 0.5 seconds per iteration for a 200x200 image[3]).

A preliminary glance at SG's potential performance in MR-regularized DBT is given in the bottom rows of Fig. 2, where the breast attenuation phantom is a breast CT slice taken from [2]. The fictitious priors are simulated using linear as well as non-linear intensity transformations of the original phantom (both information preserving and non-preserving). Next, we examine SG's robustness to missing regions in the prior and to misregistration.

Robustness to Missing Regions in Prior
The first three columns of Fig. 3 demonstrate that the absence of a region in the anatomical prior tends to decrease the contrast of that region in the reconstruction, when compared to the ground truth. However, the resulting reconstruction is still much improved compared to the unregularized case. This behavior can also be observed in the breast slice with the binarized inverse prior shown in Fig. 2, where some of the finer structures not visible in the prior are rendered in the reconstruction. It is postulated that a distance measure which is more tolerant of outliers in the joint histogram than the quadratic relations used in the basic definition of the variance may improve the robustness of the algorithm. An obvious choice for this would be the Huber penalty function [6], which we intend to investigate in future work.

In the case of MR-regularized DBT, an increased robustness may be important to accommodate microcalcifications and other high-resolution structures which are visible in the x-ray sets but not in the MRI. (It is currently an open question whether it is possible for larger regions visible in the x-ray projections not to be visible in the MRI.) Even without the use of a more robust SG prior, it is hoped that bulk correspondences between fatty and fibroglandular tissue will already improve the quality of DBT reconstructions substantially.

Robustness to Misregistration
The effects of a 2-pixel misregistration between the blob phantom and its prior (both of size 200x200) are shown in the top right of Fig. 3. The variation of RMS error with horizontal misregistration is shown below it. The degradation with increasing misalignment is obvious, but we note again that all of the original

---

[3] Implemented in MatlabR2008 on a Dell Precision PWS 390, with 2CPU at 2.39GHz, and 3.25GB of RAM.

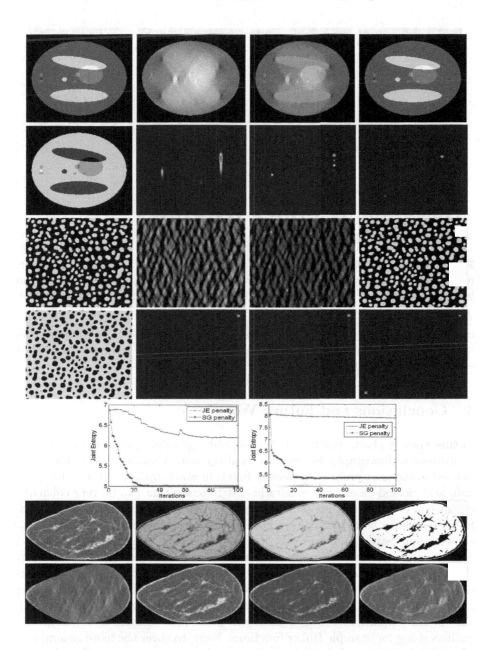

Fig. 2. Converged reconstructions from 16 noiseless views distributed evenly over ±30° from the vertical direction. Zero initial guess. The first four rows are organized in pairs: (1) original, unregularized, JE penalty, SG penalty; (2) prior and joint histograms corresponding to each reconstruction, in same order as row above. Fifth row: decrease in JE during first 100 iterations for the ellipse and blob phantoms (left to right). Sixth row: phantom, linear inverse prior, cubic inverse prior, binarized inverse prior. Seventh row: unregularized and SG regularized reconstructions, using priors on the row above.

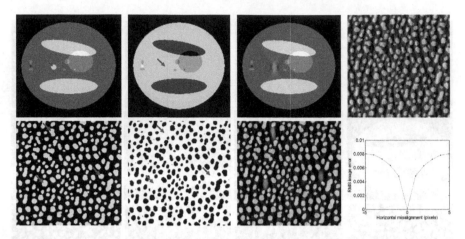

Fig. 3. Columns 1-3: Effect of missing regions in the prior. From left to right: phantom, prior, SG reconstruction. Column 4: effect of misregistration. Top: 2-pixel misalignment between phantom and prior. Bottom: RMS image error versus horizontal misalignment.

image features are still visible. Here, too, we postulate that SG's robustness to misregistration could be improved by using functions that are more tolerant of outliers in the joint histogram.

4   Conclusions and Future Work

In this work, we have shown that the joint entropy prior applied to limited view transmission tomography is prone to local optima. A single Gaussian approximation to the joint probability density function was proposed to solve this problem, and yielded an entirely quadratic cost function that can be very efficiently optimized. Our experiments showed that the single Gaussian approximation performs best for a particular class of ground truth joint histograms, namely those showing only two main clusters, or multiple ones that are more or less aligned. This suggests that the SG prior may be usable in MR-regularized DBT, where the imaged tissue is dominated by two classes (fat and fibroglandular, which are clearly distinguishable in both breast MRI's and CT's). In particular, its light computational load, high convergence rate and convexity would be highly desirable in this application. A suggestion was also made to increase robustness to outliers using for example Huber functions. Next, to cover the more general case of randomly positioned multiple clusters, we have presented a methodology for approximating joint histograms using multiple Gaussian approximations. This method retained the advantage over JE of reduced local optima by declaring only a limited number of Gaussian distributions. The method could be interpreted as a segmentation of the joint histogram, where each pixel is classified as belonging to a cluster, and then driving that pixel towards the mean of that cluster. The regularizing effects of the MG and JE priors are therefore similar;

both methods attempt to narrow clusters in the joint histogram. Due to space limitations, results of the MG approach were not presented here.

For future work, we plan further investigations of reconstruction bias, robustness to data noise, and the effect of Parzen window width on the respective priors. For the multiple Gaussian approximation, we also plan to investigate the robustness to either underdeclaration or overdeclaration of the number of classes. In the later stages of this work, we plan to investigate the robustness of simultaneous reconstruction and non-rigid registration of the pendulous MR scan to the cranio-caudally compressed DBT volume. This will be tested on clinical data, using both *a priori* and simultaneous non-rigid registration. Finally, we intend to investigate the effect of different scan sequences for the MR volume.

References

1. Nett, B., Tang, J., Leng, S., Chen, G.: Tomosynthesis via total variation minimization reconstruction and prior image constrained compressed sensing (piccs) on a c-arm system, vol. 6913, p. 69132D. SPIE (2008)
2. Boone, J.M., Nelson, T.R., Lindfors, K.K., Selbert, J.A.: Dedicated breast ct: Radiation dose and image quality evaluation. Med. Phys. 221(3), 657–667 (2001)
3. Candes, E.J., Romberg, J., Tao, T.: Robust uncertainty principles: exact signal reconstruction from highly incomplete frequency information. IEEE Transactions on Information Theory 52(2), 489–509 (2006)
4. Fessler, J.A.: Iterative methods for image reconstruction. EECS Department, The University of Michigan, ISBI Tutorial (April 2006),
   www.eecs.umich.edu/~fessler/papers/files/talk/06/isbi,p1,note.pdf (last accessed on September 7, 2007)
5. Erdogan, H., Fessler, J.A.: Accelerated monotonic algorithms for transmission tomography. In: ICIP (2), pp. 680–684 (1998)
6. Huber, P.J.: Robust Statistics. Wiley, New York (1981)
7. Dobbins III, J.T., Godfrey, D.J.: Digital x-ray tomosynthesis: current state of the art and clinical potential. Phys. Med. Biol. 45, R65–R106 (2003)
8. Kak, A.C., Slaney, M.: Principles of Computerized Tomographic Imaging. Society of Industrial and Applied Mathematics (2001)
9. Mameuda, Y., Kudo, H.: New anatomical-prior-based image reconstruction method for pet/spect. In: Nuclear Science Symposium Conference Record, NSS 2007, vol. 6, pp. 4142–4148. IEEE, Los Alamitos (2007)
10. Marroquin, J.L., Santana, E.A., Botello, S.: Hidden markov measure field models for image segmentation. IEEE Transactions on Pattern Analysis and Machine Intelligence 25(11), 1380–1387 (2003)
11. Nuyts, J.: The use of mutual information and joint entropy for anatomical priors in emission tomography. In: Nuclear Science Symposium Conference Record, NSS 2007, vol. 6, pp. 4149–4154. IEEE, Los Alamitos (2007)
12. Papoulis, A.: A new algorithm in spectral analysis and band-limited extrapolation. IEEE Transactions on Circuits and Systems 22(9), 735–742 (1975)
13. Pickalov, V., Kazantsev, D.: Iterative gerchberg-papoulis algorithm for fan-beam tomography. In: 1st IEEE Region 8 International Conference on Computational Technologies in Electrical and Electronics Engineering, pp. 218–222 (2008)

650   D. Van de Sompel and M. Brady

14. Somayajula, S., Asma, E., Leahy, R.M.: Pet image reconstruction using anatomical information through mutual information based priors. In: Nuclear Science Symposium Conference Record, pp. 2722–2726. IEEE, Los Alamitos (2005)
15. Tang, J., Tsui, B.M.W., Rahmim, A.: Bayesian pet image reconstruction incorporating anato-functional joint entropy. In: Biomedical Imaging: From Nano to Macro, ISBI 2008, May 2008, pp. 1043–1046 (2008)

Cortical Correspondence with Probabilistic Fiber Connectivity

Ipek Oguz[1], Marc Niethammer[1,3], Josh Cates[4], Ross Whitaker[4],
Thomas Fletcher[4], Clement Vachet[2], and Martin Styner[1,2]

[1] Departments of Computer Science, [2] Psychiatry, [3] Biomedical Research Imaging
Center, University of North Carolina, Chapel Hill NC
[4] Scientific Computing and Imaging Institute, University of Utah, Salt Lake City UT
ipek@cs.unc.edu

Abstract. This paper presents a novel method of optimizing point-based correspondence among populations of human cortical surfaces by combining structural cues with probabilistic connectivity maps. The proposed method establishes a tradeoff between an even sampling of the cortical surfaces (a low surface entropy) and the similarity of corresponding points across the population (a low ensemble entropy). The similarity metric, however, isn't constrained to be just spatial proximity, but uses local sulcal depth measurements as well as probabilistic connectivity maps, computed from DWI scans via a stochastic tractography algorithm, to enhance the correspondence definition. We propose a novel method for projecting this fiber connectivity information on the cortical surface, using a surface evolution technique. Our cortical correspondence method does not require a spherical parameterization. Experimental results are presented, showing improved correspondence quality demonstrated by a cortical thickness analysis, as compared to correspondence methods using spatial metrics as the sole correspondence criterion.

1 Introduction

Measurements of cerebral topographical properties such as cortical thickness and curvature are of great interest for quantitative investigations of neural development and anatomic connectivity, both for healthy populations and for clinical studies. Group analysis of such cerebral properties requires the ability to compute corresponding points across a population of cortical surfaces. Consistent computation of corresponding points on the cortical surface (defined as the boundary between the white matter (WM) and gray matter (GM) surfaces) is a difficult task, given the highly convoluted geometry of the brain and the high variability of folding patterns across subjects. It should also be noted that no generic "ground truth" definition of dense correspondence exists for the cortex. The choice of particular correspondence metric must, therefore, be application-driven.

A variety of automated cortical correspondence computation algorithms have been proposed. The FreeSurfer system [1,2] provides an entire framework for the segmentation, surface reconstruction, topology correction, cortical flattening and

J.L. Prince, D.L. Pham, and K.J. Myers (Eds.): IPMI 2009, LNCS 5636, pp. 651–663, 2009.
© Springer-Verlag Berlin Heidelberg 2009

spherical parameterization of the cortex. The correspondence across a population of cortical surfaces is established through the registration of their respective spherical representations with an average surface, based on an average convexity measure referred to as the sulcal depth, discussed in Section 3.3. Tosun et al. [3] estimate a multispectral optical flow warping procedure that aims to align the shape measure maps of an atlas and a subject brain's normalized maps, based on the shape index and curvedness metrics.

A shortcoming of these methods is that they use an atlas or a template surface to which the other surfaces are aligned in a pair-wise manner. It has been shown that group-wise correspondence methods that consider the entire population at once rather than processing one surface at a time yield better statistical population models [4,5,6]. In one of the earliest such methods by Kotcheff and Taylor [7], each shape is represented as a point in 2N-dimensional space, with associated covariance Σ. The method minimizes information content across an ensemble via a cost function $\sum_k \log(\lambda_k + \alpha)$, where λ_k are the eigenvalues of Σ and α is a regularization term. The Minimum Description Length (MDL) method proposed by Davies et al. [8] hypothesizes that the simplest description of a population is the best; in this context, they measure simplicity by the length of the code to transmit the data as well as the model parameters. MDL implementations in 3D usually rely on spherical parameterizations of the surfaces, which must be obtained through a preprocessing step, such as the method proposed in [9], that relaxes a spherical parameterization onto the input mesh. In [10], we present a gradient descent optimization method for the MDL algorithm and explore using local curvature in addition to spatial locations in the MDL cost function.

An empirical study by Styner et al.[6] demonstrates that ensemble-based statistics improve correspondences relative to pure geometric regularization, and that MDL performance is virtually the same as that of $(min \log |\Sigma + \alpha I|)$, as proposed in Kotcheff and Taylor's method described above. This last observation is consistent with the well-known result from information theory: in general, MDL is equivalent to minimum entropy [11]. Cates et al. [12,13] propose a system exploring this property; their entropy-based particle correspondence framework is the underlying technique for the methodology presented in this paper and will be discussed in more detail in Sec. 3.

We present a method that extends the entropy-based particle framework to allow the usage of additional local information, called correspondence features throughout this manuscript, for computing correspondence. Specifically, we propose a novel method for integrating fiber connectivity information into the correspondence framework. Structural MRI scans show white matter homogeneously, such that it is impossible to infer the orientation of the fiber tracts within each voxel. The understanding of the WM structure, however, can be significantly improved by additional information on fiber tracts that can be extracted from diffusion weighted imaging (DWI) scans. One of the main contributions of this manuscript is a suitable mapping of the fiber tract structure to the cortical surface. Connectivity maps, which represent whether each voxel on the cortical surface is connected via fiber tracts to a given region of interest (ROI), is the proposed solution to this problem.

Various tractography algorithms have been proposed in recent years to extract fiber tract paths from DWI scans. Streamline tractography [14] generates tracts by following the direction of maximal diffusion at each voxel. While these methods have low computation costs and simplify the visualization of the extracted fiber tracts, they cannot deal with noisy input images, regions of high isotropy, or partial volume effect. In contrast, stochastic tractography methods [15,16,17] take the uncertainty of fiber orientations into account, and therefore yield results that are more suitable for our purposes, as discussed in Sec. 2.

In the next section, a summary of our proposed approach is provided. Then, in Sec. 3, we discuss in detail the entropy-based particle correspondence framework and its extension to incorporate local correspondence features. Sec. 4 presents the two main novel contributions of this manuscript, namely, the methodology followed for projecting DWI-based connectivity information to the cortical surface and the surface deflation algorithm proposed for overcoming the problems associated with fiber tracking near the WM/GM boundary. We then define our evaluation criteria in Sec. 5 and present experimental results in Sec. 6. Fig.1 summarizes our pipeline.

2   Methodology Overview

In this work, we are presenting a cortical correspondence system that incorporates various local functions of spatial coordinates. We choose to use a particle-based entropy minimizing system, as introduced by Cates et al.[12,13], for the correspondence computation in a population-based manner. Specifically, we use the extension to this methodology we presented in [5] that allows the use of *correspondence features* for establishing correspondence. These features are locally defined functions that provide additional information about the surface, such as curvature. This extension is critical for the application of the entropy-based particle correspondence framework to populations of cortical surfaces, as additional information sources can have significant impact on correspondence quality. Structural features such as sulcal depth and local curvature provide additional information about the geometry of the brain; DWI-based fiber connectivity features provide augmented knowledge about the white matter structure. Furthermore, given the highly folded and curved nature of the cortex surface, Euclidean distances measured in 3D space between points do not reflect the actual distance along the cortical sheet (e.g. in the case of two points lying on different banks of a sulcus); it therefore makes little sense to use spatial proximity as a standalone measure of correspondence strength.

The particle framework uses a point-based surface sampling to optimize surface correspondence in a population-based manner. Like-numbered samples, named particles, define correspondence across the population. The optimization consists of moving the particles along the surfaces in the direction of the gradient of an energy functional that strikes a balance between an even sampling of each surface (characterized by shape entropy) and a high spatial similarity of the corresponding samples across the population (ensemble entropy). Local measurements on the object surfaces, referred to as correspondence features, are incorporated into the ensemble entropy to provide a generalized correspondence definition.

One of the main contributions of this work is the use of fiber connectivity patterns for optimizing cortical correspondence. This is achieved by using connectivity of the cortex to various ROI's as correspondence features. A stochastic tractography algorithm, described in Sec. 4.1, generates connectivity maps that represent the probability of each voxel being connected to these ROI's. A separate feature channel is used for connectivity to each individual ROI.

There is, however, a major obstacle to using these connectivity maps for cortical correspondence: the connectivity probabilities typically decrease drastically near the WM/GM boundary, as the diffusion gets too isotropic and noisy near the surface. This effect is more emphasized at the ridges of the gyri (as opposed to the valleys of the sulci). Thus, the tractography values at the cortical boundary voxels are more of a function of local sulcal depth than of actual connectivity. A major contribution of this work is a method of computing the connectivity probability at the cortical surface using a surface deflation algorithm, as described in Sec. 4.2. This produces a new, smoother surface that follows the cortical boundary closely while leaving out the gyri. Then, the connectivity probability at each cortical voxel is defined as the connectivity probability value at the corresponding inner-surface voxel.

A major challenge in using the particle framework for solving the cortical correspondence problem is the highly convoluted geometry of the human cortex. In the current implementation, the particles are assumed to be living on the local tangent planes of the surfaces for computational efficiency purposes; highly convoluted surfaces present a challenge to this assumption due to the rapidly changing tangent planes. We solve this problem by defining an alternative domain to the problem, by 'inflating' the cortical surface. This results in much smoother surfaces. A one-to-one mapping between this surface and the original cortical surface is necessary, as the particles live on the inflated surface, whereas the correspondence features (such as the sulcal depth or the probabilistic connectivity) are only defined on the original surface. A set of automated tools distributed as part of the FreeSurfer [1,2] package are used for preprocessing the data as well as for the cortical inflation, as described in Sec. 3.3.

3   Entropy-Based Cortical Correspondence with Local Features

3.1   Entropy-Based Shape Correspondence

Entropy-Based Surface Sampling. In this work, we use a surface sampling technique, described in [13], using a discrete set of points called particles. These particles move away from each other under a repulsive force, while constrained to lie on the surface. The repulsive forces are weighted by a Gaussian function of inter-particle distance; interactions are therefore local for sufficiently small σ.

It is noteworthy that the current formulation computes Euclidean distance between particles, rather than the geodesic distance on the surface, for computational efficiency purposes. Thus, a sufficiently dense sampling is assumed, so that nearby particles lie in the tangent planes of the zero sets of a scalar function F which provides the implicit object surface. This is an important consideration for the application to the cortical surface; the highly convoluted surface challenges this assumption, and the distribution of particles may be affected by neighbors that are outside of the true manifold neighborhood. As discussed in Sec. 2, we overcome this problem by transforming the domain of the problem to a smoother one, obtained by cortex inflation.

Ensemble Entropy of Correspondence Positions. An ensemble $\mathcal{E}$ is a collection of M surfaces, each with their own set of particles, i.e. $\mathcal{E} = z^1, \ldots, z^M$. The ordering of the particles on each shape implies a correspondence among shapes, and thus we have a matrix of particle positions $P = x_j^k$, with particle positions along the rows and shapes across the columns. We model each surface $z^k \in \Re^{Nd}$ as an instance of a random variable Z (where N is the number of particles and d is the surface dimension), and propose to minimize the combined ensemble and shape cost function

$$Q = H(Z) - \sum_k H(P^k), \tag{1}$$

which favors a compact ensemble representation balanced against a uniform distribution of particles on each surface as discussed in the previous paragraph. The different entropies are commensurate so there is no need for ad-hoc weighting of the two function terms.

Given the low number of examples relative to the dimensionality of the space, we must impose some conditions in order to perform the density estimation. For this work we assume a normal distribution and model $p(Z)$ parametrically using a Gaussian with covariance Σ. The entropy is then given by

$$H(Z) \approx \frac{1}{2} \log |\Sigma| = \frac{1}{2} \sum_{j=1}^{Nd} \log \lambda_j, \tag{2}$$

where $\lambda_1, \ldots, \lambda_{Nd}$ are the eigenvalues of Σ.

Since, in practice, Σ will not have full rank, the covariance is estimated from the data, letting Y denote the matrix of points minus the sample mean for the ensemble, which gives $\Sigma = (1/(M - 1))YY^T$. The negative gradient $-\partial H/\partial P$ gives a vector of updates for the entire system, which is recomputed once per system update. This term is added to the shape-based updates described in the previous section to give the update of each particle.

3.2   Using Local Features for Improving Correspondence

In the case of computing entropy of vector-valued functions of the correspondence positions P, we now consider the more general case where $\tilde{P} = f(x_j^k)$, where

$f : \Re^d \to \Re^q$, where d is the dimensionality of the surface and q is the dimension of f (number of correspondence features). $\tilde{Y}$ becomes a matrix of the function values at the particle points minus the means of those functions at the points, and we compute the general cost function simply as

$$\tilde{H}(\tilde{P}) = \log \left| \frac{1}{M-1} \tilde{Y}^T \tilde{Y}, \right| . \tag{3}$$

Then, the gradient of $\tilde{H}$ with respect to each shape k can be computed using the chain rule, by introducing the Jacobian of the functional data for shape k.

3.3   Surface Reconstruction and Cortex Inflation

In this work, we use FreeSurfer for the cortical surface reconstruction as well as surface inflation. We initialize the FreeSurfer algorithm with the output of the atlas based tissue segmentation tool itkEMS, which uses an Expectation-Maximization approach to segment the major brain tissue classes and correct for intensity inhomogeneity using both T1 and T2 weighted images[18].

The inflation algorithm of FreeSurfer[1] provides a much smoother surface than the cortical surface while minimizing metric distortions. This is achieved via the optimization of an energy functional consisting of the weighted sum of a spring force that works towards 'inflating' the surface and a metric preservation term that ensures that as little metric distortion as possible is introduced. The inflation process is such that points that lie in convex regions move inwards while points in concave regions move outwards over time. Thus, the average convexity/concavity of the surface over a region, referred to as sulcal depth, can be computed as the integral of the normal movement of a point during inflation.

4   Using Probabilistic Fiber Connectivity for Cortical Correspondence

4.1   Stochastic Tractography

In this work, we use an open-source implementation of a modification of Friman's stochastic tractography algorithm[15]. In this approach, fiber tracts are modeled as sequences of unit vectors whose orientation is determined by sampling a posterior probability distribution. The posterior distribution is given by a prior likelihood of the fiber orientation multiplied by the likelihood of the orientation given the DWI data. Friman uses a tensor model constrained to be linearly anisotropic to lower the computational cost of the algorithm; deviations from this distribution are modeled as uncertainty in the fiber orientation. At each step, the orientation of the previous vector in the sequence affects the prior, ensuring no backtracking occurs. The tracking stops when the tract reaches a voxel with a low posterior probability of belonging to the white matter. We use the output of the itkEMS algorithm described above, co-registered with the DWI data (by registering the T2-weighted image with the DWI baseline using an affine transformation with 15 dof's), as the necessary soft WM segmentation input. The ROI's are obtained from the FreeSurfer segmentation.

A high number of sample fibers are tracked from each voxel included in the input ROI; the probabilistic connectivity of a voxel to the ROI is defined as the ratio of fiber samples that travel through a voxel over the total number of samples. As described in the next section, the connectivity values on the WM/GM boundary are discarded, and the values at the corresponding deflated surface location are used instead, to compensate for the fading DWI signal at the boundary. Finally, to normalize for various effects such as number of voxels in the ROI's and brain size, we perform a histogram equalization on the connectivity feature values read on the deflated surface, for each individual and for each ROI.

4.2   Surface Deflation for Connectivity Mapping

In order to get accurate readings of fiber connectivity probability values, an inner white matter surface with one-to-one correspondence to the WM/GM boundary is necessary. This surface should be not only sufficiently away from the boundary, but also without the convolutions caused by sulci and gyri. Without such a deflated surface, the probabilistic fiber connectivity values become heavily

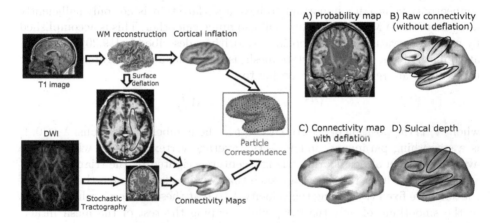

Fig. 1. *Left,* pipeline overview. We use T1 images to generate WM surfaces and inflated cortical surfaces, as well as local sulcal depth. Selected ROI's and the DWI image are input to the stochastic tractography (ST) algorithm. WM surface deflated using proposed algorithm is used to construct connectivity maps on the surface from ST results. Inflated cortical surfaces and the connectivity maps are used to optimize correspondence. *Right,* impact of brain deflation algorithm on surface connectivity values. The stochastic tractography algorithm gives connectivity probabilities for the brainstem for this subject *(A).* The noisy tracking around temporal lobe is reflected on the connectivity map that uses simple averaging *(B).* The surface deflation method ignores the noisy signal and reflects a more accurate connectivity map *(C).* Note how strongly the averaging method depends on sulcal depth *(D),* illustrated in highlighted regions.

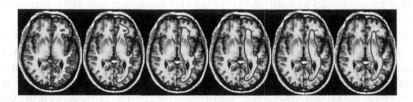

Fig. 2. Brain deflation progress for one subject. The surface outline is shown in contrasting colors overlayed on an axial slice of the brain. The leftmost image shows the original WM surface, and the consequent images show the progress of the deflation at 1000 iteration intervals. The second rightmost surface is used for retrieving probabilistic connectivity images after a final scaling step, shown on the far right. Note the progressive smoothing of the gyri as the surrounding regions become flat, which relaxes the velocity constraint on these vertices.

dependent on the local sulcal depth, yielding high connectivity values near sulci and low connectivity values near the gyri, as the fibers must be tracked a longer distance through the isotropic boundary region to reach the gyri (see Fig. 1). We propose a surface evolution method that evolves the WM surface by progressively smoothing out the gyri. To prevent the local sulcal depth from dominating the connectivity values, it's important to have a surface that is not only sufficiently away from the WM-GM boundary but also much smoother. This is accomplished by a mean-curvature-based smoothing algorithm, described in [19,20]. This iterative method smoothes the surface mesh using a relaxation operator, such that the vertices are repositioned according to

$$V_i^{t+1} = (1 - \lambda)V_i^t + \lambda \bar{V}_i^t,$$

where V_i is the position of the ith vertex, t is the number of iterations, $\lambda \in [0, 1]$ is a smoothing parameter, and $\bar{V}_i$ is the average vertex position, which is the average position of neighboring triangle centers weighted by the triangle areas.

However, we alter this algorithm such that vertices located near the valleys of the sulci are fixed (by forcing the velocity λ to 0 at these vertices), which results in the smoothing of only the gyri, while keeping the rest of the mesh intact. The fixed locations are progressively released, to avoid creating singular points on the surface due to the hard constraints posed. The progressive relaxation is based on thresholding of the L_2 norm of the mean curvature H, defined as

$$\|H\|_2 = \sqrt{\frac{1}{4\pi} \int H^2 dA}.$$

The vertices to be fixed initially are determined based on the sulcal depth. All positive local maxima of the sulcal depth are marked as fixed, and all vertices of the mesh that are located between already fixed locations are also fixed, in order to create merged surface patches rather than standalone points. It is preferable to start with too many fixed vertices rather than too few, as the progressive relaxation stage ensures no vertices remain fixed for more than necessary. Constraining the fixed points to positive sulcal depth values ensures vertices located on the gyri are free to move at all times, whereas the sulci can start moving only after the surrounding gyri have been smoothed out.

The progressive relaxation of the fixed locations is necessary to avoid any patches from remaining fixed indefinitely despite the fact that the rest of the mesh around it has sufficiently deflated. Once the fixed sulcal region becomes flat (detected by the mean curvature threshold), the zero-velocity constraint on the vertex is released, and the vertex is free to move.

As a final step in the deflation, we shrink the entire surface inwards by about one voxel, to ensure that the vertices at the sulci move away from the WM/GM boundary. Without this shrinking step, the probabilistic connectivity values at the sulci and gyri would be treated differently, which would introduce unwanted bias by only moving the gyri away from the WM/GM boundary. Note that the shrinking has to be done in small increments to avoid introducing topological changes to the surface. Fig. 2 shows intermediate results of the surface deflation on an axial slice of the brain scan as well as the final scaling.

5   Evaluation Criteria for Correspondence Quality

To compare the results of the various correspondence methods, evaluation metrics are needed. The choice of evaluation metrics is important since the definition of a "good" correspondence can greatly vary among different applications. In this work, we are using the well established generalization and specificity metrics[6], based on the cortical thickness and sulcal depth measures. It should be noted that sulcal depth based evaluation is biased, since sulcal depth is used for optimization both by FreeSurfer and partially by our method. Cortical thickness based metrics provide an unbiased evaluation. We also use the mean variance (averaged across the surface) of cortical thickness and sulcal depth given the various correspondence results as an additional evaluation criterion.

Given a statistical shape model, generalization is a measure of how well the model can describe unseen objects of the same class. The generalization ability $G(M)$ is computed by performing a leave-one-out principal components analysis (PCA), reconstructing the left-out object, and averaging the reconstruction error for each object, where M is the number of shape eigenmodes used in reconstruction. A good model should exhibit low generalization values.

Specificity is a metric of how well the model fits the object class, in that it measures the distance between measurements in the training set and new measurements generated using the model. A specific model should only generate measurements similar to those in the training set. The specificity $S(M)$ is computed via generating a large number of random measurement vectors (such as cortical thickness) from the model PCA shape space and comparing them to the measurement vectors in the training set.

6 Results and Discussion

We applied our methodology to a dataset of 9 healthy subjects with 1.5T DTI scans as well as structural MRI scans. The DTI scans had 60 gradient directions and 10 baselines, with $b = 700s/mm^2$ and $(2mm)^3$ voxel size. Cortical surfaces were reconstructed via FreeSurfer from T1 images that have been corrected for bias via the itkEMS tool using both T1 and T2 scans. No manual interventions were made to the FreeSurfer pipeline. Only left hemispheres were used.

We compare three methods of correspondence computation: FreeSurfer, xyz-based particle system, and connectivity-based particle system. For the latter, we used probabilistic connectivity measurements to the corpus callosum, the brain-stem and the left caudate, with the ROI segmentations provided by FreeSurfer. We also use sulcal depth as an additional feature channel. Each feature channel was weighted such that the variance of the features across the population would have a mean value of 1.0 across the surface. This is necessary to prevent features with large absolute values (such as spatial location, typically in the range $[-128..128]$) from dominating the features with small absolute values (such as connectivity probabilities, in the range $[0..1]$).

In general, we expect our method to produce improved correspondence over certain regions (for instance, the ones that are strongly identifiable by fiber tract connections to subcortical regions chosen as ROI's) and smaller improvement in other regions where no relevant additional local information is provided. The goal of our approach is to improve local cortical correspondence in given regions by using relevant data. Note that it would be up to each individual application to define what regions are important for the given context, and what additional data can be used to improve the correspondence in these critical regions.

In particular, for this study, since we observed fiber connections to the temporal lobe from both the corpus callosum and the left caudate, we expect to see significantly improved correspondence in this region. Therefore, in addition to the cortical thickness variance averaged across the entire surface, we also report the same values computed over the temporal lobe only.

The results are summarized in Fig. 3. FreeSurfer yields a much tighter sulcal depth distribution than our method, which is to be expected as this is a biased evaluation metric. The sulcal depth based generalization and specificity plots (not shown) also show better results for FreeSurfer. However, the unbiased

	Sulcal depth	Cortical thickness	Cortical thickness in temporal lobe
FreeSurfer	0.039	0.312	0.343
XYZ entropy	0.109	0.262	0.275
Connectivity + XYZ + SD entropy	0.108	0.260	0.259

Fig. 3. Average variances of cortical thickness and sulcal depth measurements across the whole cortical surface as well as across the temporal lobe, given different correspondence maps

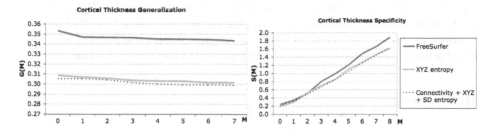

Fig. 4. Cortical thickness based generalization and specificity comparison. For both evaluation metrics, a lower value indicates a better correspondence. Therefore, we see that our method outperforms the other two algorithms regarding these two metrics.

cortical thickness measurements show, as seen in Fig. 4, that the connectivity-based entropy system has better generalization and specificity properties, independent of the number of shape eigenmodes used (M). Our method also yields tighter cortical thickness distribution overall compared to both FreeSurfer and the spatial location based particle system. In particular, the correspondence quality was significantly enhanced in the temporal lobe, which appears to present a 'problem area' for the other two algorithms (as evidenced by higher than average cortical thickness variance). The incorporation of additional connectivity information clearly improves correspondence. Our results are also in agreement with the previous findings [4,5,6] that group-wise approaches tend to be more efficient than pair-wise correspondence optimization methods.

7   Conclusion

We present a novel method that allows using data from diffusion weighted images along with structural MRI scans in a cortical correspondence setting. Our algorithm allows for the fiber connectivity information extracted from the DWI to be effectively projected on the cortical surface using a novel surface deflation technique. We then use our entropy-based dynamic particle framework to seamlessly integrate this information with geometrical cues, such as spatial location and sulcal depth, in order to improve cortical correspondence.

Our results illustrate the powerful generalizability of this technique: the user can improve the correspondence in all regions of the cortical surface, as long as strongly identifiable local features can be provided. Such local features can be extracted from structural images, DTI, or other imaging modalities such as magnetic resonance angiography (MRA). Future work includes exploring additional features to be used for this purpose as well as applying the technique to group analysis studies.

Acknowledgements. This work is part of the National Alliance for Medical Image Computing (NAMIC), funded by the NIH through the NIH Roadmap for Medical Research, Grant U54 EB005149. Information on the National Centers for Biomedical Computing can be obtained from http://nihroadmap.nih.gov/bioinformatics.

This research is also funded by UNC Neurodevelopmental Disorders Research Center HD 03110. We are thankful to Randy Gollub and the MIND Clinical Imaging Consortium for the data, and Tri Ngo, Carl-Fredrik Westin and Polina Golland for the stochastic tractography software implemented as a 3D Slicer module.

References

1. Fischl, B., Sereno, M.I., Dale, A.M.: Cortical surface-based analysis II: Inflation, flattening, and a surface-based coordinate system. NeuroImage 9, 195–207 (1999)
2. Fischl, B., Sereno, M., Tootell, R., Dale, A.: High-res. intersubject averaging and a coordinate system for the cortical surface. Human Brain Mapping, 272–284 (1999)
3. Tosun, D., Prince, J.: Cortical surface alignment using geometry driven multi-spectral optical flow. In: Christensen, G.E., Sonka, M. (eds.) IPMI 2005. LNCS, vol. 3565, pp. 480–492. Springer, Heidelberg (2005)
4. Styner, M., Xu, S., El-Sayed, M., Gerig, G.: Correspondence evaluation in local shape analysis and structural subdivision. In: ISBI, pp. 1192–1195 (2007)
5. Oguz, I., Cates, J., Fletcher, T., Whitaker, R., Cool, D., Aylward, S., Styner, M.: Cortical correspondence using entropy-based particle systems and local features. In: IEEE Symposium on Biomedical Imaging, ISBI 2008, pp. 1637–1640 (2008)
6. Styner, M., Rajamani, K., Nolte, L., Zsemlye, G., Székely, G., Taylor, C., Davies, R.: Evaluation of 3D correspondence methods for model building. In: Taylor, C.J., Noble, J.A. (eds.) IPMI 2003. LNCS, vol. 2732, pp. 63–75. Springer, Heidelberg (2003)
7. Kotcheff, A.C., Taylor, C.J.: Automatic construction of eigenshape models by direct optimization. Medical Image Analysis 2(4), 303–314 (1998)
8. Davies, R., Twining, C., Cootes, T., Waterton, J., Taylor, C.: A minimum description length approach to statistical shape modeling. TMI 21(5), 525–537 (2002)
9. Brechbühler, C., Gerig, G., Kübler, O.: Parametrization of closed surfaces for 3-D shape description. CVIU 61, 154–170 (1995)
10. Styner, M., Oguz, I., Heimann, T., Gerig, G.: Minimum description length with local geometry. In: Proc. ISBI, pp. 283–1286 (2008)
11. Cover, T.M., Thomas, J.A.: Elements of Information Theory. Wiley-Intersc., Chichester (1991)
12. Cates, J., Fletcher, T., Whitaker, R.: Entropy-based particle systems for shape correspondence. In: MFCA Workshop, MICCAI 2006, pp. 90–99 (2006)
13. Cates, J., Fletcher, T., Styner, M., Shenton, M., Whitaker, R.: Shape modeling and analysis with entropy-based particle systems. In: Karssemeijer, N., Lelieveldt, B. (eds.) IPMI 2007. LNCS, vol. 4584, pp. 333–345. Springer, Heidelberg (2007)
14. Basser, P.J., Pajevic, S., Pierpaoli, C., Duda, J., Aldroubi, A.: In vivo fiber tractography using DT-MRI data. Magnetic Resonance in Medicine 44, 625–632 (2000)
15. Friman, O., Westin, C.F.: Uncertainty in white matter fiber tractography. In: Duncan, J.S., Gerig, G. (eds.) MICCAI 2005. LNCS, vol. 3749, pp. 107–114. Springer, Heidelberg (2005)
16. Behrens, T., Woolrich, M., Jenkinson, M., Johansen-Berg, H., Nunes, R., Clare, S., Matthews, P., Brady, J., Smith, S.: Characterization and propagation of uncertainty in diffusion-weighted MR imaging. Mag. Res. Med. 50, 1077–1088 (2003)
17. Jones, D., Pierpaoli, C.: Confidence mapping in DT-MRI tractography using a bootstrap approach. Mag. Res. Med. 53, 1143–1149 (2005)

18. Prastawa, M., Gilmore, J., Lin, W., Gerig, G.: Automatic segmentation of MR images of the developing newborn brain. Medical Image Analysis, 457–466 (2005)
19. Tosun, D., Rettmann, M., Prince, J.: Mapping techniques for aligning sulci across multiple brains. Medical Image Analysis 8(3), 295–309 (2004)
20. Meyer, M., Desbrun, M., Schroder, P., Barr, A.: Discrete differential-geometry operators for triangulated 2-manifolds. VisMath, 35–57 (2003)

A Variational Image-Based Approach to the Correction of Susceptibility Artifacts in the Alignment of Diffusion Weighted and Structural MRI

Ran Tao, P. Thomas Fletcher, Samuel Gerber, and Ross T. Whitaker

School of Computing, University of Utah
Scientific Computing and Imaging Institute, University of Utah

Abstract. This paper presents a method for correcting the geometric and greyscale distortions in diffusion-weighted MRI that result from in-homogeneities in the static magnetic field. These inhomogeneities may due to imperfections in the magnet or to spatial variations in the magnetic susceptibility of the object being imaged—so called *susceptibility artifacts*. Echo-planar imaging (EPI), used in virtually all diffusion weighted acquisition protocols, assumes a homogeneous static field, which generally does not hold for head MRI. The resulting distortions are significant, sometimes more than ten millimeters. These artifacts impede accurate alignment of diffusion images with structural MRI, and are generally considered an obstacle to the joint analysis of connectivity and structure in head MRI. In principle, susceptibility artifacts can be corrected by acquiring (and applying) a field map. However, as shown in the literature and demonstrated in this paper, field map corrections of susceptibility artifacts are not entirely accurate and reliable, and thus field maps do not produce reliable alignment of EPIs with corresponding structural images. This paper presents a new, image-based method for correcting susceptibility artifacts. The method relies on a variational formulation of the match between an EPI baseline image and a corresponding T2-weighted structural image but also specifically accounts for the physics of susceptibility artifacts. We derive a set of partial differential equations associated with the optimization, describe the numerical methods for solving these equations, and present results that demonstrate the effectiveness of the proposed method compared with field-map correction.

1 Introduction

Echo-planar imaging (EPI), used in virtually all diffusion-weighted MRI acquisition protocols, including diffusion tensor imaging (DTI), assumes a homogeneous static magnetic field, which generally does not hold for head MRI. These field inhomogeneities are caused in large part by spatial variation in the magnetic susceptibility of the objects being scanned. Thus, these *susceptibility artifacts* are image dependent, and will be different for each subject being scanned.

J.L. Prince, D.L. Pham, and K.J. Myers (Eds.): IPMI 2009, LNCS 5636, pp. 664–675, 2009.

The effect of static field inhomogeneities is described by a physical model of the distortions in k-space. These distortions result in both a spatial warp of the image geometry as well as a change in the image intensities. The geometric distortion is a nonlinear warping along the phase-encoding direction, which is typically the same for the baseline ($b = 0$) and diffusion weighted images (DWIs). Conventionally, this direction is along the coronal axis of the patient, and is denoted as the y coordinate. The image intensities are preserved as *densities* in this transformation, and thus the intensities of EPIs are affected locally, proportional to the Jacobian of the corresponding transformation.

The effects of susceptibility artifacts on clinical images are significant. The geometric distortions can be more than a centimeter, and the effects on EPI-acquired intensities in brain tissue can be more than 100% of the original signal. The example in Figure 2 shows a pair of images, an EPI (baseline from a DTI sequence) of a brain and a coregistered, structural T2 image of the same patient. Here we see the obvious distortion in frontal cortex (and associated changes in intensity), but the entire head is also distorted (shortened) in this case. These artifacts impede accurate alignment of diffusion images with structural MRI, and are generally considered an obstacle to the joint analysis of connectivity and structure in head MRI. This joint analysis is one of the primary motivations for the work in this paper. However, even analysis of DTI alone is impaired by these artifacts, because tensor estimates depend on the distorted intensities of the each of the DWIs (with an inhomogeneous relationship), and subsequent geometric analysis, such as tractography, depends on the distorted geometric relationships between nearby tensors. Thus, susceptibility artifacts are an important problem in the analysis of diffusion weighted MRI.

Susceptibility artifacts can be corrected, to a certain extent, by the acquisition of a corresponding field map, as described in [1]. However, the literature shows [2] and we will further demonstrate in this paper, that field map corrections of susceptibility artifacts are not entirely accurate and reliable, and thus field maps do not produce reliable alignment of EPI to corresponding structural MRI. The reasons for this discrepency are not entirely understood, but noise in the field map reconstructions as well as small inaccuracies in the associated physical model can lead to significant artifacts. Fundamentally, however, any attempt to correct EPIs so that they align with structural data must explicitly account for geometry of the structural data (e.g., T1, T2, PD) in order to overcome inevitable noise and inaccuracies in the physical model as well as distortions in the structural data itself. This is the motivation for the image-driven EPI correction proposed in this paper.

The literature does show several examples of image-driven EPI correction [3,4]. However, the methods in [3] employ low-dimensional, relatively smooth warps, which are not adequate for many of the examples in this paper. The methods presented in [4], while using higher-order deformations, do not explicitly account for the intensity transformations in the signal that result from local expansion or contraction of the corresponding transformation. Thus, these methods are not adquate for the very nonlinear distortions that we have observed in practice, particularly in the frontal cortex.

The proposed method uses an image-based correction for susceptibility artfacts. We formulate the correction as an optimization of a penalty that captures the intensity differences between the *Jacobian corrected* EPI baseline images and a corresponding T2-weighted structural image. The penalty includes a penalty on the dervative of the transformation, to ensure smoothness in the final warp. We derive the first variation of this expression, including the Jacobian term, and show that this formulation reduces to a novel PDE for intensity-conserving image registration. We present a numerical method that allows the method to solve for the optimal registration in practical times and we show results on phantoms and real head data that demonstrates the effectiveness of the method relative to corrections based solely on the field map.

2   Related Work

There is a significant body of work in the area of correcting susceptibility artifacts in echo-planar MRI. Here we review some of that work, for context, with an emphasis on approaches that are technically and strategically related to the proposed method.

The physical model of susceptibility-related distortion is described by Jezzard et al. [1], and they present a method for correcting these distortions using an associated field map. The correction of EPI distortion by field maps is, in principle, correct. However, a variety of researchers have noted that such field maps are not always available, and, when they are, often fail to completely correct geometric distortions. This was most recently observed by Wu et a. [2], and will be confirmed by results presented later in this paper.

Therefore, a variety of researchers have proposed image-based methods for correcting EPI artifacts. For instance, Kybic et al. [5] present a method that uses a deformable registration, represented by B-splines and minimize the mean-squared-difference between a B0 (baseline) EPI image and a T2 weighted, anatomically correct MRI. They optimize by a gradient descent using analytical derivatives and coarse-to-fine multiresolution framework. They do not account for the significant changes in image intensity that occur, due to the conservation of the EPI signal when deformed, which is particularly important with more recent imaging acquisitions that use higher field strengths. Studholme et al. [3] use a spline-based deformation and include the signal amplitude correction (which is proportional to the Jacobian of the transformation). They use the log of the signal to accentuate the impact of low-amplitude image regions, and optimize mutual information using a gradient descent with a finite difference scheme for the updates. Wu et al. [2] also propose a B-spline registration between EPI and structural MRI, and make quantitative comparisons with field maps.

With modern imaging systems, which employ larger magnetic fields to improve noise characteristics, EPI distortions can be quite severe. Thus, there is a need for EPI-structural registration technologies that incorporate a more versatile set of transformations, such as those described by dense displacement fields. For instance, Hellier et al. [6] describe an elastically-regularized displacement field for EPI-structural registration, based on mutual information, but without a correction for signal conservation. Likewise, Tao et al. [4] describe a dense, regularized warp between structural images and EPI, without a Jacobian correction.

The contribution of this paper is to describe a complete variational approach to the registration of EPI images to structural data which gives a gradient descent on dense displacement fields with a proper correction for the conservation of the EPI signal. The result is novel partial differential equation for signal-preserved image registration with some unique characteristics. We present the derivation, describe a numerical scheme for solving this equation, and demonstrate its effectiveness at EPI susceptibility-artifact correction relative to a state-of-the art field-map correction.

3 EPI Susceptibility Artifact Correction

3.1 Variational Formulation

The correction of susceptibility artifacts, which is the subject of this paper, is a necessarily part of a processing pipeline [2] for DWI processing, which corrects for head motion, eddy current artifacts, and coordinate system inconsistencies between scans. We begin with the methodology for susceptibility correction, and then describe the entire pipeline which we use for the subsequent experiments.

Generally, we denote the transformation between the EPI and structural coordinate systems as $x_E = \phi(x)$, where $x = (x, y, z)$ is a shorthand for vectors, and the "E" subscript indicates the EPI coordinate system. The coordinate transformation associated with field inhomogeneities is usually approximated as a displacement along the phase direction of the scan (e.g. as described in [3]). For most protocols this is along the posterior-anterior axis, Thus we denote, without a loss of generality, this displacement direction as y. The displacement is $v(x, y, z)$ and EPI image coordinates are

$$(x_E, y_E, z_E) \approx (x, y + v(x, y, z), z). \tag{1}$$

The relationship between the uncorrected and corrected EPI images must account for the conservation of signal [3], and thus the expression of the EPI image, I_E, in structural coordinates is:

$$I_{E-S}(x, y, z) = J_\phi(x, y, z)I_E(x, y + v(x, y, z), z), \tag{2}$$

where J_ϕ is the Jacobian of ϕ, which, in this case, has a conventient form:

$$J_\phi(x, y, z) = 1 + \frac{\partial v(x, y, z)}{\partial dy}. \tag{3}$$

The strategy we use in this paper is to register the B0 image in an DWI acquisition with a T2-weighted structural image. Because these two images are correlated, we contruct a squared-error penality between the T2 and the corrected EPI, and include an elastic penalty on v. That is,

$$\mathcal{E}_v = \frac{1}{2} \int_{\mathcal{D}} \left[\left(1 + \frac{\partial v}{\partial y}\right) I_{\mathrm{E}}(x, y + v, z) - I_{\mathrm{S}}(x, y, z) \right]^2 dx\, dy\, dz$$

$$+ \frac{\lambda}{2} \int_{\mathcal{D}} |\nabla v|^2 dx\, dy\, dz,$$

where we have left out the formal dependency of v on x to keep the expressions concise. We optimize with gradient descent, which we derive from the first variation. Thus we have

$$\delta \mathcal{E}_v = I_{\mathrm{E}}(x, y + v, z) \frac{\partial}{\partial y} \left[I_{\mathrm{E}}(x, y + v, z) - I_{\mathrm{S}}(x, y, z) \right]$$

$$- I_{\mathrm{E}}(x, y + v, z) \frac{\partial}{\partial y} \left[I_{\mathrm{E}}(x, y + v, z) \frac{\partial v}{\partial y} \right] - \lambda \nabla \cdot \nabla v.$$

We introduce a dummy variable, t, and let v descend the energy $\mathcal{E}_v$ as a function of t, and thus we have the PDE which describes the evolution of v as we optimize the EPI-structural alignment. This gives

$$\frac{\partial v}{\partial t} = \tilde{I}_{\mathrm{E}} \frac{\partial}{\partial y} \left[I_{\mathrm{S}} - \tilde{I}_{\mathrm{E}} \right] + \tilde{I}_{\mathrm{E}} \frac{\partial}{\partial y} \left[\tilde{I}_{\mathrm{E}} \frac{\partial v}{\partial y} \right] + \lambda \nabla \cdot \nabla v, \qquad (4)$$

$$= E(v) + F(v) + G(x), \qquad (5)$$

where $\tilde{I}_{\mathrm{E}} = \tilde{I}_{\mathrm{E}}(x, y, z) = I_{\mathrm{E}}(x, y + v, z)$ is a shorthand for the unwarped EPI image, without the Jacobian correction.

We have factored the first variation into three terms; E, F, and G; so that Equation 5 has a particular form that demonstrates its unique nature. The equation differs from many other elastic-registration PDEs in two ways. The first term (on the right hand side), which is often considered as a *forcing* term that drives the two images to correspond, depends on the derivative of the image residual rather than the image residual itself, as is typical with elastically regularized registration methods. Second, besides the regularization in the third term, there is an extra heterogeneous diffusion in the second term, which is a result of the Jacobian correction. This second term has important implications for the numerical implementation of this PDE.

3.2   Numerical Implementation

The numerical approach is to iterate with discrete time steps, Δt, on the transformation v until $\partial v / \partial t$ falls below some threshold, and we have reached some approximate steady state. The time steps should be chosen so that the updates in v are smaller than the grid spacing and the solution does not *jump over* image data in our attempt to find a minimum. We use a coarse-to-fine multiresolution minimization strategy in order to overcome this computational burden of these relatively small steps and to alleviate the tendency toward local minima.

With this limitation on Δt, the first term in Equation 5, $E(v)$, can be treated as a reaction term and implemented with finite forward differences. The third term, $G(v)$, is a diffusion term, but it is stationary and is usually implemented as convolution. The second term, however, must be treated with care. The F term is a nonstationary diffusion. Because this diffusion is proportional to the square of the image intensity, it results in a very large diffusion number for this equation. Thus, the time steps required for this equation to be stable in a forward difference scheme are so small it becomes impractical.

For this reason, we solve for the second term using a semi-implicit method. Here we describe briefly the numerical scheme, in *one dimension*; that is, the y axis along which the diffusion takes places. Subsequently we describe how the regularization (third term in Eq. 5), which is the only part of this equation that depends on $x - z$, is solved for the 3D case.

Let v_i^k be the ith grid point of the displacement for the kth time step. We denote the discretely sampled input images, the EPI and the structural images, as e_i and s_i, respectively. Let $\tilde{e}_i^k$ denote the deformed EPI image, which is computed by sampling the discrete image e_i at position $i + v_i^k$ using a linear interpolation. We denote the discrete forms of intermediate quantities in Eq. 5 as E_i, F_i, and G_i.

Now we consider the three terms in Eq. 5 one by one. For the first term we have:

$$E_i \approx \frac{\tilde{e}_i^k}{2} \left((s_{i+1} - s_{i-1}) - (\tilde{e}_{i+1}^k - \tilde{e}_{i-1}^k) \right) \tag{6}$$

The second and third terms are linear operations on v^{k+1}, which forms the implicit part of the update:

$$F_i + G_i \approx + \left(\lambda + \tilde{e}_i^k \frac{\tilde{e}_i^k + \tilde{e}_{i-1}^k}{2} \right) v_{i-1}^{k+1} \tag{7}$$

$$- \left(2\lambda + (\tilde{e}_i^k)^2 + \tilde{e}_i^k \frac{\tilde{e}_{i+1}^k + \tilde{e}_{i-1}^k}{2} \right) v_i^{k+1} + \left(\lambda + \tilde{e}_i^k \frac{\tilde{e}_{i+1}^k + \tilde{e}_i^k}{2} \right) v_{i+1}^{k+1}$$

We treat this as a linear system, letting the grid quantities without subscripts denote the vector forms of the corresponding grid data and the linear operator in Eq. 7 be A. For the update of v, we have the following

$$v^{k+1} = (I - \Delta t A)^{-1} \left(v^k + \Delta t E \right). \tag{8}$$

The matrix $(I - \Delta t A)$ is tridiagonal, and we can efficiently solve this system using a two-pass Gaussian elimination. We choose Δt so that $\max[\Delta t E] < 0.4$.

For three dimensions, the discrete method is the same, except that we have two extra terms in Eq. 7 that are proportional to second derivatives in x and z, which result from the 3D Laplacian. There are several ways to include these. Because λ is usually small relative to $\max(\tilde{I}^2)$, this regularization term is not time-step limiting, and we can include the second derivatives from regularization in the explicit part of the equation, which we do in the results that follow. Alternatively, one could treat all of these second order terms implicitly, and use some type of splitting scheme to solve this system [7].

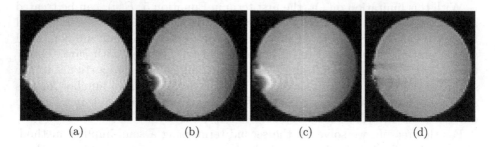

       (a)   (b)   (c)   (d)

Fig. 1. Phantom data EPI correction. (a) Structural image. (b) squashed EPI image. (c) field map corrected EPI image. (d) Proposed method corrected EPI image.

3.3   EPI-Structural Processing Pipeline

The proposed EPI distortion correction is, in practive, the final step in a combined diffusion and structural image processing pipeline. This full pipeline for aligning a set o DWI images with structural data consists of the following steps:

1. Preprocess structural images (T1 and T2) to remove skull, correct bias field, normalize intensities, and segment tissue classes (to provide a white matter mask) [8].
2. Correct diffusion weighted images for eddy currents and head motion [9].
3. Rigidly align the T1, T2, and segmentation label images to the B0 image based on mutual information metric.
4. Calculate the deformation field v using the proposed method.
5. Concatenate the eddy current transformation and the deformation field v and apply the resulting transformation to all DWIs. By sampling the original images using the composed transformations, we interpolate the images only once.

4   Results

In this section we present results of the proposed method for EPI distortion correction on real data. The first experiment is applying the correction to phantom data, and the second experiment is to apply the method to diffusion imagery of the human brain. In each experiment we compare the results of our method to field-map correction, which was done using the Statistical Parametric Mapping (SPM) field map toolbox [1,10,11,12] [1].

4.1   Phantom Data Results

We applied our method and field-map correction to a phantom dataset provided with the SPM field map toolbox [2]. The phantom is a gel phantom with a spherical

---

[1] Statistical Parametric Mapping : http://www.fil.ion.ucl.ac.uk/spm/
[2] ftp://ftp.fil.ion.ucl.ac.uk/spm/toolbox/FieldMap2/FieldMapExampleData.tar.gz

geometry. Figure 1 shows a slice from the original phantom dataset. Notice that the geometry of the phantom has been globally squashed as well as a smaller local change on the left. The results from the field-map correction (Figure 1(c)) show that the field map does a good job correcting the global squashing in the image, but it does not do a good job correcting the local "dimple" on the left side. The results from our proposed method (Figure 1(d)) show a correction of both global and local distortions. The field map correction may be unable to handle small scale geometric distortions because the field map must be blurred to remove noise.

4.2   Data Acquisition

Head data were acquired on a 3 Tesla Siemens scanner. Diffusion weighted images were acquired with a single-shot spin-echo EPI sequence with high-resolution $(2 \times 2 \times 2.5mm^3)$, which was performed using bipolar gradients with dual-echo refocusing to reduce eddy currents. This consisted of one image with $b = 0s/mm^2$ and 12 images with $b = 1000s/mm^2$ with different gradient orientations. An

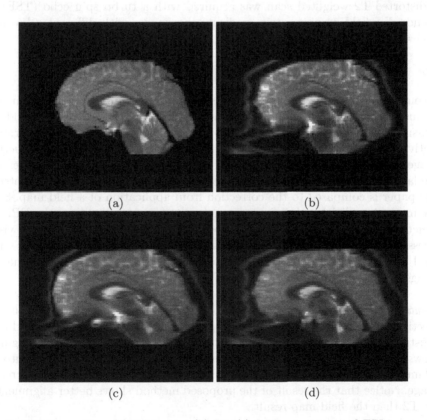

Fig. 2. EPI Correction. (a) T2 Image. (b) B0. (c) field map corrected EPI image. (d) Proposed method corrected EPI image.

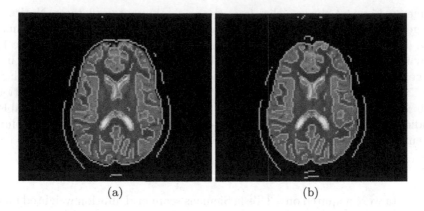

(a)   (b)

Fig. 3. EPI Correction. (a)field map overlay T2. (b) Proposed method corrected EPI image overlay T2.

undistorted T2 weighted scan was acquired with a turbo spin echo (TSE) sequence. For field mapping, two gradient-echo images with different echo times (TE = 4 and 6.46 ms) were collected.

4.3   Validation Methods

A common problem in validating results from non-rigid image registration algorithms, is the lack of ground truth. Therefore, we are limited to using indirect measures to establish the reliability of our variational approach. Since a primary motivation for this work is to facilitate joint analysis of diffusion and structural imagery, we will use the fit of the diffusion images to the structural images as a validation measure. In each experiment the result of the correction presented in this paper is compared to the correction from application of a field map. Since our method explicitly minimizes the mean-squared error between the EPI and structural T2 image, we use two independent measures for comparison: visual assessment of edges and mutual information between the DWIs and a T1 structural image. First, we show the results of our EPI distortion correction method alongside the field-corrected image in Figure 2.

Visual Assessment of Edges. As an initial check, we confirm through visual inspection that the DWIs and the corresponding T2 image are well aligned after registration by superimposing the contour of the EPIs onto the T2. Figure 3 shows the resulting edge map of the corrected baseline image overlaid onto the T2 image. Also shown for comparison is the edge map for the field-map corrected image. Notice that the result of the proposed method shows better alignment to the T2 than the field map result.

Mutual information of DWIs and T1. We compared the corrected DWIs with the structural T1 image using mutual information. The T1 image has been

Table 1. Mutual Information Comparison

Measure	B_0	Average DWIs
Before	0.725	0.731
Proposed	0.839	0.814
Fieldmap	0.736	0.718

Table 2. B-spline Mutual Information Comparison

Measure	B_0	Average DWIs
B-spline (8x10x15)	0.764	0.762
B-spline (16x20x10)	0.781	0.780
B-spline (24x30x15)	0.795	0.786

coregistered with the T2 image in step 3 of the pipeline described in Section 3.3. Mutual information to T1 was chosen because it gives a good metric of alignment of the diffusion images to the structural image, but it is independent of the registration metric used in the proposed method (mean-squared error to T2). Table 1 gives the results of the comparison for both our method and for field map correction. The table shows a comparison of mutual information of the T1 to corrected B0 image as well as the average mutual information of the T1 to each of the diffusion-weighted images. Notice that the mutual information improves for our method in all cases, while it actually decreases on average for the field-map corrected DWIs.

Comparison to Low-Order Deformation. In order to test the need for the high-order deformation (dense displacement field) that we use, we compared the results to a B-spline representation of the deformation. To do this we projected the final deformation field onto a cubic B-spline basis with control point spacings of increasing resolution. These lower-order deformations were then applied to the diffusion images in the same way. The results of a mutual information comparison to the T1 image are shown in Table 2. The high-order deformation of the proposed method achieves the best mutual information, and mutual information increases monotonically with increased resolution. This suggests that the local deformations present in the EPI are best handled with a dense displacement field.

5 Discussion

We have presented a variational image registration framework for correcting the geometric distortions from susceptibility artifacts in EPI, which has application to the alignment of diffusion and structural imaging. We have shown results on phantom data as well as a clinical DTI dataset that our method compares favorably to field map correction. Because of the variability of field maps and the dependence of field distortions on the geometry of the objects being imaged, this method will need to be tested on further data to thoroughly compare it to field maps. Another area of future investigation is the interaction between the various geometric corrections required in DTI, including head motion, eddy current, and susceptibility artifacts. Currently, we perform a head motion and eddy current correction jointly, followed by the EPI distortion correction presented in this paper. Since performing the head motion and eddy current corrections changes the phase-encoding direction, this should be accounted for in the EPI distortion correction. Future work will investigate a joint correction model that includes all three models of geometric distortion inherent in DTI. Finally, another useful improvement would be a formulation that uses mutual information rather than image correlation as an image match function. This would allow registration directly to a T1 image in cases where an undistorted structural T2 image is not available.

Acknowledgments

We would like to thank Molly DuBray and Dr. Janet Lainhart for providing the image data. This work was supported by an Autism Speaks Mentor-based Postdoctoral Fellowship, Grant Number RO1 MH080826 from the National Institute Of Mental Health, and the National Alliance for Medical Image Computing (NAMIC): NIH Grant U54 EB005149.

References

1. Jezzard, P., Balaban, R.: Correction for geometric distortion in echo planar images from B0 field variations. Magnetic Resonance in Medicine 34, 65–73 (1995)
2. Wu, M., Chang, L.C., Walker, L., Lemaitre, H., Barnett, A.S., Marenco, S., Pierpaloi, C.: Comparison of EPI distortion correction methods in diffusion tensor mri using a novel framework. In: Metaxas, D., Axel, L., Fichtinger, G., Székely, G. (eds.) MICCAI 2008, Part II. LNCS, vol. 5242, pp. 321–329. Springer, Heidelberg (2008)
3. Studholme, C., Constable, R., Duncan, J.: Accurate alignment of functional epi data to anatomical mri using a physics based distortion model. IEEE Trans. Med. Imaging, 1115–1127 (2000)
4. Tao, G., He, R., Poonawalla, A.H., Narayana, P.: The correction of epi-induced geometric distortions and their evaluation. In: Proc. ICIP (2007)
5. Kybic, J., Nirkko, A., Unser, M.: Unwarping of unidirectionally distorted epi images. IEEE Trans. on Medical Imaging 19, 80–93 (2000)
6. Hellier, P., Barillot, C.: Multimodal non-rigid warping for correction of distortions in functional MRI. In: Delp, S.L., DiGoia, A.M., Jaramaz, B. (eds.) MICCAI 2000. LNCS, vol. 1935, pp. 512–520. Springer, Heidelberg (2000)
7. Tai, X.C., Lie, K.A., Chan, T., Osher, S.: Image Processing Based on Partial Differential Equations. Springer, Heidelberg (2007)
8. Leemput, K.V., Maes, F., Vandermeulen, D., Suetens, P.: Automated model-based tissue classification of MR images of the brain. IEEE Trans. on Medical Imaging 18(10), 897–908 (1999)

9. Rohde, G., Barnett, A., Basser, P., Marenco, S., Pierpaoli, C.: Comprehensive approach for correction of motion and distortion in diffusion-weighted MRI. Magnetic Resonance in Medicine 51, 103–114 (2004)
10. Andersson, J., Hutton, C., Ashburner, J., Turner, R., Friston, K.: Modelling geometric deformations in epi time series. NeuroImage 13, 903–919 (2001)
11. Hutton, C., Bork, A., Josephs, O., Deichmann, R., Ashburner, J., Turner, R.: Image distortion correction in fmri: A quantitative evaluation. NeuroImage 16, 217–240
12. Jenkinson, M.: Fast, automated, N-dimensional phase-unwrapping algorithm. Magnetic Resonance in Medicine 49, 193–197

4D MAP Image Reconstruction Incorporating Organ Motion

Jacob Hinkle[1], P. Thomas Fletcher[1], Brian Wang[2], Bill Salter[2],
and Sarang Joshi[1]

[1] Scientific Computing and Imaging Institute, University of Utah
Salt Lake City, Utah
[2] Huntsman Cancer Institute, University of Utah, Salt Lake City, Utah

Abstract. Four-dimensional respiratory correlated computed tomography (4D RCCT) has been widely used for studying organ motion. Most current algorithms use binning techniques which introduce artifacts that can seriously hamper quantitative motion analysis. In this paper, we develop an algorithm for tracking organ motion which uses raw time-stamped data and simultaneously reconstructs images and estimates deformations in anatomy. This results in a reduction of artifacts and an increase in signal-to-noise ratio (SNR). In the case of CT, the increased SNR enables a reduction in dose to the patient during scanning. This framework also facilitates the incorporation of fundamental physical properties of organ motion, such as the conservation of local tissue volume. We show in this paper that this approach is accurate and robust against noise and irregular breathing for tracking organ motion. A detailed phantom study is presented, demonstrating accuracy and robustness of the algorithm. An example of applying this algorithm to real patient image data is also presented, demonstrating the utility of the algorithm in reducing artifacts.

1 Introduction

Four-dimensional respiratory-correlated computed tomography (4D RCCT) has been widely used for studying organ motion. The current standard practice is to use phase binned images [1]. However, the phase binning algorithm assumes that the patient has a periodic breathing pattern. When the patient's breathing is irregular, this assumption breaks down and significant image artifacts like those shown in Fig. 1 are introduced. In a recent extensive study, Yamamoto et al. [2] found that 90% of 4D RCCT patients had at least one artifact. Amplitude binning algorithms have been developed as a way to alleviate these artifacts by assuming that the underlying anatomical configuration is correlated to the amplitude of the breathing signal. This method reduces binning artifacts but since data is not acquired at all breathing amplitudes the images often have some missing slices [1]. Deformable image registration has been shown to be useful in tracking organ motion in artifact-free 4D RCCT images [3]. Such methods may be used with either phase or amplitude binned images, but are challenged in the presence of binning artifacts.

J.L. Prince, D.L. Pham, and K.J. Myers (Eds.): IPMI 2009, LNCS 5636, pp. 676–687, 2009.

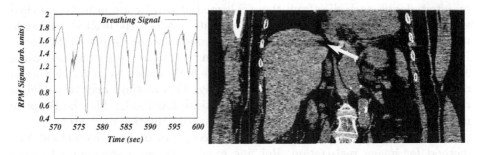

Fig. 1. Non-periodic patient breathing pattern (left) and image artifacts introduced by phase binning (right)

In this paper, we develop a maximum a posteriori (MAP) algorithm for tracking organ motion that uses raw time-stamped data to reconstruct the images and estimate deformations in anatomy simultaneously. The algorithm eliminates artifacts as it does not rely on a binning process and increases signal-to-noise ratio (SNR) by using all of the collected data. In the case of CT, the increased SNR provides the opportunity to reduce dose to the patient during scanning. This framework also facilitates the incorporation of fundamental physical properties such as the conservation of local tissue volume during the estimation of the organ motion. We show that this formulation is accurate and robust against noise and irregular breathing for tracking organ motion and reducing artifacts in a detailed phantom study. An improvement in image quality is also demonstrated by application of the algorithm to data from a real liver stereotactic body radiation therapy patient.

1.1   Previous Work in Motion Artifact Elimination

Previous attempts at reducing 4D RCCT motion artifacts do not offer all the advantages of our proposed method, which incorporates a fully diffeomorphic motion model into the reconstruction process. For instance, Yu and Wang [4] model rigid 2D motion during acquisition to alleviate in-plane artifacts in fan-beam CT. Their motion model is not valid for imaging of the torso, where respiratory-induced motion causes highly non-linear deformation with a significant component in the superior-inferior direction. Another method, presented by Li et al. [5], reconstructs a full 4D time-indexed image using a B-spline motion model and a temporal smoothing condition. Zeng et al. [6] and Li et al. [7] present other B-spline-based methods that require an artifact-free reference image (such as a breath-hold image) in addition to a 4D fan-beam or cone-beam scan. These approaches address difficulties caused by slowly-rotating cone-beam scanners. However the acquisition of an artifact-free reference image is impractical for many radiotherapy patients. While the B-spline model guarantees smooth deformations, it cannot guarantee the diffeomorphic properties for large deformations ensured by our method and it does not directly enforce local conservation of tissue volume. Erhardt et al. [8] reconstruct 3D images at arbitrary amplitudes by interpolating each slice from those collected at nearby amplitudes and then stacking them. Two slices are used to interpolate a slice at the desired amplitude using an optical flow algorithm, so only 2D motion can be estimated. Recently, Rit et al. [9] have used a 4D cone-beam scan to estimate organ motion using an optical flow approach. The motion estimate is then used to correct for organ motion during subsequent 3D scans on the fly. This method may be useful in reducing artifacts in a 3D image, but the optical flow model, like the B-Spline model, does not ensure diffeomorphic incompressible motion estimates.

As early as 1991, Song and Leahy [10] used an incompressible optical flow method for image registration. Rohlfing et al. [11] use a spline-based model which penalizes tissue compression to perform incompressible image registration. Saddi et al. [12] study incompressible fluid-based registration of liver CT. Their approach requires solution of Poisson's equation via a multigrid method at each iteration. An efficient Fourier method of incompressible projection similar to the one presented in this paper is presented by Stam [13]. His approach applies a result from the continuous domain to discrete data without alteration, while our method directly accommodates the discrete nature of our image data. Despite these efforts in image registration, the incompressible nature of internal organs has not previously been incorporated into the image reconstruction process.

2   RCCT Data Acquisition

During a typical 4D RCCT fan-beam scan, the patient passes through the scanner on an automated couch that pauses at regular intervals to collect data. At each couch position slices are acquired repeatedly 15–20 times. Each slice is acquired by collecting a series of projections at different angles. The slices are then reconstructed individually using filtered back-projection [14]. The speed of acquisition of each slice is dependent on the scanner and for current generation multi-slice scanners is generally on the order of 0.5 s. The X-ray detection process used to acquire slices is subject to Poisson noise [15]. However, at the x-ray tube currents typically used in clinical practice the signal is strong enough that the noise is approximately Gaussian. The patient's breathing is monitored during acquisition using an external surrogate for internal organ motion. The resulting breathing trace, $a(t)$, is used to tag the acquired projection retrospectively with a breathing amplitude. For the studies presented in this paper breathing is monitored via the Real-time Position Management (RPM) system (Varian Oncology Systems, Palo Alto, CA), which uses a camera to track infrared-reflective markers attached to the patient's torso. The methods presented herein are general and can be applied to signals recorded by breathing monitoring systems such as spirometry [16] or chest circumference tracking [17]. Although developed with 4D RCCT of liver as the main application, the methods may be applied to other motion such as cardiac using the ECG signal in place of a breathing monitor.

3   4D Imaging Model

The 4D image reconstruction problem is to estimate the time-indexed image $I(t, x)$ that best represents the patient's anatomy during image acquisition. In order to obtain a maximum a posteriori estimate of organ motion we derive the data likelihood and define a prior model incorporating the physical constraints. We estimate the 4D image that maximizes the posterior probability combining the data likelihood and the prior.

CT image acquisition is described by a projection operator, P_θ, which can represent fan-beam or cone-beam projections at angle θ. At sufficiently high signal-to-noise ratio, the acquisition of a single projection p_i is subject to Gaussian noise of variance σ^2. The data log-likelihood then becomes

$$\mathcal{L}(\{p_i\}|I(t, x)) = -\frac{1}{2\sigma^2} \sum_i \int_s |P_{\theta_i}\{I(t_i, x)\}(s) - p_i(s)|^2 ds, \qquad (1)$$

where the integration with respect to s is over a one or two-dimensional domain depending on the projection operator used.

Due to the sparsity of the imaging data, the full 4D image reconstruction problem is ill-posed, so it is necessary to constrain the estimation. We assume that no metabolic changes or local tissue density variations occur during acquisition and that the only dynamic process is the motion of the anatomy due to breathing. Under this assumption, the 4D image is described by a time-indexed deformation field and a single representative static 3D image, $I_0(x)$, as

$$I(t, x) = I_0(h(t, x)), \qquad (2)$$

where for each time t, $h(t, \cdot)$ is a volume-preserving diffeomorphic deformation capturing the respiratory-induced motion of the underlying anatomy.

We assume that organ motion is correlated with breathing amplitude, so the deformation may be indexed by amplitude only. Under this assumption the deformations take the form $h(a(t), x)$. The velocity of a point in the patient's anatomy is then described by the ordinary differential equation

$$\frac{d}{dt} h(a(t), x) = v(a(t), h(a(t), x)) \frac{da}{dt}, \qquad (3)$$

where v is indexed by amplitude and may be thought of as a velocity with respect to changes in amplitude rather than time. The deformation from zero amplitude to any other amplitude is given by the associated integral equation

$$h(a, x) = x + \int_0^a v(a', h(a', x)) da'. \qquad (4)$$

If the velocities are constrained to be smooth, this formulation guarantees that the resulting estimates of patient anatomy are at all times diffeomorphic to one another. This is important as it ensures that organs do not tear or disappear during breathing [18]. The diffeomorphic deformations provide a one-to-one correspondence between points in images from different breathing amplitudes, enabling tracking of tissue trajectories. We enforce smoothness by introducing a prior on the velocities via a Sobolev norm $\|v\|_V^2$, defined by

$$\|v\|_V^2 = \langle v, v \rangle_V = \int_0^1 \int_{\boldsymbol{x} \in \Omega} \|Lv(a, \boldsymbol{x})\|_{\mathbb{R}^3}^2 d\boldsymbol{x} da, \tag{5}$$

where L is a differential operator chosen to reflect physical tissue properties. Although in this paper we use a homogeneous operator, L can be spatially-varying reflecting the different material properties of the underlying anatomy.

Deformations defined by the flow along smoothly-varying vector fields as described in Eq. 3 have been well studied [19]. In particular, if the divergence of the velocity field is zero the resulting deformation is guaranteed to preserve volume locally and have unit Jacobian determinant. This is a necessary constraint when modeling the breathing induced motion of incompressible fluid-filled organs such as liver. In fact, if L is the Laplacian operator and the velocities are constrained to be divergence-free, the velocities simulate Stokes flow of an incompressible viscous fluid [20].

With the data log-likelihood and the prior model described above, the log-posterior probability of observing our data becomes

$$\mathcal{L}(I_0, v | p_i) = -\|v(a)\|_V^2 - \frac{1}{2\sigma^2} \sum_i \int_s |P_{\theta_i}\{I_0 \circ h(a_i, x, y, z_i)\}(s) - p_i(s)|^2 ds,$$

$$\text{subject to div } v = 0. \quad (6)$$

4   Model Estimation

Having defined the posterior, the 4D image reconstruction problem is to estimate the image and deformations parameterized by the velocity field that maximize Eq. 6,

$$(\hat{I}_0, \hat{v}) = \underset{I_0, v}{\operatorname{argmax}} \, \mathcal{L}(I_0, v | p_i) \qquad \text{subject to div } v = 0. \tag{7}$$

A MAP estimate that maximizes Eq. 6 is obtained via an alternating iterative algorithm which at each iteration updates the estimate of the deformation in a gradient ascent step then updates the image using the associated Euler-Lagrange equation. The continuous amplitude-indexed velocity field is discretized by a set of equally-spaced amplitudes a_k with the associated velocities v_k, with spacing Δa. Note that this amplitude discretization is independent of the amplitudes at which data is acquired. The deformation from amplitude a_k to a_{k+1} is approximated by the Euler integration of Eq. 4,

$$h(a_{k+1}, \boldsymbol{x}) = h(a_k, \boldsymbol{x}) + v_k(h(a_k, \boldsymbol{x})) \tag{8}$$

and the deformation for an amplitude a_i between a_k and a_{k+1} is linearly interpolated as

$$h(a_i, \boldsymbol{x}) = h(a_k, \boldsymbol{x}) + \frac{a_i - a_k}{\Delta a} v_k(h(a_k, \boldsymbol{x})). \tag{9}$$

Note that higher order integration schemes such as Runge-Kutta may also be used in place of the simpler Euler method.

The first variation of Eq. 6 with respect to v_k under the inner product in Eq. 5 is given by

$$\delta_{v_k} \mathcal{L}(I_0, v_k | p_i) = -2v_k - \frac{1}{\sigma^2}(L^\dagger L)^{-1} \sum_i P_{\theta_i}^\dagger \left(P_{\theta_i}\{I_0 \circ h(a_i, \cdot)\} - p_i \right) b_i(k, \cdot),$$

(10)

where b_i is the contribution to the variation due to a single projection and $P_{\theta_i}^\dagger$ is the adjoint of the projection operator, which acts by backprojecting the data discrepancy back into the 3D volume. The adjoint operators for various imaging geometries have been well studied. For parallel-beam CT geometry, the adjoint projection operator is the familiar backprojection operator. Conventional filtered backprojection CT slice reconstruction involves applying the adjoint operator, after filtering the 1D data [14]. Let $I_k(x) = I_0 \circ h(a_k, x)$ be the 3D reference image pushed forward to amplitude a_k, the factors b_i are given by

$$b_i(k, x) = \begin{cases} 0 & a_i \leq a_k \\ \frac{a_i - a_k}{\Delta a} \nabla I_k(x + \frac{a_i - a_k}{\Delta a} v_k(x)) & a_k < a_i \leq a_{k+1} \\ \left| D(h_{a_{k+1}} \circ h_{a_i}^{-1})(x) \right| \nabla I_k(x + v_k(x)) & a_i > a_{k+1}. \end{cases}$$

(11)

If the deformations are constrained to be incompressible, implying that the Jacobian determinant is unity, this simplifies to

$$b_i(k, x) = \begin{cases} 0 & a_i \leq a_k \\ \frac{a_i - a_k}{\Delta a} \nabla I_k(x + \frac{a_i - a_k}{\Delta a} v_k(x)) & a_k < a_i \leq a_{k+1} \\ \nabla I_k(x + v_k(x)) & a_i > a_{k+1}. \end{cases}$$

(12)

Following the approach of Beg et al. [21], efficient computation of $(L^\dagger L)^{-1}$ is implemented in the Fourier domain, requiring only a matrix multiplication and Fourier transforms of v_k at each iteration of the algorithm.

The Helmholtz-Hodge decomposition allows us to implement the incompressibility constraint by simply projecting the unconstrained velocity fields onto the space of divergence-free vector fields at each iteration of the algorithm [22]. In order to efficiently implement the Helmholtz-Hodge decomposition of a time-varying velocity field, we use the discrete divergence operator as it operates in Fourier domain. We write the discrete Fourier transform of a central difference approximation to the derivative of a function f as

$$\mathrm{DFT}\{\Delta_x f\}(\omega) = \mathrm{DFT}\left\{ \frac{f(x + k_x) - f(x - k_x)}{2k_x} \right\}(\omega) = \frac{i}{2k_x} \sin \omega \, \mathrm{DFT}\{f\}(\omega).$$

(13)

In the Fourier domain the divergence of a vector field takes the following form:

$$\mathrm{DFT}\{\mathrm{div}\, v\}(\omega) = W(\omega) \cdot \mathrm{DFT}\{v\}(\omega),$$

(14)

where

$$W(\boldsymbol{\omega}) = \frac{i}{2} \begin{pmatrix} \frac{1}{k_x}\sin\frac{\omega_x}{N_x} \\ \frac{1}{k_y}\sin\frac{\omega_y}{N_y} \\ \frac{1}{k_z}\sin\frac{\omega_z}{N_z} \end{pmatrix}. \tag{15}$$

This allows us to remove the divergent component easily in Fourier space via the projection

$$\text{DFT}\{v\}(\boldsymbol{\omega}) \mapsto \text{DFT}\{v\}(\boldsymbol{\omega}) - \frac{W(\boldsymbol{\omega}) \cdot \text{DFT}\{v\}(\boldsymbol{\omega})}{\|W(\boldsymbol{\omega})\|_{\mathbb{C}^3}^2} W(\boldsymbol{\omega}). \tag{16}$$

Since the operator $(L^\dagger L)^{-1}$ is implemented in the Fourier domain there is little computational overhead in performing this projection at each iteration of the algorithm described in Sec. 4.

The first variation of Eq. 6 with respect to I_0 is

$$\delta_{I_0}\mathcal{L}(I_0, v|p_i) = \frac{1}{\sigma^2}\sum_i |Dh^{-1}(a_i, \cdot)| \left(P_{\theta_i}^\dagger P_{\theta_i}\{I_0 \circ h(a_i, \cdot)\} - P_{\theta_i}^\dagger p_i \right) \circ h^{-1}(a_i, \cdot). \tag{17}$$

If organ motion is slow compared to single slice acquisition time, individual slices can be reconstructed with minimal motion artifacts using filtered back projection. In this case the 4D image is estimated from the reconstructed 2D slices $S_i(x, y)$. Note that this assumption holds reasonably well in the case of 4D RCCT. Under the slow motion assumption, the velocity field variation becomes

$$\delta_{v_k}\mathcal{L}(I_0, v_k|p_i) = -2v_k - \frac{1}{\sigma^2}(L^\dagger L)^{-1}\sum_i (I_0 \circ h(a_i, \cdot) - S_i)\, b_i(k, \cdot). \tag{18}$$

For slice data, S_i, and an incompressible deformation estimate Eq. 17 is solved by the mean of the deformed data,

$$\hat{I}_0(\boldsymbol{x}) = \frac{1}{N} \sum_{i, h^{-1}(a_i, \boldsymbol{x})_z = z_i} S_i \circ h^{-1}(a_i, \boldsymbol{x}), \tag{19}$$

which is equivalent to solving the Euler-Lagrange equation for Eq. 6.

Algorithm 1. Pseudocode for 4D reconstruction of slice data

$I_0 \leftarrow 0$
for each k **do**
  $v_k \leftarrow 0$
end for
repeat
  $I_0 \leftarrow \frac{1}{N}\sum S_i \circ h^{-1}(a_i, \boldsymbol{x})$
  for each k **do**
    $v_k \leftarrow v_k + \epsilon\delta_{v_k}\mathcal{L}(I_0, v_k)$
  end for
  Perform divergence-free projection on each v_k
until algorithm converges or maximum number iterations reached

---

Note that as soon as the velocity field is updated, the image estimate must also be updated. The change of image estimate in turn alters the velocity gradients leading to a joint estimation algorithm in which, at each iteration, the velocity fields are updated and then the image recalculated.

Algorithm 1 summarizes the 4D reconstruction procedure for slice data. The velocity fields are initialized to zero, so that the initial estimate of the base image is simply the result of averaging all of the data. This yields a quite blurry image that sharpens upon further iterations as the motion estimate improves.

5   Results

5.1   Phantom Study

In order to validate the accuracy of the 4D reconstruction algorithm, a phantom study was performed using the CIRS anthropomorphic thorax phantom (CIRS Inc., Norfolk, VA) and a GE Lightspeed RT scanner (GE Health Care, Waukesha, WI). The phantom includes a simulated chest cavity with a 2 cm spherical object representing a tumor that is capable of moving in three dimensions. A chest marker is also included in the phantom which moves in a pattern synchronized to the tumor and allows simulation of a real patient 4D RCCT scan. The scans used in this study were driven to simulate a breathing trace collected from a real patient.

Figure 2 shows the experimental setup, with the recorded RPM trace and the stationary spherical CIRS lung tumor phantom imaged with helical CT. The 4D phase binned dataset generated by the GE Advance Workstation is shown in the top row of Fig. 3. Notice the binning artifacts including mismatched slices in the phase binned data when compared with the image of the stationary phantom. Also shown in Fig. 3 bottom row are images from an amplitude binned dataset at peak-inhale, mid-range amplitude, and peak-exhale. The images do not show signs of mismatched slices and more closely resemble the static phantom image but suffer from missing data artifacts.

Because we did not have access to the raw projection data, we applied the slow motion assumption described in the previous section when using the CINE

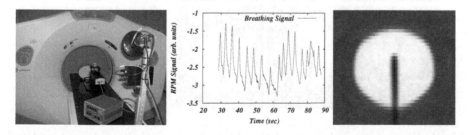

Fig. 2. (left) CIRS phantom during scan setup with Varian RPM camera and GE Lightspeed RT scanner, (center) breathing trace recorded during phantom acquisition and (right) a helical CT scan of the stationary phantom

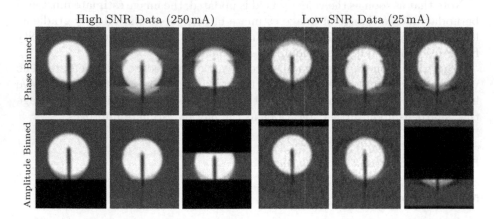

Fig. 3. Binned images of the moving CIRS phantom. The top row shows phase binned images at three different phases for the high SNR data (left) and the low SNR (10% tube current) data (right). The bottom row shows amplitude binned images at end-inhale, mid-range, and end-exhale amplitudes for both the high and low SNR data.

slice data along with the recorded RPM trace in the 4D reconstruction algorithm. In order to demonstrate robustness against noise, an initial scan was taken with an X-ray tube current of 250 mA then repeated with a tube current of 25 mA. Shown in Fig. 4 are the 4D reconstructed images generated using the same raw data as the phase and amplitude binned images in Fig. 3. Notice that the reconstructed image does not have any artifacts associated with either the

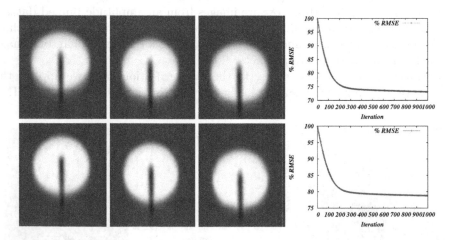

Fig. 4. 4D reconstructed images of the phantom at end-inhale, mid-range, and end-exhale amplitudes. The top row shows the 4D reconstruction of the high SNR data, while the bottom row shows that of the low SNR data. Also shown are plots of the posterior indicating the convergence of the algorithm.

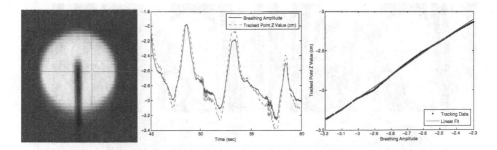

Fig. 5. Tracked point (left) with RPM signal and superior-inferior (z) coordinate (center) and plot of tracked point z coordinate versus RPM signal (right) showing strong linear correlation

phase binning or amplitude binning. Notice also the increase in SNR in the 4D reconstructed images. Reconstructed 4D images from 25 mA data have higher signal-to-noise ratio (SNR=76.5) than binned images reconstructed using 250 mA data (SNR=53.9). The similarity in images between the two 4D reconstructions shows the robustness of the image estimation to increasing noise.

To validate the estimated deformation model, a single point at the center of the phantom indicated by the cross hair in Fig. 5 was tracked by integrating the estimated velocity fields according to Eq. 4. The physical construction of the phantom dictates that the superior-inferior displacement is linearly correlated to the RPM signal. Shown in Fig. 5 is a plot of the estimated displacements versus the RPM signal. Notice the excellent linear correlation ($r = 0.9988$) between them, validating the deformation estimation process.

5.2 Real Patient Study

The 4D reconstruction algorithm was also applied to data collected from a real patient undergoing hypo-fractionated radiation therapy treatment of the liver at the Huntsman Cancer Institute at the University of Utah. A comparison between phase

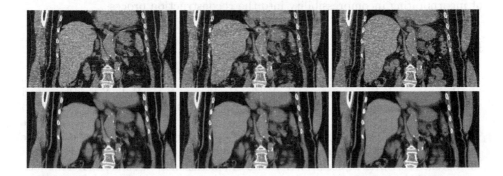

Fig. 6. Phase binned images (top) along with 4D reconstructed images (bottom) at peak-exhale, mid-range, and peak-inhale

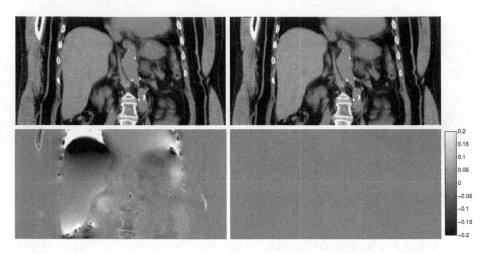

Fig. 7. 4D reconstructed images and log Jacobian determinant images (bottom) for compressible flow reconstruction (left) and with incompressibility constraint (right). Negative log Jacobian values indicate local compression, while positive values indicate expansion.

binning and the 4D reconstruction is shown in Fig. 6. In addition to improving SNR, slice mismatch artifacts are absent in the 4D reconstructed image.

The 4D reconstruction algorithm was run with and without the incompressibility constraint. Analysis of the incompressibility projection is shown in Fig. 7. The reconstructed images are extremely similar, while the Jacobian maps are quite different. In particular, it is seen that without the incompressibility constraint, the estimated motion indicates compression and expansion of the top and bottom of the liver, while the incompressible reconstruction shows no local expansion or contraction. This illustrates the fact that although the two methods produce very similar images, the motion estimates are quite different. Given that liver is a blood-filled organ, physiologically it does not undergo any appreciable local changes in volume due to breathing. This exemplifies the necessity of incorporating incompressibility into the reconstruction process.

References

1. Abdelnour, A.F., Nehmeh, S.A., Pan, T., Humm, J.L., Vernon, P., Schöder, H., Rosenzweig, K.E., Mageras, G.S., Yorke, E., Larson, S.M., Erdi, Y.E.: Phase and amplitude binning for 4D-CT imaging. Phys. Med. Biol. 52(12), 3515–3529 (2007)
2. Yamamoto, T., Langner, U., Billy, W., Loo, J., Shen, J., Keall, P.J.: Retrospective analysis of artifacts in four-dimensional CT images of 50 abdominal and thoracic radiotherapy patients. Int. J. Radiat. Oncol. Biol. Phys. 72(4), 1250–1258 (2008)
3. Pevsner, A., Davis, B., Joshi, S., Hertanto, A., Mechalakos, J., Yorke, E., Rosenzweig, K., Nehmeh, S., Erdi, Y.E., Humm, J.L., Larson, S., Ling, C.C., Mageras, G.S.: Evaluation of an automated deformable image matching method for quantifying lung motion in respiration-correlated CT images. Med. Phys. 33(2), 369–376 (2006)

4. Yu, H., Wang, G.: Data consistency based rigid motion artifact reduction in fan-beam CT. IEEE Trans. Med. Imag. 26(2), 249–260 (2007)
5. Li, T., Schreibmann, E., Thorndyke, B., Tillman, G., Boyer, A., Koong, A., Goodman, K., Xing, L.: Radiation dose reduction in four-dimensional computed tomography. Med. Phys. 32(12), 3650–3660 (2005)
6. Zeng, R., Fessler, J.A., Balter, J.M.: Respiratory motion estimation from slowly rotating X-ray projections: Theory and simulation. Med. Phys. 32(4), 984–991 (2005)
7. Li, T., Koong, A., Xing, L.: Enhanced 4D cone-beam CT with inter-phase motion model. Med. Phys. 34(9), 3688–3695 (2007)
8. Ehrhardt, J., Werner, R., Säring, D., Frenzel, T., Lu, W., Low, D., Handels, H.: An optical flow based method for improved reconstruction of 4D CT data sets acquired during free breathing. Med. Phys. 34(2), 711–721 (2007)
9. Rit, S., Wolthaus, J., van Herk, M., Sonke, J.J.: On-the-fly motion-compensated cone-beam CT using an a priori motion model. In: Metaxas, D., Axel, L., Fichtinger, G., Székely, G. (eds.) MICCAI 2008, Part I. LNCS, vol. 5241, pp. 729–736. Springer, Heidelberg (2008)
10. Song, S.M., Leahy, R.M.: Computation of 3-D velocity fields from 3-D cine CT images of a human heart. IEEE Trans. Med. Imag. 10(3), 295–306 (1991)
11. Rohlfing, T., Calvin, R., Maurer, J., Bluemke, D.A., Jacobs, M.A.: Volume-preserving nonrigid registration of MR breast images using free-form deformation with an incompressibility constraint. IEEE Trans. Med. Imag. 22(6), 730–741 (2003)
12. Saddi, K.A., Chefd'hotel, C., Cheriet, F.: Large deformation registration of contrast-enhanced images with volume-preserving constraint. In: Proceedings of International Society for Optical Engineering (SPIE) Conference on Medical Imaging 2007, vol. 6512 (2007)
13. Stam, J.: A simple fluid solver based on the FFT. Journal of Graphics Tools 6(2), 383–396 (2001)
14. Prince, J.L., Links, J.M.: Medical imaging signals and systems. Prentice-Hall, Englewood Cliffs (2006)
15. Guan, H., Gordon, R.: Computed tomography using algebraic reconstruction techniques (ARTS) with different projection access schemes: a comparison study under practical situations. Phys. Med. Biol. 41(9), 1727–1743 (1996)
16. Hoisak, J.D.P., Sixel, K.E., Tirona, R., Cheung, P.C.F., Pignol, J.P.: Correlation of lung tumor motion with external surrogate indicators of respiration. Int. J. Radiat. Oncol. Biol. Phys. 60(4), 1298–1306 (2004)
17. Bosmans, G., van Baardwijk, A., Dekker, A., Öllers, M., Boersma, L., Minken, A., Lambin, P., Ruysscher, D.D.: Intra-patient variability of tumor volume and tumor motion during conventionally fractionated radiotherapy for locally advanced non-small-cell lung cancer: A prospective clinical study. Int. J. Radiat. Oncol. Biol. Phys. 66(3), 748–753 (2006)
18. Joshi, S.C., Miller, M.I.: Landmark matching via large deformation diffeomorphisms. IEEE Trans. Imag. Proc. 9(8), 1357–1370 (2000)
19. Arnold, V.I.: Mathematical Methods of Classical Mechanics, 2nd edn. Springer, Heidelberg (1997)
20. Panton, R.L.: Incompressible Flow, 2nd edn. Wiley-Interscience, Hoboken (1996)
21. Beg, M.F., Miller, M.I., Trouvé, A., Younes, L.: Computing large deformation metric mappings via geodesic flows of diffeomorphisms. Int. J. Comp. Vis. 61(2), 139–157 (2005)
22. Cantarella, J., DeTurck, D., Gluck, H.: Vector calculus and the topology of domains in 3-space. Amer. Math. Monthly 109(5), 409–442 (2002)

Incorporating Patient Breathing Variability into a Stochastic Model of Dose Deposition for Stereotactic Body Radiation Therapy

Sarah E. Geneser[1], Robert M. Kirby[1], Brian Wang[2], Bill Salter[2], and Sarang Joshi[1]

[1] Scientific Computing and Imaging Institute, University of Utah, Salt Lake City, UT, USA
[2] Huntsman Cancer Institute, University of Utah, Salt Lake City, UT, USA
`geneser@sci.utah.edu`

Abstract. Hypo-fractionated stereotactic body radiation therapy (SBRT) employs precisely-conforming high-level radiation dose delivery to improve tumor control probabilities and sparing of healthy tissue. However, the delivery precision and conformity of SBRT renders dose accumulation particularly susceptible to organ motion, and respiratory-induced motion in the abdomen may result in significant displacement of lesion targets during the breathing cycle. Given the maturity of the technology, sensitivity of dose deposition to respiratory-induced organ motion represents a significant factor in observed discrepancies between predictive treatment plan indicators and clinical patient outcome statistics and one of the major outstanding unsolved problems in SBRT. Techniques intended to compensate for respiratory-induced organ motion have been investigated, but very few have yet reached clinical practice. To improve SBRT, it is necessary to overcome the challenge that uncertainties in dose deposition due to organ motion present. This requires incorporating an accurate prediction of the effects of the random nature of the respiratory process on SBRT dose deposition for improved treatment planning and delivery of SBRT. We introduce a means of characterizing the underlying day-to-day variability of patient breathing and calculate the resulting stochasticity in dose accumulation.

Keywords: stochastic dose deposition modeling, respiratory-induced organ motion, stereotactic body radiation therapy, polynomial chaos, stochastic collocation.

1 Introduction

Hypo-fractionated stereotactic body radiation therapy (SBRT) employs three-dimensional conformal therapy and stereotactic targeting to reduce treatment volumes as well as the number of fractions necessary to deliver extremely large ablative doses and dramatically increase the likelihood of tumor control [1]. The precision and conformity of SBRT-predicted dose to physician-defined tumor target

J.L. Prince, D.L. Pham, and K.J. Myers (Eds.): IPMI 2009, LNCS 5636, pp. 688–700, 2009.

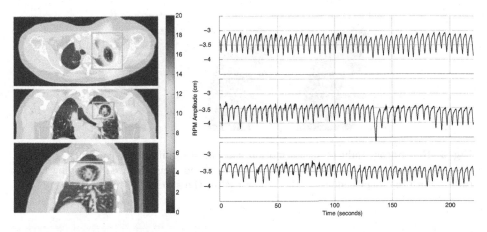

Fig. 1. The static dose plan and Real-time Position Management^{TM} (RPM) traces for a typical SBRT lung cancer patient illustrates the high spatial gradients of target-conforming dose and day-to-day variations in breathing. The static deposited dose (in units of Gray) is color-mapped for the anatomy for axial, sagittal, and coronal views according to the colorbar of the axial view. The RPM breathing traces are recorded for the same patient and time interval on different days.

geometry (evident in the static-dose calculation depicted in Figure Fig. 1) reduce the collateral damage inflicted upon surrounding healthy tissue, particularly in cases where the tumor is stationary during treatment.

State-of-the-art commercial treatment-planning systems are currently capable of calculating accurate dose distributions for only the static case in which the tumor and surrounding tissues are unmoving for the duration of the dose-delivery. However, respiratory-induced organ motion results in significant movement of lesion targets during the breathing cycle [2,3] as evidenced in Fig. 2. Because SBRT is particularly susceptible to motion of the targeted tumor, patient respiration can lead to significant dose-delivery errors. Several studies have investigated the dosimetric consequences of respiratory-induced tissue motion on SBRT and found variations between planned and delivered dose distributions as significant as 20% [4].

Controlling patient breathing during treatment and restricting beam-on times to windows of low variation in patient anatomy are two means of minimizing the variability in dose deposition due to respiratory-induced motion. A number of methods exist to reduce dose variation (e.g., respiratory gating [5], breath-hold [6], and coached breathing [7]). However, such techniques have drawbacks and none are appropriate for all patients as they either induce an unacceptable level of patient discomfort (e.g., due to their compromised respiratory function, many lung cancer patients cannot tolerate breath-hold methods), significantly increase the treatment time (e.g., during respiratory-gated treatment, the beam is only on for a small fraction of the treatment period, necessitating a much extended treatment time), or may be impractical (e.g., in the case of coached

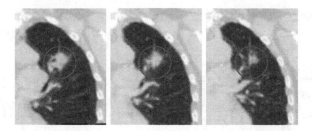

Fig. 2. Respiratory-induced organ motion can cause significant movements of the tumor. These coronal slices represent anatomy corresponding to three breathing amplitudes. Note the displacement of the tumor within the stationary red outline.

breathing, some patients are not trainable). While some radiation oncologists employ these methods, most instead design a treatment based on simple mechanisms, e.g., the inclusion of a border or "margin" around the defined target volume. This technique is widely employed to limit the impact of motion on dose deposition; however, it ensures a complete treatment of the target at the expense of irradiating adjacent healthy tissues. Indeed, breathing motion remains one of the major obstacles to reducing the irradiation volume while maintaining a high probability of tumor control.

Patients may exhibit markedly different breathing patterns between treatment fractions. The fundamentally random nature of respiration can result in delivered doses that significantly vary from treatment to treatment. Failure to accommodate for patient-specific breathing stochasticity can result in under-dosing of the target and deposition of dangerous dose levels to surrounding healthy tissue. When limiting variability of patient organ-motion during treatment is impossible or unreasonable, it is essential to incorporate an accurate prediction of the effects of the stochastic respiratory process on SBRT dose deposition for safe and effective treatment-planning and delivery of SBRT. Though several groups have worked to develop accurate models that incorporate the effect of respiratory-induced organ motion on dose deposition [8], we know of no studies that incorporate a patient-specific stochastic model of breathing variability into dose calculations and no computational tools yet exist to accomplish this goal. The aim of this work is to compute the stochasticity in dose accumulation for SBRT treated lesions resulting from stochastic organ motion induced by variations in day-to-day patient breathing patterns.

We begin by developing a framework for modeling patient specific breathing as a stochastic process. To quantify the stochasticity in patient breathing patterns we parametrize the recorded patient breathing traces and model the resulting breathing parameters as random variables. Once we estimate the underlying distributions of the random variables, we incorporate our stochastic breathing model into a calculation of the stochastic dose that accounts for variations in organ motion during treatment. We may then calculate any pertinent statistics of the stochastic dose.

2   Methods

To account for stochastic respiratory-induced tumor motion, we must first accurately quantify the impact of organ motion on dose deposition over the course of a treatment. This necessitates an accurate patient specific anatomical model over the course of the treatment and the ability to calculate the dose deposition at each anatomical configuration observed during treatment. Commercially available respiratory-correlated CT (RCCT) [9,10] tools provide a means of visualizing four-dimensional organ motion, and clinicians currently rely on the detailed images produced from such scans to generate the contours of targeted volumes to be irradiated. However, tumor volumes and margins for treatment-planning are generated from images obtained on a single day, and fail to consider the stochastic nature of breathing. Using deformable image registration techniques, the anatomical data from all different anatomical conformations during breathing can be mapped onto a common geometry. The mapping can further be used to compute the dose deposition resulting from any observed or simulated respiratory-induced organ motion during treatment [11,12]. By analyzing patient respiratory patterns, we generate a stochastic model of breathing variability. We then incorporate this into an estimate of the stochasticity in total deposited energy resulting from a distribution of breathing-induced organ motion.

2.1   Incorporating Organ Motion into Dose Calculation

To calculate the effect of respiratory-induced organ motion on dose deposition, we first build an explicit model of tissue deformation from anatomical patient images that depict respiratory-induced organ motion. Our motion model and subsequent dose calculations rely on the well-justified and widely accepted assumption that the position of the anatomy is a function of breathing pattern (measured by some external signal e.g., Varian's Real-Time Position Management (RPM) system). Several groups have investigated the correlation between external and internal motion markers [13,14] and reported high correlation between them.

From the patient images, it is essential to construct a deformation field, $h(x, a(t))$, which maps each spatial point, x, in a base image according to the deformation of the anatomy as a function of breathing amplitude. Generating deformation fields that model organ motion is a well-studied problem and several groups have developed techniques that produce accurate deformation fields from artifact-free CT images [15,16]. We employ these well-established image registration methods to construct an amplitude-indexed high-dimensional transformation that maps sequential CT images to a base anatomy on which we calculate dose.

The dynamic dose deposition, D, accounting for the organ motion during a treatment is integrated over the treatment time interval $[0, T]$ as follows:

$$D = \int_0^T d(h(x, a(t)), a(t))dt,$$

where $d(h(x, a(t)), a(t))$ is the static dose corresponding to the amplitude of the breathing signal during treatment, $a(t)$, and mapped to the base image according to the deformation field $h(x, a(t))$. A change of variables yields the total deposited dose over a treatment period as an integral over the amplitudes,

$$D = \int_{min(a)}^{max(a)} d(h(x, a), a)w(a)da, \tag{1}$$

where $w(a)$ is the time density of the breathing amplitudes. Given a set of amplitude-binned CT images and a model of the organ deformation as described above, we estimate delivered dose by discretizing Eq. 1 to obtain a weighted sum of amplitude-indexed dose images as follows:

$$D = \sum_{i=0}^{N} w_i d(h(a_i), a_i), \quad w_i = \int_{a_i - \delta a}^{a_i + \delta a} f(x)dx,$$

where $f(x)$ is a quantification of the relative density of breathing amplitudes over treatment time and $\delta a = \frac{1}{2}(a_{i+1} - a_i)$ is the size of the amplitude discretization. The term $d(h(a_i), a_i)$ corresponds to the calculated dose deposited at a particular breathing amplitude, a_i, and the weights, w_i, account for the relative amount of time the tissue spends at the anatomical configuration corresponding to the amplitude, a_i, during the treatment period.

It is important to stress that the model of dose distribution, D, as presented above accounts only for the respiratory-induced organ motion observed during a single treatment. As such, it includes none of the observed day-to-day variability in a patient's breathing motion. For D to give insight to the effects of day-to-day variability, one must incorporate a model of patient breathing variability as the input to the dose deposition calculation. In the following sections, we provide the framework to determine the stochasticity in daily breathing patterns and to apply our stochastic model to determine the resulting variations in dose distribution.

2.2   Parametrization of Breathing Amplitude Density

The extent of breathing variability differs from patient to patient, necessitating patient-specific models of breathing variability to generate accurate predictions of dose deposition resulting from variations in day-to-day breathing patterns. In particular, because the time density of breathing amplitudes is sufficient to calculate dose distribution, we need only determine the day-to-day variations in amplitude density as a function of time, which we model as a stochastic process.

To parametrize and estimate the amplitude density of each patient breathing trace, we fit a Gaussian Mixture Model (GMM) to the set of recorded amplitudes from each patient breathing trace [17]. Given the parameters of the individual breathing trace amplitudes, we can then analyze the characteristics of variability for the patients and build a model to capture the patient-specific stochasticity in breathing amplitudes.

GMMs provide a means of parametrizing the probability density of a random process and thus the amplitude density of RPM breathing traces. Such models are convex combinations of M Gaussian probability distributions as follows,

$$m(x, p_i, \mu_i, \sigma_i) = \sum_{i=1}^{M} p_i \frac{1}{\sigma_i \sqrt{2\pi}} e^{\frac{-(x-\mu_i)^2}{2\sigma_i^2}} \qquad (2)$$

where μ_i and σ_i are the mean and standard deviation of the ith Gaussian distribution and p_i are positive weighting factors that sum to one. We fit these parameters to patient RPM breathing traces using the well-known Expectation Maximization (EM) algorithm [18,17]. Because patients pause at inhale and exhale and the amplitudes for both are typically consistent over time, one observes peaks in the amplitude density function at both locations. As a consequence, one might conjecture that a two Gaussian mixture model is appropriate for estimating and parametrizing the amplitude density of RPM breathing traces.

2.3   Model of Breathing Variability

In order to quantify the daily variability in the patient specific dose accumulation, we first characterize the variability in the patient's breathing patterns. Because we have parametrized the estimates of the daily amplitude density of patient breathing, we require a formulation of the variation of these parameters from day-to-day. To accomplish this, we performed principal component analysis (PCA) [19] on the model parameters. A two-Gaussian mixture model has five parameters. Using PCA, we identify the components of greatest variation in the GMM parameters.

We formulate the stochasticity in the GMM model parameters as a function of independent and uncorrelated Gaussian random variables, $\boldsymbol{\xi} = (\xi_1, \ldots, \xi_P)$ where P is the number of principal components necessary to accurately capture the breathing variability. This analysis allows us to formulate the variability as a stochastic function of the Gaussian distributed principal components.

2.4   Variations in Dose

Given a model of patient-specific variability in respiratory-induced organ motion and dose calculation, we can now compute statistics of the deposited dose from a single fraction. With the variation in the GMM parameters expressed in terms of a P-dimensional random variable, $\boldsymbol{\xi}$, we incorporate the stochastic model into a statistical characterization of the dose distribution, D, resulting from variations in respiratory-induced organ motion. Because the dose distribution is a direct consequence of anatomical configuration, the dose is expressed as a function of $\boldsymbol{\xi}$, and we denote the dose as $D(\boldsymbol{\xi})$. In our study, we are interested in computing statistics (e.g., mean and variance) on the stochastic dose deposition, $D(\boldsymbol{\xi})$. Based upon these quantities, we can assess the impact of respiratory-induced organ motion variability on generation and interpretation of predicted SBRT dose distributions.

Monte Carlo (MC) techniques are an obvious first choice for computing statistics of a random field like $D(\boldsymbol{\xi})$. Such an approach requires sampling the stochastic GMM parameter space to obtain dose deposition for each treatment realization. However, because Monte Carlo requires a very large number of samples for sufficient convergence of computed statistics, and each dose calculation requires sufficiently long computing time, the inordinate time necessary to calculate accurate statistics using Monte Carlo renders the approach infeasible, especially for clinical use.

2.5   Generalized Polynomial Chaos-Stochastic Collocation

We employ the generalized polynomial chaos-stochastic collocation (gPC-SC) method [20,21] as a computationally efficient and easily implemented alternative to MC sampling. Unlike traditional MC, in which very large numbers of collocation points are required to compute accurate statistics, only a limited number of samples are necessary. The gPC-SC approach requires that the stochastic aspects of the system be mathematically characterizable stochastic processes to take advantage of quadrature rules to integrate the stochastic process of interest over the appropriate domain. Like MC methods, gPC-SC is a sampling method in that it does not require derivation of the stochastic approximating system. In contrast to MC, where the deterministic system must be solved at a very large set of randomly chosen sample values of the stochastic input process, gPC-SC exploits assumptions concerning the mathematical nature of the stochastic system of interest to minimize the number of samples necessary for accurate statistics. Under assumptions of smoothness of the system with respect to inputs, which in this case equate to the recognition that the dose distributions vary smoothly as a function of the breathing patterns, we gain exponential convergence in the statistical accuracy as a function of the number of dose distribution forward simulations we compute. This process yields a sequence of solutions for a small and far more computationally tractable number of specific realizations of the stochastic field. These solutions are then used to obtain highly accurate estimates of the mean, variance, and higher statistical moments of the system.

The generalized polynomial chaos (gPC) method provides a means of representing stochastic processes as a linear combination of orthogonal stochastic polynomials [22]. In our case, the GMM parameters are Gaussian distributed, and are represented exactly by two Hermite polynomials. Because dose calculation is a non-linear process with respect to the GMM parameters and patient anatomy, the distribution of dose will be non-Gaussian. Stochastic processes with arbitrary or non-Gaussian distributions are represented using weighted sums of Hermite polynomials as follows: $\boldsymbol{\xi}(\omega) = \sum_{i=0}^{N} \alpha_i H_i(\omega)$, where ω is a random variable and α_i is a weight obtained by projecting the stochastic process onto the ith Hermite polynomial.

The stochastic collocation approach consists of selecting a collection of points at which to sample the random field and corresponding weights that account for the underlying stochastic characteristics of the system. Each collocation point, $\boldsymbol{\xi}_i$, represents a particular breathing amplitude density for the duration of a treatment selected from the set of likely breathing patterns. We compute the dose deposition for each collocation realization, $D(\boldsymbol{\xi}_i)$, by the method described in Sec. 2.1.

For Gaussian distributed random variables, ψ, of mean zero and unit variance, the collocation points, ψ_i, are the roots of the Hermite polynomials and the weights, c_i, are given by $c_i = \frac{2^{n-1}n!\sqrt{\pi}}{n^2(H_{n-1}(\psi_i))^2)}$. Though polynomial roots can be approximated using a root-finding method like Newton's method, it is faster to use the Golub-Welsch algorithm [23] in the case of Hermite polynomials [24]. We obtain the Hermite roots by calculating the eigenvalues of the Jacobi matrix, J, composed of the recurrence relation coefficients of the Hermite polynomials, and the weights are equivalent to the first component of the normalized eigenvectors of the Jacobi matrix J [24]. To accommodate Gaussian random variables, $\boldsymbol{\xi}$, of arbitrary mean, μ, and variance, σ^2, we map the collocation points as follows: $\boldsymbol{\xi}_i = \sigma\psi_i + \mu$. The collocation weights and points can be extended to multiple stochastic dimensions using tensor products for lower dimensions or the Smolyak construction [20,21] for higher dimensions.

For each collocation point, $\boldsymbol{\xi}_i$, representing a particular breathing amplitude density for the duration of a treatment we calculate the corresponding dose deposition, $D(\boldsymbol{\xi}_i)$. The mean and variance of the deposited dose are calculated using the forward dose computations and the collocation weights as follows:

$$\mathbb{E}[D(\boldsymbol{\xi})] \approx \sum_{i=0}^{N} c_i D(\xi_i) \quad \text{and} \quad \mathbb{E}[(D(\boldsymbol{\xi}) - \mathbb{E}[D(\boldsymbol{\xi})])^2] \approx \sum_{i=0}^{N} c_i (D(\xi_i) - \mu(D(\boldsymbol{\xi})))^2.$$

3   Results

In this section we present results for a lung cancer patient undergoing stereotactic body radiation treatment (SBRT) of 60 Gy total dose over 3 fractions at the Department of Radiation Oncology at the Huntsman Cancer Institute. The static dose plan for the patient is depicted for axial, sagittal, and coronal CT slices in Fig. 1 along with three representative RPM traces recorded for the patient on different days.

We collected 4DCT images on a 16-slice large bore LightSpeed RT CT scanner (Ge Health Care, Waukesha, WI) using the 4D RCCT [9,10] scan protocol described below. Scans at each couch position were continuously acquired in the axial cine mode for a period of time equal to the maximum breathing cycle plus one second with a 0.5 second per revolution gantry rotation speed and slice thickness of 1.25 mm at 120 kVp and 436 mA. A total of roughly 2900 CT slices were acquired at 187 couch positions. The patient's chest amplitude was continuously recorded during CT acquisition using Varian's RPM system. A total of six RPM traces were recorded during CT imaging on different treatment days and subsequently analyzed to determine the variability in patient breathing behavior.

To generate a set of amplitude indexed three-dimensional images from the CT slices, we first generated two amplitude binned images near the minimum and

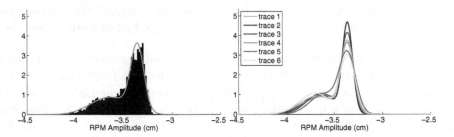

Fig. 3. The Gaussian mixture model provides an estimation of amplitude densities of the RPM breathing traces. The GMM fit for a single RPM trace overlays the histogram of amplitudes in the left image. The day-to-day variations in amplitude density of the RPM breathing traces recorded on several different days are evident on the right image.

maximum of the RPM signal. We then performed deformable image registration using the method of Keall et al., [12] to obtain a deformation field and linearly interpolated along that field to produce anatomical images corresponding to any chosen amplitude between the minimum and maximum. In a similar manner, we construct dose depositions for arbitrary amplitude by applying the deformation field to the base image dose deposition calculated using the BrainScan v5.31 treatment-planning system (BrainLAB AG, Munchen, Germany).

Figure 3 depicts the normalized histogram of and GMM fit to the amplitudes of the middle RPM trace depicted in Fig. 1. By visually comparing the GMM fit with the histogram of the breathing amplitudes, it is evident that the model provides an appropriate fit for the data. The six GMM estimations of amplitude density recorded for the same patient on different days depicted in the right image of Fig. 3 clearly illustrate the day-to-day variability in breathing amplitude density.

Examination of the eigenvalues corresponding to variation in the parameters depicted in the right image of Fig. 4 suggests that only three PCA components

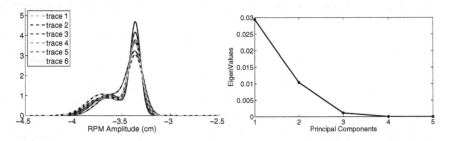

Fig. 4. The PCA reduction of the Gaussian mixture models gives very close reconstructions to the original mixture models with only three independent and uncorrelated eigenvectors. The eigenvalues of the principal components of the Gaussian Mixture Model parameters are negligible for the fourth and fifth components, confirming that only three are necessary to accurately capture the variation observed in the breathing traces.

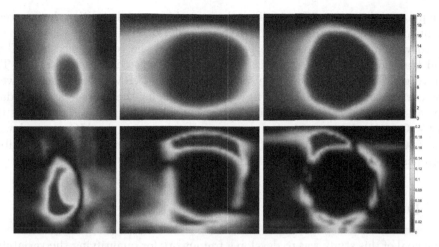

Fig. 5. The average (top row) and standard deviation (bottom row) of stochastic dose deposition (in Gray) is depicted in axial, sagittal, and coronal views, respectively. The regions of interest correspond to those in Fig. 1.

are necessary to accurately capture the variability in breathing. This enables a reduction of the stochastiSc dimensionality from five to three with at most, a 1.46×10^{-3} root mean squared error between the original and reduced GMMs. For visual comparison, the reconstruction of the GMM models for the six RPM breathing traces is depicted in left image of Fig. 4. The close correspondence between the original fitted GMMs and the GMMs reconstructed from a reduced dimensionality via PCA allows significant reduction in the complexity of the stochastic system owing to the correspondingly reduced dimensionality of the stochastic space.

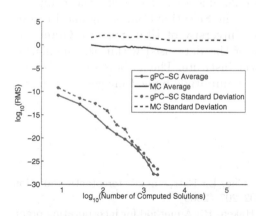

Fig. 6. The convergence rates for MC and gPC-SC methods as used to compute average and standard deviation of the deposited dose.

Figure 5 depicts the average and standard deviations of deposited dose over a single treatment for axial, sagittal, and coronal views. A comparison of the average dose depositions to the static-dose deposition calculation in Fig. 1 shows little difference. However, examination of the standard deviation in dose shows non-trivial high values (greater than 0.2 Gray) occurring near the boundaries of the lesion. We observed that large standard deviations in dose often correspond to regions of high dose gradient that undergo large respiratory-induced organ deformation. Such areas are significant because they indicate regions in which the planned dose may differ significantly from the actual deposition during treatment and are likely candidates for over- or under-dosing.

To validate our approach, we present in Fig. 6 the convergence in gPC-SC and traditional MC dose statistics for the patient case depicted in Fig. 5. The convergence data depicted is the root mean squared (RMS) difference between the current and final number of forward solutions for the average and standard deviation of dose calculations. It is clear that with only 2,744 realizations the gPC-SC method has reached greater convergence than the MC method with 155,000 forward dose solutions. Thus, for this particular model, gPC-SC exhibits significantly faster convergence than MC.

4   Discussion

The goal of this study was to develop a framework for quantifying the variability in respiratory-induced organ motion and incorporate that stochastic model into the calculation of dose deposition for SBRT treatment-planning. In contrast to Monte Carlo methods which are clinically infeasible because they require days or even weeks to compute accurate dose deposition statistics, the efficiency of the proposed approach enables physicians to perform statistical studies of dose response to breathing induced organ motion on a clinically realistic time scale. Statistical dose computations are particularly useful in planning because they allow physicians to identify and avoid dose plans in which high standard deviations in dose coincide with radiation sensitive tissues e.g., the spinal cord. We propose that accurate statistical models of predicted dose deposition resulting from organ motion will enable physicians to better assess the impact of SBRT dose plans on normal tissue and tumor lesions.

Acknowledgements. The authors would like to acknowledge the computational support and resources provided by the Scientific Computing and Imaging Institute. This work was funded by a University of Utah Synergy Grant No. 51003269. Support for the acquisition of the data used within the simulation studies came from the Huntsman Cancer Institute. The authors would also like to thank Jacob Hinkle for providing the amplitude-binned images used in this work.

References

1. Timmerman, R., Forster, K., Chinsoo Cho, L.: Extracranial stereotactic radiation delivery. Semin. Radiat. Oncol. 15, 202–207 (2005)
2. Lujan, A., Larsen, E., Balter, J., Ten Haken, R.: A method for incorporating organ motion due to breathing into 3D dose calculations. Med. Phys. 26, 715–720 (2003)
3. Brandner, E., Wu, A., Chen, H., Heron, D., Kalnicki, S., Komanduri, K., Gerszten, K., Burton, S., Ahmed, I., Shou, Z.: Abdominal organ motion measured using 4D CT. Int. J. Radiat. Oncol. Biol. Phys. 65, 554–560 (2006)

4. Wu, Q., Thongphiew, D., Wang, Z., Chankong, V., Yin, F.: The impact of respiratory motion and treatment technique on stereotactic body radiation therapy for liver cancer. Med. Phys. 35(4), 1440–1451 (2008)
5. Keall, P., Kini, V., Vedam, S., Mohan, R.: Potential radiotherapy improvements with respiratory gating. Australas. Phys. Eng. Sci. Med. 25, 1–6 (2005)
6. Hanley, J., Debois, M., Raben, A., et al.: Deep inspiration breath-hold technique for lung tumors: The potential value of target immobilization and reduced lung density in dose escalation. Int. J. Radiat. Oncol. Biol. Phys. 36(1), 188 (1996)
7. Neicu, T., Berbeco, R., Wolfgang, J., Jiang, S.: Synchonized moving aperture radiation therapy (SMART): Improvement of breathing pattern reproducibility using respiratory coaching. Phys. Med. Biol. 51, 617–636 (2006)
8. Boldea, V., Sharp, G., Jiang, S., Sarrut, D.: 4D-CT lung motion estimation with deformable registration: Quantification of motion nonlinearity and hysteresis. Med. Phys. 35(3), 1008–1018 (2008)
9. Ford, E., Mageras, G., Yorke, E., Ling, C.: Respiration-correlated spiral ct: A method of measuring respiratory-induced anatomic motion for radiation treatment planning. Med. Phys. 30, 88–97 (2003)
10. Vedam, S., Keall, P., Kini, V., Mostafavi, H., Shukla, H., Mohan, R.: Acquiring a four-dimensional computed tomography dataset using an external respiratory signal. Phys. Med. Biol. 48(1), 45–62 (2003)
11. Foskey, M., Davis, B., Goyal, L., Chang, S., Chaney, E., Strehl, N., Tomei, S., Rosenman, J., Joshi, S.: Large deformation three-dimensional image registration in image-guided radiation therapy. Phys. Med. Biol. 50, 5869–5892 (2005)
12. Keall, P., Joshi, S., Vedam, S., Siebers, J., Kini, V., Mohan, R.: Four-dimensional radiotherapy planning for DMLC-based respiratory motion tracking. Med. Phys. 32, 942–951 (2005)
13. Beddar, A., Kainz, K., Briere, T., Tsunashima, Y., Pan, T., Prado, K., Mohan, R., Gillin, M., Krishnan, S.: Correlation between internal fiducial tumor motion and external marker motion for liver tumors imaged with 4D-CT. Int. J. Radiat. Oncol. Biol. Phys. 67(2), 630–638 (2007)
14. Ionascu, D., Jiang, S., Nishloka, S., Shirato, H., Berbeco, R.: Internal-external correlation investigations of respiratory induced motion of lung tumors. Med. Phys. 34(10), 3893–3903 (2007)
15. Pevsner, A., Davis, B., Joshi, S., et al.: Evaluation of an automated deformable image matching method for quantifying lung motion in respiration-correlated CT images. Med. Phys. 33(2), 369–376 (2006)
16. Wijesooriya, K., Weiss, E., Dill, V., Dong, L., Mohan, R., Joshi, S.: Quantifying the accuracy of automated structure segmentation in 4D CT images using a deformable image registration algorithm. Med. Phys. 35(4), 1251–1260 (2008)
17. McLachlan, G., Peel, D.: Finite Mixture Models. John Wiley & Sons, Inc., New York (2000)
18. Dempster, A., Laird, N., Rubin, D.: Maximum likelihood from incomplete data via the EM algorithm. J. Roy. Stat. Soc. B. Met. 39(1), 1–38 (1977)
19. Pearson, K.: On lines and planes of closest fit to systems of points in space. Philos. Mag. 2(6), 559–572 (1901)
20. Xiu, D., Hesthaven, J.: High-order collocation methods for differential equations with random inputs. SIAM Journal on Scientific Computing 27(3), 1118–1139 (2005)
21. Xiu, D.: Efficient collocational approach for parametric uncertainty analysis. Comm. Comput. Phys. 2(2), 293–309 (2007)

22. Xiu, D., Karniadakis, G.: The Wiener-Askey polynomial chaos for stochastic differential equations. SIAM J. Sci. Comput. 24, 619–644 (2002)
23. Golub, G., Welsh, J.: Calculation of Gauss quadrature rules. Math. Comput. 10, A1–A10 (1969)
24. Press, W., Teukolsky, S., Vetterling, W., Flannery, B.: Gaussian Quadratures and Orthogonal Polynomials. In: Numerical recipes in C: The art of scientific computing, 2nd edn., pp. 147–161. Cambridge University Press, New York (1992)

Estimation of Inferential Uncertainty in Assessing Expert Segmentation Performance from STAPLE

Olivier Commowick and Simon K. Warfield

Computational Radiology Laboratory, Department of Radiology,
Children's Hospital, 300 Longwood Avenue, Boston, MA, 02115, USA
{Olivier.Commowick,Simon.Warfield}@childrens.harvard.edu

Abstract. The evaluation of the quality of segmentations of an image, and the assessment of intra- and inter-expert variability in segmentation performance, has long been recognized as a difficult task. Recently an Expectation Maximization (EM) algorithm for Simultaneous Truth and Performance Level Estimation (STAPLE), was developed to compute both an estimate of the reference standard segmentation and performance parameters from a set of segmentations of an image. The performance is characterized by the rate of detection of each segmentation label by each expert in comparison to the estimated reference standard.

This previous work provides estimates of performance parameters, but does not provide any information regarding their uncertainty. An estimate of this inferential uncertainty, if available, would allow estimation of confidence intervals for the values of the parameters, aid in the interpretation of the performance of segmentation generators, and help determine if sufficient data size and number of segmentations have been obtained to accurately characterize the performance parameters.

We present a new algorithm to estimate the inferential uncertainty of the performance parameters for binary segmentations. It is derived for the special case of the STAPLE algorithm based on established theory for general purpose covariance matrix estimation for EM algorithms. The bounds on performance estimates are estimated by the computation of the observed Information Matrix. We use this algorithm to study the bounds on performance estimates from simulated images with specified performance parameters, and from interactive segmentations of neonatal brain MRIs. We demonstrate that confidence intervals for expert segmentation performance parameters can be estimated with our algorithm. We investigate the influence of the number of experts and of the image size on these bounds, showing that it is possible to determine the number of image segmentations and the size of images necessary to achieve a chosen level of accuracy in segmentation performance assessment.

1 Introduction

The evaluation of image segmentation has long been recognized as a difficult problem. Many methods have been proposed in the literature to deal with it. These can be classified into two groups. First, the evaluation can be based

J.L. Prince, D.L. Pham, and K.J. Myers (Eds.): IPMI 2009, LNCS 5636, pp. 701–712, 2009.
© Springer-Verlag Berlin Heidelberg 2009

on distances between surfaces extracted from the automatic and the manual segmentation. For example, these can be the Hausdorff distance [1] or a mean distance between the two surfaces [2]. The other class of measures are voxel-based measures, i.e. overlap measures based on voxel-wise computations. Among those, the Dice similarity coefficient [3] or the Jaccard similarity coefficient [4,5] have been widely used to measure the overlap between two segmentations.

These two classes of measures have their advantages and drawbacks, and both may be used to provide insight into the quality of a segmentation [6] and to compare segmentations. The evaluation of different experts or algorithms for a particular task can be done quantitatively, with performance characterized by rates of detection of labels, when a reference standard segmentation is available.

Segmentation performance characterization can also be achieved when no external reference standard segmentation is available by estimating the reference standard. One algorithm for this, called STAPLE [7], uses an Expectation-Maximization (EM) algorithm to estimate iteratively, from a set of N expert segmentations, the hidden reference standard segmentation and performance parameters for each segmentation. These parameters characterize the agreement of a given expert with the underlying reference standard.

The STAPLE algorithm generates only point estimates of the performance parameters, and provides no information about the uncertainty in the values of the parameters. Precise knowledge of the inferential uncertainty would enhance our ability to interpret the performance of segmentation generators, and could be used to determine if sufficient data size and number of segmentations have been obtained to accurately characterize the performance parameters. An estimate of this inferential uncertainty, if available, would describe confidence intervals for the values of the parameters. Such a confidence interval describes the certainty with which we know the value of the parameter. A different concept is the confidence interval for rater performance, which describes the range of performance we expect to see across repeated segmentations by the same rater. If the inferential uncertainty of the values of performance parameter estimates are very small, then a confidence interval for rater performance can be estimated simply by the sample variance over repeated segmentations.

We describe here an algorithm to estimate the inferential uncertainty of the performance parameters. We demonstrate this can be achieved by estimating the covariance matrix of the performance parameters from STAPLE by calculation of the observed Information Matrix. The computation of the observed Information Matrix has been described in the general EM framework [8]. In this paper we derive analytic closed form expressions necessary to compute the covariance of the performance parameters obtained from STAPLE in the case of binary segmentations. We then demonstrate factors that influence the uncertainty in the estimated performance parameters with simulated segmentations of images, and apply our algorithm to characterize the segmentation of unmyelinated white matter from MRI of brains of newborn infants.

2   Method

2.1   The STAPLE Algorithm

We first recall briefly the principle of the STAPLE algorithm [7]. This method uses as an input a set of segmentations from J experts (either manual delineations or automatic segmentations). These segmentations are available as decisions d_{ij}, indicating the label given by each expert j for each voxel i. The goal of STAPLE is to estimate both the reference segmentation $\mathbf{T}$ underlying the expert segmentations, and parameters $\theta = \{\theta_1, \ldots, \theta_j, \ldots, \theta_J\}$ describing the agreement between the experts and the hidden reference standard. In the general case, each of the parameters θ_j is an $L \times L$ matrix, where L is the number of labels in the segmentation, and $\theta_{js's}$ is the probability that the expert j gave the label s' to a voxel i instead of the label s, i.e. $\theta_{js's} = P(d_{ij} = s'|T_i = s)$.

If the reference standard was known, then estimating the performance parameters for each expert would be straightforward. However, as it is unknown, an EM approach [9,8] is used to estimate the reference standard $\mathbf{T}$ and the performance parameters of the experts. The EM algorithm proceeds iteratively, alternating two steps:

- E-Step: Compute the expected value of the complete data log-likelihood $Q(\theta|\theta^{(k)})$ knowing the expert parameters at the preceding iteration: $\theta^{(k)}$. Evaluating this expression requires the knowledge of the posterior probability of the true score T: $P(T|D, \theta^{(k)})$, which is sufficient in this case to perform the Maximization step.
- M-Step: Estimate the performance parameters at iteration $k+1$, $\theta^{(k+1)}$ by maximizing the expected complete data log-likelihood $Q(\theta|\theta^{(k)})$, knowing the current estimate of the reference standard.

2.2   Covariance and Information Matrix

We are interested in the computation of the covariance matrix $C(\theta)$ of the expert parameters obtained by the STAPLE algorithm. This is done via the computation of the observed Information Matrix $I(\theta)$ of the parameters obtained after convergence of the EM algorithm. Then, the covariance matrix is obtained using the well-known result [10]: $C(\theta) = I^{-1}(\theta)$.

If all the data was known, the Information Matrix would be simply the matrix of the second derivatives of the log-likelihood function. However, in the case of an EM algorithm such as STAPLE, the hidden variables are unknown and their value may only be estimated. As some variables are hidden, only the observed Information Matrix $I(\theta)$ can be computed. The expression of $I(\theta)$ has been derived for a general EM algorithm in [8] (page 100).

We proceed by first computing the expected complete data Information Matrix $I_c(\theta)$ using the expected complete data log-likelihood $Q(\theta|\theta^{(k)})$ estimated in the EM algorithm. Then, to account for the uncertainty from the missing data, the expected missing data Information Matrix $I_m(\theta)$ is subtracted from $I_c(\theta)$ to obtain the observed Information Matrix, i.e. $I(\theta) = I_c(\theta) - I_m(\theta)$.

2.3   Computation of the Observed Information Matrix

We derive here the expression of the observed Information Matrix for the STA-PLE algorithm in the binary case. In this case, each expert has delineated one structure by attributing the value 1 to a voxel belonging to the structure and 0 otherwise (background). In this particular case, the θ parameters can be represented entirely by two parameters for each expert j: $p_j = P(d_{ij} = 1|T_i = 1)$ and $q_j = P(d_{ij} = 0|T_i = 0)$. p_j is also known as the sensitivity of the expert j while q_j is also known as the specificity. To simplify as much as possible the notation for the following equations, we use the general notation $\theta_{js's}$ for the performance parameters, keeping in mind that only $p_j = \theta_{j11}$ and $q_j = \theta_{j00}$ are the meaningful parameters (θ_{j01} and θ_{j10} being completely determined as $\theta_{j01} = 1 - p_j$ and $\theta_{j10} = 1 - q_j$). Then, the EM algorithm is used to compute iteratively the expected value of the complete data log-likelihood function $Q(\theta|\theta^{(k)})$:

$$Q(\theta|\theta^{(k)}) = \sum_j \sum_i \left(W_i^{(k)} \log(\theta_{j,d_{ij},1}) + (1 - W_i^{(k)}) \log(\theta_{j,d_{ij},0}) \right) \tag{1}$$

where $\theta_{j,d_{ij},s}$ corresponds to either θ_{j0s} or θ_{j1s} depending on the decision d_{ij}. $W_i^{(k)}$ corresponds to the probabilistic estimate at the voxel i and the iteration k of the reference standard segmentation. Using this function, we now derive the observed Information Matrix of the parameters θ.

Derivation of the Expected Complete Data Information Matrix. This matrix, denoted $I_c(\theta)$, is expressed as the second derivatives of the expected value of the complete data log-likelihood function [8], i.e.

$$\mathbf{I}_c(\theta) = -\frac{\partial^2}{\partial\theta\partial\theta^T} Q(\theta|\theta^{(k)}) \tag{2}$$

Eq. (1) and Eq. (2) demonstrate that the non-diagonal terms of I_c are zero as the parameters are independent of each other. Therefore, I_c is a diagonal matrix composed of the following terms:

$$\mathbf{I}_{c;p_j} = \sum_i \frac{W_i^{(k)}}{\theta_{j,d_{ij},1}^2} \tag{3}$$

$$\mathbf{I}_{c;q_j} = \sum_i \frac{1 - W_i^{(k)}}{\theta_{j,d_{ij},0}^2} \tag{4}$$

Derivation of the Expected Missing Data Information Matrix. Once I_c has been computed, the observed Information Matrix is obtained by subtracting from it the expected missing data Information Matrix I_m. This matrix is generally more difficult to compute than $I_c(\theta)$. When no analytical expression can be derived, it can be estimated using the EM algorithm itself to compute the Jacobian matrix via numerical differentiation (see [10,8]). In the general case of any EM algorithm, an analytic expression of I_m may also be obtained by the following equation [11] if the required derivatives exist:

$$\mathbf{I}_m(\theta) = \frac{\partial^2 Q(\theta|\theta^{(k)})}{\partial\theta^{(k)}\partial\theta^T} \tag{5}$$

In the case of the STAPLE algorithm, the expected value of the complete data log-likelihood function $Q(\theta|\theta^{(k)})$ can be differentiated. We have therefore derived the analytic expression of I_m elements as follows:

$$\frac{\partial^2 Q}{\partial\theta_{jtt}\partial\theta_n^{(k)}} = \sum_i \frac{(-1)^{1+d_{ij}}}{\theta_{j,d_{ij},t}} \frac{\partial W_i^{(k)}}{\partial\theta_n^{(k)}} \tag{6}$$

where t is either 1 or 0, to derive the expressions for p_j and q_j. Interestingly, it can also be shown that the obtained I_m matrix is symmetric, therefore minimizing the number of computations required. This expression gives I_m as a function of the derivatives of the probabilistic ground truth $W_i^{(k)}$. These $W_i^{(k)}$ have been derived by Warfield et al. [7] as:

$$W_i^{(k)} = \frac{f(T_i = 1)\prod_j \theta_{j,d_{ij},1}^{(k)}}{\sum_{m=0}^1 \left(f(T_i = m)\prod_j \theta_{j,d_{ij},m}^{(k)}\right)} \tag{7}$$

For simplicity of notations, we will consider that the prior probability $f(T_i = 1)$, respectively $f(T_i = 0)$, is constant over the entire image and will abbreviate it by π_1, respectively π_0. However, all the derived expressions are still valid for spatially varying prior probabilities by replacing π_m in the following equations by $\pi_m(i)$. Knowing the expression of W_i, its derivative with respect to the expert parameters $p_n^{(k)} = \theta_{n11}^{(k)}$ and $q_n^{(k)} = \theta_{n00}^{(k)}$ can be derived:

$$\frac{\partial W_i^{(k)}}{\partial\theta_{ntt}^{(k)}} = (-1)^{1+d_{in}}\pi_0\pi_1 \frac{\left(\prod_{l\neq n}\theta_{l,d_{il},t}^{(k)}\right)\left(\prod_l \theta_{l,d_{il},1-t}^{(k)}\right)}{\left(\sum_{m=0}^1 \pi_m \prod_l \theta_{l,d_{il},m}^{(k)}\right)^2} \tag{8}$$

where t is either 0 or 1. Therefore, $I_m(\theta)$, defined in Eq. (5), is computed by replacing $\frac{\partial W_i^{(k)}}{\partial\theta_n^{(k)}}$ by its value in Eq. (6). In practice, these values are computed easily by evaluating the different expressions at each voxel.

3   Results

To illustrate our formulation for deriving bounds on the value of the estimated segmentation parameters, we will present two applications. First, we show results with a simulated database, with specified parameters. Then, we present the application of our framework to provide insight into the confidence of the estimated parameters on a manually segmented neonate database.

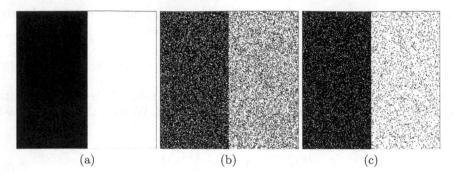

Fig. 1. Simulated Image Database. Simulated images used for the validation of our bounds estimation method : (a): known reference standard, (b): example of simulated segmentation of group 1 (sensitivity: 0.7, specificity: 0.8), (c): example of simulated segmentation of group 2 (sensitivity: 0.9, specificity: 0.9).

3.1 Simulated Experiments

To evaluate our framework with respect to a known ground truth, we created a database of ten segmentations (image size 256×256), illustrated in Fig. 1, divided into two groups. From the ground truth in Fig. 1(a), we have therefore simulated a first group of 5 images with a sensitivity parameter of 0.7 and a specificity parameter of 0.8 (illustrated in image (b)). Then, a second group, illustrated in image (c), was generated with different parameters : sensitivity and specificity of 0.9. In order to test for the influence of the image size on the confidence in the parameters, we have also generated a second database with the same parameters but with image size of 128×128.

We have then run STAPLE on those databases to estimate a reference standard and utilized our framework to estimate bounds on the estimated parameter values. The results are presented in Table 1 for the two databases. Our first observation on all our examples, including the following experiments on neonate data, was that the non diagonal terms of the covariance matrix were always much smaller than the diagonal terms. We have therefore chosen to present in this article the standard deviations obtained for each parameter, therefore neglecting the non-diagonal terms of the covariance matrix. The figures in Table 1 show that almost all the estimated parameters are correct, up to one standard deviation as estimated in our formulation. Deriving the bounds on these parameters therefore allows us to show that the estimation performed by STAPLE is accurate. The second observation that can be made on these figures is on the influence of the image size on the variability of the parameters. Our experiments indeed show a clear correlation between the image size and the variability, the standard deviations increasing when the image is subsampled.

3.2 Evaluation of Variability Parameters on a Neonate Database

Image Database. We have then applied our algorithm to five datasets of neonate MRI segmentation (one of them illustrated in Fig. 2) selected from

Table 1. Simulated Evaluation of the Expert Parameters and their Bounds. Simulated experiments results showing the estimated parameters for each segmentation and its variability (one standard deviation). Results are shown for 256 × 256 images and 128 × 128 images, showing increased variability with decreasing image size.

Segmentation #	256 × 256 Data		128 × 128 Data	
	Sens. (± StDev)	Spec. (± StDev)	Sens. (± StDev)	Spec. (± StDev)
1	0.7036 ± 0.0025	0.8011 ± 0.0022	0.6980 ± 0.0051	0.7988 ± 0.0045
2	0.7005 ± 0.0025	0.7964 ± 0.0022	0.6998 ± 0.0051	0.7960 ± 0.0045
3	0.7012 ± 0.0025	0.7909 ± 0.0023	0.6995 ± 0.0051	0.7980 ± 0.0045
4	0.6968 ± 0.0026	0.8003 ± 0.0022	0.6975 ± 0.0051	0.8007 ± 0.0044
5	0.7029 ± 0.0025	0.8010 ± 0.0022	0.6989 ± 0.0051	0.7964 ± 0.0045
6	0.9017 ± 0.0017	0.8973 ± 0.0017	0.8976 ± 0.0034	0.8998 ± 0.0034
7	0.9002 ± 0.0017	0.8995 ± 0.0017	0.8992 ± 0.0034	0.9012 ± 0.0034
8	0.8998 ± 0.0017	0.8986 ± 0.0017	0.9038 ± 0.0033	0.9027 ± 0.0033
9	0.8982 ± 0.0017	0.9018 ± 0.0017	0.8943 ± 0.0035	0.8960 ± 0.0034
10	0.8997 ± 0.0017	0.9007 ± 0.0017	0.8976 ± 0.0034	0.9036 ± 0.0033

MRI scans from previous studies. Each of these datasets consisted of a T1 and a T2 weighted image. After registration of the T2 image to the T1 image, five tissue classes were delineated interactively: cortical gray matter, sub-cortical gray

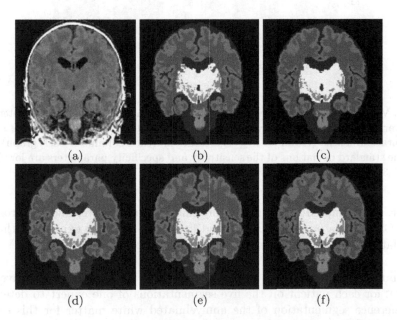

Fig. 2. Illustration of one image from the database. Coronal slice of (a) newborn T1 MRI and (b-f) its repeated manual segmentation in 5 classes done by one expert (cortical gray matter - grey, sub-cortical gray matter - white, unmyelinated white matter - red, myelinated white matter - orange - and CSF - blue).

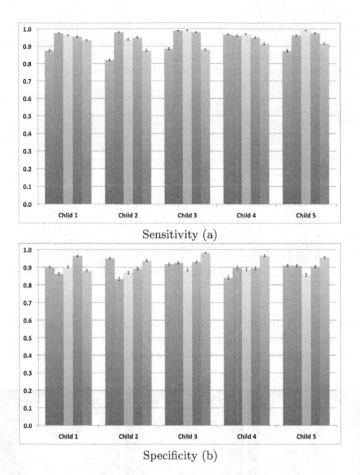

Sensitivity (a)

Specificity (b)

Fig. 3. Variability of the sensitivity and specificity parameters. Expert parameters and their variability ((a): Sensitivity, (b): Specificity) for the unmyelinated white matter segmentation. These results on five segmentations (each column of each graph) show that the standard deviations of the sensitivity and specificity parameters are low (going up to 1.3 % of the parameters values).

matter, unmyelinated white matter, myelinated white matter and cerebrospinal fluid (CSF). This process was repeated five times by three experts so that for each dataset, 15 segmentations of five structures were finally available.

Evaluation of the Bounds on the Estimated Parameters. We have used STAPLE for each patient on the five segmentations of one expert to determine the reference segmentation of the unmyelinated white matter for this expert, together with parameters of sensitivity and specificity for each manual segmentation. We have then used our analytical formulation to efficiently compute the observed Information Matrix for these parameters, and evaluated the covariance matrix of the parameters by simply inverting the Information Matrix.

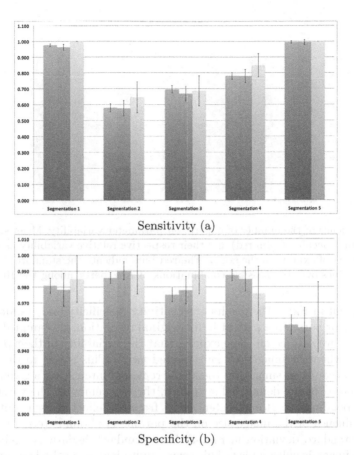

Sensitivity (a)

Specificity (b)

Fig. 4. Influence of the image dimension on parameter variability. Standard deviation of the estimated values (bars: parameter values, error bars: standard deviations) of the sensitivity (a) and specificity (b) parameters for the image at original size (blue), subsampled once (red), and subsampled twice (green). An increase in the standard deviation values is shown as the image is subsampled.

The parameters variabilities were computed on all patients and all structures but, for clarity, we only present in Fig. 3 the results on the unmyelinated white matter, showing for each parameter its standard deviation as an error bar. This figure shows that even with only five segmentations to estimate the ground truth, the estimation of the expert parameters is very precise. The maximum relative standard deviation is indeed of 1.3 %. This however seems logical as the parameters are computed from all the voxels of the considered image.

Influence of the Image Size on Parameter Variability. We also wanted to confirm in a real case previous simulated results on the influence of image size on the estimated variability of the parameters. We therefore subsampled the segmentations of one patient (again using the five segmentations of one expert) and evaluated the quality parameters as well as their variability.

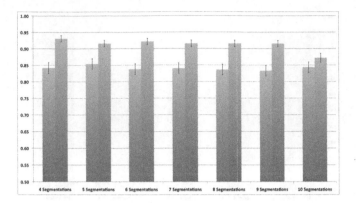

Fig. 5. Influence of the number of experts on parameter variability. Mean sensitivities (in blue) and specificities (in red) and their respective relative variability as a function of the number of experts in the study. The red bars indicate the standard deviation of the mean values over the possible combinations of K experts among the 10 available.

We present in Fig. 4 the results of sensitivity, specificity and standard deviations (as error bars) on a patient in its original resolution, subsampled once and twice. First, we can see on some experts that the variability of their parameters becomes 0 when the images are subsampled twice. This is due to the fact that the image becomes so small that the whole region of interest for a given expert is only composed of the delineated structure, thereby removing the variability for the corresponding expert parameter. Apart from this effect, these results confirm a clear influence of the image size on the parameters bounds (error bars represent one standard deviation in Fig. 4). The standard deviations again increase when the image is subsampled. This seems quite logical as the less information is known about each expert, the more variable the parameters are.

Influence of the Number of Segmentations on Parameter Variability. Finally, another potential cause of parameter variability is the number of segmentations used as an input to compute the reference segmentation. We have studied this property using binary segmentation performance estimates on ten manual segmentations of one subject. We present the evaluation of the results using from 4 segmentations up to 10 segmentations (using less experts would indeed not be meaningful for the statistical estimation of the hidden segmentation). For each number K of manual segmentations, we have performed the study over all the combinations of K images among the ten available.

We present in Fig. 5 the average parameters (blue: sensitivity, red: specificity) computed over the combinations of K images. We also show (error bars on the figure) the average standard deviations for each number of experts. These results show no significant change of the variability of the parameters. This suggests that, using 4 or more experts, the size of the structure to be delineated as well as the size of the region of interest for the STAPLE computation is more influential upon the variability of the estimated parameters than the number of experts.

4 Conclusion

We have presented in this article the expression of confidence bounds on the values of the expert performance parameters computed by the STAPLE algorithm for the binary case. These formulations are based on the derivation of analytic expressions for the observed Information Matrix of the underlying EM algorithm. Such confidence bounds will be very important as they will aid in the interpretation of the performance of segmentation generators, and determine if sufficient data size and number of segmentations have been obtained to accurately characterize the performance parameters.

We have presented examples of the application of these expressions for the evaluation of confidence intervals on the estimated values of the expert parameters first in simulated experiments, showing the ability of STAPLE to obtain accurate estimates of known performance parameters. We have also utilized these expressions in the context of neonate brain segmentation, showing a dependence of the bounds with respect to the number of voxels in the region of interest for the segmentation. However, in our particular example, no correlation was detected between the number of experts and the variability of their quality parameters when using 4 or more experts in STAPLE.

This work may be further improved in the future by extending the expression of the observed Information Matrix to the multi-category case, i.e. when several structures have been segmented by each expert. This will require to take into account the interdependency between the estimated performance parameters, for example by considering only $L - 1$ label independent parameters, the last one being computed from the others.

These expressions may then have many applications in terms of validation of segmentation or evaluation of intra-expert segmentation variability in a clinical context. In addition to the help to the clinician team in the assessment of the parameters determined by the STAPLE validation algorithm, this work could also be used in the future for the development of a local implementation of the STAPLE algorithm. This would allow to determine the minimal size of the region of interest required to obtain meaningful results for a given structure. Future work will then examine using this approach to evaluate spatially varying performance parameters and their bounds.

Acknowledgments

This investigation was supported in part by a research grant from CIMIT, grant RG 3478A2/2 from the NMSS, and by NIH grants R03 CA126466, R01 RR021885, R01 GM074068, R01 EB008015 and P30 HD018655.

References

1. Huttenlocher, D., Klanderman, D., Rucklige, A.: Comparing images using the Hausdorff distance. IEEE Transactions on Pattern Analysis and Machine Intelligence 15(9), 850–863 (1993)

2. Chalana, V., Kim, Y.: A methodology for evaluation of boundary detection algorithms on medical images. IEEE Transactions on Medical Imaging 16(5), 642–652 (1997)
3. Dice, L.: Measures of the amount of ecologic association between species. Ecology 26(3), 297–302 (1945)
4. Jaccard, P.: The distribution of flora in the alpine zone. New Phytologist 11, 37–50 (1912)
5. Zou, K.H., Warfield, S.K., Bharatha, A., Tempany, C.M.C., Tempany, C., Kaus, M.R., Haker, S.J., Wells, W.M., Jolesz, F.A., Kikinis, R.: Statistical validation of image segmentation quality based on a spatial overlap index. Acad. Radiol. 11(2), 178–189 (2004)
6. Gerig, G., Jomier, M., Chakos, M.: Valmet: A new validation tool for assessing and improving 3D object segmentation. In: Niessen, W.J., Viergever, M.A. (eds.) MICCAI 2001. LNCS, vol. 2208, pp. 516–523. Springer, Heidelberg (2001)
7. Warfield, S.K., Zou, K.H., Wells, W.M.: Simultaneous truth and performance level estimation (STAPLE): an algorithm for the validation of image segmentation. IEEE Transactions on Medical Imaging 23(7), 903–921 (2004)
8. McLachlan, G., Krishnan, T.: The EM Algorithm and Extensions. John Wiley and Sons, Chichester (1997)
9. Dempster, A., Laird, N., Rubin, D.: Maximum likelihood from incomplete data via the EM algorithm. Journal of the Royal Statistical Society (Series B) 39 (1977)
10. Meng, X., Rubin, D.: Using EM to obtain asymptotic variance-covariance matrices: the SEM algorithm. Journal of the American Statistical Association 86, 899–909 (1991)
11. Oakes, D.: Direct calculation of the information matrix via the EM algorithm. J. R. Statistical Society 61(2), 479–482 (1999)

Detection of Arterial Calcification in Mammograms by Random Walks

Jie-Zhi Cheng, Elodia B. Cole, Etta D. Pisano, and Dinggang Shen

Biomedical Research Imaging Center, University of North Carolina at Chapel Hill
106 Mason Farm Road, Chapel Hill, NC 27599, USA
{jzcheng, dgshen}@med.unc.edu

Abstract. A fully automatic algorithm is developed for breast arterial calcification extraction in mammograms. This algorithm is implemented in two major steps: a random-walk based tracking step and a compiling and linking step. With given seeds from detected calcification points, the tracking algorithm traverses the vesselness map by exploring the uncertainties of three tracking factors, i.e., traversing direction, jumping distance, and vesselness value, to generate all possible sampling paths. The compiling and linking algorithm further organizes and groups all sampling paths into calcified vessel tracts. The experimental results show that the performance of the proposed automatic calcification extraction algorithm is statistically close to that obtained by manual delineations.

Keywords: Breast arterioal calcification, Mammogram, Vessel detection, Random walk.

1 Introduction

Breast arterial calcification (BAC) is a phenomenon of calcium deposition along breast vessel lumens. Recently, it has been studied that BAC is potentially associated with cardiovascular disease, bone mineral density reduction, diabetes, and hypertension [1-3]. However, in these studies [1-3], the severity of BAC was evaluated subjectively by human experts. To further prove that BAC can actually be an effective indicator of women's risk for cardiovascular and other related diseases [4], more objective and quantitative evidence should be exploited. Accordingly effective means of quantification and assessment of BAC severity are extremely crucial for hypothesis validation and the systematic study of the vast amount of data. In this paper, an automatic BAC detection algorithm is proposed to serve as a tool for quantitative measurement of calcifications in mammograms.

In mammograms, lumens of calcified vessels are expected to show relatively high intensity values due to significant degree of attenuation of the X-ray signal as it passed through tissues with high calcium densities. As illustrated in Fig. 1(b)-(e), calcification deposition appear in various patterns along the vessel, subject to the varying amount of calcium deposition along the calcified vessel. Fig. 1(a) shows a craniocaudal (CC) view of part of a mammogram. Calcification may appear as bright spots (Fig 1(b) and (d)), or bright walls (Fig. 1(e)) on one or both sides of the vessel tube boundaries. Calcified

J.L. Prince, D.L. Pham, and K.J. Myers (Eds.): IPMI 2009, LNCS 5636, pp. 713–724, 2009.

vessels may also sometimes appear in the form of tubular structure with high interior intensity values (Fig. 1(c)). Moreover, in mammograms, one calcified vessel, other than appearing in a wide range of size, may appear to be disconnected, crossed by other vessels, and self-intersected, due to the effect of 2D projection and the occlusion by other breast structures. This can be observed in Fig. 1(a). Therefore, developing an automatic calcification detection scheme is not a trivial task, as it involves tackling all the aforementioned difficulties.

Recently, Ge et al. [5] proposed a method for detection of calcified vessels based on calcifi-

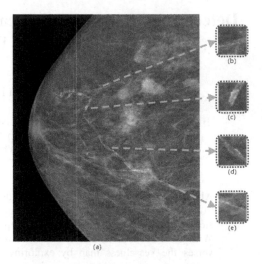

Fig. 1. An illustration of BACs from a clipped mammogram CC view. (a) A mammogram. (b)-(e) Examples of different appearance patterns of calcified vessels.

cation clues. Basically, they were able to detect calcified arterial "segments" by applying principle curve clustering on the detected calcification points. However, segments belonging to the same vessel were not assured to be grouped together, especially for highly-winding tracts. This could be problematic in providing useful information, such as lengths of the individual vessel tracts, for measurement and evaluation of calcification severity. It can hence be argued that, fragmented calcification clues may still fall short for the purpose of identifying the entire calcified vessels.

In this paper, the extraction of calcified vessel tracts is formulated as a problem of vessel tracking, seeded by calcification points. Since a calcified vessel may have various appearance patterns along the tract, the vessel extraction procedure may not function very well if it is directly based on intensity/appearance cues. Instead, we compute the *vesselness* measure [7] for each point in image as a guide for vessel extraction. To further identify individual vessel tracts, a tracking scheme is needed to extract a representative line for each vessel tract of interest. As calcified vessels may be bifurcated, overlapped/crossed by other ones, or surrounded with cluttering pseudo-vessels (like breast tissues or ducts), deterministically finding ONE representative line [8-10] for each vessel tract might not be sufficient. Accordingly, we explore the uncertainties of tracking process and generate multiple *sampling paths* by random walking. As shown in the context of DTI fiber tracking [11, 12] and sulci detection in cortical surfaces [13], the desired tract can be obtained when sufficient sampling paths are exploited. The details of random walking mechanism will be discussed in section 2.

To systematically organize the sampling paths, all these paths are further compiled into several super-paths according to the proximity of their two ending points. Some sampling paths with low calcification features or appearing to be pre-maturely terminated are eliminated to facilitate the latter processing. As described before, one calcified vessel might be disconnected or blurred by occlusion from the surrounding tissues. This problem makes the task of extracting complete vessel tracts more difficult. To assure that all segments of the same vessel tract are grouped together, a hierarchical linking scheme based on curvilinear feature is further developed for selectively linking up the tracked vessel segments into a whole tract.

The novelty of the proposed algorithm consists of (1) a random-walk based tracking scheme to detect multiple candidate sampling paths and (2) a compiling and linking scheme to complete the whole vessel tracts. By using these two strategies, the calcified vessels in mammograms can be effectively detected, even for the cases that two calcified vessels are crossing to each other. The results of the proposed algorithm will be compared with manual delineations, and the false and missing detection rates will also be reported.

2 Method

The problem of detecting calcified vessels in mammography is formulated as vessel extraction with priors from the detected calcifications. In particular, the vesselness probability map [7] is first generated to serve as a roadmap for the random-walk based tracking scheme. To extract calcified vessels, the seeding points for the random-walk based tracking are set as those suspicious calcification points detected by the method proposed in [6]. Following that, the compiling and linking schemes are performed to organize and group the sampling paths (generated from the tracking scheme) into the desired vessel tracts.

2.1 Generation of Vesselness Probability Map

The vesselness probability map is generated by a multiscale vesselness filter [7]. The vesselness filter consists of two exponential functions, which describe "the second order structureness" and "the tubular-like structure" [7], respectively. First, Hessian matrix at scale s is calculated for each pixel p. Eigenvalues of the Hessian matrix are then derived and sorted according to their magnitudes. Denoting that the two eigenvalues of the Hessian matrix at scale s are λ_1 and λ_2, $|\lambda_1| \leq |\lambda_2|$, respectively, the vesselness function of a pixel p at scale s can be expressed as:

$$\mathcal{V}_p(s) = \begin{cases} 0 & \text{if } \lambda_2 > 0 \\ \exp\left(-\frac{\mathcal{R}_B^2}{2\beta^2}\right)\left(1 - \exp\left(-\frac{s^2}{2c^2}\right)\right) & \text{otherwise} \end{cases} \tag{1}$$

where $\mathcal{R}_B$ is defined as λ_1/λ_2. S is the Frobenius matrix norm of the Hessian matrix and can be calculated as $\sqrt{\lambda_1^2 + \lambda_2^2}$. Since the intensity of calcified vessels appears higher than background, λ_2 is expected to be smaller than 0 in (1). Parameters β and c are set, respectively, to 0.5 and half value of the maximum Hessian norm throughout this study. To integrate the vesselness from every scale, the vesselness of each pixel p, $V(p)$, is sought as the maximum response of (1) over all scales.

2.2 Vessel Tracking by Random Walk

A standard vessel tracking algorithm detects the tract of interest by iteratively finding next candidate tracking element point (TEP). Basically, the estimation of next TEP is influenced by three major factors, i.e., traversing direction, jumping distance, and vesselness value (i.e., image intensity or other vesselness features). These three factors were often controlled by parameter setting/estimation [8], or could be described by probabilistic models [9 10]. Traversing direction and jumping distance configure the settings of the peeping window, which defines the search range of the next TEP. In particular, the traversing direction specifies the projection direction of the peeping window, while the jumping distance suggests how far to search the next candidate points in the neighborhood. The peeping window is usually defined as a fan-shape area, projected from the current TEP. The configuration of the peeping window can be observed in Fig. 2. In Fig. 2, the radius of the dashed circle represents the jumping distance. The fan-shape peeping window at the current TEP ε_t is spanned along the traversing direction Ψ_t with an angle θ_t. The spanning angle θ_t of the peeping window can be adaptively changed or fixed by a predefined value. The spanning angle is usually expected to be smaller than $180°$ for avoiding the back-tracking. The location of next TEP ε_{t+1} is selected from a pool of candidate points, e.g., $\{\delta_{t+1}^j, 1 \leq j \leq 4\}$ as shown in Fig. 2, according to the vesselness values. The selection criteria for the next TEP can be simply to choose the candidate point with the largest vesselness value. For example, the local maximum (in a ridge) is always selected as the next TEP [8].

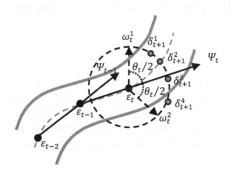

Fig. 2. Illustration of the configuration of peeping window. Bold grey curves represent the vessel boundaries, and the dashed grey curve denotes the medial axis of the vessel. Solid arrow Ψ_t indicates the traversing direction, and a black solid point ε_t is the current TEP. The peeping window is defined by two dash arrows $\overrightarrow{\varepsilon_t \omega_t^1}$ and $\overrightarrow{\varepsilon_t \omega_t^2}$ and arc $\overarc{\omega_t^1 \omega_t^2}$ of angle θ_t. The grey points, δ_{t+1}^j, $1 \leq j \leq 4$, are the candidate points for next TEP ε_{t+1}.

Generally speaking, the strategy of finding ONE local maximum/minimum of vesselness works well if the distribution of vesselness values within the vessel is relatively homogeneous, or follows a regular pattern. However, as indicated before, the appearance of calcified vessel may vary highly along the vessel tract. Thus, even in the vesselness probability map, multiple local maxima may exist due to the irregular deposition of calcium on the lumens, partial occlusion from other breast tissue, and also overlapping and branching issues, which can be observed in Fig. 3. Figs. 3(a) and 3(c) are the selected parts of mammograms, and Figs. 3(b) and 3(d) are the corresponding vesselness maps. In Figs. 3(b) and 3(d), the tracking directions are indicated by the red arrows, and possible tracking options are marked by the yellow dotted arrows. As shown in Fig. 3(b), the tracking direction Ψ_1 has two options to go, i.e., directions i and ii. According to the original image in Fig. 3(a), two calcified vessels are overlapped together in this case. Since the vesselness map cannot provide any information to distinguish between two vessels at the same location of Ψ_1, both tracking options *i* and *ii* should be explored. Also, multiple local maxima can be observed for two tracking directions, Ψ_2 in Fig. 3(b) and Ψ_3 in Fig. 3(d). The tracking options *iv* (in Fig. 3(b)) and *vi* (in Fig. 3(d)) are undesired, which are actually caused by partial occlusion of other breast tissues and the false-detected vesselness. These undesired tracking options can be easily selected by mistake if no appropriate jumping distance is given. Moreover, sometimes the medial area of one vessel may not appear to be at the local maxima of vesselness, as shown by a red dotted circle in Fig. 3(b). Accordingly, if only ONE solution is allowed in each iterative estimation of next TEP during the extraction of calcified vessels, the tracking path can be easily deviated from the desired one. To address this problem, we extract multiple sampling paths for more robust estimation of vessel tracts, as detailed below.

A novel random walk scheme is developed in this study to derive multiple sampling paths by exploring the uncertainties of the three tracking factors: traversing direction, jumping distance, and vesselness value. A random walk randomly selects one solution with equal probability when encountering uncertainty. These three tracking factors are crucial in determining a correct tracking path. If one of the three tracking factors is biased or wrongly estimated, the error may be propagated and the tracking may *no longer* get back to the correct tract. On the other hand, with sufficient sampling paths, the effect of error propagation can be mitigated.

Traversing Direction. The traversing direction models the direction of current tracking, and indicates where to find next TEP. It can be modeled *explicitly* by linearly combining the local estimated vessel direction (from Hessian matrix) with the previous traversing directions [8], or *implicitly* by a state-space model [10]. In our problem, as the interior intensity profile of calcified vessel is peaked in the calcification locations, the estimation of local vessel direction from eigen-analysis of Hessian

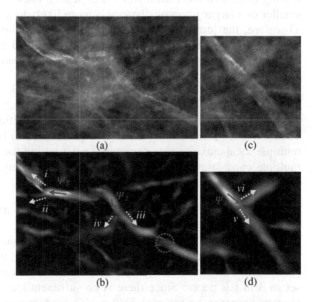

(a)

(c)

(b)

(d)

Fig. 3. Multiple local maxima in vesselness probability map. (a) and (c) are the parts of mammograms, and (b) and (d) are the corresponding vesselness maps. In (b) and (d), the red arrows indicate the tracking directions, while the yellow dotted arrows are the next possible tracking options.

matrix can be noisy and may not be applicable. Here, we propose to track the traversing direction based on a Kalman filter [14], for predicting the traversing direction according to previous ones. The traversing direction is modeled in a prediction-update fashion. In particular, at a current TEP ε_t, the current traversing direction $\Psi_{t|t-1}$ is predicted as

$$\Psi_{t|t-1} = \Psi_{t-1|t-1} \tag{2}$$

Assuming that the next TEP ε_{t+1} is estimated, the updated traversing direction can be obtained as

$$\Psi_{t|t} = \Psi_{t|t-1} + \kappa_t(\varphi_t - \Psi_{t|t-1}) \tag{3}$$

where κ_t is a Kalman gain and φ_t is a measured direction. φ_t can be calculated by $\varepsilon_{t+1} - \varepsilon_t$. The Kalman gain is served as a confidence weighting between the tracking model and the current estimation. It is usually determined by the prediction error covariance and the measurement error covariance. As we do not know the accuracy of the current estimation, the Kalman gain is uncertain. Instead of spending efforts on calculating the Kalman gain, we take the gain as an equally distributed random variable, ranging from 0 to 1. By exploring the uncertainty in the Kalman gain, various sampling paths can be exploited.

Jumping Distance. The jumping distance is one of the factors that will affect the finding of desired local maxima from undesired ones. It is an issue to argue whether a smaller or a larger jumping distance is more likely to lead to undesired local maxima. Therefore, the jumping distance is another uncertainty in the random-walk based tracking scheme. The jumping distance is described by another equally-distributed random variable, which ranges from 6 to 10 in pixel unit.

Vesselness Value. A good estimation of next TEP is substantial to stay in the right track. As shown in Fig. 2, the candidates of next TEP can be estimated from the peeping window. Due to the special characteristics of calcified vessel, the vesselness in the medial axis or the vicinities cannot be guaranteed to be local maxima. Particularly, multiple local maxima may sometimes exist within the peeping window. As a result, multiple candidates of next TEP should be considered. Thus, the candidates of TEP ε_{t+1} are selected as follows:

$$\{\delta_{t+1}^j\} = \arg\max_{\varrho_{t+1}}^n V(\varrho_{t+1}) \, ; \, \forall j, 1 \leq j \leq n \text{ and } \forall \varrho_{t+1} \in \mathcal{W} \tag{4}$$

$\mathcal{W}$ is the region of interest within the fan-shape peeping window. In this paper, $\mathcal{W}$ is defined as a ring region dilated from the periphery of the fan-shape peeping window (i.e., the dashed circle in Fig. 2). n is the number of candidates to be selected, and is set as 3 in this paper. Since there is no sufficient knowledge about which candidate is more proper to be the next TEP ε_{t+1}, a random selector with equal opportunity is adopted to pick a candidate as ε_{t+1}.

Termination of Tracking Scheme. The random-walk based tracking procedure iterates until there is no strong vesselness in the current TEP. The vesselness threshold for termination of random-walk based tracking scheme is set as 0.1.

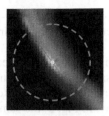

Fig. 4. Relocation of a seeding point toward the center of vessel. Blue dashed circle denotes the vicinities of the original seeding point, marked as a yellow dot in the figure. The green dot is the relocated position of the seeding point. Red crossed lines represent the two eigenvectors of PCA on the local vesselness map.

Seeding Strategy and Initialization. As only calcified vessels are interested, the seeding points for the random-walk based tracking should be set as the calcification points, which can be detected by globally thresholding a calcification-enhanced image [6]. The detected calcification points are further clustered, and the clusters with sparse calcification points are discarded as noises in the calcification detection results. For each remaining cluster, the point with the highest intensity is served as a seeding point for the random-walk based tracking scheme. As the seeding point may not locate at the center of vessel, i.e., a yellow dot in Fig. 4, Principle Component Analysis (PCA) is applied to analyze the spatial distribution of vesselness in the vicinities of the seeding point. The derived eigenvector with higher magnitude of eigenvalue is taken as an initial tracking direction (the longer red line in Fig. 4), with the positive direction for forward tracking and the negative direction for backward tracking. Along the other eigenvector, the shorter red line in Fig. 4, the seeding points can be relocated approximately toward the center of vessel, which can be observed as a green dot in Fig. 4. One example of the tracked sampling paths is depicted in Fig. 5, which will be explained in detail below.

2.3 Hierarchical Compiling and Linking of Sampling Paths

As many sampling paths from different seeding points may correlate to each others, a compiling step is developed to parcel up the sampling paths (with the close ending points in both ends) into sets of "super-paths". Before linking step, the undesired super-paths, such as incomplete, wrongly-tracked paths, and those of non-calcified tubular structures, are eliminated. Since it is not assured that the disconnected vessels could be extracted as a whole in the tracking scheme, a hierarchical linking procedure is developed to link up those super-paths that belong to the same vessel tract.

Compiling the Sampling Paths into Super-paths. To facilitate the later processing of the derived sampling paths, the sampling paths are further compiled into sets of super-paths. The super-paths here can be interpreted as conceptual vessel tracts or segment entities. Consequently, the sampling paths of the same super-path can be taken as

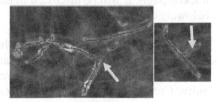

Fig. 5. An example on generation of sampling paths. Sampling paths are depicted in the mammograms. The paths generated from the same seeding point are drawn in the same color in each panel. The green dots denote the ending points of sampling paths. A super-path is defined by a bunch of sampling paths with their two ending points in the same clusters. The yellow arrows indicate the incomplete and wrongly-tracked paths.

possible representative lines of this entity. The hierarchical concept of the super-paths and the sampling paths can scale down the search space when building up the linkage information for the linking step.

A super-path is defined as a parcel of the sampling paths that have close ending points in both ends. Accordingly, the ending points of all sampling paths should be clustered in L_2 distance metric first. All sampling paths connected by two clusters of ending points are grouped into the same super-path. As shown in Fig. 5, the sampling paths connecting the same two clusters of ending points, i.e., the clusters of green dots in Fig. 5, belong to the same super-path.

Elimination of Undesired Sampling Paths. The derived sampling paths may consist of paths without calcification, or some incomplete, wrongly-tracked paths, as shown in Fig. 5. The incomplete paths generally end at the undesired locations when tracking along the highly-winding vessels. Also, some false-detected calcification points will lead to the detection of non-calcified tubular structures, which will affect the latter linking procedure and should be removed. The incomplete paths can be easily discarded if they are highly covered by other longer paths at high percentage, i.e., 95%. For differentiating non-calcified tubular structures from calcified vessels, local contrast within the detected structures is measured. As shown in Fig. 6, non-calcified tubular structures have less local contrast as compared to the calcified ones (although they may appear to be bright). Based on this observation, we can identify those non-calcified tubular structures and further remove them. As for elimination of wrongly-tracked paths, it will be discussed in the linking step below.

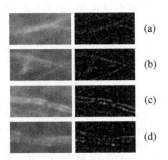

Fig. 6. Comparison of local contrast feature in calcified vessels and non-calcified tubular structures. Left column shows the original image, and right column shows the corresponding local contrast map. (a-b) are non-calcified tubular structures, and (c-d) are calcified vessels.

Hierarchical Linking of Super-Paths. To further link up the super-paths from the same vessel, a hierarchical linking framework is developed based on a concept of curvilinear continuity. Curvilinear continuity is the contextual cue for mid-level inference in human visual perception [15]. The contextual cue is usually measured by turning angle [15] or curvature after filling the gap between two curves (see Fig. 7). In this paper, we calculate the turning angle as our measurement of the curvilinear continuity.

The main idea of our hierarchical linking framework is to link the super-paths at multiple distance scales under different levels of angle constraint. At the lower distance scale, i.e., in the case where the super-paths are close to each other within a given distance threshold, a looser angle constraint is applied. When the distance scale goes higher and distant super-paths are considered, a more rigorous angle constraint is employed. At each distance scale d, a linking graph $G_d = \{U, E\}$ is built by setting

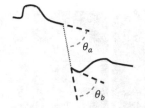

Fig. 7. An illustration of turning angle. The two solid curves are the two sampling paths, and the dotted line is the gap-filling line. The turning angle can be calculated as $\theta_a + \theta_b$.

each super-path as a graph node, u_l. The graph edge $e_{i,j}$ is established if the length and angle constraints, $\ell_{i,j} \leq L_d$ and $\rho_{i,j} \leq \Theta_d$, are satisfied. Here, L_d and Θ_d are, respectively, the distance and angle thresholds at the current distance scale d. $\ell_{i,j}$ is calculated as

$$\ell_{i,j} = \frac{1}{p_i + q_j} \sum_{\varsigma^i}^{p_i} \sum_{\tau^j}^{q_j} dist(\varsigma^i, \tau^j), \qquad (5)$$

where p_i and q_j are the respective numbers of sampling paths within the super-paths u_i and u_j. The function $dist(\varsigma^i, \tau^j)$ is the L_2 distance between the two connecting ending points of the two sampling paths ς^i and τ^j. $\rho_{i,j}$ is sought as

$$\rho_{i,j} = \min_{\varsigma^i, \tau^j} \vartheta(\varsigma^i, \tau^j). \qquad (6)$$

The function $\vartheta(\varsigma^i, \tau^j)$ denotes the turning angle between the sampling paths after completion of the gap filling as shown in Fig. 7. The linking graph G_d is a forest with several connected components. A depth-first traversing scheme is applied on each connected component to find all possible path combinations, which will be interpolated to be new super-paths for the next distance scale. Before going up to a larger distance, those wrongly-tracked super-paths are eliminated according to the length and the partial overlap criteria. Comparing to the desired super-paths, the wrongly-tracked paths will not grow up. Consequently, they can be removed from the pool of super-paths when other super-paths of vessel tracts grow sufficiently long (see Fig. 8). The loop of iteratively increasing the distance scale is terminated when no possible linking between super-paths exists. In the final, a threshold for the length of super-path is also used to discard those short super-paths. The representative line in each remaining super-path is determined as the one with the maximum integral of vesselness along the tract.

3   Results

The performance of each significant step of our proposed method is demonstrated in Fig. 8. There are three major calcified vessels in the mammogram shown in Fig. 8, with the two longest ones crossing each other. Fig. 8(g) is the final result by our method, which indicates that all major calcified vessels are effectively extracted. The manual delineation result is provided in Fig. 8(h).

For performance evaluation, our method is tested on 20 mammograms, and the obtained results are compared with two sets of manual delineations. The difference between computer-detected delineations and manual delineations is evaluated by five assessment metrics: mutual distance (Diff_Dist), difference of the total vessel length (Diff_Ln), difference of the average vessel diameter (Diff_Diam), length of the missing segments (Miss_Ln), and length of the false-detected segments (FD_Ln). In particular, the distance metric (Diff_Dist) measures the specific difference of vessel tracts in two comparing sets R and Q, and is defined as $\frac{1}{R_m + Q_n} [\sum_j^{R_m} e(r_j, Q) +$

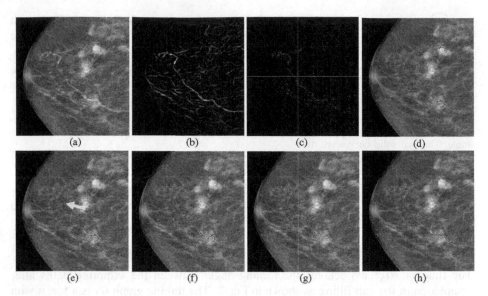

Fig. 8. A step-by-step demonstration of the propose method. (a) Original mammogram; (b) vesselness map; (c) detected calcification points; (d) initially extracted super-paths; (e) refined super-paths after removing incomplete and non-calcified tubular structures; (f) intermediate result after linking paths and removing wrong ones; (g) final result; (h) a manual delineation. It can be observed that the wrongly-tracked path, as indicated by a yellow arrow in (e), is eliminated by the linking scheme, with the further result shown in (f).

$\sum_{i}^{Q_n} e(q_i, R)$], where The function $e(r_j, Q)$ represents the distance between a point r_j in the set R to the nearest point in the set Q. Similarly, $e(q_i, R)$ finds the nearest distance from the point q_i in the set Q to the set R. R_m and Q_n are the total numbers of points in the sets R and Q, respectively. The Diff_Diam metric measures the difference of average diameter between the corresponding vessel tracts in the two comparing sets. The diameter of vessel can be estimated as the length of profile (yellow lines in Fig. 9) in the vesselness map, with the direction of profile determined by PCA as similarly done for the estimation of red short axis in Fig. 4.

The difference of the total vessel length (Diff_Ln) is measured by simply calculating the difference of the total lengths of vessels in two sets under comparison. The missing segments are checked if they are missed in one set (R) but exist in other set (Q), when comparing the set R to the set Q, denoted as R-Q. Similarly, those segments that exist in R but not in Q are regarded as false-detected segments during R-Q comparison. The total lengths of missing and false-detected segments in each testing mammogram are taken as Miss_Ln and FD_Ln metrics, respectively.

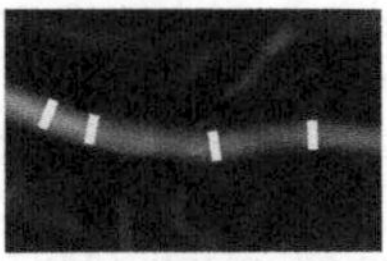

We compare the difference between computer-detected delineations (CD) and each of two sets of manual delineations (MD), denoted as CD-MD1 and CD-MD2, as well as the difference between two sets of manual delineations, i.e., MD1-MD2. Table 1 summarizes the assessment results of CD-MD1, CD-MD2, and MD1-MD2 using all five

Fig. 9. Estimation of diameters along the vessel tract

Table 1. Summary of five assessment metrics in the three pairs of comparison, i.e., CD-MD1, CD-MD2, and MD1-MD2

Assessment Metric	CD-MD1 (mm)	CD-MD2 (mm)	MD1-MD2 (mm)
Diff_Dist	0.27 ± 0.08	0.31 ± 0.08	0.24 ± 0.08
Diff_Diam	0.03 ± 0.03	0.03 ± 0.02	0.02 ± 0.02
Diff_Ln	$\mathbf{5.55 \pm 7.05}$	$\mathbf{5.33 \pm 5.54}$	$\mathbf{5.06 \pm 5.01}$
Miss_Ln	1.96 ± 2.08	3.38 ± 3.18	2.99 ± 3.86
FD_Ln	4.37 ± 5.14	4.21 ± 4.33	1.57 ± 1.63

metrics. The means and the standard deviations of all five metrics in 20 mammograms are also reported. It can be observed that the performance of the proposed method is statically very close to that by manual delineations.

Moreover, we performed the Friedman test [16] on the same 20 mammograms, to test the null hypothesis if there is no significant difference among the three comparing pairs, CD-MD1, CD-MD2, and MD1-MD2. The p-values of the Friedman test for five assessment metrics are 0.05, 0.29, **0.42**, 0.2, and 0.04, respectively. The length of the false-detected segments (FD_Ln) slightly rejects the hull hypothesis in 0.05 significance level, while all other four indicate no significant difference among CD, MD1, and MD2. The false-detected segments come from the non-calcified tubular structures in our method, and also by human experts who missed some subtle calcified vessels. The length ratios of the false-detected segments against the overall vessels in CD-MD1 and CD-MD2 are 2.72% and 2.57%, respectively, which are relatively small and thus acceptable for practical application. On the other hand, the total length of calcified vessels (with p-value **0.42**) is very consistently measured in three sets of delineations. Since this is the most important measure to assess the calcification severity in practical application, it further confirms the close performance of our proposed method to manual experts.

4 Conclusion

A fully automatic breast arterial calcification detection method is proposed in this paper. Experimental results show that the performance of our method is statistically comparable to the manual delineations. With extraction of calcified vessel tracts, the BAC measurements, i.e., major diameters and lengths of calcified vessels, as well as severity of calcification, can provide quantitative information to further investigate the association between BAC and women cardiovascular diseases. To further eliminate the false-detected tubular structures, we may train a classifier to indentify calcified vessels. This classifier can provide priors to constrain the random walking.

Acknowledgments. The authors would like to thank GE Healthcare for sponsorship with Grant R21CA140841.

References

1. Kemmeren, J.M., et al.: Breast Arterial Calcifications: Associations with Diabetes Mellitus and Cardiovascular Mortality. Radiology 201, 75–78 (1996)
2. Reddy, J., Bilezikian, J.P., Smith, S.J., Mosca, L.: Reduced Bone Mineral Density Is Associated with Breast Arterial Calcification. J. Clin. Endocrinol. Metab. 93, 208–211 (2008)

3. Rotter, M.A., et al.: Breast Arterial Calcifications (BACs) Found on Screening Mammography and Their Association with Cardiovascular Disease. Menopause 15, 276–281 (2008)
4. Dale, P., Mascarhenas, C., Richards, M., Mackie, G.: Mammography as a Screening Tool for Coronary Artery Disease. Journal of Surgical Research 148, 1–6 (2008)
5. Ge, J., et al.: Automated Detection of Breast Vascular Calcification on Full-Field Digital Mammograms. In: Proc. SPIE Med. Img. 2008, 691517, pp. 1–7 (2008)
6. Ge, J., et al.: Computer Aided Detection of Clusters of Microcalcifications on Full Field Digital Mammograms. Medical Physics 33, 2975–2988 (2006)
7. Frangi, A., Niessen, W., Vincken, K., Viergever, M.: Multiscale Vessel Enhancement Filtering. In: Wells, W.M., Colchester, A.C.F., Delp, S.L. (eds.) MICCAI 1998. LNCS, vol. 1496, pp. 130–137. Springer, Heidelberg (1998)
8. Aylward, S.R., Bullitt, E.: Initialization, Noise, Singularities, and Scale in Height Ridge Traversal for Tubular Object Centerline Extraction. IEEE TMI 21, 61–75 (2002)
9. Wong, W.C.K., Chung, A.C.S.: Probabilistic Vessel Axis Tracing and Its Applications to Vessel Segmentation with Stream Surfaces and Minimum Cost Paths. MedIA 11, 567–587 (2007)
10. Schaap, M., et al.: Bayesian Tracking of Elongated Structures in 3D Images. In: Karssemeijer, N., Lelieveldt, B. (eds.) IPMI 2007. LNCS, vol. 4584, pp. 74–85. Springer, Heidelberg (2007)
11. Lazar, M., Alexander, A.L.: Bootstrap White Matter Tractography (BOOT-TRAC). NeuroImage 24, 524–532 (2005)
12. Jones, D.K.: Tractography Gone Wild: Probabilistic Fibre Tracking Using the Wild Bootstrap with Diffusion Tensor MRI. IEEE TMI 27, 1268–1274 (2008)
13. Shi, Y., et al.: Joint Sulci Detection Using Graphical Models and Boosted Priors. In: Karssemeijer, N., Lelieveldt, B. (eds.) IPMI 2007. LNCS, vol. 4584, pp. 98–109. Springer, Heidelberg (2007)
14. Doucet, A., Godsill, S., Andrieu, C.: On Sequential Monte Carlo Sampling Methods for Bayesian Filtering. Statistics and Computing 10, 197–208 (2000)
15. Ren, X., Fowlkes, C.C., Malik, J.: Learning Probabilistic Models for Contour Completion in Natural Images. Int. J. Comput. Vis. 77, 47–63 (2008)
16. Daniel, W.W.: Applied Nonparametric Statistics. Houghton Mifflin, Boston (1978)

Author Index

Printed in the United States
by Bookmasters

Printed in the United States
By Bookmasters